PNEUMOCYSTIS CARINII PNEUMONIA

SECOND EDITION, REVISED AND EXPANDED

LUNG BIOLOGY IN HEALTH AND DISEASE

Executive Editor

Claude Lenfant
*Director, National Heart, Lung and Blood Institute
National Institutes of Health
Bethesda, Maryland*

1. Immunologic and Infectious Reactions in the Lung, *edited by Charles H. Kirkpatrick and Herbert Y. Reynolds*
2. The Biochemical Basis of Pulmonary Function, *edited by Ronald G. Crystal*
3. Bioengineering Aspects of the Lung, *edited by John B. West*
4. Metabolic Functions of the Lung, *edited by Y. S. Bakhle and John R. Vane*
5. Respiratory Defense Mechanisms (in two parts), *edited by Joseph D. Brain, Donald F. Proctor, and Lynne M. Reid*
6. Development of the Lung, *edited by W. Alan Hodson*
7. Lung Water and Solute Exchange, *edited by Norman C. Staub*
8. Extrapulmonary Manifestations of Respiratory Disease, *edited by Eugene Debs Robin*
9. Chronic Obstructive Pulmonary Disease, *edited by Thomas L. Petty*
10. Pathogenesis and Therapy of Lung Cancer, *edited by Curtis C. Harris*
11. Genetic Determinants of Pulmonary Disease, *edited by Stephen D. Litwin*
12. The Lung in the Transition Between Health and Disease, *edited by Peter T. Macklem and Solbert Permutt*
13. Evolution of Respiratory Processes: A Comparative Approach, *edited by Stephen C. Wood and Claude Lenfant*
14. Pulmonary Vascular Diseases, *edited by Kenneth M. Moser*
15. Physiology and Pharmacology of the Airways, *edited by Jay A. Nadel*
16. Diagnostic Techniques in Pulmonary Disease (in two parts), *edited by Marvin A. Sackner*
17. Regulation of Breathing (in two parts), *edited by Thomas F. Hornbein*
18. Occupational Lung Diseases: Research Approaches and Methods, *edited by Hans Weill and Margaret Turner-Warwick*
19. Immunopharmacology of the Lung, *edited by Harold H. Newball*
20. Sarcoidosis and Other Granulomatous Diseases of the Lung, *edited by Barry L. Fanburg*

21. Sleep and Breathing, *edited by Nicholas A. Saunders and Colin E. Sullivan*
22. *Pneumocystis carinii* Pneumonia: Pathogenesis, Diagnosis, and Treatment, *edited by Lowell S. Young*
23. Pulmonary Nuclear Medicine: Techniques in Diagnosis of Lung Disease, *edited by Harold L. Atkins*
24. Acute Respiratory Failure, *edited by Warren M. Zapol and Konrad J. Falke*
25. Gas Mixing and Distribution in the Lung, *edited by Ludwig A. Engel and Manuel Paiva*
26. High-Frequency Ventilation in Intensive Care and During Surgery, *edited by Graziano Carlon and William S. Howland*
27. Pulmonary Development: Transition from Intrauterine to Extrauterine Life, *edited by George H. Nelson*
28. Chronic Obstructive Pulmonary Disease: Second Edition, Revised and Expanded, *edited by Thomas L. Petty*
29. The Thorax (in two parts), *edited by Charis Roussos and Peter T. Macklem*
30. The Pleura in Health and Disease, *edited by Jacques Chrétien, Jean Bignon, and Albert Hirsch*
31. Drug Therapy for Asthma: Research and Clinical Practice, *edited by John W. Jenne and Shirley Murphy*
32. Pulmonary Endothelium in Health and Disease, *edited by Una S. Ryan*
33. The Airways: Neural Control in Health and Disease, *edited by Michael A. Kaliner and Peter J. Barnes*
34. Pathophysiology and Treatment of Inhalation Injuries, *edited by Jacob Loke*
35. Respiratory Function of the Upper Airway, *edited by Oommen P. Mathew and Giuseppe Sant'Ambrogio*
36. Chronic Obstructive Pulmonary Disease: A Behavioral Perspective, *edited by A. John McSweeny and Igor Grant*
37. Biology of Lung Cancer: Diagnosis and Treatment, *edited by Steven T. Rosen, James L. Mulshine, Frank Cuttitta, and Paul G. Abrams*
38. Pulmonary Vascular Physiology and Pathophysiology, *edited by E. Kenneth Weir and John T. Reeves*
39. Comparative Pulmonary Physiology: Current Concepts, *edited by Stephen C. Wood*
40. Respiratory Physiology: An Analytical Approach, *edited by H. K. Chang and Manuel Paiva*
41. Lung Cell Biology, *edited by Donald Massaro*
42. Heart–Lung Interactions in Health and Disease, *edited by Steven M. Scharf and Sharon S. Cassidy*
43. Clinical Epidemiology of Chronic Obstructive Pulmonary Disease, *edited by Michael J. Hensley and Nicholas A. Saunders*
44. Surgical Pathology of Lung Neoplasms, *edited by Alberto M. Marchevsky*

45. The Lung in Rheumatic Diseases, *edited by Grant W. Cannon and Guy A. Zimmerman*
46. Diagnostic Imaging of the Lung, *edited by Charles E. Putman*
47. Models of Lung Disease: Microscopy and Structural Methods, *edited by Joan Gil*
48. Electron Microscopy of the Lung, *edited by Dean E. Schraufnagel*
49. Asthma: Its Pathology and Treatment, *edited by Michael A. Kaliner, Peter J. Barnes, and Carl G. A. Persson*
50. Acute Respiratory Failure: Second Edition, *edited by Warren M. Zapol and Francois Lemaire*
51. Lung Disease in the Tropics, *edited by Om P. Sharma*
52. Exercise: Pulmonary Physiology and Pathophysiology, *edited by Brian J. Whipp and Karlman Wasserman*
53. Developmental Neurobiology of Breathing, *edited by Gabriel G. Haddad and Jay P. Farber*
54. Mediators of Pulmonary Inflammation, *edited by Michael A. Bray and Wayne H. Anderson*
55. The Airway Epithelium, *edited by Stephen G. Farmer and Douglas Hay*
56. Physiological Adaptations in Vertebrates: Respiration, Circulation, and Metabolism, *edited by Stephen C. Wood, Roy E. Weber, Alan R. Hargens, and Ronald W. Millard*
57. The Bronchial Circulation, *edited by John Butler*
58. Lung Cancer Differentiation: Implications for Diagnosis and Treatment, *edited by Samuel D. Bernal and Paul J. Hesketh*
59. Pulmonary Complications of Systemic Disease, *edited by John F. Murray*
60. Lung Vascular Injury: Molecular and Cellular Response, *edited by Arnold Johnson and Thomas J. Ferro*
61. Cytokines of the Lung, *edited by Jason Kelley*
62. The Mast Cell in Health and Disease, *edited by Michael A. Kaliner and Dean D. Metcalfe*
63. Pulmonary Disease in the Elderly Patient, *edited by Donald A. Mahler*
64. Cystic Fibrosis, *edited by Pamela B. Davis*
65. Signal Transduction in Lung Cells, *edited by Jerome S. Brody, David M. Center, and Vsevolod A. Tkachuk*
66. Tuberculosis: A Comprehensive International Approach, *edited by Lee B. Reichman and Earl S. Hershfield*
67. Pharmacology of the Respiratory Tract: Experimental and Clinical Research, *edited by K. Fan Chung and Peter J. Barnes*
68. Prevention of Respiratory Diseases, *edited by Albert Hirsch, Marcel Goldberg, Jean-Pierre Martin, and Roland Masse*
69. *Pneumocystis carinii* Pneumonia: Second Edition, Revised and Expanded, *edited by Peter D. Walzer*
70. Fluid and Solute Transport in the Airspaces of the Lungs, *edited by Richard M. Effros and H. K. Chang*

ADDITIONAL VOLUMES IN PREPARATION

Airway Secretion: Mucous Hypersecretion, *edited by Tamotsu Takishima and Sanae Shimura*

Sarcoidosis and Other Granulomatous Disorders, *edited by D. Geraint James*

Epidemiology of Lung Cancer, *edited by Jonathan Samet*

Pulmonary Embolism, *edited by Mario Morpurgo*

Sleep and Breathing: Second Edition, Revised and Expanded, *edited by Nicholas A. Saunders and Colin E. Sullivan*

The opinions expressed in these volumes do not necessarily represent the views of the National Institutes of Health.

PNEUMOCYSTIS CARINII PNEUMONIA

SECOND EDITION, REVISED AND EXPANDED

Edited by

Peter D. Walzer

Cincinnati Veterans Affairs Medical Center
and University of Cincinnati College of Medicine
Cincinnati, Ohio

Marcel Dekker, Inc. New York • Basel • Hong Kong

Library of Congress Cataloging-in-Publication Data

Pneumocystis carinii pneumonia / edited by Peter D. Walzer. -- 2nd ed., rev. and expanded.
    p. cm. -- (Lung biology in health and disease ; v. 69)
    Includes bibliographical references and indexes.
    ISBN 0-8247-8854-0 (alk. paper)
    1. Pneumocystis carinii pneumonia. I. Walzer, Peter D.
  II. Series.
    [DNLM: 1. Pneumonia, Pneumocystis carinii. W1 LU62 v.69 1994 / WC 209 P738 1994]
RC772.I56P57 1994
616.2'41--dc20
DNLM/DLC
for Library of Congress   93-11338
                                                                                     CIP

The publisher offers discounts on this book when ordered in bulk quantities. For more information, write to Special Sales/Professional Marketing at the address below.

This book is printed on acid-free paper.

Copyright © 1994 by Marcel Dekker, Inc. All Rights Reserved.

Neither this book nor any part may be reproduced or transmitted in any form or by any means, electronic or mechanical, including photocopying, microfilming, and recording, or by any information storage and retrieval system, without permission in writing from the publisher.

Marcel Dekker, Inc.
270 Madison Avenue, New York, New York 10016

Current printing (last digit):
10 9 8 7 6 5 4 3 2 1

PRINTED IN THE UNITED STATES OF AMERICA

To Eileen and Eugene Walzer
for their love of words and medicine

INTRODUCTION

Life is short and the Art long; the occasion fleeting; experience fallacious, and judgement difficult.
—Hippocrates

Were Hippocrates alive today, would he say this about the acquired immunodeficiency syndrome (AIDS)? Probably! As Dr. Walzer states in his preface to this volume, "*Pneumocystis carinii* is an organism of major medical, scientific, and public health importance." Despite the early identification of the organism in 1910, progress in understanding it has been very slow. Indeed, it took the appearance and evolution of the AIDS epidemic to stimulate research on *P. carinii*.

Today, lung disease associated with HIV-1 infection continues to be the leading cause of death in people with AIDS. It was reported in 1989 that *P. carinii* pneumonia (PCP) was the AIDS-defining illness in 60% of the cases, and that it accounted for 59% of the deaths. Since that time, significant advances have been made in the prevention and treatment of PCP—largely because the magnitude of the research enterprise has increased markedly and new drugs have been developed and used in prophylactic and therapeutic (albeit palliative) regimens. As well, our ability to diagnose PCP has advanced.

Despite significant recent progress, it is likely that this form of pneumonia will continue to be responsible for much morbidity in persons with AIDS and in other immunosuppressed patients. However, the continued strides in our knowledge of *Pneumocystis* and its relationship to the lung should improve our ability to develop and screen more drugs with potential activity against the organism.

This volume provides an up-to-date account of our knowledge about this condition. There is no doubt that it will be of considerable interest to its readership of clinicians and researchers: in addition to describing what we know today, it identifies questions and avenues of investigation that are waiting to be explored.

PCP is a terrible condition with a frightening toll. It does indeed remind us that the experience is fallacious and the judgment difficult . . . but also that the art is long.

This volume is a major contribution to the field and a true asset to the series of monographs Lung Biology in Health and Disease. I am grateful to Dr. Walzer and the contributors for having given so much time and talent to this contribution.

Claude Lenfant, M.D.
Bethesda, Maryland

FOREWORD

More than a decade and a half ago, I set out to organize a book on what was then considered an esoteric disease entity: namely, *Pneumocystis carinii* pneumonia (1). In the 1960s and 1970s, there had been growing clinical recognition of a nosological entity caused by this putative protozoan that was almost exclusively associated with the immunocompromised host. Investigators like Karl Western and Peter Walzer had sorted out some of the basic epidemiology during their tenures at the Centers for Disease Control, Beryl Jameson had studied the circulating humoral response against this agent, Henry Masur evaluated the interaction of pneumocysts with phagocytic cells, and Walzer and James Smith (among others) had tried to propagate these organisms ex vivo and in immunosuppressed animal models such as the nude mouse. However, when it was time to put the final book together, we felt that what we had been working on was indeed a curiosity that was unlikely to affect the mainstream of American or international medicine.

Just as the first edition of *Pneumocystis carinii Pneumonia* was about to be published in 1982, I received a call from the publisher suggesting that we add a chapter. About a year earlier, clinicians had begun to see pneumocystosis in an extraordinary new group of patients, unlike those previously linked to this complication. I am, of course, referring to the now well-established association between *P. carinii* infection and the acquired immunodeficiency syndrome (AIDS). Since I was at UCLA in the early 1980s, I thought it logical to ask my fellow clinicians Michael Gottlieb, Jerome Groopman, and Philip Zakowski to contribute a chapter to the book summarizing the salient features about the presentation of the disease and the clinical significance of pneumocystosis in what was then the "gay-related immune deficiency syndrome" (now clearly appreciated as a more global problem and appropriately called AIDS).

In the 10 years that have elapsed since the first publication of *Pneumocystis carinii Pneumonia*, a breathtaking amount of new knowledge has accumulated about this pathogen. I need not reiterate the table of contents of this new volume, but I am simply overwhelmed by the productivity of so many new workers who have been drawn into the field. Their interest in studying basic *P. carinii* taxonomy, immunology, pathology, clinical expression, and clinical management has been fueled by the appreciation of the AIDS pandemic worldwide. AIDS is surely the greatest health crisis of modern times. I see no end in sight, but I also realize that crisis is the parent of invention in science and medicine as well as in warfare. The urgent need to understand this pathogen and to develop new treatments has spawned breathtaking advances in molecular biology, meticulous epidemiological studies, further valuable studies of host defense, and seminal studies of the treatment and prevention of *P. carinii* pneumonia in the immunocompromised host, using agents that have never previously been used to treat this opportunistic infection.

Tremendous progress has been made, yet there are some astonishing failures in our approaches toward understanding this ubiquitous pathogen. I speak of our inability to cultivate this organism for extended passage in artificial media and our helplessness in trying to estimate, ex vivo, what drugs might be active against this organism. It is hoped that the combined efforts of so many individuals and laboratories who have contributed to this extraordinary volume of knowledge will provide answers. Surely this must be one of the most common infectious disease pathogens of mankind, and an understanding and effective treatment and prophylaxis of pneumocystosis will have many dividends not only to the field of clinical immunology and AIDS care, but to cancer treatment, organ transplantation, and virtually every clinical state where individuals are immunosuppressed. I can only say, as one who has become inactive in this field (preferring to turn my attention to organisms that are more easily cultivated in the laboratory), that I respect the tenacity of the enthusiastic investigators who have contributed to this volume and will watch with interest as the insights of knowledge they provide herein will further fuel much-needed research in the future.

Lowell S. Young, M.D.
Director
Kuzell Institute for Arthritis and
Infectious Diseases
San Francisco, California

Reference

1. Young LS, ed. *Pneumocystis carinii* Pneumonia. New York: Marcel Dekker, 1984.

PREFACE

Pneumocystis carinii is an organism of major medical, scientific, and public health importance. The first edition of this book, published in 1984 and edited by Dr. Lowell Young, was widely acclaimed as a valuable and authoritative reference. The dramatic changes since that time in our concepts of *P. carinii*, stemming from its association with the acquired immunodeficiency syndrome (AIDS), created the need for a second edition. To better understand these events and the revisions that have been made in the new edition, it is appropriate to briefly review the history of *P. carinii* and the conferences and publications that have been devoted to this organism.

P. carinii was discovered in the early 1900s but did not attract attention until the 1940s and 1950s, when it was found to be the etiological agent of interstitial plasma cell pneumonia. This was a disorder that afflicted premature, malnourished infants in orphanages in Europe during World War II, but has also been reported in other parts of the world where such conditions exist. In the 1960s and 1970s, *P. carinii* became recognized as a major cause of pneumonia in the immunocompromised host and thus represented a complication of medical progress. Increasing numbers of cancer patients and organ transplant recipients were being kept alive by more aggressive immunosuppressive or cytotoxic therapy; advances in immunology led to the identification and characterization of primary immune deficiency disorders. Research on *P. carinii* was inhibited by the lack of a reliable in vitro cultivation system. With the discovery of safe, effective therapy and prophylaxis for *P. carinii*, the lack of basic knowledge about the biology of the organism did not seem to be an urgent problem.

In the 1980s, *P. carinii* became recognized as the leading cause of opportunistic infection and mortality in patients with AIDS in the United States and many countries in Western Europe. Pneumocystosis in AIDS patients was characterized by new clinical features, such as subtle presentation, extrapulmonary manifestations, and high frequency of recurrence. Major new problems for the use of standard anti–*P. carinii* drugs developed in terms of efficacy, toxicity, and cost. The tens of thousands of cases of *P. carinii* pneumonia that occurred each year created an enormous burden on the health care system, and "PCP" became well known in the media as a rallying point for activist groups demanding more government action on AIDS. These events stimulated new initiatives in basic and clinical *P. carinii* research, such as the National Cooperative Drug Discovery Groups, the AIDS Clinical Trials Units, and special grants and contracts.

The first international conference on *P. carinii* was held in December 1973, at the National Institutes of Health. Emphasis was placed on the clinical aspects of *P. carinii* pneumonia and on tracing the development of the disease from its occurrence in debilitated infants to the compromised host. The proceedings of this meeting were published as the *National Cancer Institute Monograph #43* in 1976. Fifteen years elapsed before the second conference, which was held at the University of Bristol, England, in July 1988, under the auspices of the Society of Protozoologists. This meeting focused on research and attracted physicians and basic scientists from all over the world. There were some truly startling revelations (e.g., ribosomal RNA data suggesting that *P. carinii* is a member of the fungi), which led to major changes in our concepts of the organism. Collaborative projects developed involving subjects ranging from molecular biology to drug therapy. The proceedings of this meeting were published in the January/February 1989 issue of the *Journal of Protozoology*. The third international conference, also sponsored by the Society of Protozoologists, was held at Montana State University, Bozeman, Montana, in July 1991, and the proceedings appeared in the November/December 1991 issue of the *Journal of Protozoology*. The meeting built on the success of its predecessor and, judging by the increased attendance and number of papers presented, enthusiasm for gatherings of this type will remain high for the foreseeable future.

Three books have been devoted exclusively to *P. carinii*. The first was the original edition of *Pneumocystis carinii Pneumonia*, edited by Dr. Young. This book was conceived before the AIDS epidemic became widely known; although a chapter on AIDS was included, most of the text was devoted to the pre-AIDS era. The book consisted of eight chapters written by nine contributing authors who were given considerable freedom in chapter length and content. *Pneumocystis carinii Pneumonitis*, a two-volume text written by Dr. Walter Hughes in 1987, was a systematic and thorough analysis of *P. carinii* since its discovery and included some material on AIDS. *Pneumocystis carinii*, written by Dr. Julian Hopkin in 1991, is a concise review of our current clinical and basic knowledge of the organism.

The second edition of *Pneumocystis carinii Pneumonia* has undergone major changes. Since Dr. Young was no longer actively engaged in *P. carinii* research, I was asked to become the editor. I had been a contributor to the first edition and had also served as the editor of another Marcel Dekker book, *Parasitic Infections in the Compromised Host*, published in 1989. Dr. Young's Foreword provides continuity beween the two editions.

The second edition consists of 31 chapters written by more than 40 contributors. This marked increased over the first edition reflects the dramatic rise in the general level of interest in and understanding of this organism. The authors who participated in this endeavor are among the leaders in *P. carinii* clinical care and research. The book has been designed to present a balanced and comprehensive examination of the latest advances in this field, and to contain the most up-to-date references. There has also been an attempt to include topics (e.g., drug development) that have received little formal attention in the past.

Chapters in the book have been arranged according to the traditional subject headings. A major effort has been made to allow the authors latitude to express their opinions while at the same time giving careful attention to issues of clarity, continuity, and avoidance of duplication. However, as with any multiauthored text, some areas of controversy and overlap were unavoidable.

Although this book is intended as a reference text on *P. carinii*, I believe it will have wide appeal to clinicians and basic scientists who are interested in AIDS and opportunistic infections.

Peter D. Walzer

CONTRIBUTORS

Donald Armstrong, M.D.   Chief, Infectious Disease Service, Memorial Sloan–Kettering Cancer Center, and Professor of Medicine, Cornell University Medical College, New York, New York

Martine Y. K. Armstrong, M.D.   Senior Research Scientist, Department of Epidemiology and Public Health, Yale University School of Medicine, New Haven, Connecticut

Marilyn S. Bartlett, M.S.   Professor of Pathology, Indiana University School of Medicine, Indianapolis, Indiana

Robert P. Baughman, M.D.   Associate Professor of Medicine, Division of Pulmonary and Critical Care Medicine, Department of Internal Medicine, University of Cincinnati College of Medicine, Cincinnati, Ohio

Constance A. Bell, M.S.P.H., Ph.D.   Division of Experimental Therapeutics, Walter Reed Army Institute of Research, Washington, D.C.

John R. Black, M.D. Clinical Associate Professor, Department of Internal Medicine, Indiana University School of Medicine, Indianapolis, Indiana

Samuel A. Bozzette, M.D. Department of Medicine, University of California, San Diego, and Health Sciences Program, RAND, Santa Monica, California

Melanie T. Cushion, Ph.D. Assistant Professor of Medicine, Division of Infectious Diseases, Department of Internal Medicine, University of Cincinnati College of Medicine, Cincinnati, Ohio

Michael N. Dohn, M.D. Assistant Professor of Clinical Medicine, Division of Pulmonary and Critical Care Medicine, Department of Internal Medicine, University of Cincinnati College of Medicine, Cincinnati, Ohio

Jeffrey C. Edman, M.D. Assistant Professor, Department of Laboratory Medicine, University of California, San Francisco, San Francisco, California

Jay A. Fishman, M.D. Assistant Professor of Medicine, Infectious Disease Unit and Transplantation Unit, Massachusetts General Hospital and Harvard Medical School, Boston, Massachusetts

Peter T. Frame, M.D. Professor of Clinical Medicine, Division of Infectious Diseases, Department of Internal Medicine, University of Cincinnati College of Medicine, Cincinnati, Ohio

Francis Gigliotti, M.D. Associate Professor of Pediatrics and of Microbiology and Immunology, Department of Pediatrics, University of Rochester School of Medicine and Dentistry, Rochester, New York

Don C. Graves, Ph.D. Professor of Microbiology and Immunology, Department of Microbiology and Immunology, University of Oklahoma Health Sciences Center, Oklahoma City, Oklahoma

Julian Hopkin, M.D. Consultant Physician, Osler Chest Unit, Churchill Hospital, Oxford, England

Walter T. Hughes, M.D. Chairman, Department of Infectious Diseases, St. Jude Children's Research Hospital, Memphis, Tennessee

Roger W. Jelliffe, M.D. Professor of Medicine, Laboratory of Applied Pharmacokinetics, Department of Medicine, University of Southern California School of Medicine, and Los Angeles County–University of Southern California Medical Center, Los Angeles, California

Contributors

Edna S. Kaneshiro, Ph.D. Professor, Department of Biological Sciences, University of Cincinnati, Cincinnati, Ohio

Joseph A. Kovacs, M.D. Head, AIDS Section, Critical Care Medicine, National Institutes of Health, Bethesda, Maryland

Gregg Y. Lipschik, M.D. Director, Medical Intensive Care Unit, Philadelphia Veterans Affairs Medical Center, and Assistant Professor, Departments of Medicine and Microbiology, Medical College of Pennsylvania, Philadelphia, Pennsylvania

Willliam J. Martin II, M.D. Floyd and Reba Smith Professor of Medicine, Department of Medicine, Indiana University Medical Center, Indianapolis, Indiana

Henry Masur, M.D. Chief, Critical Care Medicine, Warren G. Magnuson Clinical Center, National Institutes of Health, Bethesda, Maryland

Edward L. Pesanti, M.D. Chief, Medical Service, Veterans Affairs Medical Center, and Professor of Medicine, University of Connecticut, Newington, Connecticut

Dianne C. Polsen, M.D. Fellow, Critical Care Medicine, National Institutes of Health, Bethesda, Maryland

Scott T. Pottratz, M.D. Assistant Professor of Medicine, Division of Pulmonary and Critical Care Medicine, Indiana University Medical Center, Indianapolis, Indiana

Sherry F. Queener, Ph.D. Professor, Department of Pharmacology and Toxicology, Indiana University School of Medicine, Indianapolis, Indiana

John B. Roths, Ph.D. Research Associate, Department of Molecular Genetics, Biochemistry, and Microbiology, University of Cincinnati College of Medicine, Cincinnati, Ohio

John J. Ruffolo, Ph.D. Director of Sponsored Programs, Henry M. Jackson Foundation for the Advancement of Military Medicine, Rockville, Maryland

Fred R. Sattler, M.D. Associate Professor, Department of Medicine, University of Southern California School of Medicine, and Los Angeles County–University of Southern California Medical Center, Los Angeles, California

Dennis M. Schmatz, Ph.D. Director, Department of Parasite Biochemistry and Cell Biology, Merck Research Laboratories, Rahway, New Jersey

Charles L. Sidman, Ph.D.   Professor, Department of Molecular Genetics, Biochemistry, and Microbiology, University of Cincinnati College of Medicine, Cincinnati, Ohio

Richard G. Sleight, Ph.D.   Associate Professor, Department of Molecular Genetics, Biochemistry, and Microbiology, University of Cincinnati College of Medicine, Cincinnati, Ohio

James W. Smith, M.D.   Professor and Chairman, Department of Pathology, Indiana University School of Medicine, Indianapolis, Indiana

A. George Smulian, M.D.   Staff Physician, Cincinnati Veterans Affairs Medical Center, and Assistant Professor of Clinical Medicine, Division of Infectious Diseases, Department of Internal Medicine, University of Cincinnati College of Medicine, Cincinnati, Ohio

Mitchell L. Sogin, Ph.D.   Senior Scientist, Molecular Evolution Center, Marine Biological Laboratory, Woods Hole, Massachusetts

James R. Stringer, Ph.D.   Associate Professor, Department of Molecular Genetics, Biochemistry, and Microbiology, University of Cincinnati College of Medicine, Cincinnati, Ohio

Edward E. Telzak, M.D.   Chief, Division of Infectious Disease, Bronx–Lebanon Hospital Center, and Albert Einstein College of Medicine, Bronx, New York

Richard R. Tidwell, Ph.D.   Professor, Departments of Pathology and Medicinal Chemistry, School of Medicine, University of North Carolina at Chapel Hill, Chapel Hill, North Carolina

William D. Travis, M.D.   Chief, Pulmonary Pathology Section, Laboratory of Pathology, National Cancer Institute, National Institutes of Health, Bethesda, Maryland, and Armed Forces Institute of Pathology, Washington, D.C.

Ann E. Wakefield, D.Phil.   Royal Society University Research Fellow, Molecular Infectious Diseases Group, Institute of Molecular Medicine, University of Oxford, Oxford, England

Robert E. Walker, M.D.   Medical Officer, Laboratory of Immunoregulation, National Institute of Allergy and Infectious Diseases, National Institutes of Health, Bethesda, Maryland

Peter D. Walzer, M.D.   Chief, Infectious Disease Section, Cincinnati Veterans Affairs Medical Center, and Professor of Medicine, University of Cincinnati College of Medicine, Cincinnati, Ohio

CONTENTS

Introduction Claude Lenfant   *v*
Foreword Lowell S. Young   *vii*
Preface   *ix*
Contributors   *xiii*

PART ONE: BASIC BIOLOGY

1. In Vitro Cultivation   **3**

Martine Y. K. Armstrong and Melanie T. Cushion

    I. Introduction   3
    II. Historical Background   4
    III. Problems Surrounding *Pneumocystis carinii* Culture   4
    IV. Culture Systems in Current Use: Their Limitations and Application   17
    V. Conclusions and Future Approaches   20
        References   22

xvii

2. *Pneumocystis carinii* Cell Structure — 25

John J. Ruffolo

    I. Introduction — 25
   II. Trophic Stages — 27
  III. Encystment (Sporogenesis) — 31
  IV. Excystation (Spore Release) — 34
   V. Endogeny (Thin-Walled Cysts) — 35
  VI. Relation of Structure to Function and Taxonomy — 35
 VII. Conclusions — 38
      References — 39

3. Biochemistry and Metabolism — 45

Edna S. Kaneshiro and Richard G. Sleight

    I. Introduction — 45
   II. Intermediary and General Metabolism — 46
  III. Nucleic Acids — 49
  IV. Proteins — 52
   V. Lipids — 55
  VI. Carbohydrates — 58
 VII. Conclusions — 64
      References — 65

4. Molecular Genetics of *Pneumocystis carinii* — 73

James R. Stringer

    I. Introduction — 73
   II. The Genome of *Pneumocystis cariniii* — 74
  III. *Pneumocystis carinii* Genes — 83
  IV. Transcription and Translation — 87
   V. Conclusion — 88
      References — 89

5. Molecular Phylogeny of *Pneuocystis carinii* — 91

Jeffrey C. Edman and Mitchell L. Sogin

    I. Introduction and Background — 91
   II. Relevance — 92
  III. Previous Attempts at Classification — 94

IV. Phylogenetic Relations Based on Molecular Biological Information	94
V. Additional Genes that Could Be Studied	101
VI. Conclusions	102
References	103

6. Antigenic Characteristics of *Pneumocystis carinii*   107

Francis Gigliotti

I. Introduction	107
II. Surface Glycoprotein A (Mannosylated Surface Glycoprotein, gp120, gp95)	108
III. Other Antigens	114
IV. New Directions	115
V. Conclusion	116
References	117

PART TWO: EPIDEMIOLOGY

7. Transmission and Epidemiology   123

Melanie T. Cushion

I. Introduction	123
II. Evidence for an Airborne Mode of Transmission	124
III. Origin of Infection	125
IV. Epidemiology	130
References	137

8. Serological Studies of *Pneumocystis carinii* Infection   141

A. George Smulian and Peter D. Walzer

I. Introduction	141
II. Complement Fixation Assays	145
III. Indirect Immunofluorescent Assay	145
IV. Enzyme Immunoassay	146
V. Immunoblotting	147
VI. Serology of *Pneumocystis carinii* Outbreaks	149
VII. Conclusion	149
References	149

PART THREE: PATHOPHYSIOLOGY

9. Pathological Features   155

William D. Travis

I. Introduction	155
II. Classic Histopathology	157
III. Unusual Histological Features	158
IV. Concomitant Processes	171
V. Treated *Pneumocystis carinii* Pneumonia	171
VI. Disseminated (Extrapulmonary) *Pneumocystis carinii* Infection	173
VII. Immunohistochemistry	173
VIII. Conclusion	173
References	174

10. Animal Models   181

Martine Y. K. Armstrong and Melanie T. Cushion

I. Introduction	181
II. The Classic Corticosteroid-Treated Rat Model of *Pneumocystis carinii* Pneumonia	182
III. *Pneumocystis carinii* Infection in Mice	187
IV. Development of Inoculated Rodent Models	190
V. *Pneumocystis carinii* Infection in Immunodeficient Mice and Rats	193
VI. *Pneumocystis carinii* Infection in Other Mammals	202
VII. *Pneumocystis carinii* Strain and Species Variations	209
VIII. Conclusion	213
References	215

11. New Animal Models for *Pneumocystis carinii* Research: Immunodeficient Mice   223

Charles L. Sidman and John B. Roths

I. Introduction: Advantages of Mutant Mouse Models	223
II. *scid* Mice and Mechanisms of Immunity to *P. carinii*	225
III. Non-*scid* Mouse Models of *P. carinii*	227
IV. *P. carinii* Derived from Mouse Versus Other Species	230
V. Synergy Between *P. carinii* and Other Organisms	231
VI. Considerations for Colony Maintenance	232

VII.	Conclusions	233
	References	233

12. Mechanisms of *Pneumocystis carinii* Attachment to Lung Cells 237

Scott T. Pottratz and William J. Martin II

I.	Introduction	237
II.	Pathogen Attachment Mechanisms	237
III.	*Pneumocystis carinii* Attachment	240
IV.	Fibronectin-Mediated *Pneumocystis carinii* Attachment	241
V.	Lectin-Mediated *Pneumocystis carinii* Attachment	245
VI.	Conclusion	246
	References	246

13. Pathogenic Mechanisms 251

Peter D. Walzer

I.	Introduction	251
II.	Establishment of the Infection	251
III.	Organism Proliferation	253
IV.	Changes in the Alveolar Microenvironment	256
V.	Host Inflammatory or Immune Response	260
VI.	Conclusion	261
	References	261

14. Humoral and Cellular Immunity 267

Don C. Graves, A. George Smulian, and Peter D. Walzer

I.	Introduction	267
II.	Humoral Immunity	269
III.	Cellular Immunity	275
IV.	Conclusion	281
	References	281

15. Host Defense Effector Mechanisms and *Pneumocystis carinii* 289

Edward L. Pesanti

I.	Introduction	289
II.	Background	289
III.	Functions of Phagocytic Cells Against *Pneumocystis carinii*	291

IV.	Nonphagocytic Mechanisms of Host Defense Against *Pneumocystis carinii*	293
V.	Cellular Immunity, Cytokines, and Epithelial Cells	298
VI.	Evasion of Host Defense Effectors by *Pneumocystis carinii*	303
VII.	Conclusions	305
	References	306

PART FOUR: CLINICAL FEATURES

16. Clinical Manifestations in Children   319

Walter T. Hughes

I.	Introduction	319
II.	Asymptomatic Infection	320
III.	Infantile Interstitional Plasma Cell Pneumonitis	320
IV.	Child–Adult Sporadic Pneumonitis in the Immunocompromised Host	321
V.	Extrapulmonary *Pneumocystis carinii* Infection	326
VI.	Treatment	326
VII.	Prevention	327
	References	327

17. Clinical Manifestations in Adults   331

Michael N. Dohn and Peter T. Frame

I.	Introduction	331
II.	Risk Groups for *Pneumocystis carinii* Pneumonia	332
III.	Clinical Presentation and Markers for Disease Severity and Prognosis	336
IV.	Clinical Course of *Pneumocystis carinii* Pneumonia	345
V.	Conclusion	349
	References	349

18. Extrapulmonary Infection and Other Unusual Manifestations of *Pneumocystis carinii*   361

Edward E. Telzak and Donald Armstrong

I.	Introduction	361
II.	Extrapulmonary Infection	362
III.	Frequency of Extrapulmonary *Pneumocystis carinii*	362
IV.	Clinical Presentation	363
V.	Case Reports	364

VI. Diagnosis and Pathology	371
VII. Outcome	372
VIII. Risk Factors	372
IX. Unusual Pulmonary Manifestations of *Pneumocystis carinii* Pneumonia	373
X. Pneumothorax	374
XI. Summary	375
References	375

PART FIVE: DIAGNOSIS

19. Current Methods of Diagnosis   381

Robert P. Baughman

I. Introduction	381
II. Obtaining Specimens	382
III. Stains	388
IV. Indirect Diagnostic Measures	392
V. Conclusion	394
References	395

20. A Molecular Approach to the Diagnosis of *Pneumocystis carinii* Pneumonia   403

Ann E. Wakefield and Julian Hopkin

I. Introduction	403
II. *Pneumocystis carinii*–Specific DNA Sequences	404
III. Clinical Studies	408
IV. Epidemiology	411
V. Conclusions	412
References	412

21. Radiological Approaches to the Diagnosis of *Pneumocystis carinii* Pneumonia   415

Jay A. Fishman

I. Introduction	415
II. The Chest Radiograph in *Pneumocystis carinii* Pneumonia: Acute Infection	416
III. Computed Tomography and Magnetic Resonance Imaging	423
IV. Ultrasound	427
V. "Inflammation Imaging"	427

VI.	Resolution of Infection	430
VII.	Conclusions	431
	References	431

PART SIX: TREATMENT AND PREVENTION

22. Current Regimens of Therapy and Prophylaxis   439

Robert E. Walker and Henry Masur

I.	Introduction	439
II.	Treatment	440
III.	Adjunctive Corticosteroids	449
IV.	Prophylaxis	450
V.	Treatment and Prophylaxis in Pediatric Patients with Human Immunodeficiency Virus Infection	458
VI.	Conclusion and Future Directions	459
	References	461

23. Pharmacokinetic and Pharmacodynamic Considerations for Drug Dosing in the Treatment of *Pneumocystis carinii* Pneumonia   467

Fred R. Sattler and Roger W. Jelliffe

I.	Introduction	467
II.	Trimethoprim–Sulfamethoxazole	468
III.	Pentamidine	473
IV.	Trimethoprim–Dapsone	478
V.	Clindamycin–Primaquine	481
VI.	Experimental Therapies	482
VII.	Summary	482
	References	483

24. Development of Models and Their Use to Discover New Drugs for Therapy and Prophylaxis of *Pneumocystis carinii* Pneumonia   487

James W. Smith, Marilyn S. Bartlett, and Sherry F. Queener

I.	Introduction	487
II.	Culture Method	488
III.	Culture Screen	489
IV.	In Vitro Evaluations of Folate Pathway Antagonists	494

V. Animal Models	494
VI. Conclusions	505
References	506

25. Development of New Anti–*Pneumocystis carinii* Drugs: Cumulative Experience at a Single Institution 511

Peter D. Walzer

I. Introduction	511
II. Review of the Literature	512
III. The University of Cincinnati Experience	514
IV. Conclusions	537
References	539

26. Folate Antagonists in the Treatment of *Pneumocystis carinii* Pneumonia 545

Dianne C. Polsen, Joseph A. Kovacs, and Gregg Y. Lipschik

I. Introduction	545
II. Folate Metabolism: Overview	546
III. *Pneumocystis carinii* Dihydropteroate Synthase	548
IV. *Pneumocystis carinii* Dihydrofolate Reductase	549
V. Methods of Identifying New Agents	550
VI. Dihydropteroate Synthase Inhibitors	550
VII. Dihydrofolate Reductase Inhibitors	554
VIII. Summary and Conclusions	556
References	557

27. Pentamidine and Related Compounds in the Treatment of *Pneumocystis carinii* Infection 561

Richard R. Tidwell and Constance A. Bell

I. Introduction	561
II. Structure–Activity Studies	563
III. Pharmacology	569
IV. Toxicity	571
V. Mechanism of Action	573
VI. Drug Resistance	577
VII. Conclusions	577
References	578

28. Primaquine, Other 8-Aminoquinolines, and Clindamycin — 585

Sherry F. Queener, John R. Black, Marilyn S. Bartlett, and James W. Smith

    I. Introduction — 585
    II. In Vitro Data — 586
   III. Studies in Animal Models — 589
   IV. Treatment Studies of Clindamycin and Primaquine for *Pneumocystis carinii* Pneumonia in Humans — 597
    V. Summary — 599
       References — 600

29. Hydroxynaphthoquinones — 603

Walter T. Hughes

    I. Introduction — 603
    II. Initial Studies to Determine Anti–*Pneumocystis carinii* Activity of a 1,4-Hydroxynaphthoquinone — 604
   III. Pharmacokinetics and Safety — 604
   IV. Therapeutic Efficacy — 609
    V. Conclusion — 612
       References — 612

30. The Use of β-1,3-Glucan Synthesis Inhibitors for the Treatment and Prevention of *Pneumocystis carinii* Pneumonia — 615

Dennis M. Schmatz

    I. History of β-1,3-Glucan Synthesis Inhibitors — 615
    II. Mechanism of Action — 616
   III. Antipneumocystis Activity of β-1,3-Glucan Synthesis Inhibitors — 618
   IV. Structure–Activity Relationships and Chemically Modified Echinocandins — 619
    V. Development and Evaluation of Water-Soluble Prodrug L-693,989 — 623
   VI. Antipneumocystis Activity of Aerosolized Echinocandins — 624
  VII. Conclusion and Future Prospects — 625
       References — 626

31. Corticosteroids and Other Adjunctive Agents	**633**
Samuel A. Bozzette	
I. Introduction	633
II. Rationale	634
III. Clinical Trials	635
IV. Controversies	641
V. Other Agents	643
References	644
Author Index	*649*
Subject Index	*701*

PNEUMOCYSTIS CARINII PNEUMONIA

SECOND EDITION, REVISED AND EXPANDED

Part One

BASIC BIOLOGY

1

In Vitro Cultivation

MARTINE Y. K. ARMSTRONG

Yale University School of Medicine
New Haven, Connecticut

MELANIE T. CUSHION

University of Cincinnati College of Medicine
Cincinnati, Ohio

I. Introduction

Much of the basic biology of *Pneumocystis carinii* remains unknown because of the absence of a standard source of plentiful organisms free from host contamination. As sustained growth of *P. carinii* in vitro has yet to be achieved, investigators are still heavily dependent for their studies on organisms derived from animal models of *P. carinii* pneumonia. The lack of a reproducible culture system was identified as the key obstacle to progress in the management of *P. carinii* pneumonia by the National Institutes of Health (NIH) workshop on future directions in discovery and development of therapeutic agents for opportunistic infections associated with the acquired immunodeficiency syndrome (AIDS) (1). The workshop, convened in September 1989, recommended as a first priority the development of in vitro cultivation of *P. carinii*, to advance understanding of its biology and to foster drug discovery. As a direct result of this recommendation, the National Heart, Lung, and Blood Institute and the National Institute of Allergy and Infectious Diseases jointly organized and sponsored the formation of a working group on the cultivation of pneumocystis, which met in September 1990. Some of the material presented in this chapter is based on the document developed by this working group (2) and represents a synthesis of the participants' experience with *P. carinii* culture.

II. Historical Background

After the etiological relation of *P. carinii* to interstitial plasma cell pneumonitis of premature and marasmic infants was established in the 1950s (3), several reports were published describing the isolation and growth of yeast-life forms from the lungs of such patients, using fungal media. These reports have been reviewed in some detail (4–6), and the consensus seems to be that there is no convincing proof that the fungal-like forms isolated were *P. carinii*. Subsequent attempts to cultivate *P. carinii* in a cell-free environment using a wide variety of media formulations for isolating and growing either bacteria, fungi, or parasites, were all unsuccessful. It was not until 1977 that the propagation of *P. carinii* was first reported (7), using cultures of primary embryonic chick epithelial lung cells. In the years that have elapsed since then, numerous other cell types have been investigated for their potential to support the growth of *P. carinii* in vitro. Although modest growth has been reported by various investigators using a number of different cell cultures, there is general agreement that no reproducible, continuous culture system for *P. carinii* currently exists (1,2,6).

III. Problems Surrounding *Pneumocystis carinii* Culture

Table 1 summarizes several studies reporting growth of *P. carinii* in cell culture (7–16). It is evident from the reports that some *P. carinii* growth has been observed at one time or another in all of these cell culture systems. However, such growth has been unpredictable, difficult to document, not readily reproducible, and generally limited to an initial modest multiplication of the organisms, with little or no growth on subsequent transfer.

Problems encountered during attempts to culture *P. carinii* are best appreciated when some of the properties of the organism and the milieu in which it proliferates in vivo are considered. *Pneumocystis carinii* exists as a saprophyte in the lungs of the healthy host. However, under certain conditions of immunosuppression, it may express its potential as an opportunistic pathogen, leading to the development of *P. carinii* pneumonia. Observation of *P. carinii* pneumonia development in the immunosuppressed rat model (17) has shown that *P. carinii* organisms propagate relatively slowly. Initially, a few scattered cysts are detected along alveolar septa. The establishment of *P. carinii* infection in the lungs appears to require attachment of the organism to a specific alveolar lining cell, the type I pneumocyte (18). As the organisms multiply, the alveoli gradually fill with trophozoites and cysts, set in a frothy exudate. More and more alveoli become

Table 1 Cell Cultures Reported to Support Some *P. carinii* Growth

Investigators	Source of *P. carinii*	Cell type used	Quantitation	Maximum increase in *P. carinii* number
Pifer et al. (7,8)	Sprague–Dawley rat lungs shaken in PBS	Chicken embryonic lung (CEL), Vero	Cysts only counted	Tenfold[a]
LaTorre et al. (9)	Ground Sprague–Dawley rat lung	Vero, Chang liver, MRC-5	Trophozoites and cysts stained but not counted	2^{16}-fold[b] (estimate)
Bartlett et al. (10)	Ground Sprague–Dawley rat lung	WI-38, MRC-5	Giemsa-stained organisms counted	16-fold[c]
Cushion et al. (11,12)	Homogenized Sprague–Dawley rat lung	A549, WI-38 VA 13-2RA	Trophozoites and cysts stained, nuclei and cysts counted	Tenfold[a]
Armstrong et al. (13,14)	Sprague–Dawley rat lungs washed in PBS or minced finely	Mv 1 Lu	Trophozoites and cysts stained, nuclei counted	Sixfold[d]
Durkin et al. (15,16)	Ground Sprague–Dawley rat lung	WI-38, Mv 1 Lu, A549, human embryonic lung (HEL)	Giemsa-stained organisms counted	Eightfold[a]

[a]Compared with the number of *P. carinii* organisms counted in the inoculum.
[b]Based on similar density of clumps of *P. carinii* organisms appearing in the supernatant of cultures split approximately 1:2 every week and subcultured for 4 months
[c]Compared with the number of *P. carinii* organisms counted in the culture supernatants on day 1
[d]Based on an increase in *P. carinii* organisms counted in culture supernatants between days 4 and 5 and days 7 and 8
Source: Modified from Ref. 6.

involved, and the intra-alveolar material acquires a classic honeycomb appearance. The alveolar material contains numerous *P. carinii* organisms enmeshed in a variety of host components. These include fibronectin, immunoglobulins and complement, surfactant lipids and proteins, as well as alveolar macrophages and other immune cells, their secreted products, and serum proteins that filter into the alveoli (19–22). Such alveolar contents reflect the continuing interaction between the proliferating *P. carinii* population and the alveolar lining cells, the host response to the infection, and the inherent stickiness of the organisms themselves. This stickiness underlies the cohesiveness of alveolar aggregations and is a property of the abundant, carbohydrate-rich *P. carinii* cell surface glycoprotein (23), an excess of which is also released extracellularly by the organisms (Radding JA, unpublished observation). Characteristically, *P. carinii* clump together and readily adhere to or become coated by whatever material is present in their environment. As a result, it has proved remarkably difficult to free *P. carinii* from host lung components and, once in culture, from culture components.

The inherent variability in *P. carinii* culture systems revolves around three major factors: (1) the nature of the inoculum, (2) the properties of the culture system, and (3) the assessment of *P. carinii* growth.

A. Nature of the Inoculum

A variable, but significant, proportion of *P. carinii* preparations fail to grow in a particular cell culture system that supports modest growth of other *P. carinii* preparations. Why this is, remains unclear. It could reflect (1) the influence of certain host contaminants, (2) the presence or absence of a critical number of viable *P. carinii* organisms at a specific stage in their life cycle, or (3) *P. carinii* strain differences.

Influence of Host Contaminants

Organisms inoculated into cell culture are always contaminated, to some degree, with material from host airways. Such material frequently includes other infectious agents that thrive in the setting of immune suppression. Although the effects of infectious agents such as viruses or mycoplasmas may be inapparent, contamination of the *P. carinii* inoculum with bacteria and fungi is of particular concern because of their potential to overgrow and destroy the culture. Contaminating host substances that are biologically active, such as cytokines, also have the potential to influence *P. carinii* cultivation. Their effect could be either stimulatory or inhibitory, depending on their relative presence in a particular *P. carinii* preparation. Different procedures have been used, with various degrees of success, in an attempt to maximize the yield of *P. carinii* from infected lungs and to minimize the amount of host contaminants. What has not been established is the degree to which diverse isolation procedures, such as enzyme digestion and homogenization of infected lungs, may affect the viability of the *P. carinii* organisms in the culture inoculum.

Pneumocystis carinii *Viability and Stage Specificity*

It is clear from published reports that a minimum number of *P. carinii* are required to achieve some growth of the organism in culture. The number ranges from 10^4 to 10^8, depending on the culture method used and the form of organism counted. This may reflect substantial variability in *P. carinii* viability and in the proportion of specific developmental stages from preparation to preparation. The severity of the *P. carinii* infection in the host lung from which the *P. carinii* inoculum is derived also appears to be a factor. For example, several modestly successful culture systems depend on the use of a sizeable *P. carinii* inoculum, of about 1–2 $\times$ 10^7 *P. carinii* nuclei per milliliter of medium (11–14). Furthermore, the chances for successful culture appear to be greater when the *P. carinii* preparation is obtained from rats that have developed moderate or severe *P. carinii* pneumonia. Organisms isolated from rats that develop only a mild infection often perform poorly in culture (Armstrong MYK, unpublished observation). A striking increase in the trophozoite population accompanies increasing severity of the *P. carinii* pneumonia and, in most of the cultures supporting some *P. carinii* growth, trophozoites appear to be the major proliferating population (2,13,15,24). One interpretation of these observations is that culture conditions may be conducive to only the proliferation of trophozoites and, additionally, that such proliferating trophozoites may first require to be activated in vivo. It is possible that a proportional increase in cyst forms over the culture period may reflect adverse culture conditions, since encystation is a mechanism that has evolved in many microorganisms to ensure survival in an unfavorable milieu.

Pneumocystis carinii *Strain Differences*

Strain differences among different *P. carinii* isolates may determine the success or failure of a particular culture. Recent studies of *P. carinii* karyotypes identified by pulsed-field gel electrophoresis have demonstrated strain variation among rodent *P. carinii* isolates (25–27). Although there appeared to be little genetic heterogeneity among organisms within a given isolate, a shift in the strains of *P. carinii* infecting rats occurred over an 18-month period in one of the studies (25). Of relevance is that the rats used were all Sprague–Dawley rats and that they were obtained from the same vendor. In the other study, a characteristic, but distinct, karyotype was identified in *P. carinii* isolated from each of four different colonies of infected rats, two of which consisted of Sprague–Dawley rats and two of which were Lewis rats (26). The latter study led to a further survey of *P. carinii* karyotypes in eight rat strains obtained from several vendors (27). Four of the eight rat groups produced a similar *P. carinii* karyotype, two of the groups were infected with another karyotype, and each of the two remaining rat groups harbored unique karyotypes. These data indicate that a given *P. carinii* strain can infect rats of different genetic backgrounds, and that it is not restricted to a single rat strain. Whether or not certain *P. carinii* karyotypes can adapt more readily to the culture environment awaits evaluation.

It is noteworthy that the inoculated material in those studies reporting some reproducible *P. carinii* growth in cell culture (see Table 1) have all been prepared from rats, and principally from rats of the outbred Sprague–Dawley strain. It is possible that such rats harbor specific *P. carinii* strains that adapt more readily to in vitro conditions, or that the *P. carinii* pneumonia that they develop is more severe. This latter situation might well reflect the sensitivity of these rats to immunosuppression or the nature and influence of other opportunistic infections in the colony, factors more fully discussed in the chapter on animal models (see Chap. 10). The number of *P. carinii* organisms recovered from the lungs of an individual rat with severe *P. carinii* pneumonia may reach 10^{10}, a relatively good yield for the size of the animal. Such preparations are also rich in actively proliferating trophozoites. Attempts to reproducibly culture *P. carinii* obtained from human sources (7,11,28), and particularly from patients with AIDS, have been thwarted because of problems that include an increased frequency of microbial contamination, insufficient numbers of organisms, particular quantitation difficulties, and a decrease in viability owing to therapy. Attempts to culture mouse-derived *P. carinii* have generally met with a similar lack of success, but the problem here has usually been a lack of sufficient organisms.

B. Properties of Culture Systems

Cell Monolayer Systems

Until quite recently, culture systems in which some growth of *P. carinii* has been reported have required the presence of a feeder cell layer on the culture vessel surface or on carrier beads within the culture vessel (6,15). This could reflect the necessity for interaction between the organism and a feeder cell, or that feeder cells may provide a conditioned environment conducive to short-term growth of *P. carinii*. The most widely used feeder cells have been mammalian lung-derived cells (29). These have included the following cell lines: A549 (ATCC no. CCL185, human presumptive type 2 cells derived from a lung carcinoma); MRC-5 (ATCC no. CCL171, human fibroblast-like cells derived from a 14-week fetus); WI-38 (ATCC no. CCL75, human fibroblast-like cells derived from a 3-month fetus), and WI-38 VA13-2RA (ATCC no. CCL75.1, WI-38 cells transformed by SV_{40}); HEL (human embryonic lung); Mv 1 Lu (ATCC no. CCL64, mink fibroblast-like cells, derived from near-term fetuses); L2 (ATCC no. CCL149, rat presumptive type 2 cells, derived from an adult Lewis rat).

What is the function of the feeder cells in successful *P. carinii* cultures?

Sequential observations of cell cultures following the inoculation of *P. carinii* preparations show that, within several hours, components of the inoculum become adherent to the feeder cells and that adherent organisms can be detected on feeder cell monolayers throughout the culture period (13). Although this phenomenon may merely reflect the natural adhesiveness of *P. carinii*, it may also be indicative of an active and obligatory process by which the organism must interact with an appropriate cell for its survival and growth. Such interaction may permit the transfer of essential nutrients from feeder cell to organism and could trigger proliferative activity in a susceptible form of the organism. In successful cultures, over the course of a week or so following inoculation, clumps of *P. carinii* become more clearly discernible floating freely in the culture supernatant, and these clumps become larger and more numerous (11,13,14). This apparently proliferating subpopulation consists principally of trophozoites (13–15,24). What is not clear is whether such proliferative activity is dependent on interaction with feeder cells. The degree to which *P. carinii* organisms associate with feeder cells appears to be a function of the feeder cells used. A recent report documents the variation in degree of association between *P. carinii* and three different cell lines: MRC-5, WI-38, and A-549 (30). Whether or not the intensity of *P. carinii* association with the feeder cells influences the growth of the organism in culture has not been established. In practice, those cell lines that allow *P. carinii* to be more readily released into the culture supernatant have been more useful and more widely used because the organisms harvested from the supernatant are relatively free of feeder cell contamination. The freeing of adherent organisms from the feeder cells poses the same sort of difficulties as the original isolation of *P. carinii* from infected lungs. Additionally, even though the *P. carinii* released into the supernatant are relatively easy to quantitate, enumeration of cell-associated organisms has proved too cumbersome to document readily and reproducibly.

The usefulness of certain cell types for *P. carinii* cultivation may be limited by the extent to which the feeder cells are shed into the culture medium, thereby contaminating the organisms harvested from culture supernatants. Thus, although WI-38, Mv 1 Lu, and A549 cells may, under optimal conditions, support a similar, modest increase in *P. carinii*, the A549 cells tend to slough off more readily into the culture medium (Armstrong MYK, unpublished observation).

Pifer et al. observed a cytopathic effect on primary embryonic chick epithelial lung cells, a phenomenon the severity of which increased as the ratio of organisms to lung cells was increased (7). Although overt cytopathic effects have not been observed in several different cell lines following *P. carinii* inoculation, evidence of minor damage is not uncommon. Impairment of A549 cell growth in the presence of *P. carinii* organisms has been documented (31). The degree of growth impairment was directly proportional to the number of organisms added to the culture and occurred in the absence of detectable cytopathic effects. Such cryptic damage, with subsequent repair of monolayer integrity, may underlie the scavenging property exhibited by Mv 1 Lu cells, whereby not only *P. carinii* organisms but also host cells and debris, become incorporated into the cell sheet (Armstrong MYK, unpublished observation).

Cell-Free Systems

Two culture systems devoid of mammalian cells have been reported to produce increases in rat-derived *P. carinii* similar to those obtained using monolayer-based cell culture systems (32,33). In the study by Tegoshi et al. (32), organisms obtained from the lungs of nude mice increased fourfold (by enumeration of nuclei per milliliter) in a primary culture that comprised Dulbecco's MEM or L-15 medium, 10% fetal bovine serum, 2-mercaptoethanol, bathocuprine sulfonate, and cysteine. Four serial passages of declining numbers were observed. The authors noted that *P. carinii* did not grow in cultures without the reducing agents, which presumably prevented the oxidation of cysteine to cystine, a compound that was not used by the organism.

Cushion and Ebbets identified a medium composed of 1–2% neopeptone and 10 mM *N*-acetylglucosamine at pH 4.0, which supported up to a tenfold increase in rat-derived *P. carinii* over a 3-day period (33). The organisms were metabolically active, as evidenced by the temporal incorporation of radiolabeled methionine into specific proteins (Fig. 1). However, passage of the cultures was not supported under these conditions.

Although not reported as such, the microculture-screening system of Comley et al. could also be considered another short-term cell free culture system (34). The rat-derived *P. carinii* were shown to incorporate radiolabeled *para*-aminobenzoic acid and to de novo synthesize folates in a cell-free system consisting of RPMI-1640 and 10% fetal bovine serum in HEPES buffer with 7,8-dihydro-D-neopterin, a precursor of dehydrofolate that was shown to cause a threefold increase in *para*-aminobenzoic acid uptake in this system. Although the latter two systems differed in the composition of the media used, the investigators reached similar conclusions concerning the kinetics of the organism in each system. Organisms were most viable the first 24 hr of culture, as shown by increasing uptake of tritiated *para*-aminobenzoic acid in the system of Comley et al. and by uptake of metabolic labels in the system of Cushion and Ebbets. Both studies found that, although the numbers of organisms increased during the first few days of culture, the subsequent decrease in *P. carinii* number was gradual. This was in contrast to the sharp increase in radiolabeled uptake during the first 24 hr of culture and rapid return to baseline immediately afterward. These data suggest that organisms that are no longer viable may persist in culture and contribute to an inflated organism count.

Several implications are apparent from these studies. It is now possible to radiolabel the organism without interference from the host feeder layer. This

In Vitro Cultivation

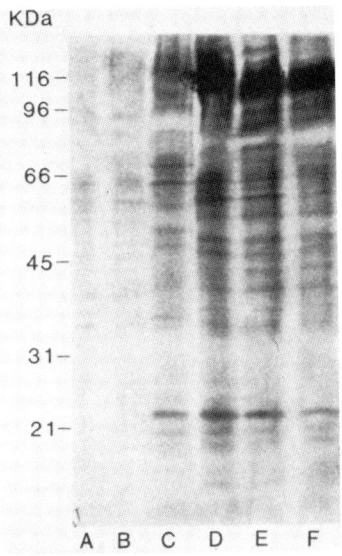

Figure 1 Autoradiogram of [^{35}S]methionine incorporation into *P. carinii* cultured in 2% neopeptone and 0.2% *N*-acetylglucosamine liquid medium over 7 days. Cultures were harvested at hour 6 (lane A), 12 (lane B), 24 (lane C), 72 (lane D), 120 (lane E), and 168 (lane F) postinoculation. Densitometric analysis revealed a fourfold increase for a protein component of relative molecular size 116 kDa. The organism density as evaluated by enumeration of nuclei per milliliter increased from an inoculum of 1.3×10^8 to 9.9×10^8. (From Ref. 33.)

should now permit investigators to evaluate uptake of nutritional compounds or metabolic precursors, providing insights into the organism's metabolic requirements. Quantification of organisms over time in culture without a viability indicator may lead to erroneous conclusions about the actual levels of growth supported by a test system. The replication of the organism in the cell-free cultures is equivalent to that observed in the monolayer-based systems, suggesting that feeder cells may not be required for the ex vivo maintenance of all developmental stages of the organism. These data also indicate that the organism "coasts" in all cultures, exhausting intracellular supplies of nutrients required for a brief burst of metabolic activity, followed by a gradual, but unrelenting, decrease in number and metabolism.

Monolayer and cell-free systems each have distinct advantages and shortcomings. It is generally believed that the infective process is mediated by attachment of *P. carinii* to the type I pneumocyte. Studies designed to identify the molecules responsible for this adherence have exploited the A549, MRC-5, and WI-38 cell lines (19,30), and further investigation into these processes will require host cells. However, problems arise when cell-based systems are used to evaluate radiolabel uptake or drug efficacy. Cell monolayers can take up radiolabeled compounds and may be affected by the experimental drugs, causing difficulties in data interpretation. In these circumstances, a cell-free system offers a better way of identifying nutritional requirements or potential therapies.

C. Assessment of *Pneumocystis carinii* Growth

Accurate assessment of *P. carinii* growth in culture has been thwarted by problems of quantitation and the lack of a standard viability assay.

Quantitation of Pneumocystis carinii Organisms

Several obstacles stand in the way of accurate quantitation of *P. carinii*. The difficulties start with the quantitation of *P. carinii* inoculated into cell culture. When *P. carinii* isolated from infected rodent lungs are stained with Giemsa or Diff-Quik, which stain trophozoites and the nuclei of intracystic bodies, both trophozoites and cysts can be identified. However, trophozoite nuclei are very small, nearly at the limit of light microscopic resolution, and their cytoplasm is often scanty and ill-defined. A trained eye is needed to distinguish such trophozoites from debris and other small structures, such as platelets. Accordingly, it is quite difficult to count accurately the total number of *P. carinii* nuclei present. In preparations from the more severely infected lungs, trophozoites are preponderant, clustered together in cloud-like masses in which their cytoplasm appears to coalesce. Such aggregates are often obscured by stained amorphous material (Fig. 2a). Because of these difficulties, some investigators choose to enumerate cysts only. Cyst wall stains, such as toluidine blue O, cresyl echt violet, and Grocott's methenamine silver nitrate, stain neither the amorphous material nor the trophozoites; the cysts generally remain discrete and, thus, are readily countable (see Fig. 2b). However, such an approach ignores the presence of a population that may be at least ten times more numerous than the cyst population. Furthermore, the cyst stains do not permit a distinction between cysts that contain intracystic bodies and cysts that are empty and presumably nonviable.

The nature of material obtained from *P. carinii*-infected human lungs makes quantitation of the human organism particularly problematic. Currently, the most common source of human *P. carinii* for in vitro studies is bronchoalveolar lavage (BAL) fluid obtained by bronchoscopy from AIDS patients with *P. carinii* pneumonia. When such BAL fluids are centrifuged and cytospin preparations of the pelleted material are stained with either Giemsa (Fig. 3a) or methenamine silver nitrate (see Fig. 3b), it can be readily appreciated that the characteristic, highly adherent aggregates of cysts and trophozoites cannot be accurately quantitated. Although cyst stains clearly delineate the wall of cysts in the preparation, the sole use of such stains discounts a major trophozoite population.

Quantitation problems continue once the *P. carinii* organisms are in culture. A major problem concerns the proportion of total organisms that are adherent to the feeder cells at any one time. This adherent population is very difficult to enumerate accurately because most procedures designed to dislodge it from the feeder cells cause the cells to detach from the surface of the culture vessel with the *P. carinii* still adherent. Although counting of adherent *P. carinii* in situ has been reported (35), a relatively accurate count is possible only when the adherent organisms remain scanty. The quantitation of *P. carinii* in the culture supernatant becomes easier as the culture proceeds, probably owing to a gradual loss of obscuring host contaminants. However, the organisms are still characteristically clumped together, a phenomenon that makes for significant sampling errors. A standard method of quantitation is as follows. An aliquot of the *P. carinii* suspension is placed within a delineated area on a glass slide and air-dried. After fixation and staining, the organisms in selected microscopic fields are counted. That count is then extrapolated to the total area/volume of the aliquot (10,12). The volume of aliquots counted by different investigators varies anywhere from 2 to 100 μL. Generally, the smaller the aliquot the greater the sampling error, although the larger aliquots tend to spread less evenly, so that the actual area counted may not be representative of the whole. It should be stressed that when enumerating *P. carinii* nuclei, the area counted is a very small portion of the whole, because adequate visualization of the minute trophozoites and intracystic bodies usually requires the use of a ×100 oil immersion objective. Replicate aliquots and replicate areas within aliquots must be counted to reduce such sampling errors, resulting in very tedious, time-consuming effort.

However, counting *P. carinii* nuclei does offer advantages over counting trophozoites or cysts, because it includes all potentially viable major life cycle stages as we currently know them: trophozoites, precysts, and intracystic bodies. Empty or spent cysts are not counted, and when the intracystic bodies are released upon cyst rupture, there is no net change in the number of organisms counted.

Viability of Pneumocystis carinii Organisms

Technical obstacles preventing accurate quantitation of *P. carinii* in its various forms are further compounded by the lack of a reproducible method for distinguishing live from dead organisms. The development of a standard, reproducible viability assay for *P. carinii* has proved elusive. This is largely due to the absence of independent, definitive criteria by which the organism's presumed viability may be confirmed. The usual criteria used to assess the significance of any one viability test are not available when that organism does not readily grow in vitro or consistently produce infection in vivo when inoculated into the airway.

Single vital stains, such as trypan blue, erythrosin B, acridine orange, and neutral red, have been used by various investigators to assess the viability of *P. carinii* in wet preparations (36). However, even if it could be established that the exclusion or uptake of a particular vital stain was unequivocal evidence that the organism was alive and well, the problem of accurately quantitating such viable organisms would remain, given their small size and tendency to clump together.

Double-staining of *P. carinii* with fluorescein diacetate and fluorescent nucleic acid-intercalating agents, such as ethidium bromide and propidium iodide

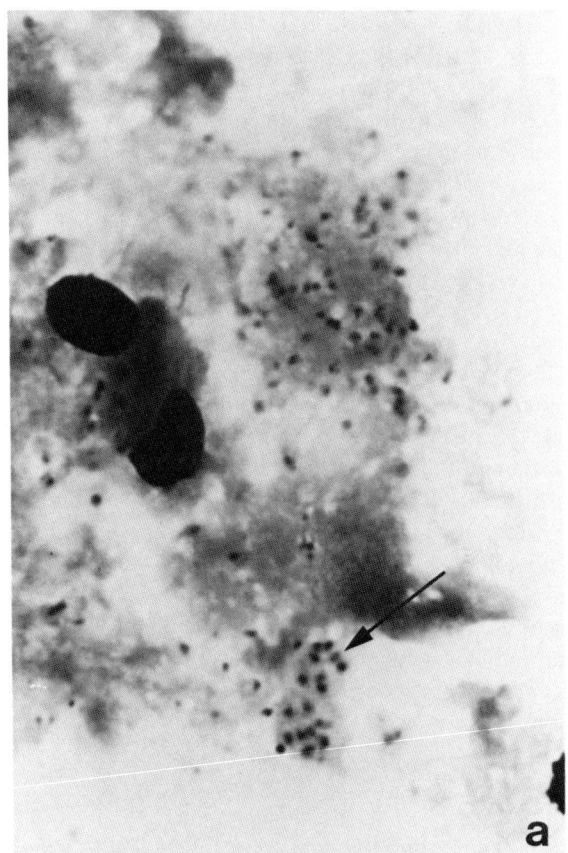

Figure 2 *P. carinii* organisms stained by two methods. (a) Giemsa-stained cytospin preparation of material washed out of the lungs of a rat with *P. carinii* pneumonia (×1000). Note the numerous tiny organism nuclei and the two large rat cell nuclei, all enmeshed in amorphous and obscuring material. The cluster of *P. carinii* nuclei (arrow) probably represents a cyst in the process of releasing its eight intracystic bodies, as does the adjacent cluster. (From Ref. 13.) (b) Cresyl echt violet (CEV)-stained cysts obtained from an infected immunosuppressed rat (×1000). Arrow indicates one of several cysts clearly visible in the field of view.

(37,38), has recently been evaluated (14,39). Esterases in the living cell covert the highly permeable, nonfluorescent fluorescein diacetate to yellow-green fluorescein. Ethidium bromide and propidium iodide are excluded by live cells, but readily penetrate dead or damaged cells where they intercalate with nucleic acids, causing such cells to fluoresce red. When stained with fluorescein diacetate and

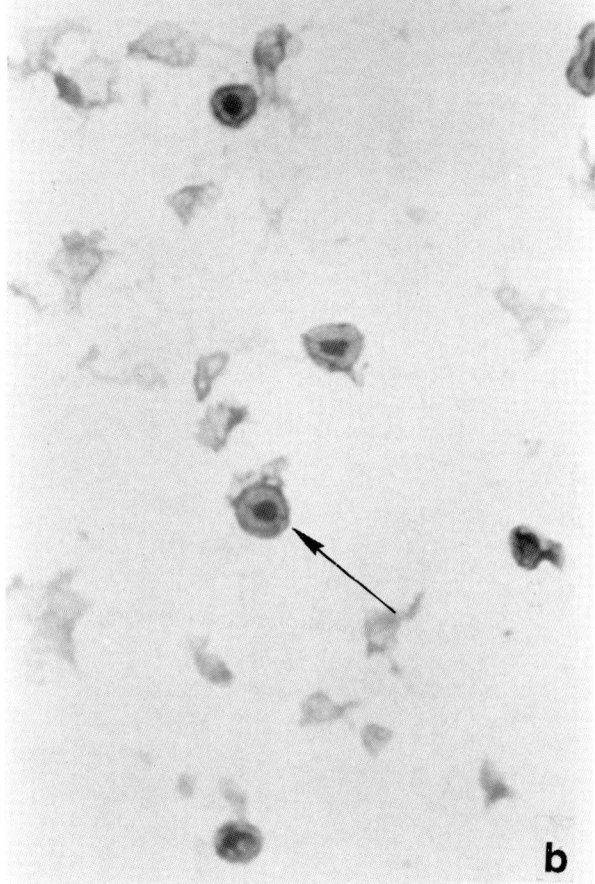

ethidium bromide or propidium iodide, most *P. carinii* in fresh preparations exhibit bright green fluorescence, whereas heat-killed organisms exhibit red fluorescence. Kaneshiro et al. (39) confirmed that cysts containing intracystic bodies that are actively motile, and hence alive, also fluoresce a bright green. Doubly stained organisms probably represent dying cells. Although there is no difficulty in distinguishing the green fluorescein from the red fluorescence of the intercalating agents, accurate quantitation of these fluorescing populations is still a problem because of the very rapid quenching of the fluorescein signal. Calcein AM (calcein acetoxymethylester; Molecular Probes, Eugene, Oregon), bleaches more slowly than does fluorescein and, when used in combination with propidium iodium iodide or ethidium homodimer, was the most reliable and interpretable

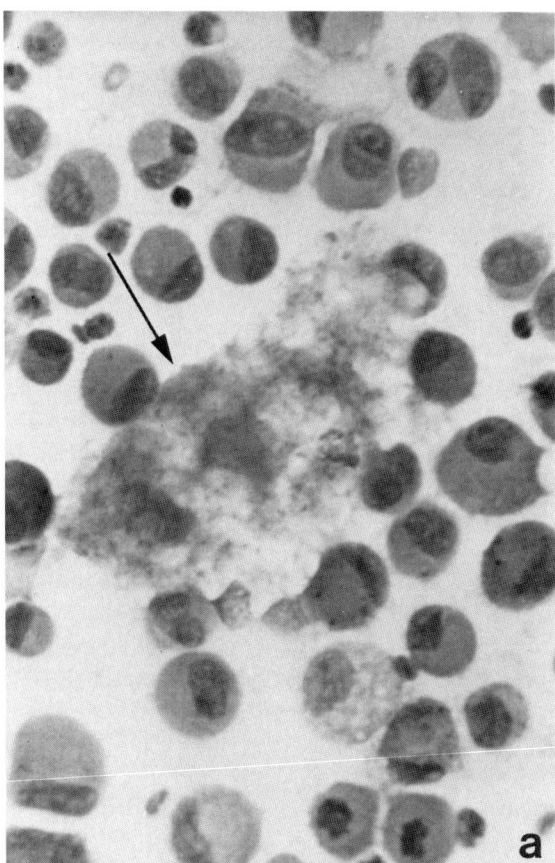

Figure 3 Cytospin preparations of pelleted bronchoalveolar lavage fluid from AIDS patients with *P. carinii* pneumonia. (a) Stained with Giemsa (×400). Note the characteristic alveolar plug (arrow), made up of highly adherent aggregates of trophic forms and cysts. (b) Stained with Grocott's methenamine silver nitrate (×400). This stain delineates only the cyst forms within an alveolar cluster (arrow).

method for *P. carinii* viability assessment by microscopy (39). Flow cytometry analysis of cultured *P. carinii* doubly stained with fluorescein diacetate and propidium iodide confirmed that over 80% of the organisms had catalyzed the conversion of fluorescein diacetate to fluorescein, and also excluded propidium iodide (14) (Fig. 4). Since the organisms in this study were sampled from culture supernatants at a time when their metabolic activity, as gauged by the level of glucan synthase activity (40), was at its peak, the flow cytometry results con-

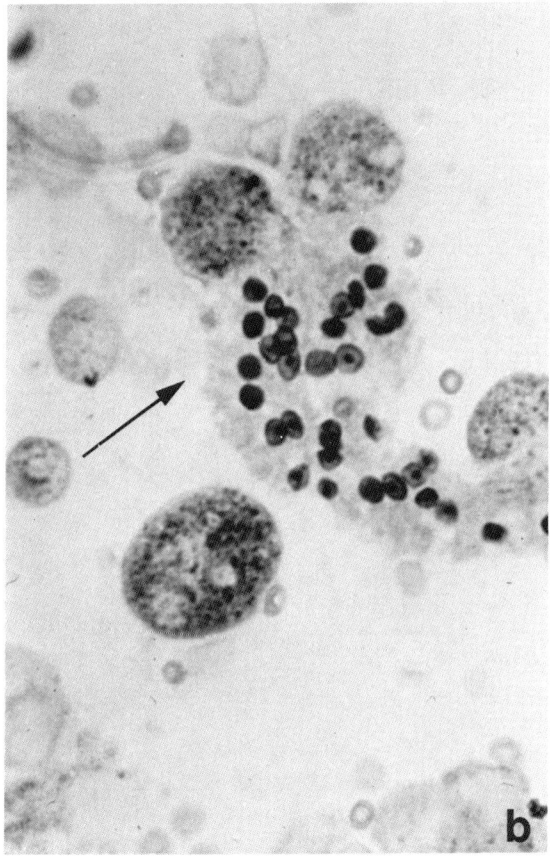

firm the validity of the double fluoregenic staining procedure as a *P. carinii* viability assay.

IV. Culture Systems in Current Use: Their Limitations and Application

The limitations of current culture systems are substantial. It is not yet possible to reproducibly document the number of viable *P. carinii* organisms inoculated into culture, nor to identify and quantitate those developmental stages in the inoculum that are capable of replicating. The difficulties are further compounded, once the culture is initiated, by the fact that a variable number of the inoculated organisms adhere to the feeder cell layer in cell culture systems where, for all practical

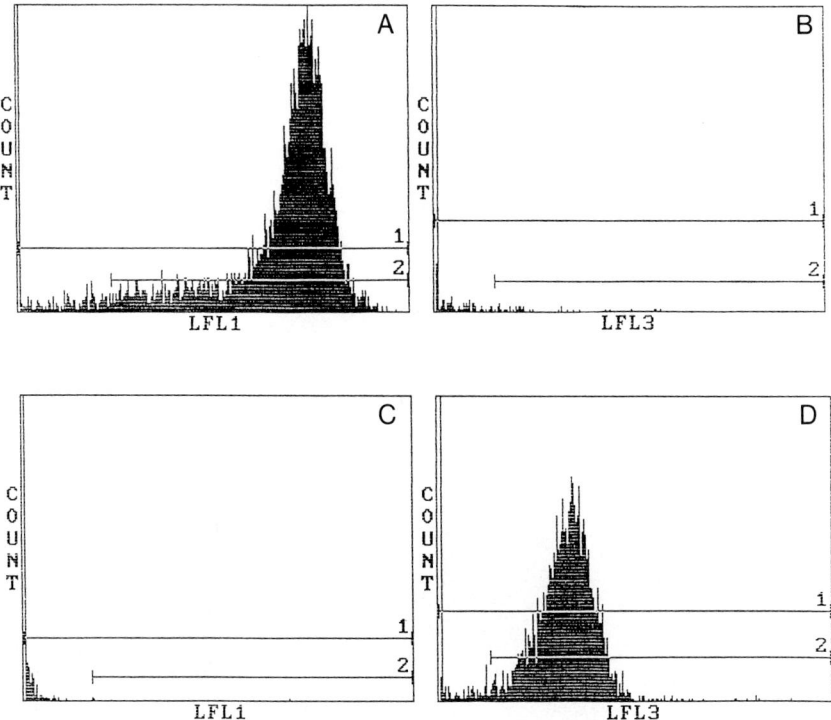

Figure 4 Flow cytometric analysis of rat *P. carinii* harvested from a 6-day culture and dually stained with fluorescein diacetate (FDA) and propidium iodide (PI), before (A,B) and after (C,D) boiling. The vertical axis represents organism number and the horizontal axis indicates log fluorescence intensity of green fluorescence (LFL1) and of red fluorescence (LFL3). As shown in A and B, over 80% of the cultured organisms exhibit FDA conversion (A), whereas fewer than 1% stain with PI (B). After boiling, the organisms no longer convert FDA to green fluorescein (C) and now stain positively with PI and fluoresce red (D). (From Ref. 14.)

purposes, they cannot be counted. Furthermore, current quantitation methods are tedious, are fraught with error, and do not distinguish live from dead organisms. Given all these circumstances, it may not be possible to unequivocally document actual growth in culture, particularly if it is modest, at best, and limited to a subpopulation of those organisms inoculated. The potential for growth in culture among *P. carinii* prepared from the lungs of different hosts remains unpredictable, bacteria and fungi from the host are a constant threat, and culture failures are all too common. Thus, any experiment utilizing *P. carinii* culture requires that the same *P. carinii* inoculum be used to assess all the study parameters. Fortunately, lung-derived *P. carinii* preparations showing some growth in culture and free of significant bacteria and fungal contaminants may be cryopreserved and successfully cultured upon thawing, without apparent loss of growth potential (13).

Despite all these limitations, investigators have capitalized on the modest and transient growth reported in the various culture systems. *Pneumocystis carinii* cell cultures have proved valuable in several ways: (1) as a source of functioning organisms relatively free of contaminating host cells and host cell products, (2) in the testing of potential anti-*P. carinii* drugs, and (3) in studies of the organism's life cycle and metabolic activity.

A. Source of Organisms for Basic Studies

Infected lungs of the immunosuppressed rat continue to be the principal source of *P. carinii* for basic studies of the organism's structure and function. Because of their adherent properties, the organisms are heavily contaminated with host material, and efforts to free them from such contamination may be damaging and often results in a significant loss of numbers. Given that *P. carinii* organisms are so much smaller than the cells of their mammalian hosts and, consequently, that their components and products are insignificant compared with those of host cells, relatively little contamination with host material suffices to compromise experimental data. A few days in an appropriate cell culture may allow enrichment of a proliferating population of *P. carinii* which, when harvested from the culture supernatant, is free of significant host cell contamination (15,16,23).

B. In Vitro Drug Testing

The responses to antimicrobial drugs by *P. carinii* in cell culture was first reported by Pifer et al. (41). Cushion et al. (42) subsequently confirmed that four antimicrobial agents used in the treatment of human pneumocystosis caused a relatively modest inhibition of the growth of rat *P. carinii* on A549 feeder cells. Investigators at Indiana University School of Medicine have made extensive use of cultures of WI-38 human embryonic lung fibroblast infected with rat *P. carinii* to test the therapeutic potential of a variety of antimicrobial agents (43–47). Unfortunately, assessment of in vitro drug sensitivity is plagued by all the technical problems that make the documentation of *P. carinii* growth so elusive. It may also be difficult to distinguish the effect that the compound under study may have on *P. carinii* organisms from the effect that it may have on the culture feeder cells. In addition, the inhibition of *P. carinii* growth in culture by certain drugs does not always correlate with the efficacy of such agents in prophylaxis and treatment of pneumocystosis in immunosuppressed rats (17).

C. Pneumocystis carinii Metabolic Activity

Pneumocystis carinii cell cultures have been used in studies of the organism's metabolic activity. Although certain metabolic and synthetic activities have been observed in short-term cell-free culture (33,48), in cell monolayer culture, such activities are greatly overshadowed by those of the feeder cells, making interpretation of the data problematic. De novo folate synthesis in *P. carinii* has recently been demonstrated (49). Because mammalian cells cannot synthesize folates de novo, this metabolic activity can be studied in the presence of feeder cells and host cell contamination. As expected, when precursor incorporation studies were carried out on *P. carinii* maintained in cultures of WI-38 cells, these feeder cells were unable to incorporate tritiated *para*-aminobenzoic acid into reduced folates, whereas the organisms did. However, under the culture conditions described (49), the incorporation by *P. carinii* of the radiolabeled precursor was short-lived and often markedly diminished after 2–3 days in culture, suggesting a loss of viability. A preliminary report (14) documents substantial and sustained *P. carinii*-specific glucan synthase activity (40) in organisms harvested from the supernatant of mink lung cell cultures. The glucan synthase activity, undetectable in uninoculated feeder cells, was observed throughout the course of 14-day cultures and peaked at a time when the number of organisms in the supernatant was maximal and when analysis of the organisms by flow cytometery confirmed their ability to catalyze the conversion of nonfluorescent fluorescein diacetate to fluorescein (14).

V. Conclusions and Future Approaches

The variability inherent in *P. carinii* cell culture systems has severely hampered efforts to identify optimal conditions for the cultivation of *P. carinii* in vitro. Simpler, more accurate ways must be developed to quantitate the organism in its various forms and to determine its viability and metabolic activity. Once growth can be unambiguously documented, systematic approaches to culturing the organism will become feasible. Without such documentation, it is very difficult to interpret the effect of any particular manipulation of the cell culture system. Lists have been published (6), and have also been compiled by members of the working group on the cultivation of pneumocystis, identifying feeder cell types, other growth matrices, and various media formulations that did not appear to support or enhance the growth of *P. carinii* in vitro (2). However, it is entirely possible that some of these modifications could be shown to be effective once all other variables are standardized.

A recent report documents a promising approach to *P. carinii* quantitation. Lapinsky et al. (50) used flow cytometric analysis to obtain reproducible quantitation of both *P. carinii* cysts and trophozoites. Purified *P. carinii*-infected rat homogenates and bronchoalveolar lavage fluids were fixed with methanol or

Formol–saline and stained with propidium iodide. By making use of the fact that propidium iodide produces as red fluorescence, the intensity of which correlates with the nucleic acid content of the cell (51), *P. carinii* organisms were identified on a flow cytometer histogram that plotted organism size against nucleic acid content. These investigators also used flow cytometry to assess the viability of fresh, unfixed *P. carinii* stained with propidium iodide alone. This they did by quantitating the number of fluorescent and presumably nonviable organisms in an aliquot of unfixed *P. carinii* suspension and using a Formol–saline-fixed aliquot of the same suspension to calculate the total number of organisms present.

Several organism-specific functions, such as glucan synthase activity (40) and de novo folate synthesis (49), are under current investigation as potential markers for *P. carinii* viability and growth. Comley et al. (34) have used *para*-aminobenzoic acid incorporation by *P. carinii* in a microtiter assay. Conditions of the assay have been optimized so that over an 18-hr period, the incorporation of *para*-[^{3}H]aminobenzoic acid into folates by *P. carinii* suspensions in 96-well microtiter plates without feeder cells is proportional to the number of organisms present. With use of such activity as an index of viability, they have developed an in vitro screening test for potential anti-*P. carinii* drugs.

The development of such readily quantifiable surrogate measures of viable *P. carinii* should facilitate the assessment of future approaches to *P. carinii* culture. One such approach might be to reproduce more precisely the complex milieu that favors *P. carinii* infection in the lung. A vital element in this milieu may well be the lipid environment at the interface between the organism and the type I pneumocyte. Although a variety of lipids have been added to *P. carinii* cultures, without enhancing effects, more physiological ways of delivering such additives need to be devised, and should be such that the organisms can also be readily separated from these lipids. Since cytokines are being increasingly incriminated in the pathogenesis of human immunodeficiency virus (HIV) infection (52), their potentially stimulatory effect on *P. carinii* cultures, both singly and in combination, should also be investigated.

At a round table discussion on the in vitro culture of *P. carinii* held during the First International Workshop on *Pneumocystis carinii* in 1988, several factors were targeted for modification that might permit the establishment of continuous culture of the organism (53). These included (1) the tissue of origin of the feeder cells; (2) the origin and preparation of serum added to the culture medium; (3) physical factors such as temperature, pH, aeration, and gas exchange; (4) supplements; and (5) growth without a feeder layer. Although there is considerable evidence that close interaction with host or feeder cells is a prerequisite for *P. carinii* growth, it is possible that sustained growth of the organism in cell-free medium can be achieved if all its nutritional requirements can be met and a proliferative stimulus is supplied. Systematic evaluation in current culture systems of the effects of various additives and metabolic precursors on defined *P. carinii*-specific functions could permit the development of continuous axenic culture. This would have decided advantages over cell monolayer culture by removing the confounding problems posed by the presence of feeder cells. Establishment of sustained *P. carinii* growth in cell-free culture would represent a major break-through in *P. carinii* research.

References

1. Laughon BE, Allaudeen HS, Becker JM, Current WL, Feinberg J, Frenkel JK, Hafner R, Hughes WT, Laughlin CA, Meyers JD, Schrager LK, Young LS. Summary of the workshop on future directions in discovery and development of therapeutic agents for opportunistic infections associated with AIDS. J Infect Dis 1991; 164:244–51.
2. Sloand E. The challenge of *Pneumocystis carinii* culture. J Euk Microbiol 1993; 40 (in press).
3. Vanek J, Jirovec O, Lukes, J. Interstitial plasma cell pneumonia in infants. Ann Paediatr 1953; 180:1–21.
4. Smith, JW, Bartlett MS. In vitro cultivation of *Pneumocystis*. In: Young L, ed. *Pneumocystis carinii* Pneumonia. New York: Marcel Dekker, 1984:107–137.
5. Hughes WT. In: *Pneumocystis carinii* Pneumonitis. vol 1. Boca Raton: CRC Press, 1987:20–32.
6. Cushion MT. In vitro studies of *Pneumocystis carinii*. J Protozool 1989; 36:45–52.
7. Pifer LL, Hughes WT, Murphy MJ. Propagation of *Pneumocystis carinii* in vitro. Pediatr Res 1977; 11:305–316.
8. Pifer LL, Woods D, Hughes WT. Propagation of *Pneumocystis carinii* in Vero cell cultures. Infect Immun 1978; 20:66–68.
9. Latorre CR, Sulzer AT, Norman LG. Serial propagation of *Pneumocystis carinii* in cell line cultures. Appl Environ Microbiol 1977; 33:1204–1206.
10. Bartlett MS, Vervanac PA, Smith JW. Cultivation of *Pneumocystis carinii* with WI-38 cell. J Clin Microbiol 1979; 10:796–799.
11. Cushion MT, Walzer PD. Growth and serial passage of *Pneumocystis carinii* in the A549 cell line. Infect Immun 1984; 44:245–251.
12. Cushion MT, Ruffolo JJ, Linke MJ, Walzer PD. *Pneumocystis carinii*: growth variables and estimates in the A549 and WI 38 VA13 human cell lines. Exp Parasitol 1985; 60:43–54.
13. Armstrong MYK, Richards FF. Propagation and purification of rat *Pneumocystis carinii* in short-term cell culture. J Protozool 1989; 36:24S–27S.
14. Armstrong MYK, Koziel H, Rose RM, Arena C, Richards FF. Indicators of *Pneumocystis carinii* viability in short-term cell culture. J Protozool 1991; 38:88S–90S.
15. Durkin MM, Bartlett MS, Queener SF, Shaw MM, Smith JW. A culture method allowing production of relatively pure *Pneumocystis carinii* trophozoites. J Protozool 1989; 36:31S–32S.
16. Durkin MM, Shaw MM, Bartlett MS, Smith JW. Culture and filtration methods for obtaining *Pneumocystis carinii* trophozoites and cysts. J Protozool 1991; 38:210S–212S.
17. Walzer PD, Kim CK, Cushion MT. *Pneumocystis carinii*. In: Walzer PD, Genta RM,

eds. Parasitic Infections in the Compromised Host. New York: Marcel Dekker, 1989: 83–178.
18. Walzer PD. Attachment of microbes to host cells: relevance of *Pneumocystis carinii*. Lab Invest 1986; 54:589–592.
19. Pottratz ST, Martin WJ II. Role of fibronectin in *Pneumocystis carinii* attachment to cultured lung cells. J Clin Invest 1990; 85:351–356.
20. Brzosko WJ, Madalinski K, Krawczynski K, Nowoslawski A. Immunochemistry in studies on the pathogenesis of pneumocystis pneumonia in infants. Ann NY Acad Sci 1971; 177:156–170.
21. Bisetti I. Pulmonary surfactant and respiratory infections. Respiration 1989; 55(suppl. 1):45–48.
22. Phelps DS, Rose RM. Increased recovery of surfactant protein A in AIDS-related pneumonia. Am Rev Respir Dis 1991; 143:1072–1075.
23. Radding JA, Armstrong MYK, Ullu E, Richards FF. Identification and isolation of a major cell surface glycoprotein of *Pneumocystis carinii*. Infect Immun 1989; 57: 2149–2157.
24. Cushion MT, Ruffolo JJ, Walzer PD. Analysis of the developmental stages of *Pneumocystis carinii*, in vitro. Lab Invest 1988; 58:324–331.
25. Lundgren B, Cotton R, Lundgren JD, Edman JC, Kovacs JA. Identification of *Pneumocystis carinii* chromosomes and mapping of five genes. Infect Immun 1990; 58:1705–1710.
26. Hong S-T, Steele PE, Cushion MT, Walzer PD, Stringer SL, Stringer JR. *Pneumocystis carinii* karyotypes. J Clin Microbiol 1990; 28:1785–1795.
27. Cushion MT, Kaselis M, Zhang J. Heterogeneity of pneumocystis isolates by pulsed field gradient electrophoresis (PFGE). Abstr Annu Meet Am Soc Microbiol. New Orleans, May 1992.
28. Blumenfeld W, Griffiss JM. In vitro differentiation of human-derived *Pneumocystis carinii*. J Clin Microbiol 1989; 27:480–485.
29. Hay RJ, Williams CD, Macy ML, LaVappa KS. Cultured cell lines for research on pulmonary physiology available through the American Type Culture Collection. Am J Respir Dis 1982; 125:222–232.
30. Jackson HC, Hancock V, Elahi N. Analysis of the dynamics of *Pneumocystis carinii* in vitro. J Protozool 1991; 38:93S–95S.
31. Limper AH, Martin WJ II. *Pneumocystis carinii*: inhibition of lung cell growth mediated by parasite attachment. J Clin Invest 1990; 85:391–396.
32. Tegoshi T. New system of in vitro cultivation of *Pneumocystis carinii* without feeder cells. J Kyoto Pref Univ Med 1988; 97:1473–1482.
33. Cushion MT, Ebbets D. Growth and metabolism of *Pneumocystis carinii* in axenic culture. J Clin Microbiol 1991; 28:1385–1394.
34. Comley JCW, Mullin RJ, Wolfe LA, Hanlon MH, Ferone R. A microculture screening assay for the primary in vitro evaluation of drugs against *Pneumocystis carinii*. Antimicrob Agents Chemother 1991; 35:1965–1974.
35. Burnstein T, Rhodes J, Turek J. Adherence of *Pneumocystis carinii* in lung cells during in vitro cultivation. J Protozool 1989; 36:35S–37S.
36. Ruffolo JJ, Cushion MT, Walzer PD. Techniques for examining *Pneumocystis carinii* in fresh specimens. J Clin Microbiol 1986; 23:17–21.

37. Jackson PR, Pappas MG, Hansen BD. Fluorogenic substrate detection of viable intracellular and extracellular pathogenic protozoa. Science 1985; 227:435–438.
38. Schupp DG, Erlandsen SL. A new method to determine giardia cyst viability: correlation of fluorescein diacetate and propidium iodide staining with animal infectivity. Appl Environ Microbiol 1987; 53:704–707.
39. Kaneshiro ES, Wu Y-P, Cushion MT. Assays for testing *Pneumocystis carinii* viability. J Protozool 1991; 38:85S–87S.
40. Williams DJ, Radding JA, Dell A, Khoo K-H, Rogers ME, Richards FF, Armstrong MYK. Glucan synthesis in *Pneumocystis carinii*. J Protozool 1991; 38:427–437.
41. Pifer LL, Pifer DD, Woods DR. Biological profile and response to anti-pneumocystis agents of *Pneumocystis carinii* in cell culture. Antimicrob Agents Chemother 1983; 24:674–687.
42. Cushion MT, Stanforth D, Linke MJ, Walzer PD. Method of testing the susceptibility of *Pneumocystis carinii* to antimicrobial agents in vitro. Antimicrob Agents Chemother 1985; 28:796–801.
43. Bartlett MS, Eichholtz R, Smith JW. Antimicrobial susceptibility of *Pneumocystis carinii* in culture. Diagn Microbiol Infect Dis 1985; 3:381–387.
44. Bartlett MS, Marr JJ, Queener SF, Klein RS, Smith JW. Activity of inosine analogs against *Pneumocystis carinii* in culture. Antimicrob Agents Chemother 1986; 30: 181–183.
45. Queener SF, Bartlett MS, Jay MA, Durkin MM, Smith JW. Activity of lipid-soluble inhibitors of dihydrofolate reductase against *Pneumocystis carinii* in culture and in a rat model of infection. Antimicrob Agents Chemother 1987; 31:1323–1327.
46. Queener SF, Bartlett MS, Richardson JD, Durkin MM, Jay MA, Smith JW. Activity of clindamycin with primaquine against *Pneumocystis carinii* in vitro and in vivo. Antimicrob Agents Chemother 1988; 32:807–813.
47. Bartlett MS, Queener SF, Tidwell RR, Milhous WK, Berman JD, Ellis WY, Smith JW. 8-Aminoquinolines from Walter Reed Army Institute for Research for treatment and prophylaxis of *Pneumocystis* pneumonia in rat models. Antimicrob Agents Chemother 1991; 35:277–282.
48. Pesanti EL, Cox C. Metabolic and synthetic activities of *Pneumocystis carinii* in vitro. Infect Immun 1981; 34:908–914.
49. Kovacs JA, Allegra CJ, Beaver J, Boarman D, Lewis M, Parrillo JE, Chabner B, Masur H. Characterization of de novo folate synthesis in *Pneumocystis carinii* and *Toxoplasma gondii*: potential for screening therapeutic agents. J Infect Dis 1989; 160: 312–320.
50. Lapinsky SE, Glencross D, Car NG, Kallenbach JM, Zwi S. Quantification and assessment of viability of *Pneumocystis carinii* organisms by flow cytometry. J Clin Microbiol 1991; 29:911–915.
51. Shapiro HM. Practical flow cytometry. New York: Alan R Liss, 1988:115–198.
52. Rosenberg ZF, Fauci AS. The immunopathogenesis of HIV infection. Adv Immunol 1989; 47:377–430.
53. Trager W, Daggett P-M. Summary of a round table discussion on the in vitro culture of *Pneumocystis carinii*. J Protozool 1989; 36:37S–38S.

2

Pneumocystis carinii Cell Structure

JOHN J. RUFFOLO

Henry M. Jackson Foundation for the Advancement of Military Medicine
Rockville, Maryland

I. Introduction

A. Overview

Pneumocystis carinii is a unicellular eukaryote that appears to be ubiquitous in geographic distribution and harmlessly present in the lungs of a wide variety of homeothermic terrestrial vertebrates. In an immune-compromised host, however, *P. carinii* is an opportunistic pathogen. Most studies of the cell structure of *P. carinii* have been carried out on human and rat infections or on short-term cultures of *P. carinii* isolated from infected lungs. No morphological differences have been detected between rat and human *P. carinii*, nor among the forms described in various other animals.

There is no general agreement on the taxonomic classification of *P. carinii*. A few investigators have asserted that *P. carinii* is a protozoon (1–3), some have proposed that it may be a protist of independent taxonomic position (4–6) and several investigators (including this author) have asserted that it is a fungus (7–14), most likely an ascomycete. The morphological descriptive terminology for *P. carinii* has been based on the assumption that it is a protozoon. Terms such as trophozoite, pellicle, cyst, and intracystic body are not appropriate to describe a yeast-like fungus or stages of its life cycle. In this chapter the traditional descriptive terminology for *P. carinii* will be accompanied by suggested alternative terms bracketed and in italics.

Several reviews that discuss various aspects of the cell structure of *P. carinii* have been published (5–8,10). Also there are several published descriptions of the life cycle stages of *P. carinii* as observed in the lung or in culture (5–8,10,14–17). The intrapulmonary life cycle of *P. carinii* involves asexual reproduction of haploid trophic forms by cell division, and the sexual formation of reproductive cysts [*sporogenesis*], involving meiosis and mitosis to form eight intracystic bodies [*spores*] within the thickened cyst wall [*spore case*]. The asexual formation of thin-walled reproductive cysts (endogeny) also has been proposed.

In this chapter I shall present the current status of knowledge about the cell structure of *P. carinii* as it pertains to the various stages of its life cycle. References cited are mostly from literature published during the past 20 years.

B. Microscopic Techniques

Morphological data have been used to address many important questions about the basic biology and pathogenesis of *P. carinii*. Several studies have made use of various forms of light optical microscopy (2,10,16,18–24). Some investigators have studied fresh specimens of living *P. carinii* (16,20,22,25), including one study that used video recording in real-time (25). There are no published studies using time-lapse video or film recording of *P. carinii*. There are no reports on the use of confocal microscopy to study *P. carinii*, nor the use of less common forms of microscopy, such as video-enhanced, computer-assisted, scanning acoustic, x-ray, or nuclear magnetic resonance.

Numerous ultrastructural studies of *P. carinii* using transmission electron microscopy of thin-sectioned material have been published (1,3–8,10,11,13,14, 17,19,26–63). Unfortunately, many of these studies have provided limited information. Often the data are scanty and the quality of fixation of the specimens was very poor, causing various artifacts. It is apparent that *P. carinii* is difficult to fix well, even under controlled conditions with experimental animals, and some investigators have called attention to the problem (7,11,14). Most studies of the ultrastructure of *P. carinii* have used glutaraldehyde in concentrations ranging from 1.25 to 6%, in either cacodylate or phosphate buffer, as the primary fixative. No one fixation technique can reveal all the ultrastructural features of a cell, so it is desirable that a variety of techniques be used. Relatively few studies have involved alternative fixation techniques (11,13,14,32,37,54,64), and there is need for more experimentation with specimen preparation techniques. To date, no one has reported use of the freeze-substitution method to fix *P. carinii*.

Recently, one research group has published the results of computed three-dimensional reconstruction of digitized data from transmission microscopy of

Pneumocystis carinii *Cell Structure*

serial thin sections of *P. carinii* (42–44). No data have been published from the use of high-voltage electron microscopy, from scanning transmission electron microscopy, or from analytical electron microscopy. Several investigators have used transmission electron imaging of freeze-fracture replicas to study membranes of *P. carinii* (6,7,28,34,56–58,61,62,65,66). There have been several studies of *P. carinii* using scanning electron microscopy (1,7,13,17,49,64,67–70).

Several investigators have used cytochemical and special staining techniques on *P. carinii* for light microscopy (7,8,10,16,18–22,71,72), for transmission electron microscopy (7,10,11,32,36,38,41,50,53,55,60,63), and for scanning electron microscopy (69,70).

II. Trophic Stages

The primary proliferative life cycle of *P. carinii* consists of small, haploid trophic forms that grow into large, diploid trophic forms and reproduce asexually by cell division (5,15,16). There is evidence for a process of binary fission from electron microscopy (6,15,31,46), but no one has reported observations on cell division in living specimens. There is no clear evidence for a yeast-like budding process, from either light microscopic or ultrastructural studies.

When describing the morphology and ultrastructure of the trophic form of *P. carinii*, most investigators have not distinguished between small and large forms. Because relatively few investigators have specifically described the small trophic form (5,14–16,18,20,41), the detailed consideration of the cell structure of trophic forms will be given in the section on the large trophic form.

A. Small Trophic Form

The small trophic form, illustrated in Figure 1, is a very small cell (1.5–2 µm) and, when living cells are viewed by light microscopy in fresh preparations (16,18,20), it is round to ellipsoid in shape. It is probably a haploid progeny cell derived asexually by binary fission from a large parent cell. Additionally, this form is likely the product of sexual reproduction and excystation [*spore release*]. Morphologically and ultrastructurally, the small trophic form closely resembles the round form of intracystic body [*spore*] (see Fig. 3). Compared with the large trophic form, the small form has few or no tubular extensions of the cell surface, it has a small nucleus (about 0.5 µm), and its cytoplasm has less glycogen and fewer other inclusions.

B. Large Trophic Form

The large trophic form (see Fig. 1) is about 3–5 µm in size and, when living cells are viewed by light microscopy in fresh preparations (16,20,22), it is more

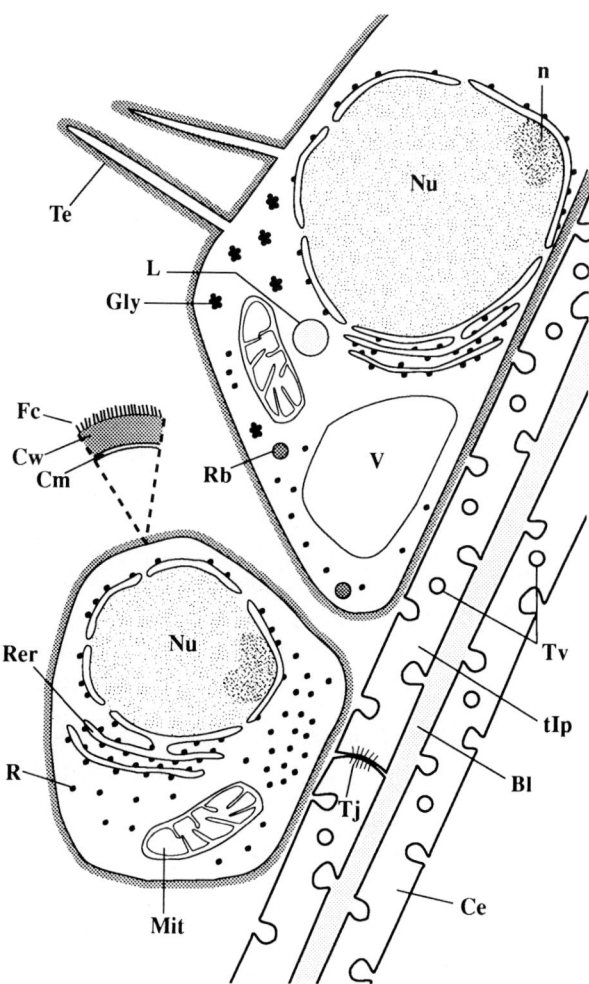

Figure 1 Trophic forms in a lung alveolus. Summary of cell structural features of a small trophic form (lower left) and a large trophic form (upper right) attached to type I pneumocytes. Labels: tIp, type I pneumocyte; Tj, tight junction; Tv, transport vesicles; Bl, basal laminae; Ce, capillary endothelium; Cw, cell wall; Fc, fuzzy coat; Cm, cell membrane; Te, tubular expansion, Nu, nucleus; n, nucleolus; Rer, rough endoplasmic reticulum; Mit, mitochondrion; R, free ribosome; Gly, glycogen rosette; Rb, round body; L, lipid droplet; V, vacuole. (Prepared by Kathleen A. Hayes.)

irregular in shape than the small trophic form. Perhaps plasticity of shape depends on a combination of the cell size, thickness of the cell wall, and the degree of cell turgor. During ultrastructural studies, many investigators have described the shape of trophic forms as "ameboid" or "pleomorphic," and frequently the shape of large trophic forms appears very irregular in electron micrographs. However, it is clear that the large trophic form of *P. carinii* is difficult to fix well. Usually, mitochondria are swollen and cristae are not preserved, and often the nuclear envelope is not well preserved. Frequently the cytoplasm appears extracted. These signs of poor fixation result from inadequate cross-linking and large fluxes of water and solutes which, in turn, lead to other artifacts during specimen dehydration and polymerization of the plastic embedding material. Efforts to improve specimen preparation and the application of a variety of staining techniques may yield additional information about the native cell structure of the large trophic form.

Surface

The cell membrane is covered externally by a thin cell wall, ranging from 20 to 50 nm in thickness, depending on the mode of fixation and staining and on the plane of section. The cell wall is a uniform, electron-dense layer of extracellular material (about 35 nm thick) (40,57,61), covered with a "fuzzy coat" (about 15 nm thick) that can be revealed by tannic acid staining (11). The outermost fuzzy coat of the cell wall is probably rich in polysaccharides, and it is a likely site for lectin binding and a source of surface antigens.

By light microscopy, the cell wall of trophic forms does not show detectable silver staining (4), but silver deposition can be observed by transmission electron microscopy (60). Weak silver staining has been reported as detectable by back-scattered imaging with the scanning electron microscope (70). There is biochemical evidence that trophic forms produce glucan (73), which is probably a component of the cell wall, and there is cytochemical evidence that chitin also is present (19,72).

A peculiar and prominent surface feature of large trophic forms, characteristically observed by electron microscopy, is the presence of numerous, long, thin, "tubular expansions" of the cell membrane and cell wall (reviewed in Ref. 6). A variety of terms have been used to describe them (71), and numerous investigators have discussed the functional significance (considered in Sec. VI). Tubular expansions are rarely seen on small trophic forms, are few or absent on cysts [*spore cases*], and are not always seen on the large trophic forms. Considering that the large trophic form is particularly difficult to preserve and is subject to artifacts and distortions, it is prudent to be cautious in interpreting the significance of these structures. It would be very helpful if tubular expansions could be demonstrated on the surface of living trophic forms.

The cell membrane appears as a typical unit membrane in thin sections, as viewed by transmission electron microscopy. The freeze-fracture technique has been used to examine the distribution of intramembranous particles (6,34,56, 57,61) and the distribution of cholesterol (65,66).

Nucleus

The nucleus of *P. carinii* is small (0.5–1 μm), as is its genome (8). It contains a conspicuous nucleolus and is bounded by a typical nuclear envelope that has pores and often shows continuity with rough endoplasmic reticulum (6,14,15,58). In electron micrographs, the chromatin generally appears diffuse. By light microscopy, the nucleus of trophic forms is readily visualized by Giemsa staining, and in some large trophic forms the nucleus is noticeably larger (20,22).

There is limited information about nuclear division in trophic forms. There is evidence for binary fission from published images of apparent cytokinesis and binucleate cells, but there are only two examples of karyokinesis showing the mitotic spindle (6,17,39,51). Each spindle pole is a dense plaque, which appears to be embedded in the nuclear envelope, and the nuclear envelope apparently persists, at least in part. It is not yet clear if mitosis in *P. carinii* is *closed*, being fully contained within the nuclear envelope, or *semiopen*, with partial breakdown of the nuclear envelope.

Cytoplasm

The mitochondria of *P. carinii* are almost always poorly preserved. Usually, they appear swollen, and the cristae are not recognizable. In the few cases where mitochondrial cristae are observed, they appear lamellar (6,11,14,21,30,37). Analysis of serial sections of a trophic form indicate that small trophic forms probably have a single mitochondrion that can be branched or irregular in shape (43).

The presence of rough endoplasmic reticulum in trophic forms is well documented (13–15,41–43). In their studies of rabbit-derived *P. carinii* Palluault et al. (41–44) have described smooth endoplasmic reticulum, Golgi-like vesicles, primary lysosomes, and endoplasmic (autophagic) saccules. Other investigators have asserted that *P. carinii* does not have a Golgi complex, nor lysosomes, nor evidence of endocytosis or intracellular digestion (2,6,11,13,14). There is a need for further study of the cytoplasmic membrane system of *P. carinii*. It is reasonable to expect the presence of functional equivalents to smooth endoplasmic reticulum and Golgi complex because of the basic biochemical roles of such membranes in eukaryotic cells. Cytoplasmic vacuoles have been observed in living trophic forms by light microscopy (22), and some investigators have described vacuoles by electron microscopy (6,13–15,50,58).

Free ribosomes, glycogen particles, and lipid droplets are commonly observed in trophic forms (2,6,7,13–15,33,40,50). Dense "round bodies" (about

100 nm in diameter) also are frequently described (2,5–7,14,15,50,58). The significance of the round bodies is unclear, and their chemical composition is unknown. Round bodies may be less frequent in large trophic forms (15). The similar-sized particles described by Wang et al. (52) as resembling the dense core of cytomegalovirus, probably are not equivalent to round bodies. Cytoskeletal elements are either poorly developed or poorly preserved in *P. carinii* (7,11,13). Neither microtubules nor microfilaments have been demonstrated in nondividing trophic forms.

III. Encystment [*Sporogenesis*]

The intrapulmonary life cycle stage from which *P. carinii* derives its name is the cyst [*spore case*]. This is a thick-walled reproductive stage consisting of eight haploid progeny cells that develop from a parent cell by meiosis and partitioning of the cytoplasm (5–8,10,14–16). It is likely that encystment [*sporogenesis*] is preceded by conjugation, a fusion (syngamy) of haploid gametic cells to form a diploid zygote that probably looks like a large trophic form. Probably the sex cells are morphologically indistinguishable (isogametes), but of complementary mating types. The current concept that the cyst represents sexual reproduction is presumptive, based on inferences from two key morphological observations: examples of binucleate trophic forms that could be conjugants, and a single observation of synaptonemal complexes in the nucleus of a precyst [*sporocyte*] (39). If mating and encystment [*sporogenesis*] of *P. carinii* follow the pattern of other protists, then the process probably is induced by unfavorable environmental factors, such as depletion of nutrients or crowding.

A. Precyst [*Sporocyte*]

The precyst (Fig. 2) is an intermediate stage of sexual reproduction during which a large parent cell (zygote) undergoes encystment [*sporogenesis*] (5–7,10,13–15,30,36,39,40,44,61–63,70). The parent cell is about 4–5 μm in diameter and has an ovoid shape and a large nucleus (about 2 μm). The cytoplasm and its complement of organelles resemble that of a large trophic form (15,39,62). Synaptonemal complexes, indicative of meiotic prophase, have been observed in this stage (39). As development progresses, the cell becomes more spherical and the cell wall becomes thicker by formation of an inner electron-lucent layer beneath the outer electron-dense layer (61,63). The surface shows few tubular expansions. The four haploid nuclei that are produced by meiosis probably divide by mitosis to form eight nuclei in the cytoplasm. As the nuclear divisions near completion, mitochondria become aggregated. The final stage of sporogenesis is the formation of eight intracystic bodies [*spores*]. The cytoplasm becomes partitioned by infoldings of the cell membrane (14,39,40,62) to enclose each nucleus

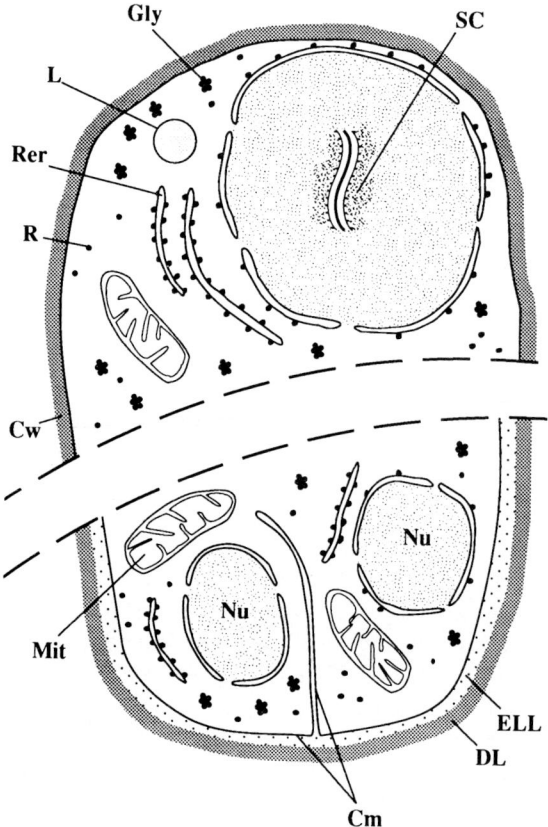

Figure 2 Encystment [*sporogenesis*]. Summary of morphological features of an early stage (upper part) and late stage (lower part) precyst [*sporocyte*]. The early precyst (zygote) undergoes meiosis and mitosis to produce eight nuclei. The cell wall becomes thick by formation of an inner layer between the cell membrane and the outer dense layer. Intracystic bodies [*spores*] are formed by partitioning of the cytoplasm by invaginations of the cell membrane to enclose a nucleus, mitochondrion, and various cytoplasmic components. Labels: Cw, cell wall; DL, outer dense layer; ELL, inner electron-lucent layer; Cm, cell membrane; Nu, nucleus; SC, synaptonemal complex; Rer, rough endoplasmic reticulum; Mit, mitochondrion; R, free ribosome; Gly, glycogen rosette; L, lipid droplet. (Prepared by Kathleen A. Hayes.)

plus a mitochondrion, some endoplasmic reticulum, and some cytoplasm to form progeny cells. During this process not all of the cytoplasm of the parent cell is incorporated into progeny cells. The unincorporated residual cytoplasm remains at the periphery of the cyst against the thickened wall.

B. Cyst [*Spore Case*]

At the completion of encystment, the mature cyst (Fig. 3) is round (about 5 μm in diameter), thick-walled, smooth (rarely shows tubular expansions (7,15,61) and contains eight intracystic bodies [*spores*]. The ultrastructure of this stage is well

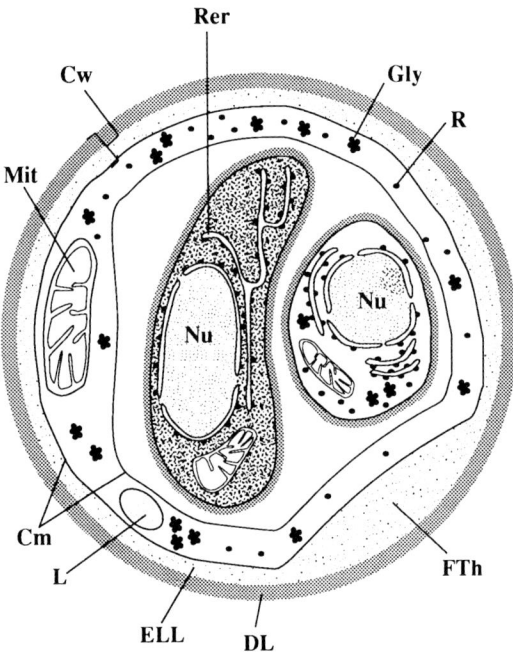

Figure 3 Composite illustration summarizing morphological features of a mature, thick-walled cyst [*spore case*]. Intracystic bodies [*spores*] can manifest a variety of morphologies of which two are illustrated, a round form that closely resembles a small trophic form and an elongated (banana-shaped) form having dense cytoplasm. For any individual cyst the intracystic bodies all have one kind of morphology (ellipsoid, round, ovoid, elongated). Residual cytoplasm, including some organelles and inclusions, forms a peripheral layer inside the cyst wall. Labels: CW, cyst wall; DL, outer dense layer; ELL, inner electron-lucent layer; FTh, focal thickening of the inner layer; Cm, cell membrane; Nu, nucleus; Rer, rough endoplasmic reticulum; Mit, mitochondrion; R, free ribosome; Gly, glycogen rosette; L, lipid droplet. (Prepared by Kathleen A. Hayes.)

characterized and extensively documented because it tends to be well preserved by various fixation techniques.

The cyst wall [*spore case*] is thick (120–160 nm) owing to the development of an electron-lucent layer inside the electron-dense layer that is found at other stages. Cysts commonly show a focal thickening of the wall caused by a patch of increased development of the electron-lucent layer. The focal thickening is visible by light microscopy in silver-stained specimens or by interference contrast microscopy of unstained specimens (20). There is considerable evidence that the thick inner layer is rich in glucan (4,28,41,53,59,60,70). De Stefano et al. (28) found evidence for a lipid membrane-like component between the inner and outer layers of the wall. The outer dense layer probably contains some chitin (19,72), and the outermost surface may consist of an irregular layer or fuzzy coat (11,14,15).

In a mature cyst, after formation of the progeny cells, residual (unincorporated) cytoplasm, including some organelles and inclusions, remains as a peripheral layer inside the cyst wall.

C. Intracystic Bodies [*Spores*]

The progeny cells within a mature, thick-walled reproductive cyst (see Fig. 3) can manifest a variety of morphologies that can be distinguished by light microscopy (16,20,22,23,25). They may be round (resembling small trophic forms), or large (irregular in shape and tightly packed), or ellipsoid, or elongated (banana-shaped) with very dense cytoplasm, perhaps caused by the loss of water. All these forms have been well documented at the ultrastructural level (3,5–7,14,15,17,21,36,37, 40,57,62). The significance of these variations is not understood. It has been suggested that the cytoplasmic densification of elongated forms might indicate dormancy, making this form suited for transmission between hosts (14,17,40). The cell surface, nucleus, and cytoplasmic components of intracystic bodies [*spores*] are essentially the same as trophic forms. There is a single report of apparent microtubules (in cross section) in an intracystic body (3).

IV. Excystation [*Spore Release*]

Very little is known about the process of excystation. Observations of the process by light microscopy are rare. Shiota (22) observed examples of excystation of spherical and of elongated intracystic bodies. It would be very informative to record excystation in living material by videomicroscopy. Ultrastructural data are very limited. Nielsen and Settnes (40) stated that an opening appears in the focal thickening of the cyst wall through which intracystic bodies are released, but they provided no documentation. Ultrastructural studies have not revealed any specialized structure in the cyst wall for spore release. The few published electron micrographs illustrating excystation indicate that the spores are released through a simple hole in the cyst wall [*spore case*] that does not show any special differentiation (14,33). It is not known how the hole is formed, nor how the intracystic bodies vacate the cyst. The stimulus for excystation also is unknown.

Empty cysts, which frequently are collapsed into a crescent shape, are commonly observed by light optical and electron microscopy. They consist of the thick wall plus residual cytoplasm retained from the mature cyst before excystation.

V. Endogeny (Thin-Walled Cysts)

Vossen et al. (17,51) described a thin-walled cyst (Fig. 4) that they considered an alternative stage of the life cycle, in which a parent cell (presumably a large trophic form) produces progeny cells asexually (presumably by multiple cell divisions) within the original cell wall, without development of the inner electron-lucent layer. They named this mode of reproduction *endogeny* (51). Yoshida et al. (5,6,63) have also documented the thin-walled cyst. In a mature thin-walled cyst, the intracystic bodies (progeny cells; number uncertain) usually resemble large trophic forms before breaking out from the confines of the thin cyst wall. The significance of this form is not understood. It is not known how it fits into the life cycle of *P. carinii*, or if the developmental process is truly asexual.

VI. Relation of Structure to Function and Taxonomy

Because function follows form, knowledge about the cell structure of *P. carinii* can be applied to significant questions about its cell physiology. Here I will consider motility, nutrition, and adhesion. The significance of morphological data for taxonomic classification of *P. carinii* also will be considered.

A. Motility

Large trophic forms frequently are described as pleomorphic or ameboid, and some investigators have inferred from this plasticity of shape that *P. carinii* is motile (15,31,33). Other investigators have asserted that trophic forms are not motile (7,8,11,13,22,24). Motility usually requires contractility and the involvement of microtubules or microfilaments, but no cytoskeletal elements have been demonstrated in nondividing trophic forms. Some investigators have noted the absence of microtubules and microfilaments (7,8,11,13). However, preservation of cytoskeletal elements requires good fixation, and their detection by electron microscopy requires high resolution and relatively high magnification. At present the ultrastructural data and direct observations of living cells indicate that trophic forms are not motile.

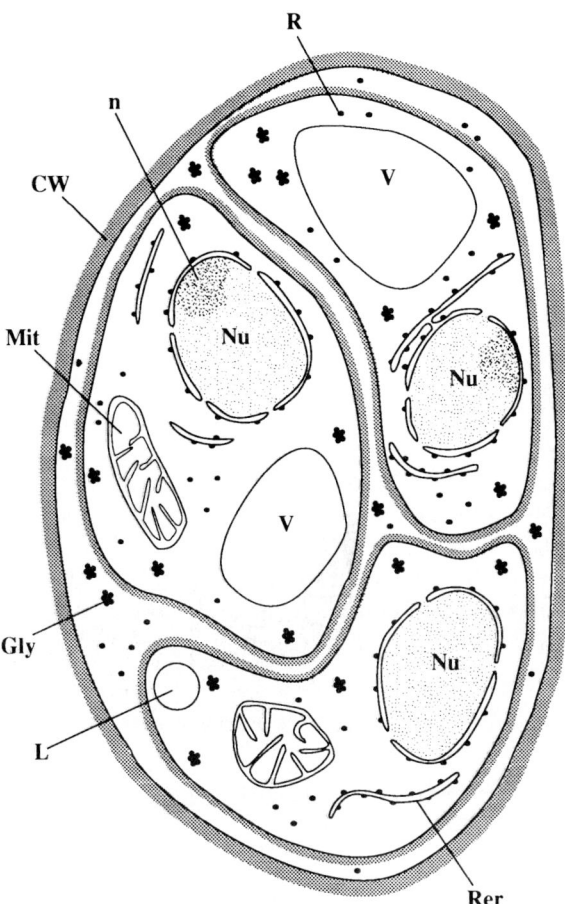

Figure 4 Endogeny, a process by which a parent cell presumably produces progeny cells asexually within the original cell wall. Summary of the morphological features of a thin-walled cyst. Labels: CW, cyst wall; Nu, nucleus; n, nucleolus; Rer, rough endoplasmic reticulum; Mit, mitochondrion; R, free ribosome; Gly, glycogen rosette; L, lipid droplet; V, vacuole. (Prepared by Kathleen A. Hayes.)

Movement of intracystic bodies within the cyst has been reported (18,22, 24,25). In the judgment of some investigators the movement is probably passive (11,18). Newsome et al. (25), after analyzing real-time video recordings, reported flexing movement in ellipsoidal forms attached at a common point in the cyst and greater movement in nonattached elongated forms. Shiota (22) observed that intracystic bodies often showed active movements, which stopped when they were heated. These direct observations of living cysts suggest that intracystic bodies may be motile, or at least contractile. Vossen et al. (3) observed apparent microtubules (in cross section) in an intracystic body, but we (11) were not able to detect any cytoskeletal elements in intracystic bodies. Further observations and experimental manipulations of living cysts may establish whether or not intracystic bodies are contractile, and if so, ultrastructural analysis may reveal the structural basis for the behavior.

B. Nutrition

The mode by which *P. carinii* takes up nutrients is not understood. Several investigators have looked for ultrastructural evidence of endocytosis. There is no evidence of overt phagocytosis or pinocytosis, nor has anyone observed coated pits or vesicles, which would be indicative of receptor-mediated endocytosis. However, Yoneda et al. (57) interpreted freeze-fracture membrane features to represent possible exocytosis or endocytosis. Palluault et al. (41–44) described primary lysosomes and endoplasmic (autophagic) saccules. Other investigators have asserted that *P. carinii* does not have lysosomes nor evidence of endocytosis or intracellular digestion (2,6,11,13,14,27,36). There is cytochemical evidence that acid phosphatase activity is present on the cell surface of trophic forms and cysts (27,36).

Regardless if autophagy occurs, the available data are consistent with a saprobic mode of nutrient uptake. This likely involves the secretion of digestive enzymes onto the cell surface and, perhaps, into the surrounding medium, and the uptake of small nutrient molecules by transport across the cell membrane. Some investigators have suggested that the tubular expansions (see Fig. 1) of the cell surface, commonly seen on large trophic forms, may be surface specializations for the saprobic uptake of nutrients (6,8,14,74).

What is the source of nutrients for *P. carinii* in lung alveoli? It is reasonable to suspect that surfactant is a food source, but Pesanti (75) found that adding surfactant to the medium did not improve growth of *P. carinii* in culture. Nielsen and Settnes (40) reported that adhesion of trophic forms to pneumocytes may induce the plasmalemmal vesicular transport system in the pneumocytes and provide nutrition for *P. carinii* from alveolar capillaries (see Fig. 1). If this were the main source of nutrients, it would explain why trophic forms adhere to type I pneumocytes. When the surface of the alveolus is covered with trophic forms and some cells cannot get access to nutrients, this would provide the stimulus for mating and encystment (33).

C. Adhesion

In lung alveoli and in vitro, there is evidence that *P. carinii* cells and cysts adhere in clusters (8,10,18,20). In vitro, large clumps are formed containing a mixture of trophic and cyst forms, but no extracellular matrix is discernible at the level of light microscopy. Clusters of *P. carinii* cells and cysts can be observed attached to feeder cells in culture (16,18,67). Some investigators have suggested that tubular expansions may be specializations for anchoring (6,7), but others have asserted that tubular expansions are not specialized for adhesion (34,36,40). Trophic forms tend to adhere to type I pneumocytes in the lung alveoli (see Fig. 1) (10,34,36,37,40,56), and this property is an important aspect of the pathogenesis of *P. carinii* infection. Interdigitation between the surfaces of trophic forms and pneumocytes has been observed (29,36), but investigations into the mechanism of adhesion have not shown any specialized junctions between trophic forms and lung cells, indicating that adhesion is likely mediated by surface polysaccharides (see Fig. 1) (11,34,36,57).

Limper and Martin (64) studied the role of cytoskeletal components in adhesion of chromium–51-labeled *P. carinii* to monolayers of feeder cells in culture. Agents that depolymerize actin filaments and microtubules caused reduced adherence by this assay, and these authors concluded that adherence requires functional integrity of both actin filaments and microtubules in *P. carinii*. If one considers that cytoskeletal elements are poorly developed or lacking in nondividing trophic forms, an alternative argument could be made that the requirement of cytoskeletal integrity for adhesion in this assay resides with the feeder cells.

D. Taxonomy

The data available on the cell structure of *P. carinii* strongly correlate with that of a yeast-like fungus. There are several areas where further light microscopic, ultrastructural, and cytochemical analyses could provide data on which taxonomic distinctions could be made (e.g., nuclear division, cytokinesis, cell wall, cytoskeletal elements and contractility, mitochondria, Golgi complex and secretion, and endocytosis and intracellular digestion).

VII. Conclusions

Morphological data can be used to address many important questions about the basic biology and pathogenesis of *P. carinii*. Despite many publications on the ultrastructure of *P. carinii*, understanding of the cell structure of the trophic form has been limited by poor fixation. There is a need to improve specimen preparation and to apply a variety of staining and imaging techniques. Knowledge about nuclear division, both mitosis and meiosis, is very limited; but such information is important for understanding the *P. carinii* life cycle. Further study of the cytoplasmic membrane system is also needed, particularly of smooth endoplasmic reticulum and Golgi complex. Cytoskeletal elements are either poorly developed or poorly preserved in *P. carinii*. Although trophic forms probably are not motile, intracystic bodies may be motile, or at least contractile. Questions about contractility require further study. Very little is known about the process of excystation. The relation of thin-walled cysts to the life cycle of *P. carinii* is not established. The mode by which *P. carinii* takes up nutrients is not understood. The significance of tubular expansions of the cell surface is uncertain. Adhesion between *P. carinii* forms to form clumps and attachment of *P. carinii* trophic forms to type I pneumocytes likely are mediated by surface polysaccharides. The data available on the cell structure of *P. carinii* strongly correlate with that of a yeast-like fungus. Appropriate alternative terminology for *P. carinii* morphology and life cycle stages is suggested.

References

1. Balachandran I, Jones DB, Humphrey DM. A case of *Pneumocystis carinii* in pleural fluid with cytologic, histologic and ultrastructural documentation. Acta Cytol 1990; 34:486–490.
2. Bouton C, Kernbaum S, Christol D, Trinh Dinh H, Vezinet F, Gutman L, Seman M, Bastin R. Diagnostic morphologique de *Pneumocystis carinii*. Pathol Biol 1977; 25:153–160.
3. Vossen MEMH, Beckers PJA, Meuwissen JHET, Stadhouders AM. Microtubules in *Pneumocystis carinii*. Z Parasitenk 1976; 49:291–292.
4. Matsumoto Y, Matsuda S, Tegoshi T. Yeast glucan in the cyst wall of *Pneumocystis carinii*. J Protozool 1989; 36:21S–22S.
5. Matsumoto Y, Yoshida Y. Advances in *Pneumocystis* biology. Parasitol Today 1986; 2:137–142.
6. Yoshida Y. Ultrastructural studies of *Pneumocystis carinii*. J Protozool 1989; 36:53–60.
7. Bedrossian CWM. Ultrastructure of *Pneumocystis carinii*: a review of internal and surface characteristics. Semin Diagn Pathol 1989; 6:212–237.
8. Cushion MT, Stringer JR, Walzer PD. Cellular and molecular biology of *Pneumocystis carinii*. Int Rev Cytol 1991; 131:59–107.
9. Edman JC, Kovacs JA, Masur H, Santi DV, Elwood HJ, Sogin M. L. Ribosomal RNA genes of *Pneumocystis carinii*. J Protozool 1989; 36:18S–20S.
10. Gutierrez Y. The biology of *Pneumocystis carinii*. Semin Diagn Pathol 1989; 6:203–211.
11. Ruffolo JJ, Cushion MT, Walzer PD. Ultrastructural observations on life cycle stages of *Pneumocystis carinii*. J Protozool 1989; 36:53S–54S.
12. Stringer SL, Hudson D, Blase M, Walzer PD, Cushion MT, Stringer JR. Sequence from ribosomal RNA of *Pneumocystis carinii* compared to those of four fungi suggests an ascomycetous affinity. J Protozool 1989; 36:14S–16S.
13. ul Haque A, Plattner SB, Cook RT, Hart MN. *Pneumocystis carinii*. Taxonomy as viewed by electron microscopy. Am J Clin Pathol 1987; 87:504–510.
14. Vavra J, Kucera K. *Pneumocystis carinii* Delanoe, its ultrastructure and ultrastructural affinities. J Protozool 1970; 17:463–483.

15. Campbell WG. Ultrastructure of *Pneumocystis* in human lung. Life cycle in human pneumocystosis. Arch Pathol 1972; 93:312–324.
16. Cushion MT, Ruffolo JJ, Walzer PD. Analysis of the developmental stages of *Pneumocystis carinii* in vitro. Lab Invest 1988; 58:324–331.
17. Vossen MEMH, Beckers PJA, Meuwissen JHET, Stadhouders AM. Developmental biology of *Pneumocystis carinii*, an alternative view on the life cycle of the parasite. Z Parasitenkd 1978; 55:101–118.
18. Cushion MT, Ruffolo JJ, Linke MJ, Walzer PD. *Pneumocystis carinii*: growth variables and estimates in the A549 and WI-38 VA13 human cell lines. Exp Parasitol 1985; 60:43–54.
19. Garner RE, Walker AN, Horst MN. Morphologic and biochemical studies of chitin expression in *Pneumocystis carinii*. J Protozool 1991; 38:12S–14S.
20. Ruffolo JJ, Cushion MT, Walzer PD. Techniques for examining *Pneumocystis carinii* in fresh specimens. J Clin Microbiol 1986; 23:17–21.
21. Schwartz, DA, Munger RG, Katz SM. Plastic embedding evaluation of *Pneumocystis carinii* pneumonia in AIDS. Am J Surg Pathol 1987; 11:304–309.
22. Shiota T. Morphology and development of *Pneumocystis carinii* observed by phase-contrast microscopy and semiultrathin section light-microscopy. Jpn J Parasitol 1984; 33:443–455.
23. Shiota T, Yamada M, Yoshida Y. Morphology, development and behavior of *Pneumocystis carinii* observed by light-microscopy in nude mice. Zentralbl Baktiol Hyg A 1986; 262:230–239.
24. Yoshida Y, Shiota T, Yamada M, Matsumoto Y. Further light microscopic studies on morphology and development of *Pneumocystis carinii*. Zentralbl Baktiol Hyg I. Abt Orig A 1981; 250:213–218.
25. Newsome AL, Durkin MM, Bartlett MS, Smith JW. Videomicroscopic recording of *Pneumocystis carinii* motion. J Protozool 1991; 38:207S–208S.
26. Barton EG, Campbell WG. Further observations on the ultrastructure of *pneumocystis*. Arch Pathol 1967; 83:527–534.
27. Barton EG, Campbell WG. *Pneumocystis carinii* in lungs of rats treated with cortisone acetate. Ultrastructural observations relating to the life cycle. Am J Pathol 1969; 54:209–236.
28. De Stefano JA, Cushion MT, Sleight RG, Walzer PD. Analysis of *Pneumocystis carinii* cyst wall. I. Evidence for an outer surface membrane. J Protozool 1990; 37:428–435.
29. Dei-Cas E, Jackson H, Palluault F, Aliouat EM, Hancock V, Soulez B, Camus D. Ultrastructural observations on the attachment of *Pneumocystis carinii* in vitro. J Protozool 1991; 38:205S–207S.
30. Dei-Cas E, Soulez B, Camus D. Ultrastructural study of *Pneumocystis carinii* in explant cultures of rabbit lung and in cultures with and without feeder cells. J Protozool 1989; 36:55S–57S.
31. Filice G, Carnevale G, Lanzarini P, Castelli F, Olliaro P, Carosi G, Rondanelli EG. Life cycle of *P. carinii* in the lung of immuno-compromised hosts: an ultrastructural study. Microbiologica 1985; 8:319–328.
32. Goheen MP, Blumershine R, Hull MT, Bartlett MS, Smith JW. Enhancement of the

fine structure of *Pneumocystis carinii* using potassium ferrocyanide and tannic acid. In: Bailey, G. W., ed. Proc Annu Meet EMSA, San Francisco: San Francisco Press, 1989:984–985.
33. Hasleton PS, Curry A, Rankin EM. *Pneumocystis carinii* pneumonia: a light microscopical and ultrastructural study. J Clin Pathol 1981; 34:1138–1146.
34. Henshaw NG, Carson JL, Collier AM. Ultrastructural observations of *Pneumocystis carinii* attachment to rat lung. J Infect Dis 1985; 151:181–186.
35. Huang S-N, Marshall KG. *Pneumocystis carinii* infection. A cytologic, histologic, and electron microscopic study of the organism. Am J Resp Dis 1970; 102:623–635.
36. Itatani CA, Marshall GJ. Ultrastructural morphology and staining characteristics of *Pneumocystis carinii* in situ and from bronchoalveolar lavage. J Parasit 1988; 74:700–712.
37. Lanken PN, Minda M, Pietra GG, Fishman AP. Alveolar response to experimental *Pneumocystis carinii* pneumonia in the rat. Am J Pathol 1980; 99:561–588.
38. Matsumoto Y, Frenkel JB, Aikawa M, Yoshida Y. Proliferation of *Pneumocystis* trophozoites in human lymph nodes and in nude mice lungs. J Protozool 1989; 36:33S–34S.
39. Matsumoto Y, Yoshida Y. Sporogony in *Pneumocystis carinii*: synaptonemal complexes and meiotic nuclear divisions observed in precysts. J Protozool 1984; 31:420–428.
40. Nielsen MH, Settnes OP. Morphology of *Pneumocystis carinii* and activation of the plasmalemmal vesicular system in alveolar epithelial cells of the host. An ultrastructural study. APMIS 1991; 99:219–225.
41. Palluault F, Dei-Cas E, Slomianny C, Soulez B, Camus D. Golgi complex and lysosomes in rabbit derived *Pneumocystis carinii*. Biol Cell 1990; 70:73–82.
42. Palluault F, Pietrzyk B, Dei-Cas E, Camus D. Application of 3-D computer-aided reconstruction in parasitology. Parasitol Today 1991; 7:215–217.
43. Palluault F, Pietrzyk B, Dei-Cas E, Slomianny C, Soulez B, Camus D. Three-dimensional reconstruction of rabbit-derived *Pneumocystis carinii* from serial-thin sections. I. trophozoite. J Protozool 1991; 38:402–407.
44. Palluault F, Pietrzyk B, Dei-Cas E, Slomianny C, Soulez B, Camus D. Three-dimensional reconstruction of rabbit-derived *Pneumocystis carinii* from serial-thin sections. II. intermediate precyst. J Protozool 1991; 38:407–411.
45. Price RA, Hughes WT. Histology of *Pneumocystis carinii* infestation and infection in malignant disease in childhood. Hum Pathol 1974; 5:737–752.
46. Richardson JD, Queener SF, Bartlett M, Smith J. Binary fission of *Pneumocystis carinii* trophozoites grown in vitro. J Protozool 1989; 36:27S–29S.
47. Shively JN, Moe KK, Dellers RW. Fine structure of spontaneous *Pneumocystis carinii* pulmonary infection in foals. Cornell Vet 1974; 64:72–88.
48. Soulez B, Dei-Cas E, Palluault F, Camus D. Morphological evaluation of *Pneumocystis carinii* after extraction from infected lung. J Parasitol 1991; 77:449–453.
49. Sueishi K, Hisano S, Sumiyoshi A, Tanaka K. Scanning and transmission electron microscopic study of human pulmonary pneumocystosis. Chest 1977; 72:213–216.
50. Tamura T, Ueda K, Furuta T, Goto Y, Fujiwara K. Electron microscopy of spontaneous pneumocystosis in a nude mouse. Jpn J Exp Med 1978; 48:363–368.

51. Vossen MEM, Beckers PJA, Stadhouders AM, Bergers AMG, Meuwissen JHET. New aspects of the life cycle of *Pneumocystis carinii*. Z Parasitenk 1977; 51: 213–217.
52. Wang N-S, Huang S-N, Thurlbeck WM. Combined *Pneumocystis carinii* and cytomegalovirus infection. Arch Pathol 1970; 90:529–535.
53. Watts JC, Chandler FW. *Pneumocystis carinii* pneumonitis. The nature and diagnostic significance of the methenamine silver-positive "intracystic bodies." Am J Surg Pathol 1985; 9:744–751.
54. Weir EC, Brownstein DG, Barthold SW. Spontaneous wasting disease in nude mice associated with *Pneumocystis carinii* infection. Lab Anim Sci 1986; 36:140–144.
55. Yoneda K, Walzer PD. Interaction of *Pneumocystis carinii* with host lungs: an ultrastructural study. Infect Immun 1980; 29:692–703.
56. Yoneda K, Walzer PD. Attachment of *Pneumocystis carinii* to type I alveolar cells studied by freeze-fracture electron microscopy. Infect Immun 1983; 40:812–815.
57. Yoneda K, Walzer PD, Richey CS, Birk MG. *Pneumocystis carinii*: freeze-fracture study of stages of the organism. Exp Parasitol 1982; 53:68–76.
58. Yoshikawa H, Morioka H, Yoshida Y. Freeze-fracture studies on *Pneumocystis carinii*. II. Fine structure of the trophozoite. Parasitol Res 1987; 73:132–139.
59. Yoshikawa H, Morioka H, Yoshida Y. Ultrastructural detection of carbohydrates in the pellicle of *Pneumocystis carinii*. Parasitol Res 1988; 74:537–543.
60. Yoshikawa H, Tegoshi T, Yoshida Y. Detection of surface carbohydrates of *Pneumocystis carinii*. J Protozool 1989; 36:63S–64S.
61. Yoshikawa H, Yoshida Y. Freeze-fracture studies on *Pneumocystis carinii*. I. Structural alteration of the pellicle during the development from trophozoite to cyst. Z Parasitenkd 1986; 72:463–477.
62. Yoshikawa H, Yoshida Y. Freeze-fracture studies on *Pneumocystis carinii*. III. Fine structure of the precyst and the cyst. Parasitol Res 1987; 74:36–42.
63. Yoshikawa H, Yoshida Y. Localization of silver deposits on *Pneumocystis carinii* treated with Gomori's methenamine silver nitrate stain. Zentralbl Baktiol Hyg A 1987; 264:363–372.
64. Limper AH, Martin WJ. *Pneumocystis carinii*: inhibition of lung cell growth mediated by parasite attachment. J Clin Invest 1990; 85:391–396.
65. Yoshikawa H, Yoshida Y. Distribution of digitonin–sterol complexes in *Pneumocystis carinii* revealed by freeze-fracture method. Int J Parasitol 1988; 18:39–45.
66. Yoshikawa H, Yoshida Y. Ultrastructure of *Pneumocystis carinii*: a freeze-fracture study. J Protozool 1989; 36:51S–52S.
67. Burnstein T, Rhodes J, Turek J. Adherence of *Pneumocystis carinii* in lung cells during in vitro cultivation. J Protozool 1989; 36:35S–37S.
68. Murphy MJ, Pifer LL, Hughes WT. *Pneumocystis carinii* in vitro. A study by scanning electron microscopy. Am J Pathol 1977; 86:387–402.
69. Schraufnagel DE, Becker RP, Balaan M, Schmid A, Claypool W. Scanning electron microscopy with backscattered electron imaging to identify *Pneumocystis carinii*. N Engl J Med 1987; 317:1541.
70. Schraufnagel DE, Becker RP, Balaan M, Schmid A, Claypool W. Silver staining of *Pneumocystis carinii* in the rat's lung. J Infect 1989; 18:39–44.

71. Beals TF. Appropriate terminology for the features of *Pneumocystis carinii*. Acta Cytol 1991; 35:250–251.
72. Walker AN, Garner RE, Horst MN. Immunocytochemical detection of chitin in *Pneumocystis carinii*. Infect Immun 1990; 58:412–415.
73. Williams DJ, Radding JA, Dell A, Khoo K-H, Rogers ME, Richards FF, Armstrong MYK. Glucan synthesis in *Pneumocystis carinii*. J Protozool 1991; 38:427–437.
74. Hughes WT. *Pneumocystis carinii*: biology and mode of transmission. In: Acquired Immune Deficiency Syndrome. New York: Alan R Liss, 1984:345–354.
75. Pesanti E. Phospholipid profile of *Pneumocystis carinii* and its interaction with alveolar type II epithelial cells. Infect Immun 1987; 55:736–741.

＃ 3

Biochemistry and Metabolism

EDNA S. KANESHIRO

University of Cincinnati
Cincinnati, Ohio

RICHARD G. SLEIGHT

University of Cincinnati College of Medicine
Cincinnati, Ohio

I. Introduction

Data currently available on the biochemistry and metabolism of *Pneumocystis carinii* require reevaluation if and when continuous axenic cultures, preferably of homogeneous life cycle stages, become available. Unlike some other aspects of the biology of this organism, conclusions made about biochemical compositional analyses and physiological experiments measuring metabolic activities are particularly subject to question. For example, if incorporation of a radiolabeled precursor into *P. carinii* molecules is detected, there still remains some degree of skepticism concerning contributions of contaminating cells or molecules. If no incorporation is detected, one is justified in interpreting the observation as a consequence of suboptimal conditions of the in vitro preparation. Data from in vitro analyses must be tentatively regarded as results obtained under nongrowth or starvation conditions, since indeed these studies have, at best, been done on short-term maintenance cultures. Under these conditions, incorporation is limited to an 18- to 24-hr period. Within this period, however, some preparations exhibit metabolic activity that can be inhibited by appropriate agents. What we discuss here, given the state of the art, is a relatively uncritical review of what has thus far been observed. Although it is clear that *P. carinii* preparations analyzed in some studies were purer, more physiological, or more representative of a specific life cycle stage of the organism than in other studies, the paucity of information on *P. carinii* biochemistry compels us to wait for a future date to select the reports containing definitive data.

II. Intermediary and General Metabolism

It has been suggested that *P. carinii* does not require phagocytic processes to feed, and that it obtains all nutrients in the form of low molecular weight substances found in the alveolar fluid (1). No lysosomes with acid phosphatase activity have been found in *P. carinii* (1,2), although lysosomes or autophagous vacuoles (3) with other hydrolytic enzymes may be present. The first direct demonstration of the metabolic and synthetic activities of *P. carinii* was reported by Pesanti and Cox (4). Organisms obtained by bronchoalveolar lavage (BAL) of immunosuppressed rats were placed in Earle's balanced salt solution containing 7 μmol/mL glucose and a trace amount of radiolabeled glucose. Under those conditions, the organisms did not replicate, but remained viable and metabolically active over the 18-hr period studied. A classic anaerobic glycolytic pathway was found operative, as indicated by the conversion of either [1-^{14}C]glucose, [6-^{14}C]glucose, or [U-^{14}C]glucose to $^{14}CO_2$ at equivalent rates. In this in vitro system, radioactivity from glucose was incorporated into CO_2 at a linear rate for 2.5 hr. At 37°C, 19.5 nmol/hr of glucose were metabolized per 10^7 organisms and an additional 7.9 nmol/hr per 10^7 organisms were incorporated into trichloracetic acid-precipitable material. Coincubation with either 0.1 mM iodoacetate or 50 mM 2-deoxy-D-glucose completely inhibited conversion of glucose to CO_2; both agents were toxic to *P. carinii* at the levels tested. Coincubation with 50 mM glucose, mannose, galactose, or fructose reduced the release of radiolabeled CO_2 by 70–95%, but 50 mM glycerol had no effect (4). These data suggest that multiple sugars can be metabolized by the organism, but that glycerol kinase is missing.

Glucose-6-phosphate dehydrogenase converts glucose-6-phosphate to 6-phosphogluconate. Detection of this enzyme suggests the ability of the organism to shunt glucose into alternative modes of glucose oxidation by the phosphogluconate pathway (pentose shunt). This pathway provides a major source of reducing power for the cell by the formation of the reduced coenzyme NADPH, and it also allows the interconversion of hexoses and pentoses. Enzyme histochemical studies using a tetrazolium dye technique indicated that this enzyme activity was low or absent in cysts; trophozoites were not analyzed (5). Subsequently, starch gel electrophoresis analysis identified a glucose-6-phosphate dehydrogenase activity in mixed life cycle stage preparations that was distinct from the rat enzyme (6).

Lactate dehydrogenase (LDH), which converts lactase to pyruvate, has been detected cytochemically in cysts (5) and is electrophoretically distinct from rat LDH (6). Taylor and Easmon (7) reported that the LDH activity of a soluble fraction of rat *P. carinii* was 85–91 nmol min^{-1} mg^{-1} protein. The preparations analyzed in their report were presumably a mixture of life cycle stages, although the authors indicated that their method was capable of separating cysts from trophozoites.

The ultrastructure of *P. carinii* predicts the presence of several compounds and activities. Mitochondria (1,2,8,9) suggest that the organism has aerobic metabolic capacities, including a functional tricarboxylic acid (TCA) cycle and β-oxidation in the matrix, as well as oxidative phosphorylation and an electron transport chain (ETC) in the cristae. The presence in *P. carinii* of aerobic metabolism and the TCA cycle was shown by the in vitro incorporation of radioactivity from pyruvate into CO_2, which was an order of magnitude faster than that from glucose (4). The TCA enzyme succinic dehydrogenase has been detected in cysts by cytochemical techniques (5). Also, the TCA enzyme malate dehydrogenase was detected by starch gel electrophoresis, but the *P. carinii* and rat enzymes had some overlap in mobilities (6). The *P. carinii* and rat cytosolic malic enzymes, which convert cytosolic malate to pyruvate while generating NADPH, were clearly resolved by starch gel electrophoresis (6). The key enzyme for entry of amino acids into the TCA cycle, glutamate dehydrogenase, was cytochemically detected in cysts (5) and differed in electrophoretic mobility, with some overlap, with that of the rat enzyme (6).

In vitro oxygen consumption of isolated *P. carinii* preparations was virtually abolished by cyanide (10), providing strong evidence for the presence of cytochromes in an ETC. Also, the organism is sensitive to the drug 566C80 (1,4-hydroxynaphthoquinone), which is a selective inhibitor of the ETC, with an apparent site of action at the cytochrome bc_1 complex (complex III) (11,12). The drug may have its effect as an analogue of ubiquinone (12). Gene sequences with homologies to those for apocytochrome *b*, subunits of cytochrome oxidase, and NADH dehydrogenase of other organisms have recently been identified (13–15), providing additional data indicating the presence of a functional ETC in *P. carinii* mitochondria.

Pneumocystis carinii uses molecular oxygen, maintaining its O_2 consumption rate in vitro as low as P_{O_2} of 8 torr and remaining viable when exposed to hypoxic conditions (10). Oxygen becomes toxic at concentrations greater than 50%, and the organism is susceptible to reactive oxygen radical-generating systems such as hydrogen peroxide and superoxide (10). The antioxidant enzymes, superoxide dismutase and catalase, in *P. carinii* preparations have been demonstrated to electrophoretically migrate separately from those in rat tissues (6). However, with the possible exception of superoxide dismutase activity, the levels of glutathione peroxidase and catalase activities examined were barely detectable above control values. The levels of antioxidant enzymes of the organism appear much lower than are typical of anaerobes (10).

Electron microscopy combined with cytochemical approaches is particularly useful for a system that does not readily lend itself to direct biochemical analysis. However, to date, this approach has identified only two enzyme activities at the ultrastructural level. Acid phosphatase activity was detected on only the surfaces of large trophozoites by Barton et al. (1), but more recently Itatani and Marshall (2) have reported also finding this activity in the cyst wall. The presence of extracellular acid phosphatase activity suggests that nutrients are degraded extracellularly for subsequent uptake of these products by the parasite. A neutral ATPase activity was detected on the pellicle by electron microscopy, suggesting to the authors that it may represent a sodium–potassium pump ATPase (1).

Another surface ATPase was recently identified by molecular genetic techniques. A proton pump ATPase gene sequence was identified in *P. carinii* (16). In other organisms, such as *Leishmania* (17,18) and yeast (19–21), there are convincing data supporting the idea that an outward-directed proton pump serves to establish a transmembrane H^+ concentration gradient that then drives a symport translocation mechanism for bringing nutrients, such as amino acids and glucose, into the cell. Consistent with the presence of a similar putative transporter system in *P. carinii*, is the observation that the pH of the medium of nongrowing, but healthy, cultures dropped with time. No pH changes were observed when the organisms were treated with metabolic inhibitors or were shown not to be metabolically active, as determined by the failure to incorporate radiolabeled precursors (4,22). The pH drop was not the result of release of organic acids by the cells, since acetate, lactate, or pyruvate could not be detected in the incubation medium (4). Furthermore, the H^+ pump inhibitor, imipramine, had a cidal action on *P. carinii* in an in vitro assay (Kaneshiro ES, et al., unpublished data). The kinetics of incorporation of the amino acid analogue [^{3}H]α-aminobutyric acid indicated that *P. carinii* takes up amino acids against a concentration gradient (uphill transport). This uptake was inhibited by chloroquine and pentamidine, but not by the protein synthesis inhibitor cycloheximide (4). The involvement of a H^+ motive force driving amino acid transport in this organism is suggested by the available evidence, but it has yet to be directly demonstrated.

Arginine metabolism results in the production of ornithine and, subsequently, the formation of the polyamines, putrescine, spermidine, and spermine. Polyamines are required for cell proliferation and differentiation, and perhaps DNA replication as well. The polyamine content of rat *P. carinii* was measured at a putrescine concentration of 1.2 μg/mg protein and that of spermidine as 10.3 μg/mg protein. Spermine was absent or present only in trace amounts (23). Although [^{14}C]arginine was incorporated into *P. carinii* putrescine and spermidine, ornithine decarboxylase activity, as determined by incorporation of [1-^{14}C]ornithine into CO_2, was not detected (23,24). Since the inhibitors of ornithine decarboxylase, difluoromethylornithine and α-monofluoromethyldihydroornithine methyl ester, are effective against *P. carinii* pneumonia, it is

Biochemistry and Metabolism 49

expected that these drugs act on the enzyme (23,25). If, however, the turnover of ornithine decarboxylase in *P. carinii* is very high, the enzyme activity may have evaded detection (23). Although data were not presented, Clarkson et al. (25) reported that they succeeded in measuring *P. carinii* ornithine decarboxylase activity.

III. Nucleic Acids

From estimates of DNA content and chromosome analyses, the *P. carinii* genome appears to be relatively small (26–31) (Table 1), and chromosome sizes are comparable with those of yeast-like fungi. The GC content of rat *P. carinii* DNA was estimated at 32–34% (32), indicating the bulk of DNA is AT-rich. Hence, the fluorescence DNA indicator 4′,6-diamidino-2-phenylindole (DAPI) would be expected to provide a more sensitive *P. carinii* DNA stain than would methramycin, which intercalates GC moieties. Yamada et al. (33) have successfully employed DAPI to quantify the relative ploidy among *P. carinii* life cycle stages. Base compositions of the *P. carinii* thymidylate synthase (34) and dihydrofolate reductase (35) genes were reported to be 30 and 29% GC, respectively. The GC content of the gene coding for the small ribosomal subunit RNA was estimated at 45%, typical of this gene in organisms representing broad phylogenetic backgrounds (36). Molecular taxonomy, mainly based on rRNA homology (36–40) and the sequences of genes coding for dihydrofolate reductase (35) and thymidylate synthase (34), the occurrence of repetitive sequences (41,42), host-specific karyotypes (30,43–47) and antigenic variation (48–52) have been identified and are topics discussed in greater detail in Chapters 4, 5, and 6 on molecular genetics, molecular approach to taxonomy, and antigenic characteristics, respectively.

Little is known about DNA and chromosome replication in *P. carinii*; however, both ATP-dependent and ATP-independent topoisomerase activities were assessed by the ability of *P. carinii* preparations to relax supercoiled DNA (53). A class of aromatic divalent cations were effective against ATP-dependent activity, but not against ATP-independent activity (53) (see also Chap. 27 on diamidines). The gene for topoisomerase I has been mapped to a 650-kb chromosome (27). Relative to understanding transcription of information encoded in DNA to RNA, about the only progress along these lines is the reported successful amplification of the *P. carinii* transcription factor IID gene (16).

There are only limited data available on such basic information as what nucleic precursors *P. carinii* can transport. Pesanti and Cox (4) used isolated organism preparations placed in a salt solution and found that they readily incorporated [^{3}H]uridine into trichloroacetic acid-precipitable material. The uptake was not inhibited by pentamidine, an anti-*P. carinii* drug. However, neither

Table 1 *Pneumocystis carinii* Nucleic Acids

	Direct analyses	Indirect methods	Ref.
Quantitation			
DNA (pg/cell, intracystic body, nucleus, or organism)			
	0.22–0.34		69,70
	0.02		42
		≥ 0.015	27
		(≥7 Mbp)[a]	
		0.017–0.035	28
		(8–16 Mbp)[a]	
		0.019	26
		(8.7 Mbp)[a]	
		0.022	29,30
		(10 Mbp)[a]	
RNA (pg/organism, nucleus, or cyst)			
	13.8		70
	0.012–0.038		71
Identification and partial characterizations			
Cytoplasmic ribosomal RNA			
26S	Isolation, electrophoresis		26,32,37,39,71,72
18S (16S-like)	Isolation, electrophoresis		26,32,39,71,72
		Hybridization/gene sequence	28,36,37,39
5.8S		Hybridization/gene sequence	28
5S	Isolation, electrophoresis		40
		Hybridization/gene sequence	28
Mitochondrial ribosomal RNA			
Small subunit		Hybridization/gene sequence	13
Large subunit		Hybridization/gene sequence	14,15

[a]Calculated DNA content of diploid organism based on estimated size of haploid genome shown in parentheses.

[³H]thymidine nor [³H]hypoxanthine was taken up or incorporated into DNA (4). Although it was reported that the organisms died at pH 5.2 in a saline solution buffered with either β-alanine or citrate phosphate (10), when the organisms were incubated in a selective pH 4 yeast medium containing some nutrients, uptake of [³H]uridine, [³H]uracil, [³H]thymidine, and [³H[hypoxanthine was observed (54). The presence of potential nutrients in the culture medium that were absent in the salt solution used in the former study, may have served to protect organism viability long enough to permit the incorporation of these radiolabeled precursors. These results exemplify the current problems in interpreting most *P. carinii* direct biochemistry and metabolism data, as discussed earlier.

The concentration of the nucleotide ATP was estimated at about 1 nmol/cell by the sensitive luciferin/luciferase assay (55). The ATP content of *Giardia*, *Trichomonas*, *Entamoeba*, and *Leishmania*, but not *P. carinii* cultures was positively correlated with cell proliferation. *Pneumocystis carinii* placed in phosphate-buffered saline had no detectable ATP after three days, whereas the ATP content of cultures placed in modified tissue culture medium was maintained for five days (55).

Studies on purine metabolism have been driven by the need for effective anti-*P. carinii* drugs. Suppression of *P. carinii* proliferation by inosine analogues suggests the presence of a purine salvage pathway and that the organism may use inosine or hypoxanthine as a purine source (56). The replication of DNA requires nucleoside triphosphates, such as dTTP. In the reactions leading to DNA synthesis, thymidylate synthase converts dUMP to dTMP by concurrent utilization of the methyl donor, 5,10-methylenetetrahydrofolate. Removal of the methyl group from the donor results in the formation of 7,8-dihydrofolate which, in turn, is reduced to tetrahydrofolate in a reaction catalyzed by dihydrofolate reductase. Inhibitors of dihydrofolate reductase were earlier shown to be effective against *P. carinii* pneumonia (57–64) (discussed further in Chap. 25). Allegra et al. (65) measured the dihydrofolate reductase activity at 3.9 nmol mm^{-1} mg^{-1} protein and showed that this was a *P. carinii*-specific activity by the absence of cross-reactivity of antibodies against rat dihydrofolate reductase. Subsequently, the dihydrofolate reductase and the thymidylate synthase genes have been sequenced (34,35) and mapped (27).

Kovacs et al. (66) demonstrated that *P. carinii* was capable of de novo folate synthesis by the incorporation of the precursor [³H]*para*-aminobenzoic acid (PABA) into reduced folates; 10-formyltetrahydrofolate and tetrahydrofolate were the major radiolabeled compounds. The de novo pathway (not present in mammalian cells) involves dihydropteroate synthase and can be inhibited by PABA analogues, including sulfonamide and sulfone classes of compounds (also see Chap. 25). Incorporation of [¹⁴C]PABA into pteroic acid by *P. carinii* was detected, and the activity of dihydropteroate synthase activity in cell homogenates was reported to be 13.5 μmol of dihydropteroate synthesized per milligram of protein, a value at least an order of magnitude lower than those measured for bacterial homogenates (67). Exogenously supplied dihydroneopterin, which feeds into the de novo pathway, was recently reported to stimulate the incorporation of PABA in the organisms (68).

Less is known about pyrimidine biosynthesis, with the only kinds of biochemical information inferred from drug studies. For example, it was suggested that 566C80, an ETC inhibitor, may inhibit pyrimidine biosynthesis, since the ETC is linked by ubiquinone to dihydroorotate dehydrogenase, the key enzyme in pyrimidine biosynthesis (12).

IV. Proteins

The ultrastructural identification of microtubules, especially clear in the spindle apparatus (8,73) and pseudopods (2), suggests that their tubulin monomers are present in *P. carinii*. With the handicaps of the system for direct biochemical analyses, molecular genetic approaches have recently been successful in identifying a gene sequence in *P. carinii* for β-tubulin (74), and the organism has been shown to be sensitive to benzimidazole drugs known to inhibit tubulin polymerization (75). Similarly, filamentous structures in pseudopods (2) may represent the ultrastructural correlate of actin, for which a gene has been mapped to a 460-kb chromosome in rat *P. carinii* by hybridization methods (27). Reports on gene sequences coding for apocytochrome *b* and several enzyme proteins have been described (Table 2).

Aside from direct and indirect evidences for proteins of known functions, very little more is known. However, several direct analyses of *P. carinii* proteins have been conducted. Whole-organism preparations (cysts plus trophozoites of various percentage compositions) have been subjected to one-dimensional sodium dodecyl sulfate–polyacrylamide gel electrophoresis (SDS–PAGE). Protein profiles have been visualized by stains such as Coomassie blue (76–79) or silver (80) (Fig. 1). Although protein resolution and detection techniques are good, numerous bands are visible, and some bands are consistently present in organism preparations; only the rat, ferret, and mouse gp105–120s (analogous and cross-reactive to the human gp90–95) have been identified with any degree of certainty as *P. carinii* proteins. That this band is not due to host proteins has been proved mainly by antigenic analyses (43,76–80) (studies on antigens are discussed in greater detail in Chap. 6). Because the band with a relative molecular mass (M_r) of about 45 kDa was not detectable in normal rat lung analyses, this band was also thought be a *P. carinii* protein (81). Recently the amino acid sequence of a portion of a rat *P. carinii* antigen with an M_r of 45–55 kDa was predicted, using cloned cDNA (82). No band has been identified as exclusive of any given life cycle stage. Two-dimensional analysis involving isoelectric focusing (IEF) has been shown only for the major antigenic component, gp105–120, which comprises six isoforms (83).

Table 2 *Pneumocystis carinii* Proteins and Enzymes

	Direct analysis	Indirect methods	Ref.
Whole organism			
Total protein	62 pg/cyst		69
Acid phosphatase		EM cytochemistry	1,2
Actin		Hybridization/ gene sequence	27
ATPase (neutral)		EM cytochemistry	1
ATPase (proton)		Hybridization/ gene sequence	16,87
Catalase	Enzyme activity		6,10
Cathepsin H-like	Enzyme activity		86
Glucose-6-dehydrogenase	Enzyme activity	Cytochemistry	6 / 5
Glutamate dehydrogenase	Enzyme activity	Cytochemistry	6 / 5
β-Glycerophosphatase		EM cytochemistry	105
Lactic dehydrogenase	Enzyme activity	Cytochemistry	6,7 / 5
Malate dehydrogenase	Enzyme activity		6
Malic enzyme	Enzyme activity		6
Superoxide dismutase	Enzyme activity		6,10
Thiamine pyrophosphatase		EM cytochemistry	105
β-Tubulin		Ultrastructure / Hybridization/ gene sequence	2,8,73 / 74
Glycoprotein 105–120 kDa	Electrophoresis/isoelectric focusing/peptide mapping/amino acid sequencing		43,63,76–80,82–85, 87–89
Mitochondria			
Apocytochrome *b*		Hybridization/ gene sequence	13
Cytochrome oxidase subunit II		Hybridization/ gene sequence	13
NADH dehydrogenase and subunits 1, 2, 3, and 6		Hybridization/ gene sequence	13
Cyst wall			
Total protein	11% of total dry weight		89
Glycoprotein 120 kDa	Electrophoresis		89

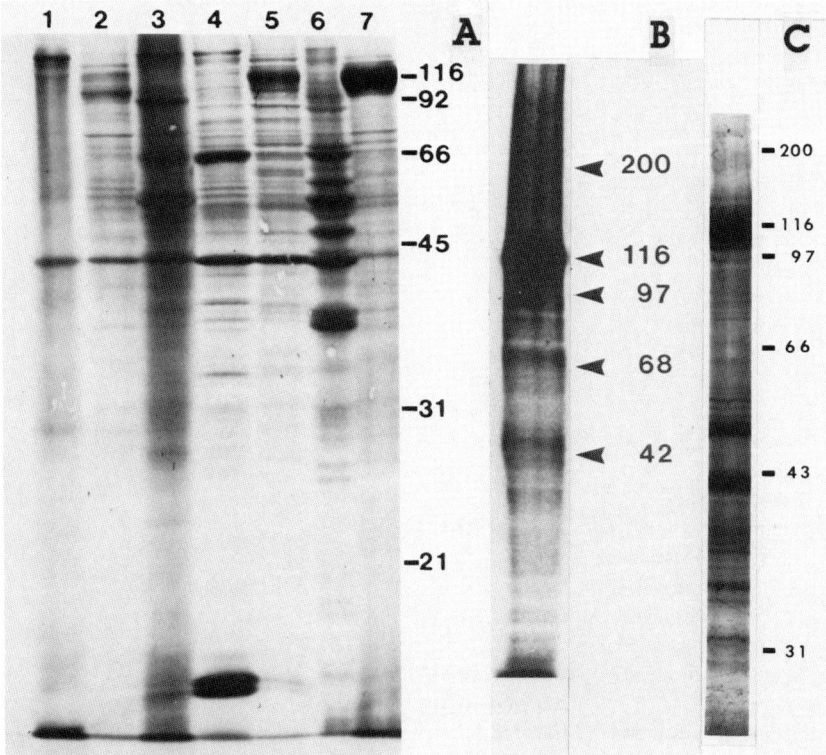

Figure 1 Polyacrylamide gel electrophoresis of *P. carinii* proteins. (A) Separated proteins in *P. carinii* and control preparations were transferred to nitrocellulose and stained with fast green. Lane 1, normal human lung; lane 2, lung-derived human *P. carinii* from an AIDS patient; lane 3, lung-derived human *Pneumocystis* from a non-AIDS patient; lane 4, normal rat lung; lane 5, lung-derived rat *P. carinii*; lane 6, A549 tissue culture cells; lane 7, A549 tissue culture-derived rat *P. carinii*. (B) Silver-stained gel of a rat *P. carinii* whole-organism preparation. (C) Silver-stained gel of proteins in a cyst wall preparation obtained by zymolyase treatment of rat *P. carinii*. The migration of the major high molecular mass band in proteins of rat *P. carinii* (gp105–120: A, lanes 5 and 7; B) is less than that of the equivalent component in human *P. carinii* (gp90–95: A, lanes 2 and 3). Comparison of fast green-stained gel blots (A) with silver-stained gels (B) indicate how the intensities of other lower molecular mass bands differ. These differences may reflect differences in the nature of the isolated organism preparations used in the two studies, or may indicate that the two procedures result in different relative intensities of protein-containing bands. Silver staining of proteins of isolated cyst walls of *P. carinii* isolated from rat lungs (C) indicate that the major component (105–120 kDa) occurs in this subcellular fraction. The profile also shows the presence of many bands not evident in whole-cell analyses. These bands may represent proteins that are enriched in this cellular component, may be due to the achievement of better electrophoretic separations, or may represent differences in the *P. carinii* preparations used in the different studies. Zymolyase used in the procedure for isolating cyst walls is not a major contaminant in this protein profile. Molecular masses are indicated in kilodaltons. (From: A, Ref. 123; B, Ref. 80; C, Ref. 89.)

Also, only the gp105–120 has been partially characterized by peptide analysis or amino acid sequencing (80,83–85).

The only kinds of data available from direct biochemical analyses of protein metabolism are that radiolabeled amino acids can incorporate into *P. carinii* proteins when the organisms are incubated under nongrowth conditions (4,54). The incorporation of radioactivity from an amino acid mixture was inhibited by cycloheximide, rifampin, tetracycline, and the anti-*P. carinii* drugs, trimethoprim plus sulfanthoxazole, had less inhibitory effects (4). By gel electrophoresis, the incorporation of [^{3}H]methionine into specific *P. carinii* proteins was demonstrated by the detection of radioactivity in bands shown to be antigens of the parasite (54). Similar results were found when using radiolabeled isoleucine and cysteine (48).

Information on protein catabolism is limited to the detection of a *P. carinii*-specific cysteine proteinase activity, similar to that of cathepsin H (86). This activity was identified by IEF gels of *P. carinii* preparations, and it was the only cysteine proteinase detected that increased in rat lungs paralleling the infection (86).

V. Lipids

Osmiophilic cytoplasmic bodies observed by electron microscopy suggest that *P. carinii* cells have significant lipid stores. These bodies are abundant in trophozoites and less evident or absent in intracystic bodies (1,8). Studies on *P. carinii* lipid compositions have as yet been only superficial (e.g., the presence of the expected general lipid classes have been reported, 90–92) (Table 3). Analyses of this group of compounds are particularly subject to doubts of accuracy, since the organisms are isolated from the lung alveolus, which is rich in surfactant lipids. Dipalmitoyl (disaturated) phosphatidylcholine, the major lung surfactant phospholipid, dominates the phospholipid profile of lipids extracted from *P. carinii* preparations, but some of this may reflect the strong adhesive properties of the organism's surface to this lung alveolar lipid (90). The presence of relatively high lysophosphatides in these analyses (90) may reflect significant degradation of complex phospholipids before extraction or analysis.

Radiolabeled choline or acetate incorporated in vitro into phosphatidylcholine and lysophosphatidylcholine, and radiolabeled ethanolamine incorporated into phosphatidylethanolamine when *P. carinii* preparations were incubated with the precursor in a salt solution. Also, less than 5% of the phosphatidylcholine molecular species synthesized in vitro had two saturated fatty acids (90). These observations suggest that *P. carinii* can synthesize complex phospholipids from head group and fatty acid precursors.

Cholesterol was the major sterol present in freshly isolated preparations from infected rat lungs (92), which explains the organism's relative insensitivity to the antifungal polyene antibiotic, amphotericin B. The sterol distribution in various

Table 3 *Pneumocystis carinii* Lipids

	Direct analyses	Indirect methods	Ref.
Neutral lipids			
Cholesterol	Major sterol		92
		EM cytochemistry	93,94
Phospholipids (% of total phospholipid P)			
Cardiolipin	+[a]		90,91
Phosphatidylcholine	64		90
Phosphatidylethanolamine	10		90
Phosphatidylglycerol	10		90
Phosphatidylinositol	+		90
Phosphatidylserine	+		90
Sphingomyelin	+		90
Lysophosphatidylcholine	10		90
Cyst wall total lipids	50% of total dry weight		89

[a]Detected, not quantified.

P. carinii membranes was indirectly evaluated by the presence of large complexes of sterol and filipin (93) or digitonin (94), as visualized by freeze-fracture electron microscopy. The number of intramembranous particles representing those complexes decreased in surface membranes as the organisms presumably developed from trophozoites to precysts and then to cysts (93,94).

The fatty acid compositions of only the total lipids extracted from mixed life cycle populations are known (Table 4); individual lipid classes have yet to be analyzed. In general, the lipid profiles grossly resemble those of the parasite's environment in the host's lung, but it is now thought that the earlier analyses (92) may have included significant lung surfactant material, which contributed to the fatty acid profiles reported. As methods for removing lung surfactant from *P. carinii* preparations improve, it appears that the relative concentrations of individual *P. carinii* fatty acids differ from those of the lung controls. Radiolabeled oleate was shown to be taken up by the organisms in vitro (95) and cysts and trophozoites took up fluorescent fatty acid analogues (Kaneshiro ES, et al., unpublished observations), indicating that *P. carinii* readily takes up exogenous fatty acids. Trophozoites, but not intact cysts, took up 1-palmitoyl-2-(*N*-4-nitrobenzo-2-oxa-1,3-diazole)aminocaproylphosphatidylcholine, a fluorescent analogue of phosphatidylcholine labeled in the fatty acid moiety. Similar observations were made using the head group-derivatized, rhodamine analogue of phosphatidylethanolamine, *N*-(Texas red sulfonyl)phosphatidylethanolamine (96,97). Thus,

Table 4 *Pneumocystis carinii* Total Lipid Fatty Acid Composition (Weight %)

	Total[b]	Ester-linked[c]			Amide-linked[d]	
	Whole organism	Whole organism		Cyst wall	Whole organism	
Fatty Acid[a]	Lung[e]	Lung[e]	A549[f]	Lung[e]	Lung[e]	A549[f]
14:0	1.1	1.4	1.5	1.8	1.5	4.0
15:0	0.4	0.3			0.5	
16:0	36.4	35.9	30.6	32.7	53.4	40.1
16:1	0.1	3.4	3.0	3.1		
17:0	0.5	0.6			0.9	
18:0	15.5	12.7	14.3	10.7	8.1	9.0
18:1	5.8	23.4	23.3	10.7	1.0	3.8
18:2	0.7	8.3	4.7	8.9		
20:0	0.5	0.3			0.6	1.0
20:4 + 22:0	9.1	6.0	10.1	10.1	4.2	4.5
24:0	3.3				14.9	12.8
26:0	1.9				9.2	2.9
28:0	6.7				0.9	
Others	18.0	7.7	12.5	22.0	4.8	21.9

[a]Number of carbon atoms:number of double bonds.
[b]Total ester-and amide-linked fatty acids of total lipids extracted from the preparation.
[c]Saponifiable plus free fatty acids of total lipids extracted from the preparation.
[d]Sphingolipid fatty acids of total lipids extracted from the preparation.
[e]Organisms freshly isolated from infected rat lungs.
[f]Organisms isolated from cultures with A549 cells after three serial passages.
Source: Kaneshiro ES, et al., unpublished.

the organism, especially the trophozoite stage, appears capable of taking up fatty acids and perhaps even complex lipids from its lipid-rich environment. *Pneumocystis carinii* probably uses many host lipids for direct incorporation into the bulk of its own lipids (e.g., cholesterol and most of the fatty acid moieties of its phospholipids), but the organism may synthesize small amounts of unique lipids necessary for its vital functions.

Only low levels of de novo fatty acid synthesis appeared to occur in vitro, as indicated by the low levels of incorporation of radiolabeled acetate into phospholipid fatty acids, but experiments thus far analyzing radiolabeled acetate incorporation gave inconsistent results in two independent laboratories (90; Kaneshiro ES, et al., unpublished observations). Thus, conclusions concerning acetate and lipid metabolism cannot yet be made. However, since ≥90% of radiolabeled palmitate that had incorporated into *P. carinii* lipids remained as palmitate (92), this observation indicates that under the in vitro nongrowth conditions employed, *P. carinii* exhibited only limited capacities to chain-elongate as well as to desaturate this fatty acid.

In a study of BAL fluids, it was concluded that phospholipase activity was elevated in *P. carinii* pneumonia, and that BAL fluids from cortisone-treated control rats were the same as those in untreated controls (98). This observation suggested an explanation for the reduced amounts of phospholipids measured in lungs infected with *P. carinii*. The enzyme may be released by the parasite, enabling the hydrolysis of complex lipids in the alveolus into smaller nutrient molecules. However, the results obtained by Sheehan et al. (99) indicated that the increase in phospholipase activity was accounted for by the steroid immunosuppression regimen alone. These workers suggested that the drop in BAL fluid phospholipids involved an effect that the parasite had on surfactant phospholipid synthesis or release. Analysis of phospholipase activities present on the outer surfaces of the organism or released into the external milieu has not yet been reported.

Masala et al. (91) have identified cardiolipin in lipids extracted from *P. carinii*, by high-performance liquid and thin-layer chromatography (HPLC and TLC). Although, anticardiolipin antibodies are known to occur in patients, such as those with autoimmune diseases like lupus, these workers reported that anticardiolipin antibodies appear to be present in acquired immunodeficiency syndrome (AIDS) patients, specifically in response to *P. carinii* infection.

Isolated cyst wall preparations obtained by zymolyase treatment were recently analyzed. Surprisingly, only 11 and 10% of the preparations were proteins and carbohydrates, respectively, and 50% of the dry weight consisted of lipids. However, the degree of possible contamination from lung surfactant material in the preparations was not established. The saponifiable fatty acid profile of total lipids extracted from these preparations grossly resembled that of whole organism total lipids (89) (see Table 4). The possibility that a large percentage of the cyst wall is made up of lipids suggests that these compounds may play an important role in the biology of this organism.

VI. Carbohydrates

Although several direct biochemical analyses have been reported (Table 5), most studies on carbohydrates in *P. carinii* thus far have employed lectins (Table 6). De Stefano et al. (100) provided some definitive data on the sugar composition of the organism, and two types of cyst wall preparations that were obtained by zymolyase treatment. Digestion for 30 min resulted in a preparation that presumably contained the surface glycocalyx material. Digestion for 60 min resulted in the

Table 5 *Pneumocystis carinii* Carbohydrates

	Direct analyses	Indirect methods	Ref.
Quantitation			
Whole organism			
Glycogen	5.3 pg/cyst		70
Hexosamines	0.002 ng/cyst		70
Ribose	Trace		89,100
Sialic acid	Trace		89,100
Uronic acids	7.5 pg/cyst		70
Cyst wall			
Total carbohydrates	75–80 µg/mg dry weight (10% of total dry weight)		70,100
Identification and partial characterization			
Whole organism			
Glycoproteins (rat gp105–120, human gp90–95)	Electrophoresis/ chromatography	Enzyme sensitivity/lectin-binding/antibody-binding	76,83,84 43,44,76,78–80,111
Glycogen		Ultrastructure	1,8,110,111
α-1,4-Glucan	α-1,4-Glucan synthase activity		112
Cyst wall, cell surface			
Glycogen		Cytochemistry	102,104,105
α-1,4-Glucan	α-1,4-Glucan synthase activity		112
β-1,3-Glucan		Zymolyase sensitivity, drug sensitivity, cytochemistry	96,100–102, 105,107,108
Chitin		Cytochemistry, chitinase sensitivity, lectin binding	116–119
Major surface antigen			
Chitin		Chitinase sensitivity	77–79
N-Acetyl-glucosamine	Chromatography	Lectin binding	76,83 43,77,78,111
Fucose	Chromatography		83
Galactose	Chromatography	Lectin binding	76,83 43,77,78,111
Glucose	Chromatography	Lectin binding	76,83 43,77,78,111
Mannose	Chromatography	Lectin binding	76,83 43,77,78,111

Table 6 Lectin Binding by *Pneumocystis carinii*

Primary sugar(s) detected	Lectin	Reactivity	Ref.
α-D-Mannose	*Wisteria floribunda* agglutinin (WFA)	Strong, partial	120,121
α-D-Mannose>α-D-glucose	Concanavalin A (Con A)	Strong	104,105,111,119–122
β-1,4-N-Acetylglucosamine	Wheat germ agglutinin (WGA)	Strong, weak	111,120–122
	Pokeweed mitogen (PWM)	Strong	111
	Solanum tuberosum agglutinin (STA)	Partial, weak	119–121
α- and β-N-acetylglucosamine	*Griffonia simplicifolia* lectin II (GS II)	Weak, nonreactive	119,120
α- and β-N-acetylgalactosamine >α- and β-galactose	Soybean agglutinin (SBA)	Strong, partial	111,119–122
α-D-N-Acetylgalactosamine	*Bauhinia purpurea* agglutinin (BPA)	Strong, partial	119–122
	Maclura pomifera agglutinin (MPA)	Strong, partial	119–122
α-1,3-N-Acetylgalactosamine	*Dolichos biflorus* agglutinin (DBA)	Partial, weak	119–122
β-1,3-N-Acetylgalactosamine >α- and β-galactose	Peanut agglutinin (PNA)	Weak, nonreactive	111,119–122
α-D-Galactose	*Griffonia simplicifolia* lectin I (GS-I)	Partial, weak	119–121
	G. simplicifolia lectin I-B$_4$ (GS-IB$_4$)	Weak, nonreactive	119–121
β-D-Galactose	*Viscum album* agglutinin (VAA)	Nonreactive	119–121
α-L-Fucose	*Ulex europeus* agglutinin I (UEA)	Strong, partial, weak	119–122
	Tetragonobolus purpureas agglutinin	Nonreactive	111
α-Neuraminic acid	*Limax flavus* agglutinin (LFA)	Weak, nonreactive	119–121

Biochemistry and Metabolism

removal of the cyst wall, including the glycocalyx, outer bilayer membrane, and probably part of the middle electron-lucent layer as well. The remaining cyst protoplast, which may also include part of the middle layer, plus the trophozoites in the preparation were also analyzed. Alditol acetate, trimethylsilyl, and deuterated derivatives of the sugars in these preparations were identified, characterized, and quantified by combinations of gas chromatographic (GC) and mass spectrometric (MS) techniques. Glucose was the major sugar in whole organisms and subcellular fractions (Fig. 2). Mannose, galactose, and N-acetylglucosamine were present in significant quantities; however, only trace or undetectable amounts of ribose and sialic acid were found in these samples.

The cyst wall can be stained with a variety of polysaccharide stains including aniline blue (101), which is specific for β-1,3-glucans. Although trophozoites did not stain positive for glycogen–mucin by Gomori's methenamine silver

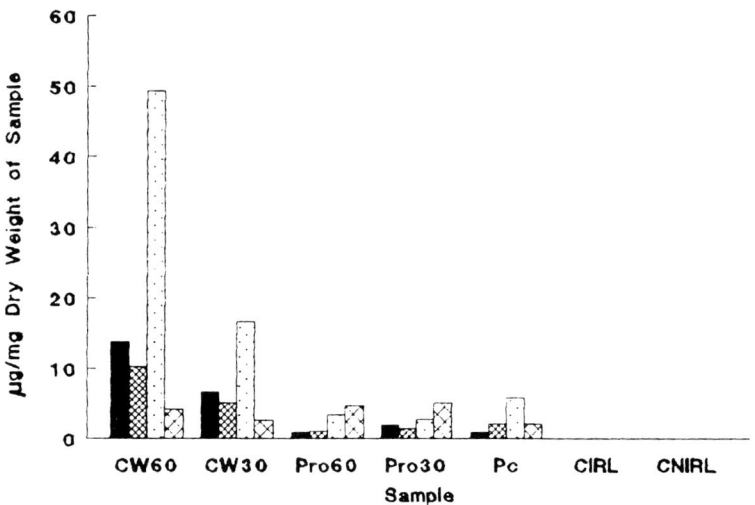

Figure 2 Sugar composition of rat *P. carinii* whole-organism and cyst wall preparations. Values are based on 1 mg dry weight of each sample. CW60, cyst wall preparation obtained from 60-min zymolyase treatment, which removes the cyst wall and leaves the inner plasma membrane of mature cysts intact. This fraction may also contain glycocalyxes from other life cycle stages present in the preparation. CW30, cyst wall sample from 30-min zymolyase treatment, which probably removes the outermost glycocalyx of all life cycle stages in the preparation. PRO60, protoplasts remaining after 60-min treatment; PRO30, protoplasts remaining after 30-min zymolyase treatment; Pc, *P. carinii* whole-organism preparation; CIRL, control lung from immunosuppressed rat; CNIRL, control lung from nonimmunosuppressed rat. Mannose ■, galactose ▧, glucose ⬚, N-acetylglucosamine ⧅. (From Ref. 89.)

nitrate (GMS), the endogenous form of trophozites (8) exhibited a thin GMS-positive layer in the parent pellicle (102). The binding of gold-labeled concanavalin A lectin on the surfaces of all life cycle forms, including intracystic bodies, was identified by electron microscopy (103–105), suggesting the presence of mannose–glucose residues on surface structures of *P. carinii*. Yoshikawa et al. (103,104) also identified similar *Macura pomifera* agglutinin (MPA) binding, which suggests that *N*-acetylgalactose–galactose terminal residues also are at these surface structures.

Cytochemistry on the electron microscopic level has been done in attempts to identify carbohydrates in cyst wall substructures. Yoshikawa et al. (104) showed that both the outer electron-dense layer and the middle electron-lucent layer of the cyst wall stained with periodic acid–methenamine silver and periodic acid thiocarbohydrazide silver–proteinate (PA-TCH-SP); the outer layer was more intensely stained with PA-TCH-SP. On the other hand, Palluault et al. (105) reported that the middle layer stained with PA-TCH-SP, but the outer layer did not. Thus, these cytochemical studies on the presence and relative concentrations of carbohydrates in cyst wall substructures using similar stains apparently gave different results. However, Yoshikawa and Yoshida (102) reported that the middle layer, especially the outer regions of this layer, stained positive for glycogen–mucin by GMS, and the outer layer was not stained.

Treatment of mature cysts with zymolyase, containing β-1,3-glucan laminaripentaohydrolase as its key activity [but also reported to have some protease activity (101,106)], results in the removal of the cyst wall (96,101). Since trophozoites and zymolyase-treated cysts are aniline blue-negative, the middle layer of the cyst wall was considered to be the site of the putative β-1,3-glucan (101). However, since the outer bilayer membrane within the outer electron-dense layer of the cyst wall became apparent by freeze-fracture only after limited (30 min) zymolyase treatment (96), this observation indicates that these types of polysaccharides may also reside in the outer layer. Concanavalin A was found to bind to both the outer and middle layers of the cyst wall by two groups (104,105). The *N*-acetylgalactose–galactose-specific lectin MPA bound to the outer, but not the middle layer (103). Together, these observations suggest that both the outer and middle layers contain β-1,3-glucan, glycogen, or mucin types of polysaccharides with terminal mannose–glucose residues. Polysaccharides with *N*-acetylgalactose–galactose terminal residues may be restricted to the outer layer.

Recently, two groups have demonstrated that inhibitors of β-1,3-glucan synthesis (aculeacin A and L-671,329) have anti-*P. carinii* activity in an immunosuppressed rat model of acute *P. carinii* pneumonia (107–109). In both studies, mature cysts were rapidly lost from infected lungs, and it appeared that the production of new cysts was halted. The effect of the agents on the trophozoite form was less dramatic, but appeared to have a static effect, since trophozoite numbers did not increase (109). These studies suggest that the development of the trophozoite to the cyst stage requires synthesis of β-1,3-glucan for cyst wall formation. Since trophozoite numbers did not increase when cysts were eliminated, these workers also suggested that the cyst form may be an obligate stage for trophozoite proliferation (109).

Although a β-1,3-glucan is apparently present in the cyst wall, synthesis of this material by *P. carinii* has not been directly demonstrated. However, α-1,4-glucan is expected to be present in *P. carinii*, since glycogen granules have been demonstrated by several electron microscopic studies to be especially abundant in trophozoites (1,8,105,110) and also present in cysts (111). Quantitation of glycogen in isolated *P. carinii* preparations has been reported by Pifer et al. (70). Furthermore, Williams et al. (112) have demonstrated that α-1,4-glucan synthesis occurred in organisms maintained in short-term maintenance cultures. When 10^6 organisms are placed in buffer containing radiolabeled UDP-glucose, approximately 0.3 nmol/hr was incorporated into polysaccharides and glycoproteins. This represents an uptake rate about five times greater than that observed in *Saccharomyces cerevisiae*. Extremely high levels of glucan synthase activity were also observed in deoxycholate extracts of *P. carinii*, which produced an α-1,4-D-glucopyranose polysaccharide. Definitive structural characterizations of the glucan synthesized in vitro employed a variety of GC and MS analytical techniques. The hexose monomers synthesized in vitro were oxidized by D-glucose oxidase and, unlike mammalian glycogen, it contained few or no branches. These workers also detected α-1,4-glucan synthase activity in cyst wall preparations of *P. carinii*, suggesting that α-1,4-glucans may also be at this site (112).

Chitin, a β-1,4-linked polymer of *N*-acetyl-D-glucosamine, is a component of the cell walls of most fungi and may occur in the cyst walls of some protozoans (113–115). *Pneumocystis carinii*, maintained in a low pH modified yeast medium, were able to take up [^{3}H]acetylglucosamine (54). Autoradiographic analysis of [^{3}H]glucosamine uptake indicated that radioactivity was present in trophozoites, intracystic bodies, and cyst walls (116). From the patchy- or faint-staining patterns obtained with picro-Sirius Red F3BA and periodic acid–Schiff reagent (PAS), it was initially reported that *P. carinii* cysts (but not trophozites) contained chitin (117). More recently, antibodies to chitin and chitin oligomers (chitotriose, chitotetraose, and chitopentaose) (118) and lectins with specificity for chitin (116) have been used to examine *P. carinii*. Both types of reagents bound to mature cysts, intracystic bodies, and trophic forms of the organism. Also, electrophoretic migration of the major surface antigen gp105–120 was reported to be slightly affected by treatment with chitinase (77,78). Although these results suggest that chitin is present, it is unlikely that chitin represents a large fraction of the cyst wall of rat *P. carinii* carbohydrate, because the amount of *N*-acetylglucosamine present there appears to be small (76,83). Direct biochemical studies for definitive chitin identification, including linkage analyses, have yet to be reported.

The major surface antigens of rat (gp105–120) (76,80) and human (gp95)

(76) *P. carinii* contain 5–9% carbohydrate, as estimated by molecular mass reduction after endoglycosidase H digestion (cleaves *O*-linked oligosaccharides) (76,80) or chemical deglycosylation with trifluoromethane sulfonic acid (80). Endoglycosidase F and α-mannosidase also cleaved these glycoproteins, indicating high mannose or mixed oligosaccharides that are *N*-linked to a core protein (76,83,84). The carbohydrate moiety of gp105–120 appears to confer the ability to separate isoforms by IEF, since endoglycosidase F and α-mannosidase treatment resulted in conversion of the six isoforms to a single focusing component (84).

There are several indications that the carbohydrate composition of *P. carinii* glycoproteins varies among isolates from different hosts and, perhaps, between different strains of the host as well. For example, Lundgren et al. (76) and Tanabe et al. (83) have shown that the major surface antigen glycoprotein derived from rats contained mainly mannose and glucose, with much lower amounts of *N*-acetylgalactosamine, fucose, galactose, and *N*-acetylglucosamine, whereas from humans it contained equimolar amounts of galactose, glucose, mannose, and *N*-acetylglucosamine, and lesser amounts of fucose and other components (76) (see Chap. 6 for detailed discussion of antigens).

VII. Conclusions

Somewhat similar to our experience, Gutteridge (124) described his frustration in preparing the biochemistry section in his recent comprehensive review on *P. carinii* as "trying to put together two jigsaw puzzles from a mixture of the two with most of the pieces missing and an indeterminate number of those actually present belonging to a third puzzle!" Given the difficulty faced in obtaining information on *P. carinii* metabolism and biochemistry, a remarkable amount of information has nonetheless been accumulated, albeit from biochemically flawed experimental conditions and from indirect evidence. The bulk of data currently available are, for the main part, expected or have been described in other eukaryotic organisms. If a molecule or metabolic pathway unique to *P. carinii* exists, the probability that it could be discovered is rather low with the current lack of good culture systems for this organism. Thus far, the identification or detection of *P. carinii*-specific or -unique molecules have relied heavily on immunochemical and molecular genetics approaches. Investigators, especially those doing direct biochemical and physiological studies, are to be commended for getting such hard-to-come-by data. It is only with good knowledge of the developmental stage of this experimental system, acceptance of the current state of the art, and heroic perseverance that this body of information has been gathered. It is important to continue such studies because these data are particularly crucial for providing a better understanding of the nutrition of this organism. Such data are needed to serve as guidelines in formulating media for the continuous cultivation of this opportunistic pathogen, the lack of which is clearly the major hindrance to all aspects of *P. carinii* research.

Acknowledgments

Supported in part by funding from the National Institutes of Health (RO1 AI29316 and UO1 AI31702).

References

1. Barton EG Jr, Campbell WG Jr. *Pneumocystis carinii* in lungs of rats treated with cortisone acetate. Am J Pathol 1969; 54:209–236.
2. Itatani CA, Marshall GJ. Ultrastructural morphology and staining characteristics of *Pneumocystis carinii* in situ and from bronchoalveolar lavage. J Parasitol 1988; 74: 700–712.
3. Palluault F, Pietrzyk B, Dei-Cas E, Slomianny C, Soulez B, Camus D. Three-dimensional reconstruction of rabbit-derived *Pneumocystis carinii* from serial-thin sections. I. Trophozoite. J Protozool 1991; 38:402–407.
4. Pesanti EL, Cox C. Metabolic and synthetic activities of *Pneumocystis carinii* in vitro. Infect Immun 1981; 34:908–914.
5. Mazer MA, Kovacs JA, Swan JC, Parillo JE, Masur H. Histoenzymological study of selected dehydrogenase enzymes in *Pneumocystis carinii*. Infect Immun 1987; 55: 727–730.
6. Pesanti EL. Enzymes of *Pneumocystis carinii*: electrophoretic mobility on starch gels. J Protozool 1989; 36:2S–3S.
7. Taylor MB, Easmon CSF. Separation of *Pneumocystis carinii* from the lung of the steroid-suppressed rat. FEMS Microbiol Lett 1990; 70:49–54.
8. Yoshida Y. Ultrastructural studies of *Pneumocystis carinii*. J Protozool 1989; 36: 53–60.
9. Palluault F, Pietrzyk B, Dei-Cas E, Slomianny C, Soulez B, Camus D. Three-dimensional reconstruction of rabbit-derived *Pneumocystis carinii* from serial-thin sections. II. Intermediate precyst. J Protozool 1991; 38:407–411.
10. Pesanti EL. *Pneumocystis carinii* oxygen uptake, antioxidant enzymes, and susceptibility to oxygen-mediated damage. Infect Immun 1984; 44:7–11.
11. Hughes WT, Gray VL, Gutteridge WE, Latter VS, Pudney M. Efficacy of a hydroxy naphthoquinone, 566C80, in experimental *Pneumocystis carinii* pneumonitis. Antimicrob Agents Chemother 1990; 34:225–228.
12. Dohn MN, Frame PT, Baughman RP, Lafon SW, Smulian AG, Caldwell P, Rogers MD. Open-label efficacy and safety trial of 42 days of 566C80 for *Pneumocystis carinii* pneumonia in AIDS patients. J Protozool 1991; 38:220S–221S.
13. Pixley FJ, Wakefield AE, Banerji S, Hopkin JM. Mitochondrial gene sequences show fungal homology for *Pneumocystis carinii*. Mol Microbiol 1991; 5:1347–1351.
14. Wakefield AE, Pixley FJ, Banerji S, Sinclair K, Miller RF, Moxon ER, Hopkin JM. Amplification of mitochondrial ribosomal RNA sequences from *Pneumocystis carinii* DNA of rat and human origin. Mol Biochem Parasitol 1990; 43:69–76.
15. Wakefield AE, Pixley FJ, Banerji S, Sinclair K, Miller RF, Moxon ER, Hopkin JM.

Detection of *Pneumocystis carinii* with DNA amplification. Lancet 1990; 336: 451–453.
16. Meade JC, Stringer JR. PCR amplification of DNA sequences from the transcription factor IID and cation transporting ATPase genes in *Pneumocystis carinii*. J Protozool 1991; 38:66S–68S.
17. Mukkada AJ. Energy coupling in active transport of substrates in *Leishmania*. In: Gilles, R., Gilles-Baillien, M. Transport Process, Iono- and Osmoregulation. New York: Springer-Verlag, 1985:326–333.
18. Zilberstein D, Dwyer DM. Protonmotive force-driven active transport of D-glucose and L-proline in the protozoan parasite *Leishmania donovani*. Proc Natl Acad Sci USA 1985; 82:1716–1720.
19. Davis CB, Hammes GG. Topology of the yeast plasma membrane proton-translocating ATPase. J Biol Chem 1989; 264:370–374.
20. Davis CB, Smith KE, Campbell BN Jr, Hammes GG. The ATP binding site of the yeast plasma membrane proton-translocating ATPase. J Biol Chem 1990; 265:1300–1305.
21. VanLeeuwen CC, Postma E, VandenBroek PJ, VanSteveninck J. Proton-motive force-driven D-galactose transport in plasma membrane vesicles from the yeast *Kluyveromyces marxianus*. J Biol Chem 1991; 266:12146–12151.
22. Pesanti EL. In vitro effects of antiprotozoa drugs and immune serum on *Pneumocystis carinii*. J Infect Dis 1980; 141:775–780.
23. Lipschik GY, Masur H, Kovacs JA. Polyamine metabolism in *Pneumocystis carinii*. J Infect Dis 1991; 163:1121–1127.
24. Pesanti EL, Bartlett MS, Smith JW. Lack of detectable activity of ornithine decarboxylase in *Pneumocystis carinii* [letter]. J Infect Dis 1988; 158:1137–1138.
25. Clarkson AB Jr, Saric M, Grady RW. Deferoxamine and eflornithine (DL-α-difluoromethylornithine) in a rat model of *Pneumocystis carinii* pneumonia. Antimicrob Agents Chemother 1990; 34:1833–1835.
26. Fishman JA, Ullu E, Armstrong MYK, Richards FF. Organization of DNA and RNA from rat *Pneumocystis carinii*. J Protozool 1989; 36:45–55.
27. Lundgren B, Cotton R, Lundgren JD, Edman JC, Kovacs JA. Identification of *Pneumocystis carinii* chromosomes and mapping of five genes. Infect Immun 1990; 58:1705–1710.
28. Yoganathan T, Lin H, Buck GA. An electrophoretic karyotype and assignment of ribosomal genes to resolved chromosomes of *Pneumocystis carinii*. Mol Microbiol 1989; 3:1473–1480.
29. Hong S-T, Steele PE, Cushion MT, Walzer PD, Stringer JR. *Pneumocystis carinii* karyotypes. J Clin Microbiol 1990; 28:1785–1795.
30. Cushion MT, Hong ST, Steele PE, Stringer SL, Walzer PD, Stringer JR. Molecular biology of *Pneumocystis carinii*. Ann NY Acad Sci 1990; 616:415–420.
31. Sinclair K, Wakefield AE, Banerji S, Hopkin JM. *Pneumocystis carinii* organisms derived from rat and human hosts are genetically distinct. Mol Biochem Parasitol 1991; 45:183–184.
32. Worley MA, Ivey MH, Graves DC. Characterization and cloning of *Pneumocystis carinii* nucleic acid. J Protozool 1989; 36:9S–11S.
33. Yamada M, Matsumoto Y, Hamada S, Fujita S, Yoshida Y. Demonstration and determination of DNA in *Pneumocystis carinii* by fluorescence microscopy with 4',6-

diamidino-2-phenylindole (DAPI). Zentralbl Bakteriol Hyg 1986; A262:240–246.
34. Edman U, Edman JC, Lundgren B, Santi DV. Isolation and expression of the *Pneumocystis carinii* thymidylate synthase gene. Proc Natl Acad Sci USA 1989; 86: 6503–6507.
35. Edman JC, Edman U, Cao M, Lundgren B, Kovacs JA, Santi DV. Isolation and expression of the *Pneumocystis carinii* dihydrofolate reductase gene. Proc Natl Acad Sci USA 1989; 86:8625–8629.
36. Edman JC, Kovacs JA, Masur H, Santi DV, Elwood HJ, Sogin ML. Ribosomal RNA sequence shows *Pneumocystis carinii* to be a member of the fungi. Nature 1988; 334:519–522.
37. Edman JC, Kovacs JA, Masur H, Santi DV, Elwood HJ, Sogin ML. Ribosomal RNA genes of *Pneumocystis carinii*. J Protozool 1989; 36:18S–20S.
38. Stringer SL, Hudson K, Blase MA, Walzer PD, Cushion MT, Stringer JR. Sequence from ribosomal RNA of *Pneumocystis carinii* compared to those of four fungi suggests an ascomycetous affinity. J Protozool 1989; 36:14S–16S.
39. Stringer SL, Stringer JR, Blase MA, Walzer PD, Cushion MT. *Pneumocystis carinii*: sequence from ribosomal RNA implies a close relationship with fungi. Exp Parasitol 1989; 68:450–461.
40. Watanabe J, Hori H, Tanabe K, Nakamura Y. 5S ribosomal RNA sequence of *Pneumocystis carinii* and its phylogenetic association with "rhizopoda/myxomycota/zygomycota group." J Protozool 1989; 36:16S–18S.
41. Stringer SL, Hong S-T, Giuntoli D, Stringer JR. Repeated DNA in *Pneumocystis carinii*. J Clin Microbiol 1991; 29:1194–1201.
42. Watanabe J, Nakata K, Nashimoto H, Ikeda H. Cloning and characterization of a repetitive sequence from *Pneumocystis carinii*. Parasitol Res 1992; 78:23–27.
43. Gigliotti F, Ballou LR, Hughes WT, Mosley BD. Purification and initial characterization of a ferret *Pneumocystis carinii* surface antigen. J Infect Dis 1988; 158:848–854.
44. Gigliotti F, Stokes DC, Cheatham AB, Davis DS, Hughes WT. Development of murine monoclonal antibodies to *Pneumocystis carinii*. J Infect Dis 1986; 154: 315–322.
45. Graves DC. Immunological studies of *Pneumocystis carinii*. J Protozool 1989; 36: 60–69.
46. Kovacs JA, Halpern JL, Lundgren B, Swan JC, Parrillo JE, Masur H. Monoclonal antibodies to *Pneumocystis carinii*: identification of specific antigens and characterization of antigenic differences between rat and human isolates. J Infect Dis 1989; 159:60–70.
47. Weinberg GA, Bartlett MS. Comparison of pulsed field gel electrophoresis karyotypes of *Pneumocystis carinii* derived from rat lung, cell culture, and ferret lung. J Protozool 1991; 38:64S–65S.
48. Cushion MT, Stringer JR, Walzer PD. Cellular and molecular biology of *Pneumocystis carinii*. Int Rev Cytol 1991; 131:59–107.
49. Gigliotti F. Antigenic variation of a major surface glycoprotein of *Pneumocystis carinii*. J Protozool 1991; 38:4S–5S.
50. Bauer NL, Paulsrud JR, Bartlett MS, Smith JW, Wilde CE III. Immunologic comparisons of *Pneumocystis carinii* strains obtained from rats, ferrets, and mice using convalescent sera from the same source. J Protozool 1991; 38:166S–168S.

51. Gigliotti F. Host-specific antigenic variation of a mannosylated surface glucoprotein of *Pneumocystis carinii*. J Infect Dis 1992; 165:329–336.
52. Lundgren B, Kovacs JA, Nelson NN, Stock F, Martizes A, Gill VJ. *Pneumocystis carinii* and specific fungi have a common epitope, identified by a monoclonal antibody. J Clin Microbiol 1992; 30:391–395.
53. Dykstra CC, Tidwell RR. Inhibition of topoisomerase from *Pneumocystis carinii* by aromatic dicationic molecules. J Protozool 1991; 38:78S–81S.
54. Cushion MT, Ebbets D. Growth and metabolism of *Pneumocystis carinii* in axenic culture. J Clin Microbiol 1990; 28:1385–1394.
55. Miyahira Y, Takeuchi T. Application of ATP measurement to evaluation of the growth of parasitic protozoa in vitro with a special reference to *Pneumocystis carinii*. Comp Biochem Physiol 1991; 100A:1031–1034.
56. Bartlett MS, Marr JJ, Queener SF, Klein RS, Smith JW. Activity of inosine analogs against *Pneumocystis carinii* in culture. Antimicrob Agents Chemother 1986; 30: 181–183.
57. Frenkel JK, Good JT, Schultz JA. Latent *pneumocystis* infection of rats, relapse and chemotherapy. Lab Invest 1966; 15:1559–1577.
58. Hughes WT, Feldman S, Chaudhary SC, Ossi MJ, Cox H, Sanyal SK. Comparison of pentamidine isethionate and trimethroprim–sulfamethoxazole in the treatment of *Pneumocystis carinii* pneumonia. J Pediatr 1978; 92:285–291.
59. Hughes WT. Animal models for *Pneumocystis carinii* pneumonia. J Protozool 1989; 36:41–45.
60. Masur H. Clinical studies of *Pneumocystis carinii* and relationship to AIDS. J Protozool 1989; 36:70–74.
61. Kovacs JA, Allegra CJ, Swan JC, Drake JC, Parrillo JE, Chabner BA, Masur H. Potent antipneumocystis and antitoxoplasma activities of piritrexim, a lipid-soluble antifolate. Antimicrob Agents Chemother 1988; 32:430–433.
62. Kovacs JA, Allegra CJ, Kennedy S, Swan JC, Drake J, Parrillo JE, Chabner B, Masur H. Efficacy of trimetraxate, a potent lipid-soluble antifolate, in the treatment of rodent *Pneumocystis carinii* pneumonia. Am J Trop Med Hyg 1988; 39:491–496.
63. Masur H, Lane HC, Kovacs JA, Allegra CJ, Edman JC. Pneumocystis pneumonia: from bench to clinic. Ann Intern Med 1989; 111:813–826.
64. Queener SF, Bartlett MS, Jay MA, Durkin MM, Smith JW. Activity of lipid-soluble inhibitors of dihydrofolate reductase against *Pneumocystis carinii* in culture and in a rat model of infection. Antimicrob Agents Chemother 1987; 31:1323–1327.
65. Allegra CJ, Kovacs JA, Drake JC, Swan JC, Chabner BA, Masur H. Activity of antifolates against *Pneumocystis carinii* dihydrofolate reductase and identification of a potent new agent. J Exp Med 1987; 165:926–931.
66. Kovacs JA, Allegra CJ, Beaver J, Boarman D, Lewis M, Parillo JE, Chabner B, Masur H. Characterization of de novo folate synthesis in *Pneumocystis carinii* and *Toxoplasma gondii*: potential for screening therapeutic agents. J Infect Dis 1989; 160:312–320.
67. Merali S, Zhang Y, Sloan D, Meshnick S. Inhibition of *Pneumocystis carinii* dihydropteroate synthetase by sulfa drugs. Antimicrob Agents Chemother 1990; 34: 1075–1078.
68. Comley JCW, Mullin RJ, Wolfe LA, Hanlon MH, Ferone R. A radiometric method

for objectively screening large numbers of compounds against *Pneumocystis carinii* in vitro. J Protozool 1991; 38:144S–146S.
69. Gradus MS, Gilmore M, Lerner M. An isolation method of DNA from *Pneumocystis carinii*: a quantitative comparison to known parasitic protozoan DNA. Comp Biochem Physiol 1988; 89B:75–77.
70. Pifer LLW, Pifer DD, Woods DR, Joyner RE, Edwards CC. Preliminary studies on the development of vaccine for *Pneumocystis carinii* I. Immunological and biochemical characterization. Vaccine 1986; 4:257–265.
71. Cushion MT, Blase MA, Walzer PD. A method for isolation of RNA from *Pneumocystis carinii*. J Protozool 1989; 36:12S–14S.
72. Essig LJ, Timms ES, Hancock DE, Sharp GC. Plasma cell interstitial pneumonia and macroglobulinemia. A response to corticosteroid and cyclophosphamide therapy. Am J Med 1974; 56:398–405.
73. Matsumoto Y, Yoshida Y. Sporogony in *Pneumocystis carinii*: synaptonemal complexes and meiotic nuclear divisions observed in precysts. J Protozool 1984; 31:420–428.
74. Edlind TD, Bartlett MS, Smith JW. Characterization of the β-tubulin gene of *Pneumocystis carinii*. J Protozool 1991; 38:62S–63S.
75. Bartlett MS, Edlind TD, Durkin MM, Shaw MM, Queener SF, Smith JW. Antimicrotubule benzimidazoles inhibit in vitro growth of *Pneumocystis carinii*. Antimicrob Agents Chemother 1992; 36:779–782.
76. Lundgren B, Lipschik GY, Kovacs JA. Purification and characterization of a major human *Pneumocystis carinii* surface antigen. J Clin Invest 1991; 87:163–170.
77. Linke MJ, Cushion MT, Walzer PD. Properties of the major antigens of rat and human *Pneumocystis carinii*. Infect Immun 1989; 57:1547–1555.
78. Linke MJ, Walzer PD. Analysis of a surface antigen of *Pneumocystis carinii*. J Protozool 1989; 36:60S–61S.
79. Linke MJ, Walzer PD. Identification and purification of a soluble species of gp120 released by zymolyase treatment of *Pneumocystis carinii*. J Protozool 1991; 38:176S–178S.
80. Radding JA, Armstrong MYK, Ullu E, Richards FF. Identification and isolation of a major cell surface glycoprotein of *Pneumocystis carinii*. Infect Immun 1989; 57:2149–2157.
81. Chatterton JMW, Joss AWL, Davidson MM, Ho-Yen DO. Why have *Pneumocystis carinii* trophozites been ignored? J Clin Pathol 1990; 43:265–268.
82. Smulian AG, Stringer JR, Linke MJ, Walzer PD. Expression cloning of *Pneumocystis carinii* antigens. J Protozool 1991; 38:8S–10S.
83. Tanabe K, Takasaki S, Watanabe J-I, Kobata A, Egawa K, Nakamura Y. Glycoproteins composed of major surface immunodeterminants of *Pneumocystis carinii*. Infect Immun 1989; 57:1363–1368.
84. Nakamura Y, Tanabe K, Egawa K. Structure of major surface determinants and DNA diagnosis of *Pneumocystis carinii*. J Protozool 1989; 36:58S–60S.
85. Paulsrud JR, Queener SF, Bartlett MS, Smith JW. Isolation and characterization of rat lung *Pneumocystis carinii* gp120. J Protozool 1991; 38:10S–11S.
86. Hayes DJ, Stubberfield CR, McBride JD, Wilson DL. Alterations in cysteine proteinase content of rat lung associated with development of *Pneumocystis carinii* infection. Infect Immun 1991; 59:3581–3588.

87. Zhang J, Cushion MT, Giuntoli D, Hong ST, Meade JC, Smulian AG, Stringer SL, Stringer JR. Analysis of the *Pneumocystis carinii* genome. J Protozool 1991; 38:69S.
88. Haidaris CG, Wright TW, Gigliotti F, Haidaris PJ. Molecular cloning and characterization of ferret *Pneumocystis carinii*. J Protozool 1991; 38:5S–6S.
89. DeStefano JA. Analysis of *Pneumocystis carinii* cyst wall. Ph.D. dissertation, University of Cincinnati. Ann Arbor, Mich.: University Microfilms International, 1990.
90. Pesanti EL. Phospholipid profile of *Pneumocystis carinii* and its interaction with alveolar type II epithelial cells. Infect Immun 1987; 55:736–741.
91. Masala C, Sorice M, DiPrima MA, Lenti L, Misasi R, Contini C, Vullo V. Anticardiolipin antibodies and *Pneumocystis carinii* pneumonia. Ann Intern Med 1989; 110:749.
92. Kaneshiro ES, Cushion MT, Walzer PD, Jayasimhulu K. Analysis of *Pneumocystis* fatty acids. J Protozool 1989; 36:69S–72S.
93. Yoshikawa H, Morioka H, Yoshida Y. Freeze-fracture localization of filipin–sterol complexes in plasma- and cyto-membranes of *Pneumocystis carinii*. J Protozool 1987; 34:131–137.
94. Yoshikawa H, Yoshida Y. Distribution of digitonin–sterol complexes in *Pneumocystis carinii* revealed by freeze-fracture method. Int J Parasitol 1988; 18:39–45.
95. Paulsrud JR, Glancy TP, Shaw MM, Bartlett MS, Smith JW. Fatty acid metabolism of *Pneumocystis carinii* in culture [abstract]. 38th Annu Meet Am Soc Trop Med Hyg 1989:246 (abstr 330).
96. DeStefano JA, Cushion MT, Sleight RG, Walzer PD. Analysis of *Pneumocystis carinii* cyst wall. I. Evidence for an outer surface membrane. J Protozool 1991; 37:428–435.
97. DeStefano JA, Sleight RG, Babcock GF, Shramkoski RM, Walzer PD. Isolation of *Pneumocystis carinii* by flow cytometry. Parasitol Res 1992 78:179–182.
98. Kernbaum S, Masliah U, Alcindor LG, Bouton C, Christol D. Phospholipase activities of bronchoalveolar lavage fluid in rat *Pneumocystis carinii* pneumonia. Br J Exp Pathol 1983; 64:75–80.
99. Sheehan, PM, Stokes DC, Yeh Y-Y, Hughes WT. Surfactant phospholipids and lavage phospholipase A_2 in experimental *Pneumocystis carinii* pneumonia. Am Rev Respir Dis 1986; 134:526–531.
100. DeStefano JA, Cushion MT, Puvanesarajah V, Walzer PD. Analysis of *Pneumocystis carinii* cyst wall. II. Sugar composition. J Protozool 1990; 37:436–441.
101. Matsumoto Y, Matsuda S, Tegoshi T. Yeast glucan in the cyst wall of *Pneumocystis carinii*. J Protozool 1989; 36:21S–22S.
102. Yoshikawa H, Yoshida Y. Localization of silver deposits on *Pneumocystis carinii* treated with Gomori's methenamine silver nitrate stain. Zentralbl Baktiol Hyg [A] 1987; 264:363–372.
103. Yoshikawa H, Morioka H, Yoshida Y. Ultrastructural detection of carbohydrates in the pellicle of *Pneumocystis carinii*. Parasitol Res 1988; 74:537–543.
104. Yoshikawa H, Tegoshi T, Yoneda Y. Detection of surface carbohydrates of *Pneumocystis carinii*. J Protozool 1989; 36:63S–64S.
105. Palluault F, Dei-Cas E, Slomianny C, Soulez B, Camus D. Golgi complex and lysosomes in rabbit derived *Pneumocystis carinii*. Biol Cell 1990; 70:73–82.

106. Kitamura K, Kaneko T, Yamamoto Y. Lysis of viable yeast cells by enzymes of *Arthrobacter luteus*. II. Purification and properties of an enzyme, zymolyase, which lyses viable yeast cells. J Gen Appl Microbiol 1974; 20:323–344.
107. Matsumoto Y, Yamada M, Amagai T. Yeast glucan of *Pneumocystis carinii* cyst wall: an excellent target for chemotherapy. J Protozool 1991; 38:6S–7S.
108. Schmatz DM, Romancheck MA, Pittarelli LA, Schwartz RE, Fromtling RA, Nollstadt KH, Vanmiddlesworth FL, Wilson KE, Turner MJ. Treatment of *Pneumocystis carinii* pneumonia with 1,3-β-glucan synthesis inhibitors. Proc Natl Acad Sci USA 1990; 87:5950–5954.
109. Schmatz DM, Powles M, McFadden DC, Pittarelli LA, Liberatar PA, Anderson JW. Treatment and prevention of *Pneumocystis carinii* pneumonia and further elucidation of the *P. carinii* life cycle with 1,3-β-glucan synthesis inhibitor L-671,329. J Protozool 1991; 38:151S–153S.
110. Goheen MP, Bartlett MS, Queener SF, Smith JW. The effect of primaquine on the ultrastructural morphology of *Pneumocystis carinii*. J Protozool 1991 38:164S–165S.
111. Pesanti EL, Shanley JD. Glycoproteins of *Pneumocystis carinii*: characterization by electrophoresis and microscopy. J Infect Dis 1988; 158:1353–1359.
112. Williams DJ, Radding JA, Dell A, Khoo K-H, Rogers ME, Richards FF, Armstrong MYK. Glucan synthesis in *Pneumocystis carinii*. J Protozool 1991; 38:427–437.
113. Avron B, Deutsch RM, Mirelman D. Chitin synthesis inhibitors prevent cyst formation by *Entamoeba* trophozoites. Biochem Biophys Res Commun 1982; 108:815–821.
114. Reiss E. Molecular immunology of mycotic and actinomycotic infections. New York: Elsevier Science Publishing, 1986:14–20.
115. Ward HD, Alroy J, Lev BI, Keusch GT, Pereira MEA. Identification of chitin as a structural component of *Giardia* cysts. Infect Immun 1985; 49:629–634.
116. Garner RE, Walker AN, Horst MN. Morphologic and biochemical studies of chitin expression in *Pneumocystis carinii*. J Protozool 1991; 38:12S–14S.
117. Waldrop FS, Younker TD, Puchtler H. Histochemical observations on *Pneumocystis carinii*: selective demonstration of honeycomb forms. Histochemistry 1979; 63:1–6.
118. Walker AN, Garner RE, Horst MN. Immunocytochemical detection of chitin in *Pneumocystis carinii*. Infect Immun 1990; 58:412–415.
119. Cushion MT, DeStefano JA, Walzer PD. *Pneumocystis carinii*: surface reactive carbohydrates detected by lectin probes. Exp Parasitol 1988; 67:137–147.
120. DeStefano JA, Cushion MT, Trinkle LS, Walzer PD. Lectins as probes to *Pneumocystis carinii* glycocomplexes. J Protozool 1989; 36:65S–66S.
121. DeStefano JA, Trinkle LS, Walzer PD, Cushion MT. Flow cytometric analysis of lectin binding to *Pneumocystis carinii* surface carbohydrates. Parasitology 1992; 78:271–280.
122. Yoshikawa H, Tegoshi T, Yoshida Y. Detection of surface carbohydrates on *Pneumocystis carinii* by fluorescein-conjugated lectins. Parasitol Res 1987; 74:43–49.
123. Walzer PD, Linke MJ. A comparison of the antigenic characteristics of rat and human *Pneumocystis carinii* by immunoblotting. J Immunol 1987; 138:2257–2265.
124. Gutteridge WE. *Pneumocystis carinii*: potential targets for chemotherapeutic attack. In: Coombs G, North M. Biochemical Protozoology. London: Taylor & Francis, 1991:35–51.

4

Molecular Genetics of *Pneumocystis carinii*

JAMES R. STRINGER

University of Cincinnati College of Medicine
Cincinnati, Ohio

I. Introduction

Although *Pneumocystis carinii* has been known to be a significant human pathogen for more than 80 years, very little is known about its basic genetic properties. The principal impediment to the study of *P. carinii* genetics has been that it has not been possible to grow the organism in culture. Molecular genetic approaches have helped overcome some of the difficulties inherent in the study of *P. carinii* genetics. By studying the *P. carinii* genome and by isolating and characterizing *P. carinii* genes, it has been possible to achieve the following advances: (1) clarification of the phylogenetic relations of the organism, (2) determination of the primary structure of important *P. carinii* enzymes and protein antigens, (3) production of pure preparations of these proteins, (4) application of nucleic acid probes to detect *P. carinii* derived from infected animals and patients, (5) identification of distinct varieties of the pathogen, and (6) exploration of the epidemiology of *P. carinii* infections in animals and in humans. This chapter will review the molecular genetic information currently available concerning analysis of the *P. carinii* genome by electrophoretic karyotyping and restriction enzyme analysis of *P. carinii* DNA and by cloning and sequencing of *P. carinii* genes and repetitive DNA elements. Further discussion of applications and implications of molecular genetic data pertaining to taxonomy, transmission, immunology, and detection of the pathogen are discussed in other chapters in this book.

II. The Genome of *Pneumocystis carinii*

The genome of *P. carinii* has been studied primarily by electrophoretic karyotyping. Other techniques, such as analysis of repeated DNA and detection of restriction fragment length polymorphisms (RFLP), are beginning to be applied. From electrophoretic karyotyping, we now have a fairly clear picture of the size and complexity of the *P. carinii* genome and how the genome is packaged into chromosomes. Most studies have focused on rat-derived organisms, but some data have been presented for organisms from humans and from ferrets. Probably the most important finding to come from studying the *P. carinii* genome has been the clear demonstration of genetic variation among *P. carinii* isolates.

A. Electrophoretic Karyotyping

Separation of *P. carinii* chromosomes by pulsed-field gradient electrophoresis (PFGE) has been reported by several laboratories. Interestingly, it was found in each case that chromosomal DNA was released from the organism by treatment with proteinase K in the presence of sarkosyl. This is in contrast with what is required to lyse other fungi and many bacteria, the sturdy cell walls of which must be removed by digestion with a glycosidase before exposure to proteinase (1). From a practical point of view, the relative fragility of *P. carinii* is advantageous because preparations of the organism are typically contaminated by other microbes, and even when such contamination is at low levels, it is always a worrisome aspect of working with *P. carinii*. In control experiments, essentially no DNA is released from a variety gram-negative and gram-positive bacteria after incubation of these organisms under the lysis conditions used for *P. carinii* (Cushion MT, personal communication). This suggests that, even if other fungi or bacteria were present in a *P. carinii* preparation, little if any of the DNA from such contaminants would enter the gel.

In an early study by Fishman et al. (2), 13 rat *P. carinii* bands were reported to be resolved by orthogonal-field gel electrophoresis (OFAGE). These bands ranged in size from 200 kilobase pairs (kbp) to 2 megabase pairs (mbp). A smear of material smaller than 200 kbp was also present. Although it seemed likely that the discrete bands migrating between 200 and 1000 kb were *P. carinii* chromosomes, it was unclear whether the largest bands or smaller fragments were from the organism or from host DNA. Yoganathan et al. (3) separated rat *P. carinii* chromosomes using OFAGE and contour-clamped homogeneous field gel electrophoresis (CHEF), and resolved 16–20 bands, ranging in size from 320 kbp to 1.5 Mbp. Edman et al. (4,5) and Lundgren et al. (6) applied the PFGE technique of transverse alternating-field electrophoresis (TAFE) to separate rat *P. carinii*. They resolved at least 13 bands that ranged in size from 295 to 710 kbp, but noted that the nonmolar ethidium bromide staining of some bands suggested comigration of chromosomes of similar sizes. Hong et al. (7) applied CHEF and field-inversion gel electrophoresis (FIGE) to organisms from four physically separate immunosuppressed rat colonies. Isolates from three of the four colonies produced patterns containing 15 bands, ranging in size from 300 to 700 kbp, with two of the bands exhibiting increased-staining intensity, suggesting comigration of at least two additional chromosomes. These investigators could occasionally resolve bands in the megabase region, but hybridization with rat and *P. carinii* probes showed these to be rat in origin. Summation of the band sizes led Lundgren et al. (6) and Hong et al. (7) to estimate the haploid genome size at between 700 and 1000 kb.

Electrophoretic karyotypes produced from rat-derived *P. carinii* have been reported to vary. Lundgren et al. (6) found variation among the band patterns produced by organisms from separate rat colonies. The band patterns were further scrutinized by hybridization to five gene probes, including dihydrofolate reductase, rRNA, topoisomerase I, thymidylate synthase, and actin. This showed that each gene could be mapped to a particular band in each karyotype. Even though there was variation in the sizes of bands that hybridized to a given probe, the size differences were slight, indicating that gross chromosomal rearrangements were not the cause of karyotypic differences seen among closely related *P. carinii* strains. Stringer et al. (8) mapped several other sequences back to *P. carinii* chromosomal bands. They too observed fairly minor size variation for each of the eight chromosomes analyzed. Hybridization to *P. carinii* chromosomes resolved by PFGE is of practical importance to researchers studying *P. carinii* genes because the technique provides a simple way to verify the identity of a putative *P. carinii*-cloned DNA fragment or polymerase chain reaction (PCR) product. This is important because of the potential for contamination of *P. carinii* DNA with that from host cells or from other microbes.

Hong et al. (7) analyzed *P. carinii* isolates from over 100 rats taken over a 6-month period. They found that the band patterns produced by *P. carinii* derived from four separate rat colonies were distinguishable one from another, and that, over a 6-month period, the same colony-specific karyotype patterns were produced whether individual or pooled isolates from a single colony were used. These data indicated that a given colony of rats could be infected with a stable population of organisms over a long period. In the Hong et al. study, isolates from three of the four colonies produced patterns containing 15 bands, ranging in size from 300 to 700 kbp. Organisms from a fourth rat colony produced a pattern that contained approximately 22 ethidium bromide-stained bands (Fig. 1). Because 15 of the 22 bands comigrated with those of another 15-band karyotype, they hypothesized that these rats may have been infected with two varieties of *P. carinii*. Hybridization of the blotted chromosome bands with an rRNA probe unique to *P. carinii*

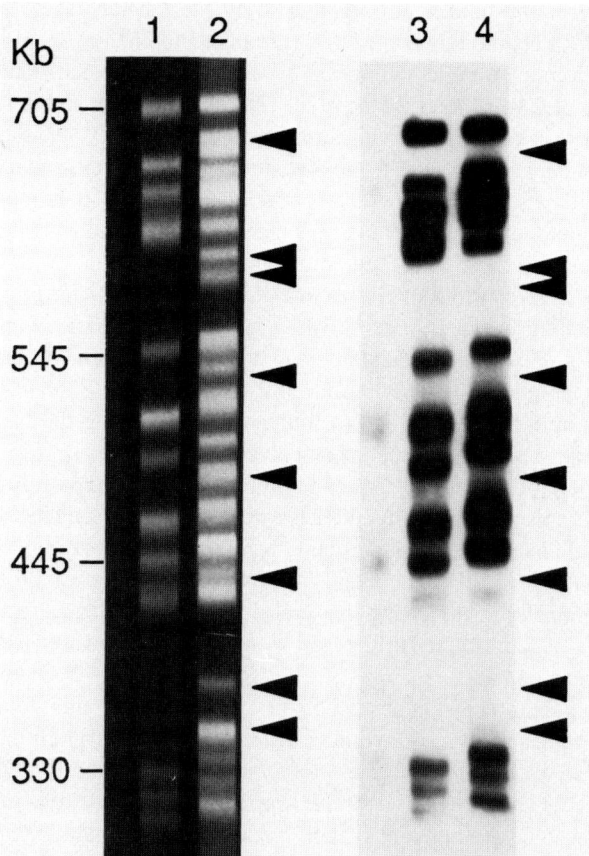

Figure 1 Two electrophoretic karyotypes from rat-derived *P. carinii*. Lanes 1 and 2 show chromosomal bands separated by field-inversion gel electrophoresis and visualized by staining with ethidium bromide. Lane 1 contains *P. carinii* showing the 15-band pattern. Lane 2 contains *P. carinii* showing the 22-band pattern. Lanes 3 and 4 show the results of an experiment in which the DNA shown in lanes 1 and 2 was hybridized to a radioactive probe containing a portion of the repeated sequence Rp3-1. The arrows in the margins indicate bands in the 22-band pattern that did not hybridize to Rp3-1.

supported this theory. Single bands of hybridization at about 500 kb were detected in the three karyotypes containing 15 bands, but in the 22-band pattern, two hybridized bands were detected at 500 and 535 kb (Fig. 2). These data suggest the presence of two types of *P. carinii* with different-sized chromosomes containing the ribosomal gene locus. Alternatively, these data may also be interpreted as being due to the presence of two chromosome homologues of different sizes in a

Molecular Genetics of Pneumocystis carinii 77

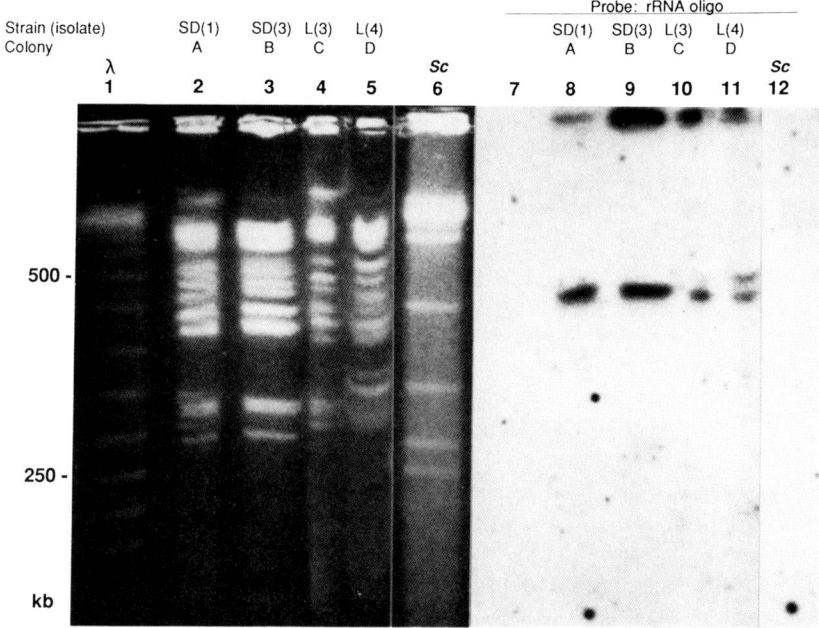

Figure 2 Mapping ribosomal RNA genes to chromosomal bands in two rat derived *P. carinii* electrophoretic karyotypes. *P. carinii* were isolated from four rat colonies and subjected to electrophoretic karyotyping by clamped homogeneous electric field gel electrophoresis. DNA bands were visualized by staining with ethidium bromide (lanes 1–6) and the DNA transferred to a nylon membrane that was hybridized to a radioactive oligonucleotide complementary to a sequence in the gene encoding the rat-*P. carinii* 18S ribosomal RNA. The results of the hybridization experiment are shown in lanes 7–12. Lanes 1 and 7 contained lambda DNA linear concatamers that served as size markers. Lanes 2 and 8, 3 and 9, and 4 and 10 contained 15-band karyotypes. Lanes 5 and 11 contained a 22-band karyotype. Lanes 6 and 12 contained chromosomes from *Saccharomyces cerevisiae*.

diploid organism. Subsequent results from my laboratory in collaboration with Cushion argue against the latter interpretation of the 22-band karyotype. We have found several other cases in which *P. carinii* preparations produced a complex band pattern similar to the 22 bands described by Hong et al. (7). The rats we used were totally unrelated to those used by Hong et al. In keeping with the original observation, some of the 22 bands comigrated with those of another 15-band karyotype. Interestingly, when the 22-band pattern was hybridized to a repeated DNA sequence from rat-derived *P. carinii*, only the 15 bands that comigrated with those of a 15-band pattern hybridized to the probe (see Fig. 1) (9). Because the repeated DNA was present in every 15-band pattern examined, the absence of the repeat suggested that the other 7 bands in the 22-band pattern may have been from a variant form of *P. carinii* that is more different from any of the *P. carinii* that produced a 15-band PFGE pattern than any of the 15-band *P. carinii* isolates are from each other. Not much is known about this putative variant, but it exhibited two features that suggest it is a form of *P. carinii*, rather than some other organism. (1) The variant could be lysed in proteinase K and sarkosyl. (2) Sequencing of a segment of the 16S-like rRNA gene of the variant *P. carinii* (Stringer JR, et al., unpublished) showed that it contained an rRNA gene similar to that described as being from rat-derived *P. carinii* (10,11). Another possibility is that some or all of the seven "extra" bands represent extra chromosomes or episomes produce by rearrangement or amplification of segments of the *P. carinii* genome. Such things have been seen in the protozoon *Trypanosoma brucei* (12).

The cumulative data from electrophoretic karyotyping indicate that the haploid genome of rat-derived *P. carinii* consists of 15–18 chromosomes containing between 700 and 1000 kbp of DNA. This is about two-thirds as large as the genome of *Saccharomyces* and is a much smaller the a previously determined value of 200,000 kbp, which was derived from earlier work that used biochemical techniques to analyze bulk DNA extracted from organisms derived either directly from rat lungs (13) or from a culture established by seeding monolayers of chick embryonic lung cells with rat lung-derived organisms (14). The disparity between the genome size estimates is too large to be accommodated by polyploidy. Rather, it seems likely that DNA content values derived from analysis of bulk DNA were overestimates because of the presence of host DNA in the samples.

An independent measure of the rat-derived *P. carinii* genome size has been obtained by analysis of a library constructed by inserting fragments of the *P. carinii* genome into a lambda phage vector. The average size of *P. carinii* DNA inserts in the library was 12 kb. The library was screened for copies of the thymidylate synthase gene by hybridization to a radioactive 600-bp fragment of the *P. carinii* thymidylate synthase gene. Plaques bearing the *P. carinii* thymidylate synthase gene composed 0.12% of the library, which is what would be expected for a unique gene in 10 Mb genome (9).

Electrophoretic karyotyping has also been performed to a limited extent on organisms isolated from humans. Hong et al. (7) were able to visualize band patterns from organisms derived from two individuals. The band patterns resembled those of rat-derived *P. carinii* in that there were about 15 bands that migrated between 200 and 700 kbp. The band patterns from human-derived *P. carinii* were different from each other and from any of the patterns produced from rat-derived *P. carinii*. Several other specimens from patients did not produce bands in these experiments, presumably because of insufficient numbers of organisms. However, it was also possible that DNA was degraded in these samples. Recently, Cushion and colleagues have obtained an additional electrophoretic karyotype from a sample of *P. carinii* derived from human lung (Fig. 3). Again, this karyotype was similar to that seen in rat-derived *P. carinii* in that the human-derived organisms contained about 15 bands that migrated between 200 and 700 kb; however, the band pattern of the human-derived karyotype was distinct from that of the rat-derived *P. carinii*. The potential of electrophoretic karyotyping as a tool for analysis of human *P. carinii* will depend on two factors. First, care must be taken to preserve the integrity of the organisms. We have found that rat-derived organisms can be preserved for karyotyping by suspension in 15% glycerol and storage at $-80°C$. Another important factor in electrophoretic karyotyping is the number of

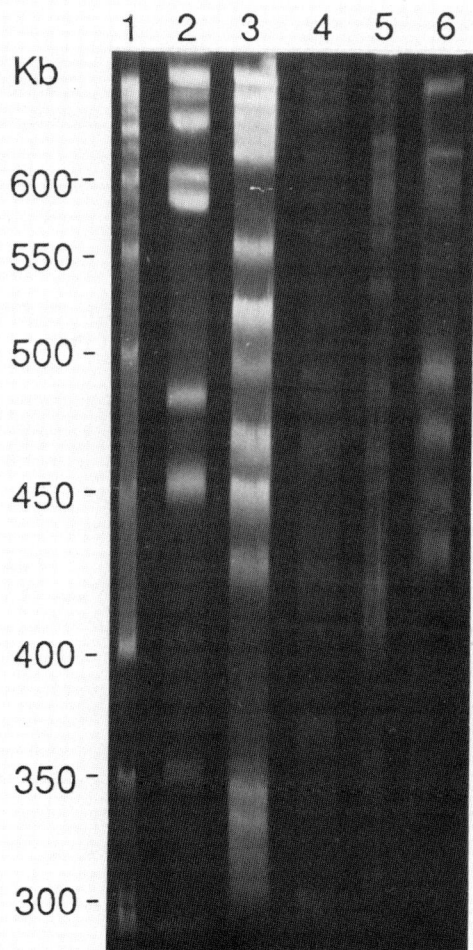

Figure 3 Comparison of electrophoretic karyotypes of *P. carinii* derived from rats, mice, and humans. Lane 1, lambda size markers; lane 2, *S. cerevisiae*; lane 3, rat-derived *P. carinii*; lane 4, human-derived *P. carinii*; lane 5, mouse-derived *P. carinii*; lane 6, *Cryptococcus diffuens*.

organisms used. At least 10^8 organisms (determined by counting the nuclei in both the trophic and cysts forms of the organism) are required to visualize bands by staining with ethidium bromide. Whether or not all the nuclei counted contribute to the DNA that migrates into the gel is unknown, nor is it known whether both the trophic forms and the cysts are lysed by treatment with proteinase K and sarkosyl.

A recent brief report presented the results of PFGE analysis of *P. carinii* derived from rat lung compared with organisms derived from ferret lung. Organisms derived from the two different host species appeared to produce different PFGE patterns (15). An electrophoretic karyotype for *P. carinii* derived from SCID mice has also been determined by Cushion (see Fig. 3). Again, the karyotype of mouse-derived *P. carinii* was different from that of rat-derived organisms.

In summary, the genome of *P. carinii* is readily visualized by electrophoretic karyotyping. This technique has provided the clearest evidence yet that, similar to other microbes, *P. carinii* occurs in many genetically distinct varieties. Further applications of the technique to examine genetic variation among *P. carinii* and to better understand the epidemiology of *P. carinii* infections will be discussed in Chapter 7.

B. Repetitive DNA

The *P. carinii* genome contains a substantial amount of repetitive DNA. Such sequences are of interest because they can serve as sensitive indices of genetic relatedness. Repeated sequences often display hypervariability when members of the family are compared one with another, presumably because of higher rates of genetic drift that occur as a consequence of the extraneous or parasitic nature of repeated DNA, which generally does not encode products essential to the organism. Hypervariability among repeated DNA sequences can also be due to movement of these elements within the host genome.

Preliminary reports suggesting that *P. carinii* might contain repetitive DNA first appeared in 1989 (16). Stringer et al. (9) characterized a repetitive DNA that was isolated from *P. carinii* by screening a genomic library for hybridization to radioactively labeled *P. carinii* DNA. Approximately 25% of the plaques bearing *P. carinii* DNA fragments hybridized strongly to the probe. DNA was extracted from several of these phages and radioactive probes prepared from each. The radioactive *P. carinii* DNAs present in each phage hybridized to all the bands resolved by PFGE of the parasite (see Fig. 1). This indicated that the sequences in these phages were distributed on most, if not all, of the *P. carinii* chromosomes.

One recombinant phage, Rp3-1, was selected for detailed analysis. Rp3-1 contained a 16-kb fragment of the *P. carinii* genome. A physical map of this fragment was produced by digestion with a battery of restriction enzymes. Hybridization experiments showed that the 16-kb *P. carinii* DNA fragment was not internally repetitious (i.e., the same sequence did not occur in more than one place in the 16-kb segment), and that repetitive DNA sequences were distributed over at least 10 kbp. Most, but not all of the rat-derived *P. carinii* genomes we have analyzed appear to contain as many as 70 copies of sequences related to those in Rp3-1. This suggested that the Rp3-1 family of sequences can compose as much as 10% of the genome. The function of members of the Rp3-1 repeat family is unknown. Its large size and high degree of sequence heterogeneity suggest that this repeat could play a structural role, such as subtelomeric sequences or centromeric sequences. However, the fact that Rp3-1 does not exist in all rat-derived *P. carinii* seems inconsistent with what would be expected for a repeated sequence playing a fundamental structural role. Also, Rp3-1 was absent in the three human-derived *P. carinii* we have analyzed to date.

The original published description of Rp3-1 included a search for RFLPs between DNA samples isolated from two rat-derived *P. carinii* isolates that had exhibited different electrophoretic karyotypes. No RFLPs were found in that study, but recently, similar analyses of additional karyotypically distinct isolates of rat *P. carinii* showed that RFLPs are detected by an Rp3-1 hybridization probe. We have recently identified another repeat in rat-derived *P. carinii*. The repeat was first found upstream of the α-tubulin gene and was named the α-repeat. Figure 4 shows that the α-repeat can be used to distinguish between different isolates of rat-derived *P. carinii* (Zhang J, Stringer JR, unpublished).

Recently, Watanabe et al. (17) described a repeated DNA isolated from rat-derived *P. carinii*. This repeat resembled Rp3-1 in that it appeared to be longer than 10 kb and was present approximately 100 times per genome. A cloned copy of the repeat contained two similar 5-kb segments lying in inverse orientation and separated by 5 kb. The relation between this repeat and Rp3-1 remains to be determined.

C. Base Composition of *Pneumocystis carinii* DNA

The genome of *P. carinii* isolated from rats is rich in adenine and thymine. Thermal denaturation studies on bulk rat-derived *P. carinii* genomic DNA indicated an average G+C content of 33%, which may be a slight overestimate owing to the presence of a small amount of rat DNA in the sample (16). The G+C contents of three protein-encoding rat-derived *P. carinii* genes, thymidylate synthase, dihydrofolate reductase, and 55-kDa antigen, were 30, 29, and 36%, respectively (4,5,18). Introns and intragenic regions were particularly rich in A and T residues. By contrast, the base composition of human-derived *P. carinii* appears to be rich in G+C. We recently determined the sequence of the α-tubulin gene from human-derived *P. carinii*, and found it to be 57% G+C (Stringer S, unpublished). The same gene from rat-derived *P. carinii* was 37%, G+C, in line with the other three genes from rat-derived *P. carinii* (Zhang J, Stringer JR, unpublished). This dramatic difference in base composition suggests that *P. carinii*

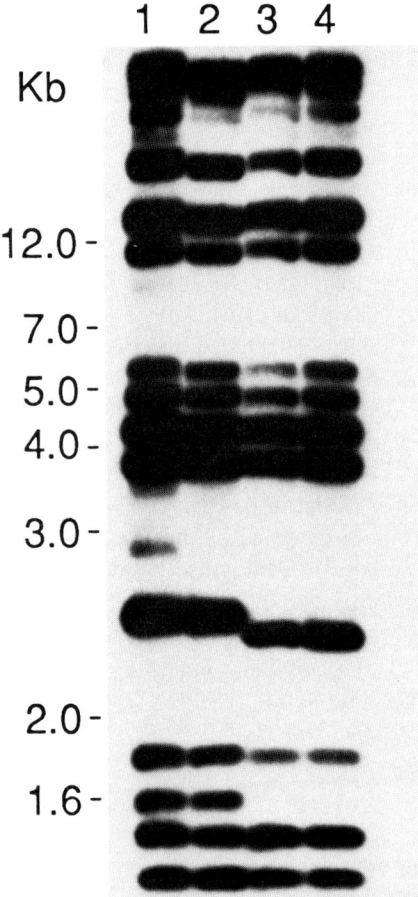

Figure 4 DNA fingerprints of rat-derived *P. carinii* using a repeated DNA sequence as a hybridization probe. DNA samples from four isolates were digested with *Eco*RI and fragments separated by electrophoresis through 1% agarose. The DNA fragments were transferred to a nylon membrane, which was hybridized to a cloned repeated DNA isolated from rat-derived *P. carinii*. Each lane contained DNA from a *P. carinii* preparation obtained from a different rat colony.

from rats and humans diverged a very long time ago. More will be said about the relation of *P. carinii* from different host species later.

D. Ploidy of the *Pneumocystis carinii* Genome

The ploidy of the various forms of *P. carinii* is unknown. Nuclear-staining assays have been applied to estimate the relative DNA contents of cysts and trophic forms of the organism (19). The data indicated that *P. carinii* cysts contain eight times more DNA than 90% of trophozooites, suggesting that the eight nuclei in a *P. carinii* cyst are haploid, as are most trophic forms. The remaining trophic forms

Molecular Genetics of Pneumocystis carinii

stained with twice the intensity of the putative haploid cells. The twofold increase in DNA content may reflect cells approaching mitosis, but it is also possible that some of the cells with a 2C DNA content represent mating events. It would seem worthwhile to reexamine the ploidy of *P. carinii* by measuring the absolute amount of DNA in a 1C nucleus and comparing this with the genome size as estimated from PFGE.

III. *Pneumocystis carinii* Genes

Pneumocystis carinii organisms have been prepared from infected rats and used to construct genomic and cDNA libraries. Although these libraries can be contaminated with DNA fragments derived from the rat genome or from the genomes of other microbes, it has been possible to isolate segments of the *P. carinii* genome and cDNA copies of *P. carinii* mRNAs. Gene cloning has allowed clarification of phylogenetic relations, which should speed progress in understanding the basic biology of the organism. Through gene cloning, it is also possible to determine the primary structure of important *P. carinii* enzymes and protein antigens. This information, coupled with the ability to produce limitless amounts of pure preparations of these proteins, will facilitate research into host–pathogen interactions and may lead to the formulation of novel therapies. Indeed, given the rapid progress in synthetic oligonucleotide technology, it is conceivable that gene-specific drugs may soon be on the horizon, in which event sequence information in and of itself would provide targets for such drugs. Finally, gene sequence information allows the development of nucleic acid probes for use in detecting *P. carinii* derived from infected animals and patients (see Chap. 20).

Several rat-derived *P. carinii* genes have now been characterized. Genes encoding the nuclear small ribosomal subunit RNA (10), 5S RNA (20), thymidylate synthase (4), and dihydrofolate reductase (5) have been isolated and completely sequenced. A deduced amino acid sequence for a mitochondrial gene, cytochrome oxidase subunit II, has been reported (21). Pixley et al. also reported cloning genes encoding five other mitochondrial genes that encode proteins, but the sequences of the genes were not included in this report. Partial sequences have been reported for a mitochondrial gene encoding the large ribosomal subunit RNA (22), and a gene encoding the 55-kDa antigen (18). Preliminary reports have appeared concerning the cloning of a β-tubulin gene (23), a transcription factor IID gene (24), and a cation translocation ATPase gene (24). The following reviews the published data available for the genes that have been most thoroughly characterized.

A. The Nuclear Ribosomal RNA Locus

The first *P. carinii* gene to be sequenced was that encoding the RNA from the cytoplasmic small ribosomal subunit (srRNA) (10). The gene was isolated by taking advantage of the conservation of rRNA genes across great phylogenetic distances. The *P. carinii* rRNA locus was identified by screening a library of genomic fragments from rat-derived *P. carinii* with a DNA fragment encoding a portion of the 16S-like rRNA gene from the ameba, *Entamoeba histolytica*. The 18S *P. carinii* gene was sequenced and found to contain 2194 bp. Comparison of the *P. carinii* sequence with that of other eucaryotes revealed the presence of what appeared to be a 390bp intron located 23 bp from the putative 3' end of the RNA. The proposed intron had the structural characteristics of the group I introns, which have previously been described in the 23S-like rRNA genes from nuclear genomes of some protozoa, the genomes of chloroplasts, and the genomes of fungal mitochondria. The *P. carinii* rRNA intron was also shown to behave as a group I intron when *P. carinii* 18S rRNAs, made by in vitro transcription, were shown to undergo self-splicing whereby the intron was removed in the absence of catalytic proteins (25). This was the first example of a group I intron in a nuclear gene. However, not all *P. carinii* contain the intron in the 18S rRNA gene. We have found a type of *P. carinii* in laboratory rats that lacks the intron, and none of the three isolates of human-derived *P. carinii* we have examined so far have the intron in the 18S rRNA gene. Excluding the intron, the *P. carinii* 18S gene sequences are most closely related to the sequences of corresponding genes from fungi (see Chap. 5).

Other ribosomal RNA genes have not yet been sequences, but the 5S rRNA was sequenced directly (20), and two laboratories have reported that the large rRNA of rat-derived *P. carinii* is approximately 26S, as determined by electrophoresis through agarose under denaturing conditions (16,26).

The rat-derived *P. carinii* rRNA locus appears to be organized in typical fashion with the 18S, 5.8S, and 26S genes arranged head-to-tail in a tandem array, each gene separated from the next by a short spacer sequence (27). The three-gene cluster is located on a chromosome of approximately 535 kb (6,7). In *S. cerevisiae*, the 5S gene is included in this cluster, but this is not a typical arrangement in eucaryotes; most carry the 5S gene unlinked to the 18S, 5.8S, and 26S genes. The rat-derived *P. carinii* 5S gene does not reside on the chromosome carrying the rRNA locus (3). Ribosomal RNA genes are typically repeated in eucaryotes and are organized as tandem arrays of the three-gene cluster. This organizational scheme may not be true for *P. carinii*. *Pneumocystis carinii* has many fewer rRNA genes. The frequency at which rRNA genes occurred in a *P. carinii* genomic library suggested that the ribosomal genes were repeated about 16 times in the *P. carinii* haploid genome (9). This is about one-eight as many rRNA genes as are present in haploid *S. cerevisiae* (28). Our more recent experiments suggest that this is an overestimate, and that the rat-derived *P. carinii* genome may contain as few as one copy of the rRNA locus per haploid complement of chromosomes (Giuntoli D, Stringer JR, unpublished). If there are multiple copies, they are spaced very far apart, compared with other eukaryotes. We have recently deter-

Molecular Genetics of Pneumocystis carinii

mined that the rRNA genes of rat-derived *P. carinii* cannot be closer than 50 kb. This contrasts with all other fungi studied so far, in which rRNA loci are typically separated by approximately 9 kb.

B. Mitochondrial Ribosomal RNA Gene

The gene encoding the large rRNA of *P. carinii* mitochondria has been isolated and partially sequenced. Sinclair et al. (22) used the sequence from rat-derived organisms to prepare oligonucleotide primers with which to amplify a 300-bp region of the gene from *P. carinii* obtained from humans. Comparison of this segment of the rRNA gene from rat and human *P. carinii* showed them to be less than 85% identical in sequence. Differences between the two sequences included base pair changes as well as several instances at which the rat *P. carinii* sequence contained bases that were missing from the human *P. carinii* sequence. These data indicated that *P. carinii* from these two host species were genetically distinct. No attempt was made to infer the degree of relatedness between the two *P. carinii* compared with the relatedness of each *P. carinii* to other organisms.

C. Protein-Encoding Genes

Thymidylate Synthase

The thymidylate synthase gene and a cDNA copy of the thymidylate synthase mRNA have both been cloned (4). The *P. carinii* gene was isolated by using the polymerase chain reaction to amplify a segment of the gene directly from the genome of rat-derived *P. carinii*. The thymidylate synthase-coding sequence spanned 1087 nucleotides and included four small introns. The 891 nucleotide open-reading frame encoded a peptide of 297 amino acids, which could be expressed in active form in *Escherichia coli*. The deduced amino acid sequence of *P. carinii* thymidylate synthase was most similar to that of thymidylate synthase from *S. cerevisiae*, with 65% identify. Codon usage was strongly biased. Seventy-eight percent of the codons contained either an A or a T in the third position. The *P. carinii* thymidylate synthase gene has been mapped to a 330-kb chromosome by hybridization to PFGE bands.

Dihydrofolate Reductase

Cloning of the *P. carinii* dihydrofolate reductase gene was accomplished by exploiting the capacity of the cDNA from that gene to confer trimethoprim resistance to *E. coli* (5). The *P. carinii* dihydrofolate reductase structural gene was sequenced and shown to span 663 nucleotides. The gene contained a single 43-bp intron. Codon usage was strongly biased, and 87% of the time an A or T occupied the third position. The deduced amino acid sequence contained 206 residues which, similar to the *S. cerevisiae* enzyme, is slightly larger than the mammalian

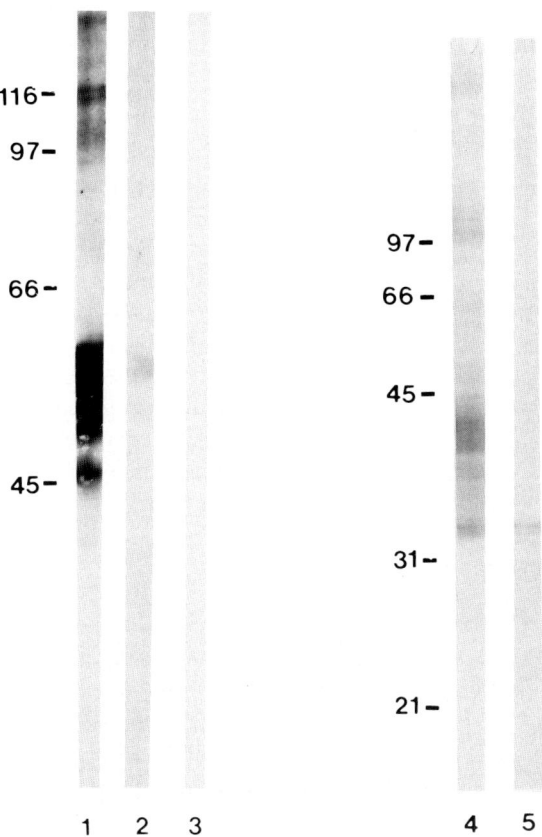

Figure 5 Identification of *P. carinii* antigen corresponding to the product of a cDNA clone isolated from rat-derived *P. carinii* by expression cloning. Antibodies were used to probe immunoblots of rat-derived and human-derived *P. carinii* proteins separated by polyacrylamide gel electrophoresis. Lane 1, rat-derived *P. carinii* probed with rabbit antirat-derived *P. carinii* antiserum; lane 2, rat-derived *P. carinii* probed with affinity-purified antibodies isolated by binding rabbit polyclonal antirat-derived *P. carinii* antiserum to preparative immunoblots of a bacterially expressed protein made from a *P. carinii* cDNA; lane 3, same as lane 2 but affinity-purified antibody was preincubated with purified bacterially expressed protein made from the *P. carinii* cDNA; lane 4, human-derived *P. carinii* probed with rabbit polyclonal antirat-derived *P. carinii* antiserum; lane 5, human-derived *P. carinii* probed with affinity-purified antibodies. Numbers in left margin are relative molecular masses in kilodaltons.

Molecular Genetics of Pneumocystis carinii

and bacterial enzymes. The *P. carinii* dihydrofolate reductase gene has been mapped to a 520-kb chromosome by PFGE.

The 55-Kilodalton Antigen Gene

Smulian and colleagues used antibodies raised against rat-derived *P. carinii* to screen an expression library made from *P. carinii* cDNA (18). They isolated a partial cDNA clone that encoded a 55-kDa protein, corresponding to a member of a major group of antigens that migrates as a broad band of 45–55 kDa on SDS–PAGE analysis of solubilized rat-derived *P. carinii* (Fig. 5). The predicted peptide sequence derived from this cDNA contained an interesting domain composed of ten copies of a seven-amino acid sequence. Each copy of the seven-amino acid sequence began with a proline residue and was rich in glutamic acid. The sequence of the cDNA ended with a poly(A) tail, which was preceded by a canonical polyadenylation signal located 46 bp upstream. Eighty percent of the codons in the 695-base open-reading frame ended in either A or T. Further analysis of the entire gene and a complete cDNA showed that the 55-kDa antigen gene contained a single 39-bp intron, an a 1245-bp open-reading frame in which 79% of the codons had either A or T in the third position. The 55-kDa antigen gene has been mapped to a 600-kbp chromosome (29).

IV. Transcription and Translation

A little is known about transcription in *P. carinii*. Several laboratories have reported success in isolating *P. carinii* RNA by standard techniques, and cDNA libraries have been constructed using oligo-dT to prime cDNA synthesis, which indicates that *P. carinii* messages are polyadenylated.

Comparison of cDNA and gene sequences for thymidylate synthase, dihydrofolate reductase, and the 55-kDa antigen allowed introns to be identified in these three genes. Thymidylate synthase has four introns, dihydrofolate reductase and 55-kDa antigen only one each. The 3' ends of the six *P. carinii* introns each contained the same trinucleotide, TAG, conforming to the YAG motif found at the 3' end of most eucaryotic introns. The 5' ends of *P. carinii* introns all featured the sequence GT; GTA is found at the 5' end of most eucaryotic introns. The distinctive branch site sequence used in *S. cerevisiae* introns was not discernible in the *P. carinii* introns.

The mechanism of *P. carinii* mRNA transcription has not been studied. *Pneumocystis carinii* promoters have not been described, and the potential for expression of *P. carinii* genes in heterologous cells has not been explored. The fact that *P. carinii* has a canonical TFIID (25) suggests that RNA polymerase II transcription occurs in the usual manner.

Analysis of the three available *P. carinii* protein-encoding gene sequences suggests that translation starts at an AUG. Sequences around the predicted translational start sites were similar in that the first base after the AUG was always a purine, a feature that is typically found at translational start sites of eucaryotic mRNAs (30).

V. Conclusion

This chapter has summarized the molecular genetic information currently available on analysis of the *P. carinii* genome by electrophoretic karyotyping and restriction enzyme analysis of *P. carinii* DNA and on cloning and sequencing of *P. carinii* genes and repetitive DNA elements. By studying the *P. carinii* genome and by isolating and characterizing its genes, it has been possible to clarify the phylogenetic position of the organism, to determine the primary structure of important *P. carinii* enzymes and protein antigens, and to identify distinct varieties of the pathogen. The stage is now set for further work based on our current understanding of *P. carinii* molecular genetics.

One important area is to better define the relationship between the pathogen and its host. *Pneumocystis carinii* was originally defined by the histopathology of *P. carinii* pneumonia, and parasites displaying these histopathological characteristics, although from diverse mammalian hosts, are all classed under this rubric. Although it has long been clear that *P. carinii* isolated from different hosts are phenotypically distinguishable, and it has been suggested that *P. carinii* nomenclature be revised to reflect these differences (31), no consensus on a more specific nomenclature has emerged. One reason for this is that it had not been possible to determine the role of genetic variation in phenotypic variation of *P. carinii*. Molecular genetic tools have begun to reveal genetic variation among rat-derived *P. carinii*. The same approaches should allow determination of the spectrum of genetic variation between organisms from diverse host species as well. Even though little published data is yet available, comparative analysis of DNA sequences from *P. carinii* derived from ferrets, mice, and humans strongly suggests that each host species harbors a different species of *P. carinii* (22; Stringer JR, et al., unpublished).

In addition to serving to better define the types of *P. carinii* in the world, molecular characterization of *P. carinii* genes provides an avenue to better understand the metabolic needs and capabilities of the organism. Such information may be necessary before it will be possible to formulate appropriate growth media. At the same time, understanding *P. carinii* enzymes at the molecular level holds promise for the development of new drugs. Gene cloning is also making *P. carinii* protein antigens available in pure form for the first time. These reagents will be vital to understanding the immune response to the pathogen. Finally, *P. carinii* DNA sequences provide targets for the molecularly based techniques that should improve detection, diagnosis, and therapy.

References

1. de Jonge P, de Jongh FCM, Meijers R, Steensma HY, Sheffers A. Orthogonal-field-alteration gel electrophoresis banding patterns of DNA from yeasts. Yeast 1986; 2:193–204.
2. Fishman JA, Ullu E, Armstrong MYK, Richards FF. Organization of DNA and RNA from rat *Pneumocystis carinii*. J Protozool 1989; 36:4S–5S.
3. Yoganathan T, Lin H, Buck GA. An electrophoretic karyotype and assignment of ribosomal genes to resolved chromosomes of *Pneumocystis carinii*. Mol Microbiol 1989; 3:1473–1480.
4. Edman U, Edman JC, Lundgren B, Santi DV. Isolation and expression of *Pneumocystis carinii* thymidylate synthase gene. Proc Natl Acad Sci USA 1989; 86:6503–6507.
5. Edman JC, Edman U, Cao M, Lundgren B, Kovacs JA, Santi DV. Isolation and expression of the *Pneumocystis carinii* dihydrofolate reductase gene. Proc Natl Acad Sci USA 1989; 86:8625–8629.
6. Lundgren B, Cotton R, Lundgren JD, Edman JC, Kovacs JA. Identification of *Pneumocystis carinii* chromosomes and mapping of five genes. Infect Immun 1990; 58:1705–1710.
7. Hong S-T, Steele PE, Cushion MT, Walzer PD, Stringer SL, Stringer JR. *Pneumocystis carinii* karyotypes. J Clin Microbiol 1990; 28:1785–1795.
8. Stringer SL, Hong S-T, Giuntoli D, Zhang J, Cushion MT, Smulian AG, Stringer JR. Analysis of repeated and unique DNA in *Pneumocystis carinii*. J Protozool 1992; (in press).
9. Stringer SL, Hong S-T, Giuntoli D, Stringer JR. Repeated DNA in *Pneumocystis carinii*. J Clin Microbiol 1991; 29:1194–1201.
10. Edman JC, Kovacs JA, Masur H, Santi D, Elwood HJ, Sogin ML. Ribosomal RNA sequence shows *Pneumocystis carinii* to be a member of the fungi. Nature 1988; 334:519–522.
11. Stringer SL, Stringer JR, Blase MA, Walzer PD, Cushion MT. *Pneumocystis carinii*: sequence from ribosomal RNA implies a close relationship with fungi. Exp Parasitol 1989; 68:450–461.
12. Gibson WC, Borst P. Size-fractionation of the small chromosomes of Trypanozoon and Nannomonas trypanosomes by pulsed field gradient gel electrophoresis. Mol Biochem Parasitol 1986; 18:127–140.
13. Gradus MS, Gilmore M, Lerner M. An isolation method of DNA from *Pneumocystis carinii*: quantitative comparison to known parasitic protozoan DNA. Comp Biochem Physiol 1988; 89B:75–77.
14. Pifer LL, Pifer DD, Woods DR, Joyner RE, Edwards CC. Preliminary studies on development of a vaccine for *Pneumocystis carinii*. I. Immunological and biochemical characterization. Vaccine 1986; 4:257–265.
15. Weinberg GA, Bartlett MS. Comparison of pulsed field gel electrophoresis karyotypes of *Pneumocystis carinii* derived from rat lung, cell culture, and ferret lung. J Protozool 1992; (in press).
16. Worley MA, Ivey MH, Graves DC. Characterization and cloning of *Pneumocystis carinii* nucleic acid. J Protozool 1989; 36:9S–11S.

17. Watanabe J, Nakata K, Nashimoto H, Ikeda H. Cloning and characterization of a repetitive sequence from *Pneumocystis carinii*. Parasitol Res 1992; 78:23–27.
18. Smulian AG, Stringer JR, Walzer PD. Isolation and characterization of a recombinant antigen of *Pneumocystis carinii*. Infect Immun 1992; (in press).
19. Yamada M, Matsumoto Y, Hamada S, Fujita S, Yoshida Y. Demonstration and determination of DNA in *Pneumocystis carinii* by fluorescence microscopy with 4',6-diamidino-2-phenylindole (DAPI). Zentralbl Baktiol Hyg 1986; 262:240–246.
20. Watanabe J-I, Hori H, Tanabe K, Nakamura Y. 5S ribosomal RNA sequence of *Pneumocystis carinii* and its phylogenetic association with "Rhizopoda/Myxomycota/Zygomycota" group. Mol Biochem Parasitol 1989; 32:163–168.
21. Pixley FJ, Wakefield AE, Banerji S, Hopkin JM. Mitochondrial gene sequences show fungal homology for *P. carinii*. Mol Microbiol 1991; 5:1347–1351.
22. Sinclair K, Wakefield AE, Banerji S, Hopkin JM. *Pneumocystis carinii* organisms derived from rat and human hosts are genetically distinct. Mol Biochem Parasitol 1991; 45:183–184.
23. Edlind TD, Bartlett MS, Smith JW. Characterization of the beta-tubulin gene of *Pneumocystis carinii*. J Protozool 1992; (in press).
24. Meade JC, Stringer JR. PCR amplification of DNA sequences from the transcription factor IID and cation transporting ATPase genes of *Pneumocystis carinii*. J Protozool 1992; (in press).
25. Sogin ML, Edman JC. A self-splicing intron in the small subunit rRNA gene of *Pneumocystis carinii*. Nucleic Acids Res 1989; 17:5349–5359.
26. Cushion MT, Blase MA, Walzer PD. A method for isolation of RNA from *Pneumocystis carinii*. J Protozool 1989; 36:12S–14S.
27. Edman JC, Kovacs JA, Masur H, Santi DV, Elwood HJ, Sogin ML. Ribosomal RNA genes of *Pneumocystis carinii*. J Protozool 1988; 36:18S–20S.
28. Petes TD. Yeast ribosomal RNA genes are located on chromosome XII. Proc Natl Acad Sci USA 1979; 76:410–414.
29. Smulian AG, Walzer PD, Stringer JR. Characterization of a gene encoding a 55 kDA antigen of *Pneumocystis carinii*. Mol Microbiol 1992; (in press).
30. Kozak M. Comparison of initiation of protein synthesis in procaryotes, eucaryotes and organelles. Microbiol Rev 1983; 47:1–45.
31. Hughes WT, Gigliotti F. Nomenclature for *Pneumocystis carinii*. J Infect Dis 1988; 157:432–433.

5

Molecular Phylogeny of *Pneumocystis carinii*

JEFFREY C. EDMAN

University of California, San Francisco
San Francisco, California

MITCHELL L. SOGIN

Marine Biological Laboratory
Woods Hole, Massachusetts

I. Introduction and Background

Pneumocystis carinii has emerged as the most significant opportunistic pathogen in patients with acquired immunodeficiency syndrome (AIDS). It stands alone among the opportunistic infections in AIDS as being the most widespread and the most frequent cause of death. It is also unique in the paucity of knowledge about the basic biology and epidemiology of the organism. Perhaps the most controversial aspect of *P. carinii* biology is its placement in the kingdom of life. Recent evidence leading to its placement among the fungi has resurrected a controversy as old as the recognition of the organism itself (1,2). A brief historical review of the controversy follows that serves to highlight our lack of understanding of the organism and the desperate need to further study this enigmatic entity.

Pneumocystis carinii was first identified in rats infected with *Trypanosoma cruzi* by Chagas (3). He mistakenly identified it as a sexual state of the kinetoplastid. Appreciation of *P. carinii* as a distinct organism was made in 1912 by the Delanöes with their discovery of *P. carinii* in Parisian sewer rats (4). The significance of the discovery of *P. carinii* was not fully appreciated until the outbreaks of plasma cell pneumonia in post-World War II orphanages. The organism remained, however, a medical curiosity and a pathogen of minor import until the outbreak of the AIDS epidemic. One wonders if *P. carinii* were not such a significant infection in patients with AIDS, whether the disease would have been recognized as soon as it was. The clustering of *P. carinii* pneumonia in male homosexuals clearly was a key piece of evidence that a new epidemic was underway (5).

In the pre-AIDS period, there were few studies that directly addressed the phylogenetic classification of the organism. Reports of culturing the organism on fungal media in the 1950s were not reproducible and are generally accepted to be the result of contamination. A detailed ultrastructural study by Vavra came to conclusion that *P. carinii* was more closely related to the fungi, based on a variety of ultrastructural features (6). A more limited study by ul Haque came to same conclusion (7). Most investigators, however, placed the organism among the protozoa, based primarily on historical reasons and its response to antiprotozoal drugs (8).

The current controversy over the proper phylogenetic placement rests largely on the molecular biological studies outlined in the following sections. Before reviewing and updating this data, it is worthwhile to point out that there are several aspects of *P. carinii* biology that are almost universally agreed on.

1. *P. carinii* is the agent that is cause of pneumocystis pneumonia. Because of the lack of an in vitro culture system, Koch's postulates remain unfulfilled.
2. *P. carinii* is a eukaryotic microorganism. Electron microscopy studies show the presence of a nuclear membrane and organelles consistent with this conclusion.
3. *P. carinii* is widespread in distribution. Not only is it found throughout the world, but it has also been reported in a wide variety of mammalian species.
4. *P. carinii* requires a perturbation of the immune system to express its pathogenic potential.

II. Relevance

There are few opportunistic pathogens that we know as little about as *P. carinii*. The relevance of phylogenetic analysis in the study of *P. carinii* biology and pathobiology has been questioned (9). What insight could possibly be offered by the phylogenetic analysis of a fungus that responds solely to antiprotozoal drugs? Is it not more worthwhile to ignore the phylogenetic issues and study the biology of *P. carinii* from an unbiased perspective?

The lack of knowledge concerning the biology of *P. carinii* is probably the foremost reason to study its phylogenetic relationships. Perhaps the most frustrating aspect in the study of this organism is the lack of a continuous in vitro culture system. It cannot be emphasized too strongly that the lack of a culture system hampers effective research on *P. carinii*. Unfortunately, to date, the placement of *P. carinii* among the fungi has not allowed the development of a culture system, and it would be naive to assume that one is forthcoming. However, the continued study of the phylogenetic relations of *P. carinii* may reveal its closest relatives in the fungal kingdom. These relations and the understanding obtained from knowledge of life cycles and metabolisms of these relatives may, in turn, shed new light on methods for the sustained in vitro culture of *P. carinii*.

The natural mode of acquisition is almost certainly by the airborne route (10,11). Yet conclusive demonstration of host–host transmission is lacking. The mode of acquisition leads one to suspect that there may be an environmental source of *P. carinii*.

If there is an environmental source, then what is it and how can we find it? Given current methods in *P. carinii* culture, it is not possible to identify an environmental source. But if such a system were available, could we expect to find the organism? The difficulty in finding environmental sources of fungal pathogens is exemplified by *Blastomyces dermatitidis* and *Cryptococcus neoformans* var *gattii*. Blastomycosis is a widespread disease of the Mississippi Valley region, yet isolation of the organism from the environment is very difficult (12). Apparently, the microenvironment supportive of *B. dermatitidis* growth is fleeting, and only on rare occasions can the fungus be isolated from the same locale twice. Recently, the ecological niche of *C. neoformans* var *gattii* was discovered by Ellis (13). This finding was the result of an exhaustive search, and it firmly established the association of the organism with flowering of a single species of eucalyptus. These data show that the identification of the ecological niche of pathogenic fungi can be elusive, and even if we were sophisticated enough to culture *P. carinii*, then it might be a long and fruitless search to uncover its ecological niche.

Is *P. carinii* an obligate fungal parasite? Many fungal plant pathogens are obligate parasites. Rusts are often obligate parasites and are restricted to single hosts. If *P. carinii* were an obligate parasite, then it would not be expected to grow in media used to cultivate fungi. It has been suggested that the lack of *P. carinii* growth in standard fungal media is indicative of its relation to the protozoa. Obviously, this feature bears no relation to the classification of the organism, but rather to our inability to determine the necessary conditions for its in vitro growth. Although it can be said that pathogenic protozoa, in general, are more difficult to cultivate than fungi and that protozoa will not grow on fungal media, there are pathogenic fungi that also do poorly on "fungal media." The pathogenic agent of lobomycosis is generally considered to be a fungus (although there is no definitive evidence for this classification) and is yet to be cultured. The human pathogenic fungus *Rhinosporidium seeberi* has only recently been cocultured in tissue culture cells (14). It is clear that the inability to culture the organism is no evidence for fungal or protozoal classification. (It is interesting to note that *R. seeberi* was originally considered to be a Sporozoa, the most favored placement of *P. carinii* by those who espouse its protozoal affinities; 12).

III. Previous Attempts at Classification

Electron microscopic studies have revealed significant ultrastructural detail of *P. carinii*. Although it is not possible to reach definitive conclusions concerning phylogenetic affinities, such studies do provide valuable insight into what features should be present to make phylogenetic placements. Some have criticized this data for being negative. Although, in fact, all the data are not entirely negative, it is their negative aspect that makes a convincing argument for the exclusion of *P. carinii* from any of the protozoal groups. Simply to dismiss the value of this data for being negative deprives us of some of the most important information on the relations of *P. carinii*. For example, characteristic structures (conoids, polar rings, rhoptries, and subpellicular tubules) found in all members of the Sporozoa are completely lacking in all forms of *P. carinii*. The detailed study by Vavra compares the features of *P. carinii* with all of the possible protozoal groups that it could feasibly be related to and comes to the conclusion that there is no ultrastructural basis to suggest that it is a protozoan (6). On the other hand, many of its features are consistent with being an ascomycetous yeast. The phylogenetic analysis of 16S-like rRNAs and other sequences (see Sec. IV.A) demonstrate a similar relation.

Other than the ultrastructural studies, there were no attempts to use known differences to address the phylogenetic placement of *P. carinii*. This was undoubtedly due to the lack of an in vitro culture system and the few investigators working with the organism. However, inferences about its protozoal affinity were made on the basis of its lack of growth on fungal media (discussed earlier) and its response to antiprotozoal drugs. The classification of organisms based on their response to various chemotherapeutic agents is tenuous, at best. Some of the antiprotozoal drugs were, in fact, developed as antibacterial agents (dihydrofolate reductase inhibitors and sulfonamides). Pentamidine does inhibit the growth of some fungi, and before introduction of amphotericin B, the diamidine hydroxystilbamidine was used for the treatment of blastomycosis (12). In addition, many of the antifungal agents inhibit the growth of pathogenic protozoa (15–17).

IV. Phylogenetic Relations Based on Molecular Biological Information

A. 16S-like Ribosomal RNA Sequences

Instead of relying upon traditional phylogenetic approaches that compare phenotypic characteristics, objective, quantitative evolutionary relations can be inferred from comparisons of macromolecular sequences that share a common ancestry. Ribosomal RNA (rRNA) sequences are particularly valuable for inferring quantitative phylogenetic frameworks. Their coding regions are found in all organisms, they are subject to similar functional constraints, and their genes do not appear to undergo horizontal transfer between evolutionary lineages. The small subunit rRNAs (16S-like rRNAs) have gained widespread acceptance for the inference of reliable phylogenetic frameworks. These molecules are essential components of the translation apparatus in all organisms, and they contain a statistically significant number of residues that can independently evolve. In eukaryotes, they range in size from 1250 nucleotides to 2305 base pairs (bp) and they can be folded into a consensus secondary structure model that contains as many as 50 helical domains. The coding regions for 16S-like rRNAs are mosaics of genetic elements that display specific rates of evolutionary change. Rapidly evolving regions are interspersed among domains that are moderately conserved or nearly invariant. This conservation pattern permits rRNA genes to function as multihanded chronometers of evolution. Evolutionary relations at the kingdom level can be estimated from comparisons of the slowly evolving sequences, whereas the nonconserved regions are valuable for resolving relations within a genus. The existing aligned data base for complete 16S-like rRNA sequences includes more than 200 species, most of which are from diverse microorganisms.

Similarities between the 16S-like rRNA-coding regions reveal that *P. carinii* is related to higher fungi (1,2). Initial analysis, similar to that shown in Figure 1, included a broad sampling of eukaryotic evolutionary lineages, but was limited by the handful of fungal sequences available at that time. The phylogenetic tree in Figure 1 is a distance matrix analysis in which fractional similarities between all pairwise comparisons of 16S-like rRNAs were converted to evolutionary distances. Alternative topologies were evaluated to identify the branching pattern in which segment lengths separating all possible pairs of organisms in the tree are in the closest agreement with a matrix of evolutionary distances between all compared organisms. Today, there are more than 270 full-length eukaryotic sequences, and the aligned data base includes more than 45 fungal taxa. The phylogeny in Figure 2 includes 20 fungal taxa, and it can be seen that *P. carinii* branches at the base of the ascomycete subtree, although a specific relative cannot be identified. Further support for placing *P. carinii* within the "higher fungi" is provided by trees that are inferred using the principles of maximum parsimony. In those analyses, topologies or branching networks are sought that require the minimal number of nucleotide changes to explain differences between sequences included in the analyses. Comparisons of parsimony and distance methods have been concisely reviewed by Swofford and Olsen (18). In both distance and parsimony analyses, statistical estimates of support for specific topological elements in the evolutionary trees can be obtained using bootstrapping procedures. For this purpose, alignment positions are randomly sampled with replacement and used to

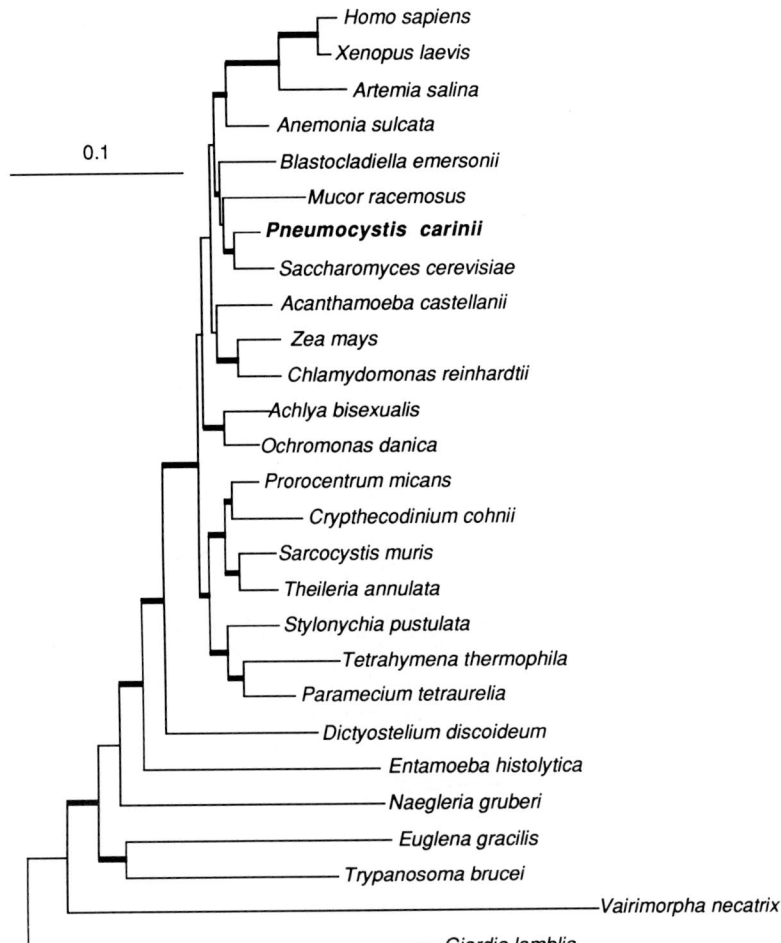

Figure 1 "Universal" phylogenetic tree inferred from 16S-like rRNA sequence similarities. Structural similarity values between the 16S-like rRNAs from the species indicated were converted into a phylogenetic tree by distance matrix methods (37). The evolutionary distance is represented in the horizontal component of their separation. The dark lines indicate statistically certain branches in the distance analyses.

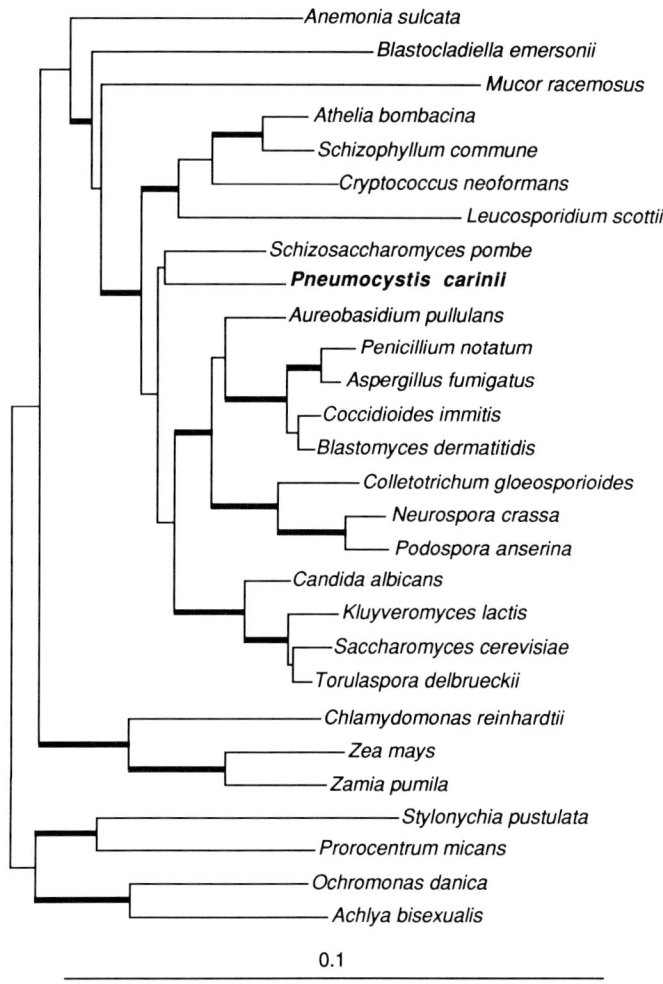

Figure 2 Phylogenetic tree inferred from 16S-like rRNA sequence similarities. Tree was constructed as described in Figure 1 and shows the relation of *P. carinii* to a variety of fungal species.

construct an input data set for distance or parsimony analyses. The number of trees that support a given topological element is taken as an estimate of support for that element in the phylogenetic branching patterns. Such estimates show that 95–100% of the bootstrap replicates place *P. carinii* at the base of the ascomycete subtree and that 100% of the time *P. carinii* branches within the higher fungi.

B. Thymidylate Synthase Sequences

Thymidylate synthase (TS) and dihydrofolate reductase (DHFR) are key enzymes in the thymidine biosynthetic cycle. The *TS* genes (and the inferred protein sequences) have been isolated and characterized from several eukaryotic organisms. A remarkable degree of similarity is seen even with distantly relatedly organisms (such as human and yeast). This degree of similarity allowed Edman et al. to design a pair of degenerate oligonucleotide primers that should be capable of amplifying (by polymerase chain reaction; PCR) fragments of *TS* genes from virtually any eukaryotic source (19). When this technique was applied to isolation of the *P. carinii TS* gene, an amplification product was indeed obtained. By using this fragment as probe, genomic and cDNA clones for *P. carinii* TS were isolated and analyzed.

A remarkable characteristic of *TS*-and *DHFR*-coding sequences in protozoa is that they are present as a single gene (20). The *DHFR* and *TS* sequences have been fused to create a bifunctional protein. Such an arrangement may allow "substrate channeling," but it is unclear why such a system should be unique to the protozoa. The *TS* and *DHFR* genes of all other organisms are present as separate genes encoding separate proteins. Although the generality of this rule remains to be established, seven protozoal TS–DHFR DNA sequences have been isolated (*Leishmania major*, *L. amazonensis*, *Trypanosoma brucei*, *Crithidia fasciculata*, *Toxoplasma gondii*, *Plasmodium chabaudi*, *P. falciparum*). In addition, bifunctional TS–DHFR proteins have been identified by protein characterization in *Euglena gracilis*, *Tetrahymena pyriformis*, *Eimeria tenella*, and *Plasmodium lophurae*. The TS and DHFR cDNAs from three fungi (*Saccharomyces cerevisiae*, *Candida albicans*, *Cryptococcus neoformans*), four mammals (*Homo sapiens*, *Rattus rattus*, *Mus musculus*, *Cricetulus longicaudatus*), and numerous bacteria show these genes and proteins are separate in these organisms. Plants may also have a bifunctional TS–DHFR, but no DNA sequences are available, and there is conflicting evidence for bifunctionality between carrot (bifunctional; 21) and soybean cells (monofunctional; 22).

Whether the absence of a bifunctional TS-DHFR can be used to exclude a close phylogenetic relationship of *P. carinii* with the protozoa remains to be proved. However, the consistency with which this characteristic bifunctional protein tracks with the protozoa is remarkable. The bifunctional gene is present in the Zoomastigophorea, the Sporozoa, the Phytomastigophorea, and the Oligohymenophorea and is absent in all other organisms, with the possible exception of plants. Given that it has been clearly demonstrated that the *P. carinii* TS and DHFR genes are separate genes on different chromosomes, it would appear by these criteria that *P. carinii* is not a member of the classic protozoan groups.

As noted earlier, TS is a highly conserved protein. This conservation allows the unambiguous alignment of TS primary sequences for diverse taxa. Such alignments, in turn, allow the construction of phylogenetic trees using the parsimony method. Figure 3 shows the results of a parsimony analysis using 12 TS sequences from a variety of organisms. Parsimony analysis demonstrates that the *P. carinii* TS sequence is most closely related to that of the fungi. The similarity of the tree generated by parsimony analysis of TS sequences and 16S-like rRNA is striking. Both trees demonstrate *P. carinii* branching off at the base of the *Ascomycete* branch.

C. Dihydrofolate Reductase Sequence

As noted earlier, DHFR genes have been isolated from a large number of organisms. Unlike TS, DHFRs are very poorly conserved at the primary sequence level, which makes the isolation of genes based on cross-hybridization or PCR difficult. Fortunately, expression of eukaryotic DHFR-coding sequences in *Escherichia coli* leads to trimethoprim resistance (23). This phenomenon was used to isolate the *P. carinii* DHFR cDNA and gene (24). The lack of extensive sequence similarity makes unambiguous alignments difficult. Nonetheless, when DHFR sequences are aligned as well as possible and subjected to parsimony analysis, a close relation to fungal DHFRs is shown (Fig. 4). The comparison of crystal structures may provide a better means for the alignment of these proteins.

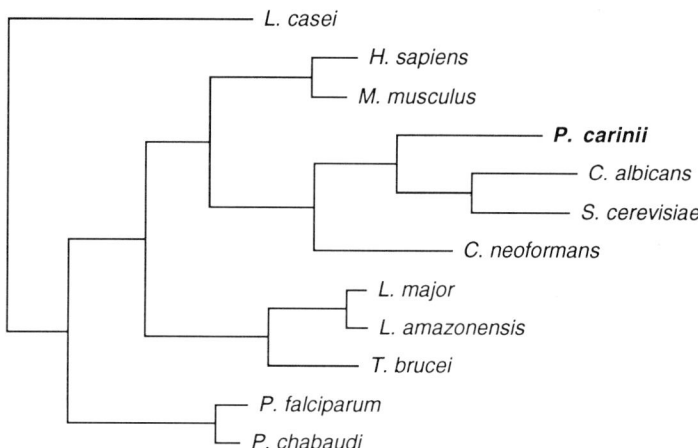

Figure 3 Phylogenetic tree inferred by parsimony analysis of TS sequences. TS protein sequences from the indicated organisms were aligned and subjected to branch-and-bound analysis using the PAUP program (38).

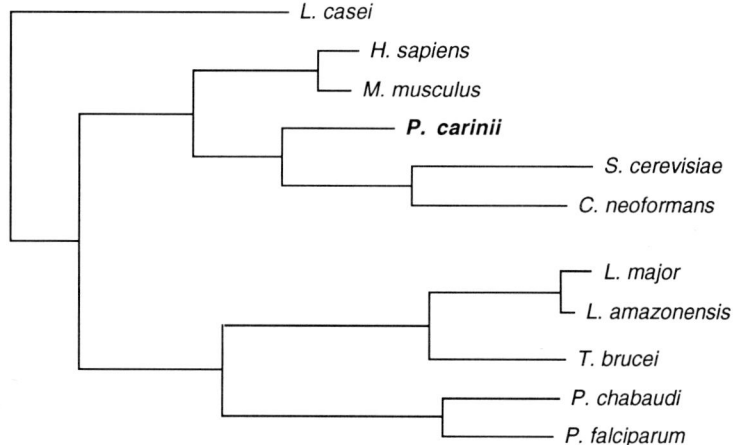

Figure 4 Phylogenetic tree inferred by parsimony analysis of DHFR sequences. DHFR protein sequences were aligned and subjected to branch-and-bound analysis using the PAUP program (38).

D. Elongation Factor 3 Sequence

Fungi possess an additional elongation factor (EF-3) required in protein synthesis (25). This protein may play a role in facilitating the interaction between other elongation factors and their substrates. The *P. carinii* EF-3 has been cloned, sequenced, and shows a high degree of similarity to *S. cerevisiae* EF-3 (Ypma-Wong, M. F., Sypherd, P. S., personal communication). This conclusively demonstrates that *P. carinii* does indeed contain EF-3, and its sequence is highly similar to that of EF-3 from *S. cerevisiae*. Previous reports of the lack of EF-3 in *P. carinii* based on Western blotting serve to demonstrate the difficulty in working with this organism and making conclusions based on the absence of detectable activity or immunoreactivity (26).

E. 5S RNA Sequence

Phylogenetic analysis of the 5S RNA gene of *P. carinii* has also been reported. The results demonstrate an association of *P. carinii* with the "*Rhizopoda/Myxomycota/Zygomycota* group" (27). However, the usefulness of 5S sequences in determining phylogenetic relations is limited by several factors. The sequence is less than 120 nucleotides and the molecule is structurally constrained into three helices. Alteration of nucleotides within these helical regions can result in "nonclock-like" changes and, hence, an overestimate of evolutionary distance. A good indication of the lack of sufficient information that can be derived from these sequences can be inferred from the fact that most workers in the field of phylogenetic analysis that once relied on 5S sequences have now switched to 16S-like rRNAs.

F. Mitochondrial DNA Sequences

Mitochondrial DNA sequences of *P. carinii* have been isolated and characterized (28). A 6785-bp fragment of *P. carinii* mitochondrial DNA was sequenced in its entirety and shown to contain the genes for apocytochrome *b*; NADH dehydrogenase subunits 1, 2, 3, and 6; cytochrome oxidase subunit II; and the small subunit of mitochondrial ribosomal RNA. Comparative analysis of these sequences with known fungal and protozoal sequences showed an average similarity of 60% with the fungi, but only 20% with the protozoa. In addition, the inferred secondary structure of small subunit ribosomal sequence of *P. carinii* shows striking similarity to that from other fungi and is dissimilar from protozoal sequences.

V. Additional Genes that Could Be Studied

A. Lysine Biosynthesis

The role of using biochemical pathways as aids in the determination of phylogenetic relations has been reviewed by Ragan (29). One of the most distinguishing metabolic pathways between the protozoa and the fungi is the lysine biosynthetic pathway. Two pathways for lysine biosynthesis are known. The diaminopimelic acid (DAP) pathway is used by bacteria, *Oomycetes*, plants, and almost all protozoa. The aminoadipic acid (AAA) pathway is used by all the true fungi (*Basidiomycetes*, *Chrytridiomycetes*, *Ascomycetes*, and *Zygomycetes*) and *Euglena gracilis*. Although the use of such pathways may offer little in terms of determining phylogenetic relations per se, the demonstration of mechanism of lysine biosynthesis in *P. carinii* may offer important corroborating evidence for its phylogenetic placement. More importantly, a novel lysine biosynthetic pathway may allow the design of new anti-*P. carinii* agents.

B. Sterol Biosynthesis

Ragan has also reviewed the sterol biosynthetic pathway in determining phylogeny (29). Although it would appear to be even less useful than the lysine biosynthetic pathway in determining phylogenetic relations, considerable interest in this subject has been demonstrated, primarily owing to the lack of response of *P. carinii* to the archetypical antifungal agent amphotericin B and other antifungals affecting the sterol biosynthetic apparatus. Many fungi contain ergosterol as the principal membrane sterol, and it is thought that the interaction of amphotericin B with ergosterol that leads to selective toxicity against fungi. Although there are no definitive reports on the sterol composition of *P. carinii*, it has been reported in preliminary form that cholesterol is the only detectable sterol. This would be consistent with *P. carinii* obtaining sterols from the host. It has also been implied that the lack of ergosterol is indicative of the lack of relation of *P. carinii* with the fungi. On the other hand, the presence of ergosterol is not restricted to the fungi, as some protozoa contain it, most notably *Trypanosoma cruzi* (16).

Not all fungi contain ergosterol as the predominant sterol component, and some lack it entirely (30). There are a wide variety of fungal sterols. Cholesterol itself is distinctly unusual for a fungus, but at least one fungus, *Penicillium funiculosum*, contains primarily cholesterol (31). Some members of the *Zygomycetes* also contain cholesterol in addition to ergosterol (32). Therefore, the presence of cholesterol does not exclude *P. carinii*. In addition, the presence of cholesterol as the major sterol component of *P. carinii* does not rule out the presence of a small quantities of ergosterol. Sterol biosynthesis requires molecular oxygen. Therefore, under oxygen-limiting conditions, facultative anaerobic fungi must and do use exogenous sterol sources. This demonstrates the widespread capability of fungi to assimilate sterols from the environment.

The ability of fungi to use cholesterol and other sterols in place of ergosterol is demonstrated by mutants in sterol biosynthesis in *S. cerevisiae* (33,34). In these mutants and in anaerobically grown cells, the exogenous addition of sterols is required. Although ergosterol is the preferred sterol, cholesterol will support the growth of sterol-starved cells to a small degree. After a short period of growth on cholesterol, these cells will adapt to presence of cholesterol; and the eventual yield of cells is similar to that seen with ergosterol as the added sterol (35,36). In the initial phase of poor growth, small amounts of ergosterol can act synergistically with cholesterol to complement this growth defect. This so-called sparking function of ergosterol allows the growth of these mutants on cholesterol with what would otherwise be noncomplementing levels of ergosterol. It is evident by these studies that normal levels of ergosterol itself are not required for the growth of these mutants, and its function can be replaced by other sterols.

VI. Conclusions

The controversy concerning the placement of *P. carinii* among the fungi seems to be somewhat like Justice Potter Stewart's famous line "I know it when I see it." The problem is that everyone is using his own local or personal standards for the definition of a fungus or a protozoan. The role of molecular biology in determining phylogenetic relations between organisms is an attempt to escape such local standards and to develop a scheme for the classification of organisms based upon quantifiable characteristics. Although the use of 16S-like rRNA sequences for the classification of microorganisms is subject to biases, as a result of unequal mutation rates and changes in base ratios, it does provide a reliable measure for those organisms that are generally agreed to be fungi or protozoa. It can be argued that a single yardstick is insufficient for the reclassification of *P. carinii*, but it remains to be shown by any molecular phylogenetic analysis that *P. carinii* has any relation to the accepted protozoan groups.

References

1. Edman JC, Kovacs JA, Masur H, Santi DV, Elwood HJ, Sogin ML. Ribosomal RNA sequences shows *Pneumocystis carinii* to be member of the fungi. Nature 1988; 334: 519–522.
2. Stringer SL, Stringer JR, Blase MA, Walzer PD, Cushion MT. *Pneumocystis carinii*: sequence from ribosomal RNA implies a close relationship with fungi. Exp Parasitol 1989; 68:450–461.
3. Chagas C. Nova tripanozomiaze humana. Mem Instit Oswaldo Cruz 1909; 1:159–218.
4. Delanoe P, Delanoe M. Sur les rapports des kystes de Carinii du poumon des rats avec le trypanosoma Lewisii. Presenter par M. Laveran. Note de Delanoe and Delanoe. CR Acad Sci (Paris) 1912; 155:658–660.
5. Gottlieb MS, Schroff R, Schanker HM, Weisman JD, Fan PT, Wolf RA, Saxon A. *Pneumocystis carinii* pneumonia and mucosal candidiasis in previously healthy homosexual men. N Engl J Med 1981; 305:1425–1431.
6. Vavra J, Kucera K. *Pneumocystis carinii* Delanoe: its ultrastructure and ultrastructural affinities. J Protozool 1970; 17:463–483.
7. ul Haque A, Plattner SB, Cook RT, Hart MN. *Pneumocystis carinii*: taxonomy as viewed by electron microscopy. Am J Clin Pathol 1987; 87:504–510.
8. Barton EG, Campbell WG. *Pneumocystis carinii* in lungs of rats treated with cortisone acetate. Am J Pathol 1969; 54:209–236.
9. Hughes WT. *Pneumocystis carinii*: taxing taxonomy. Eur J Epidemiol 1989; 5: 265–269.
10. Hughes WT. Natural mode of acquisition for the de novo infection with *Pneumocystis carinii*. J Infect Dis 1982; 145:824–848.
11. Hendley JO, Weller TH. Activation and transmission in rats of infection with *Pneumocystis carinii*. Proc Soc Exp Biol Med 1971; 137:1401–1404.
12. Rippon JW. Medical Mycology. Philadelphia: WB Saunders, 1988.
13. Ellis DH, Pfeiffer TJ. Natural habitat of *Cryptococcus neoformans* var *gattii*. J Clin Microbiol 1990; 28:1642–1644.
14. Levy MG, Meuten J, Breitschwerdt EB. In vitro cultivation of *Rhinosporidium seeberi*: interaction with epithelial cells. Science 1986; 234:474–476.
15. Urbina JA, Lazardi K, Aguirre T, Piras MM, Piras R. Antiproliferative effects and mechanism of action of ICI 195,739, a novel bis-triazole derivative, on epimastigotes and amastigotes of *Trypanosoma (Schizotrypanum) cruzi*. Antimicrob Agents Chemother 1991; 35:730–735.
16. Goad LJ, Berens RL, Marr JJ, Beach DH, Holz GJ. The activity of ketoconazole and other azoles against *Trypanosoma cruzi*: biochemistry and chemotherapeutic action in vitro. Mol Biochem Parasitol 1989; 32:179–189.

17. Croft SL, Walker JJ, Gutteridge WE. Screening of drugs for rapid activity against *Trypanosoma cruzi* trypomastigotes in vitro. Trop Med Parasitol 1988; 39:145–148.
18. Swofford DL, Olsen GL. In: Hillis, D. M., Moritz, C., eds. Phylogeny Reconstruction, Molecular Systematics. Sunderland, Mass: Sinauer Associates, 1991:p. 411–501.
19. Edman U, Edman JC, Lundgren B, Santi DV. Isolation and expression of *Pneumocystis carinii* thymidylate synthase gene. Proc Natl Acad Sci USA 1989; 86:6503–6507.
20. Garret CE, Coderre JA, Meek TD, Garvey EP, Claman DM, Beverly SM, Santi DV. A bifunctional thymidylate synthase-dihydrofolate reductase in protozoa. Mol Biochem Parasitol 1984; 11:257–265.
21. Cella R, Carbonera D, Orsi R, Ferri G, Iadarola P. Proteolytic and partial sequencing studies of the bifunctional dihydrofolate reductase–thymidylate synthase from *Daucus carota*. Plant Mol Biol 1991; 16:975–982.
22. Ratnam S, Delcamp TJ, Hynes JB, Freisheim JH. Purification and characterization of dihydrofolate reductase from soybean seedlings. Arch Biochem Biophys 1987; 255: 279–289.
23. Lagosky PA, Taylor GA, Haynes RH. Molecular characterization of the *Saccharomyces cerevisiae* dihydrofolate reductase gene (*DFR1*). Nucleic Acids Res 1987; 15:10355–10371.
24. Edman JC, Edman U, Cao M, Lundgren B, Kovacs JA, Santi DV. Isolation and expression of the *Pneumocystis carinii* dihydrofolate reductase gene. Proc Natl Acad Sci USA 1989; 86:8625–8629.
25. Riis B, Rattan SIS, Clark BFC, Merrick WC. Eukaryotic protein elongation factors. Trends Biochem Sci 1990; 15:420–424.
26. Jackson HC, Colthurst D, Hancock V, Marriott MS, Tuite MF. No detection of characteristic fungal protein elongation factor EF-3 in *Pneumocystis carinii*. J Infect Dis 1991; 163:675–677.
27. Watanabe J, Hori H, Tanabe K, Nakamura Y. Phylogenetic association of *Pneumocystis carinii* with the "*Rhizopoda/Myxomycotoa/Zygomycota* group" indicated by comparison of 5S ribosomal RNA sequences. Mol Biochem Parasitol 1989; 32: 163–168.
28. Pixley FJ, Wakefield AE, Baerji S, Hopkin JM. Mitochondrial gene sequences show fungal homology for *Pneumocystis carinii*. Mol Microbiol 1991; 5:1347–1351.
29. Ragan MA. Biochemical pathways and the phylogeny of the eukaryotes. In: Fernholm, B., Bremer, K., Jörnvall, H., eds. The Hierarchy of Life. Amsterdam: Elsevier Science Publishers, 1989.
30. Bean GA. Phytosterols. Adv Lipid Res 1973; 11:193–218.
31. Chen YS, Haskins RH. Studies on the pigments of *Penicillium funiculosum* I. Production of cholesterol. Can J Chem 1963; 41:1647–1649.
32. McCorkindale NJ, Hutchinson SA, Pursey BA, Scott WT, Wheeler, R. A comparison of the types of sterol found in species of the *Saproleginales* and *Leptomitales* with those found in other *Phycomycetes*. Phytochemistry 1969; 8:861–867.
33. Ramgopal M, Bloch K. Sterol synergism in yeast. Proc Natl Acad Sci USA 1983; 80: 712–715.

34. Rodriguez RJ, Taylor FR, Parks LW. A requirement for ergosterol to permit growth of yeast sterol auxotrophs on cholesterol. Biochem Biophys Res Commun 1982; 106: 435–441.
35. Taylor FR, Parks LW. Adaptation of *S. cerevisiae* to growth on cholesterol: selection of mutants defective in the formation of lanosterol. Biochem Biophys Res Commun 1980; 95:1437–1445.
36. Nes WR, Sekula BC, Nes WD, Adler JH. Functional importance of structural features of ergosterol in yeast. J Biol Chem 1978; 253:6218–6225.
37. Elwood HJ, Olsen GJ, Sogin ML. The small-subunit ribosomal RNA gene sequences from the hypotrichous ciliates *Oxytricha nova* and *Stylonychia pustulata*. Mol Biol Evol 1985; 2:399–410.
38. Swofford DL. Phylogenetic analysis using parsimony (PAUP-version 2.4). 1985.

6

Antigenic Characteristics of *Pneumocystis carinii*

FRANCIS GIGLIOTTI

University of Rochester School of Medicine and Dentistry
Rochester, New York

I. Introduction

Despite that *Pneumocystis carinii* has been recognized as a human pathogen for approximately 50 years, our understanding of the host–parasite interaction is still limited. One reason for this is that, until very recently, little information about specific antigens of *P. carinii* was available. In fact, the first edition of this book did not contain a chapter devoted to the antigens of *P. carinii*. The single largest impediment to identifying and characterizing the antigens of *P. carinii* is the lack of a culture system that permits repeated passage and high yield of organisms. This necessitates that organisms are generally obtained directly from a mammalian host. Unfortunately, physical means of separation from host lung tissue are less than optimal because *P. carinii* vary substantially in size and shape, depending on their stage in the life cycle. Thus, any analysis of *P. carinii* antigens is always complicated by the presence of contaminating host molecules.

In spite of these limitations, progress has been made in defining some of the antigens of *P. carinii*. The initial identification of an antigen unique to *P. carinii* was made by sodium dodecyl sulfate–polyacrylamide gel electrophoresis (SDS–PAGE) of variously solubilized *P. carinii*-infected and -uninfected lungs (1). It was not until 1986 that the first monoclonal antibodies to *P. carinii* were described

(2,3), and this technology, along with the technique of immunoblotting (Western blotting), has enabled investigators to convincingly identify *P. carinii*-specific antigens. This chapter will summarize our current understanding of the antigens of *P. carinii*.

II. Surface Glycoprotein A (Mannosylated Surface Glycoprotein, gp120, gp95)

A. Background

The application of monoclonal antibody technology to the study of the *P. carinii* has facilitated our ability to identify specific antigens of the organism. An antigen with an apparent molecular mass (M_r) of 110–120 kDa is readily identified on *P. carinii* isolated from rats and ferrets (2,3) (Fig. 1). Immunoelectron microscopy demonstrates that this molecule is distributed over the surface of the organism (2) (Fig. 2). Within a short period, numerous investigators described monoclonal and polyclonal antibodies that recognize an antigen of this approximate size on *P. carinii* obtained from a variety of hosts (4–8). From these reports, two things are readily apparent: first, antibodies to this molecule are easily produced, indicating that the molecule must be abundant, highly immunogenic, or both; second, there are differences in the size of this molecule when organisms from different mammalian hosts are used. Because of these size differences, I have chosen to use the terminology surface glycoprotein A to refer to this molecule, rather than the more conventional terminology based on molecular mass, which is cumbersome and somewhat confusing when discussing *P. carinii* from different hosts (9).

B. Isolation and Characterization

The original description of this glycoprotein (gp) was of that obtained from ferret *P. carinii* (10). Lectin-affinity chromatography was used to isolate and to demonstrate the presence of mannose (or glucose) and *N*-acetylglucosamine on this molecule. This method failed to detect *N*-acetylgalactosamine or fucose residues. The isoelectric point of surface glycoprotein A, as determined by chromatofocusing, ranges from about 5.0 to 5.7. This range of isoelectric points likely represents posttranslational modifications of the molecule (e..g, glycosylation), which is consistent with relatively broad bands seen on SDS–PAGE and immunoblots. Recently, published modifications of this isolation method (11), using heat during the elution step, permitted the easy isolation of small amounts of this glycoprotein from ferret- and mouse-derived *P. carinii*.

Analysis of the homologous molecule isolated from rat *P. carinii* has resulted in similar, although not identical, findings. With use of various chromatographic techniques and lectin-binding studies, mannose was again shown to be the major sugar component of this glycoprotein (7,12–14). The isoelectric point of rat

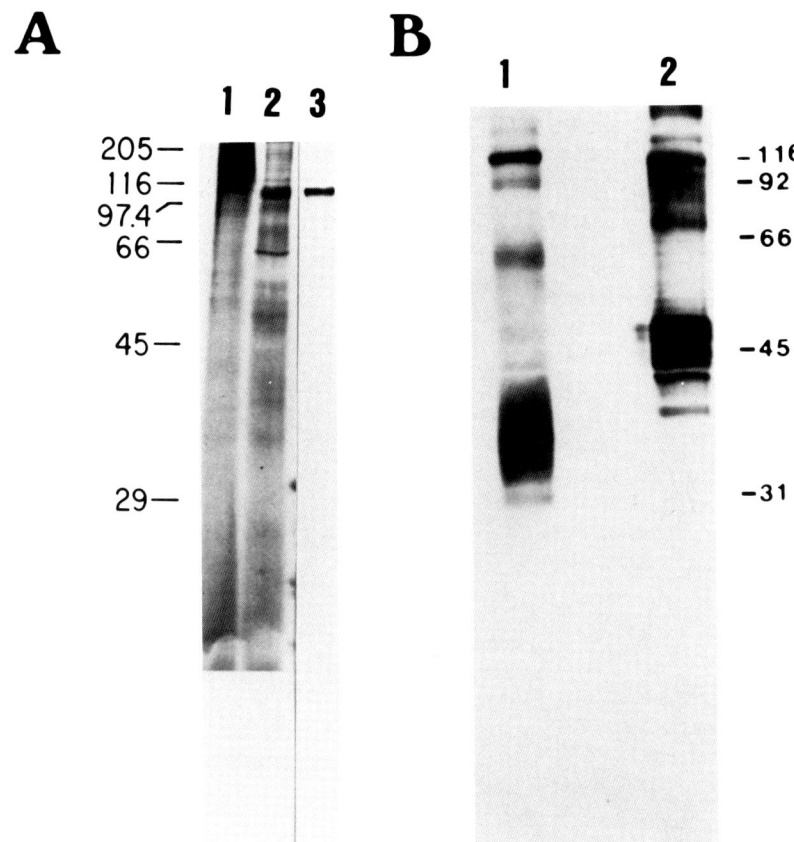

Figure 1 SDS–PAGE and immunoblot analysis of *P. carinii*. (A) SDS–PAGE followed by silver staining of equal amounts of protein from solubilized normal ferret lung (lane 1) and *P. carinii*-infected ferret lung (lane 2). A dense band with an M_r of approximately 120 kDa is readily apparent in the infected lung sample. Immunoblot using a monoclonal antibody for glycoprotein A confirms the identify of the 120-kDa band (lane 3). (B) Immunoblot of homogenates of *P. carinii*-infected human lung (lane 1) and rat lung (lane 2) using antiserum from a rabbit immunized with human *P. carinii*. *P. carinii* antigens are noted in the approximately 40–50, 60, 95–120, and >200-kDa range. (Panel B courtesy of P. D. Walzer.) (From Ref. 5.)

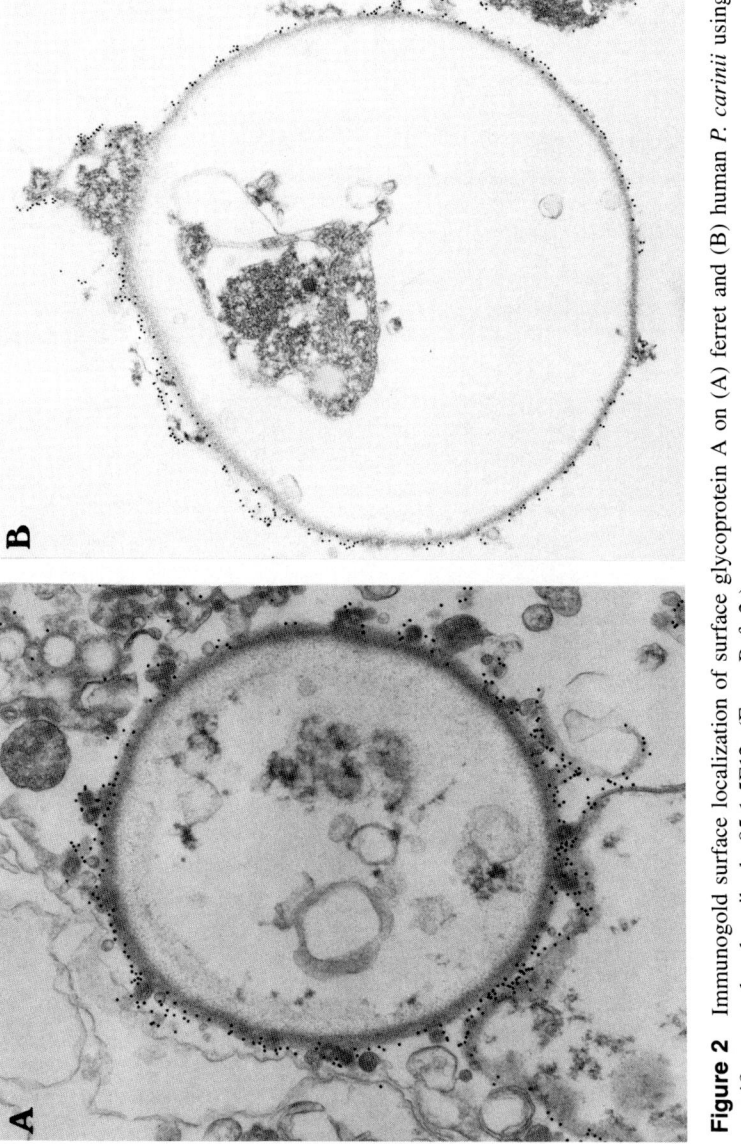

Figure 2 Immunogold surface localization of surface glycoprotein A on (A) ferret and (B) human *P. carinii* using specific monoclonal antibody 85-1-5E12. (From Ref. 2.)

P. carinii surface glycoprotein A is 6.1–6.9 (7). Two-dimensional gel analysis shows that the molecule actually exists as multiple (approximately six) isotypes, which accounts for the broad pI. It is not known whether the difference in pI of rat and ferret *P. carinii* surface glycoprotein A represents methodological differences or actual variation in the two molecules (discussed in Sec. II.C).

A similar molecule has also been isolated from human *P. carinii* (15). Albeit the molecule has a somewhat lower M_r (95 kDa), lectin-binding studies and analysis of total cell wall carbohydrate suggests that the sugar composition is similar to that of glycoprotein A isolated from other mammalian hosts. Although studied to a lesser extent, surface glycoprotein A obtained from mouse *P. carinii* also contains mannose (glucose), as defined by its binding to concanavalin A (9). Its molecular mass, however, is more variable, ranging from 100 to 140 kDa, depending on whether collagenase is used in the isolation process.

More detailed analysis of this molecule has been difficult. Amino acid analysis has been problematic, and attempts to characterize the peptide portion of the molecule have met with only limited success. The molecule tends to form large aggregates when in solution, appears to have limited solubility, and also has a propensity to adhere to membranes or solid-phase supports. Chemical deglycosylation of rat *P. carinii* surface glycoprotein A has been reported to result in a 68-kDa moiety (13). Similar treatment of human and ferret *P. carinii* surface glycoprotein A have been unsuccessful (15); Gigliotti, F, unpublished).

C. Host-Specific Antigenic Variation

It has long been suspected that *P. carinii* obtained from different host species might vary antigenically. Whereas some serological studies support this contention (16,17), others conclude that there are no significant serological differences in *P. carinii* obtained from different hosts (18,19). The development of *P. carinii*-specific monoclonal antibodies has provided the tools to more easily address this issue.

Monoclonal antibodies have been produced that bind to surface glycoprotein A of ferret, mouse, rat, and human *P. carinii* by using *P. carinii* from each species in the immunization process (9). Interestingly, with only one exception, the monoclonal antibodies fail to bind to *P. carinii* isolated from a host species other than that used in the immunization process. A summary of the binding specificity of some of these monoclonal antibodies is provided in Table 1. The one exception to the species-specific–binding pattern is antibody 85-1-5E12, which binds to the mannose portion of the molecule, indicating that this epitope is conserved among all *P. carinii* (9).

Further supporting the evidence for heterogeneity in surface glycoprotein A is the substantial size difference of the mouse and human *P. carinii*-derived molecules. Human *P. carinii* surface glycoprotein A is significantly smaller than

Table 1 Binding of Representative MAbs to Antigen 5E12 on *Pneumocystis carinii* Obtained from Various Hosts

Immunization protocol			Source of *P. carinii*				
Immunogen	Source	MAb	Rat	Mouse	Ferret	Human	Rabbit
Whole *P. carinii*	Rat	85-1-5E12	+	+	+	+	+
Whole *P. carinii*	Rat	85-1-5E8	+	−	−	−	−
Whole *P. carinii*	Mouse	90-3-2B5	−	+	−	−	ND[a]
Antigen 5E12	Ferret	88-2-1D1	−	−	+	−	ND
Antigen 5E12/ Whole *P. carinii*	Human	89-1-3H6	−	−	−	+	ND

[a]Not done
Source: Ref. 8.

the 115–120 kDa noted for ferret and rat *P. carinii*, having an M_r of about 95 kDa; whereas the mouse *P. carinii* homologue is significantly larger, with an M_r of about 130–140 kDa (9,15). In addition, after exposure to commercial collagenase preparations, mouse *P. carinii* surface glycoprotein A is cleaved to doublet of about 100 and 120 kDa, when analyzed by SDS–PAGE (9).

In summary, the recent findings just described, along with some of the earlier serological studies of *P. carinii*, are most consistent with the hypothesis that there is variation among *P. carinii* and that such variation is in some way dependent on the host of origin. Furthermore, these data suggest that various serotypes of *P. carinii* do exist. There is not yet enough experimental data to define the mechanism of this variation. Two possible explanations would be that these changes in surface glycoprotein A represent posttranslational modifications of the molecule, such as glycosylation, or that the heterogeneity is genetically determined. This latter possibility is beginning to be addressed with the recent successful cloning of *P. carinii*-specific antigens (see Sec. IV). Either possibility could be important in determining the range of host species susceptibility to infection with *P. carinii*.

D. Functional Significance of Surface Glycoprotein A in the Pathogenesis of *Pneumocystis carinii* Pneumonia

In addition to being the most well-described antigen of *P. carinii*, surface glycoprotein A is the only antigen for which data exists suggesting that it may play a role in the pathogenesis of disease caused by this organism. The first piece of evidence that suggests a role for surface glycoprotein A in the host–parasite interaction is the observation that rats recovering from *P. carinii* pneumonia develop a prominent antibody response to this molecule. A time-dependent antibody response to this molecule is also observed when healthy nonimmunosuppressed rats are cohoused with rats who have *P. carinii* pneumonia (20). It has also been demonstrated that prophylactic administration of a specific glycoprotein A monoclonal antibody to immunosuppressed rats and ferrets lessens the severity of *P. carinii* pneumonia, as judged by a reduction in the number of organisms in the lung (21). The mechanism by which this monoclonal antibody exerts its effect is unknown.

More recent information indicates that mice immunized with whole *P. carinii* develop both a T-cell and B-cell response to surface glycoprotein A. More importantly, a similar response is noted among SCID mice that have recovered from *P. carinii* pneumonia after reconstitution with normal spleen cells (11). Figure 3 shows the lymphocyte response to surface glycoprotein A by cells obtained from reconstituted SCID mice after recovery from *P. carinii* pneumonia. An interesting finding of this study was that the mice developed an immune response to mouse *P.*

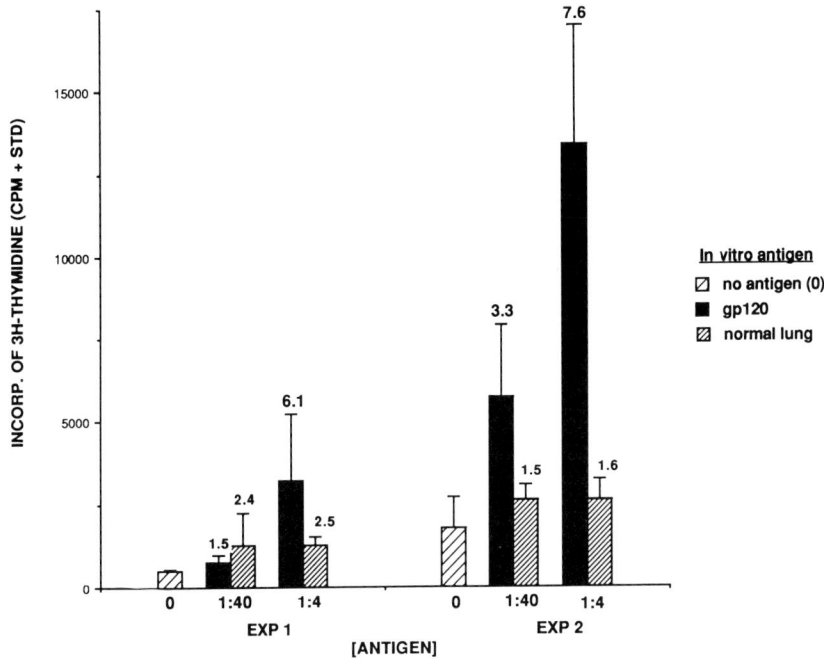

Figure 3 Response of mouse lymphocytes obtained after recovery from *P. carinii* pneumonitis to surface glycoprotein A (gp120). Numbers over the error bars indicate the calculated *stimulation index*, which is the counts per minute (cpm) of the well being assayed divided by the cpm of the no-antigen well.

carinii surface glycoprotein A, but not to that of ferret *P. carinii*. This is consistent with the observation of host-specific antigenic variation in this molecule.

An important question about the pathogenesis of *P. carinii* infection is how and why the organism attaches selectively to type I alveolar cells. A recent study (22) provides evidence that this attachment may be mediated by surface glycoprotein A by intermediary attachment to fibronectin. Furthermore, there seems to be antibody cross-reactivity between surface glycoprotein A and β-integrin, a highly conserved attachment protein (22). It is also possible that this molecule serves as the site of attachment for mannose-binding proteins (23), which could result in an innate immunity to *P. carinii*.

The pathophysiology of *P. carinii* pneumonitis is not understood. The infection results in profound hypoxia, but the mechanism is unknown. Interference with normal pulmonary surfactant physiology would produce hypoxia and diffuse atelectasis. Surfactant, a macroaggregate of phospholipids and proteins, acts in the lung to reduce surface tension, thereby maintaining the alveoli in an open state and facilitating gas exchange. Surfactant protein A has lectin-like activity and shares genetic homology with the human mannose-binding protein gene (24). One could hypothesize that *P. carinii* induces hypoxia through the interaction of the mannose residues on surface glycoprotein A with surfactant, which would, in essence, functionally deplete the lung of active surfactant. Consistent with this hypothesis is the finding that surfactant is one of the host molecules that is found adhered to *P. carinii* organisms (25). In addition, the rat model of *P. carinii* pneumonitis has been used to demonstrate a profound decrease in pulmonary surfactant in immunosuppressed rats with *P. carinii* pneumonitis, when compared with normal rats or immunosuppressed rats that do not have *P. carinii* pneumonitis (26).

In summary, direct experimental data suggests that surface glycoprotein A is involved in both immune recognition and attachment. Further study of this molecule could provide important insights into the pathogenesis and pathophysiology of *P. carinii* pneumonitis.

III. Other Antigens

Very little specific information is known about the other antigens of *P. carinii*. There are no published data on the isolation and characterization of any other *P. carinii* molecules. Most of what is known is based on immunoblot analysis of *P. carinii* preparations using monoclonal antibodies, convalescent antisera, or postimmunization antisera (4–6,8,12,14). Such studies indicate there are other antigens specific for *P. carinii* with M_r in the range of 22–24, 30–32, 40–60, and >200 kDa. Furthermore, it appears that at least the molecule(s) in the 40- to 60-kDa range is a glycoprotein. This antigen has recently been partially cloned from rat *P. carinii* (see Sec. IV). Consistent with the theme that there is host-specific variation among *P. carinii*, the immunoblot profiles of rat and human *P. carinii* preparations are not identical.

Just as has been shown for surface glycoprotein A, rats recovering from *P. carinii* pneumonia develop a strong antibody response to the 45- and 50-kDa antigens of *P. carinii* (20). Analysis of human antisera from both healthy and immunosuppressed individuals demonstrates an antibody response to many of these antigens, although the pattern of response is complex and not uniform (27). An important area for future study will be to determine the interrelation, if any, between these various antigens.

An interesting observation is that patients with *P. carinii* pneumonia develop antibodies to cardiolipin. Similar risk groups with other opportunistic infections do not have antibody to cardiolipin (28). High-performance liquid chromatography (HPLC) of *P. carinii* preparations indicates a shared peak between *P. carinii* and cardiolipin micelles. Furthermore, antisera raised against *P. carinii* also react with cardiolipin, as determined by enzyme-linked immunosorbent assay (ELISA) (29), and antisera raised against glycosphingolipids have a Western blot profile similar to antisera raised against human *P. carinii* (Fig. 4). These findings are consistent with the observation of phospholipids on *P. carinii* (25). It will be important to determine whether these results indicate true cross-reactivity with host molecules or whether the organism coats itself with host phospholipids.

In addition to possible shared epitopes with cardiolipin, *P. carinii* may also share antigens with other microorganisms. Recent studies, with monoclonal antibodies, have demonstrated the presence of cross-reactive epitopes on *P. carinii* and a wide variety of fungi (30) and *Toxoplasma gondii* (31). The nature and significance of these cross-reactions are yet to be determined.

IV. New Directions

The production and analysis of recombinant antigens is one way to gain insight about microbial antigens when they are otherwise hard to isolate. Recently, progress has been made in cloning two antigens of *P. carinii*; the 45–55-kDa antigen of rat *P. carinii* (32) and glycoprotein A of ferret *P. carinii* (33). An example of how these cloned antigens can be used to study *P. carinii* is demonstrated by Figure 5. Polymerase chain reaction (PCR) analysis of *P. carinii*-infected lung samples using primers based on the cDNA sequence of the 45–55-kDa antigen of rat *P. carinii* was positive using DNA from *P. carinii*-infected rat lung, but not with infected human or ferret lung (see Fig. 5, lanes 8–13). Similar analyses using probes specific for ferret *P. carinii* glycoprotein A resulted in the detection of target DNA in infected ferret lungs, but not in infected human or rat lungs. In contrast, probes based on the gene coding for mitochondrial ribosomal

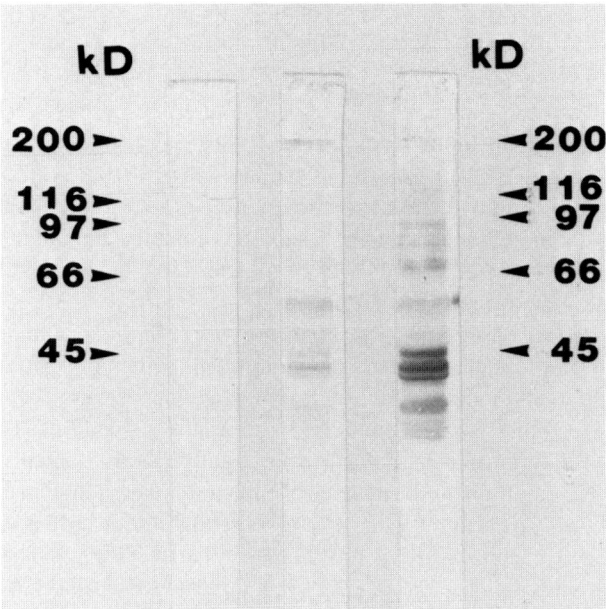

Figure 4 Western blot analysis of normal human lung (first lane) and *P. carinii*-infected human lung (second lane), using antisera to glycosphingolipid (aGM1, Wako Chemicals), and of *P. carinii*-infected human, using lung antisera raised against human *P. carinii* (third lane). The two antisera identify similar-sized antigens in the infected lung that are not present in normal lung. (Courtesy of M. Sorice.)

RNA (34) detected *P. carinii* in lungs from an infected rat, human, and ferret (see Fig. 5, lanes 1–6). Thus, the previously discussed host species–specific antigenic variation in *P. carinii* antigens can be confirmed at the molecular level. It is likely that the cloning of additional *P. carinii* antigens will facilitate notable advances in our understanding of the epidemiology, immunology, and pathogenesis of *P. carinii* pneumonia.

V. Conclusion

The antigens of *P. carinii* and their possible role in the pathophysiology of *P. carinii* pneumonitis are beginning to be defined. We hope that this information can be used in the future to define the epidemiology of infection, to improve the noninvasive diagnosis of *P. carinii* pneumonitis, and to devise methods to interrupt infection with *P. carinii*.

Antigenic Characteristics of P. carinii

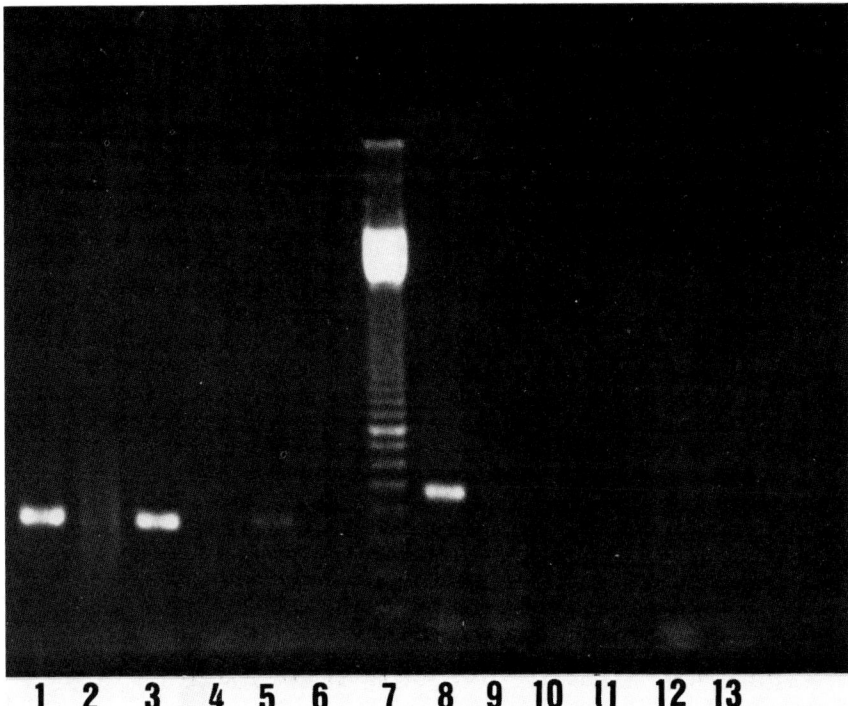

Figure 5 PCR analysis of *P. carinii*-infected and normal lung tissue. Samples are as follows: lanes 1 and 8, *P. carinii*-infected rat lung; lanes 2 and 9, normal rat lung; lanes 3 and 10, *P. carinii*-infected human lung; lanes 4 and 11, normal human lung; lanes 5 and 12, *P. carinii*-infected ferret lung; lanes 6 and 13, normal ferret lung. Size markers (in 100-bp increments) are in lane 7. Lanes 1–6 were amplified with primers based on the DNA sequence for the conserved mitochondrial rRNA sequence (34). Lanes 8–13 were amplified with primers based on the cDNA sequence for the 45–55-kDa antigen of rat *P. carinii* (32). Whereas the conserved primers amplify target DNA in infected lungs from all three hosts, the primers for the 45–55-kDa antigen appear specific for *P. carinii* of rat origin.

References

1. Maddison SE, Hayes GV, Ivey MH, Tsang VCW, Slemenda SB, Norman LG. (1982). Fractionation of *P. carinii* antigens used in an enzyme-linked immunosorbent assay for antibodies and in the production of antiserum for detecting *Pneumocystis carinii* antigenemia. J Clin Microbiol 1982; 15:1029–1035.
2. Gigliotti F, Stokes DC, Cheatham AB, Davis DS, Hughes WT. Development of murine monoclonal antibodies to *Pneumocystis carinii*. J Infect Dis 1986; 154:315–322.

3. Graves DC, McNabb SJN, Ivey MH, Worley MA. Development and characterization of monoclonal antibodies to *Pneumocystis carinii*. Infect Immun 1986; 51:125–133.
4. Kovacs JA, Halpern JL, Lundgren B, Swan JC, Parrillo JE, Masur H. Monoclonal antibodies to *Pneumocystis carinii*: identification of specific antigens and characterization of antigenic differences between rat and human isolates. J Infect Dis 1989; 159:60–70.
5. Walzer PD, Linke MJ. A comparison of the antigenic characteristics of rat and human *Pneumocystis carinii* by immunoblotting. J Immunol 1987; 138:2257–2265.
6. Kovacs JA, Halpern JL, Swan JC, Moss J, Parrillo JE, Masur H. Identification of antigens and antibodies specific for *Pneumocystis carinii*. J Immunol 1988; 140: 2023–2031.
7. Tanabe K, Takasaki S, Watanabe J, Kobata A, Egawa K, Nakamura Y. Glycoproteins composed of major surface immunodeterminants of *Pneumocystis carinii*. Infect Immun 1989; 57:1547–1555.
8. Graves DC, McNabb SJN, Worley MA, Downs TD, Ivey MH. Analyses of rat *Pneumocystis carinii* antigens recognized by human and rat antibodies using Western immunoblotting. Infect Immun 1986; 54:96–103.
9. Gigliotti F. Host species specific antigenic variation of a mannosylated surface glycoprotein of *Pneumocystis carinii*. J Infect Dis 1992; 165:329–336.
10. Gigliotti F, Ballou LR, Hughes WT, Mosley BD. Purification and initial characterization of a ferret *Pneumocystis carinii* surface antigen. J Infect Dis 1988; 158:848–854.
11. Fisher DJ, Gigliotti F, Zauderer M, Harmsen AG. Specific T-cell response to a *Pneumocystis carinii* surface glycoprotein (gp120) after immunization and natural infection. Infect Immun 1991; 59:3372–3376.
12. Pesanti EL, Shanley JD. Glycoproteins of *Pneumocystis carinii*: characterization by electrophoresis and microscopy. J Infect Dis 1988; 158:1353–1359.
13. Radding JA, Armstrong MYK, Ullu E, Richards FF. Identification and isolation of a major cell surface glycoprotein of *Pneumocystis carinii*. Infect Immun 1989; 57: 2149–2157.
14. Linke MJ, Cushion MT, Walzer PD. Properties of the major antigens of rat and human *Pneumocystis carinii*. Infect Immun 1989; 57:1547–1555.
15. Lundgren B, Lipschik GY, Kovacs JA. Purification and characterization of a major human *Pneumocystis carinii* surface antigen. J Clin Invest 1991; 87:163–170.
16. Kim HK, Hughes WT, Feldman S. Studies of morphology and immunofluorescence of *Pneumocystis carinii*. Proc Soc Exp Biol Med 1972; 141:304–309.
17. Walzer PD, Rutledge ME. Comparison of rat, mouse and human *Pneumocystis carinii* by immunofluorescence. J Infect Dis 1980; 142:449.
18. Lim SK, Eveland WC, Porter RJ. Development and evaluation of a direct fluorescent antibody method for the diagnosis of *Pneumocystis carinii* infections in experimental animals. Appl Microbiol 1973; 26:666–671.
19. Norman L, Kagan IG. Some observations on the serology of *Pneumocystis carinii* infections in the United States. Infect Immun 1973; 8:317–321.
20. Walzer PD, Stanforth D, Linke MJ, Cushion MT. *Pneumocystis carinii*: immunoblotting and immunofluorescent analyses of serum antibodies during experimental rat infection and recovery. Exp Parasitol 1987; 63:319–328.

21. Gigliotti F, Hughes WT. Passive immunoprophylaxis with specific monoclonal antibody confers partial protection against *Pneumocystis carinii* pneumonitis in animal models. J Clin Invest 1988; 81:666–668.
22. Pottratz ST, Paulsrud J, Smith JS, Martin WJ II. *Pneumocystis carinii* attachment to cultured lung cells by pneumocystis gp120, a fibronectin binding protein. J Clin Invest 1991; 88:403–407.
23. Ezekowitz RAB, Williams DJ, Koziel H, Armstrong MYK, Warner A, Richards FF, Rose RM. Uptake of *Pneumocystis carinii* mediated by the macrophage mannose receptor. Nature 1991; 351:155–158.
24. Sastry K, Herman GA, Day L, Deigan E, Bruns G, Ezekowitz RA. The human mannose-binding protein gene. Exon structure reveals its evolutionary relationship to a human pulmonary surfactant gene and localization to chromosome 10. J Exp Med 1989; 170:1175–1189.
25. Pesanti EL. Phospholipid profile of *Pneumocystis carinii* and its interaction with alveolar type II epithelial cells. Infect Immun 1987 55:736–741.
26. Sheehan PM, Stokes DC, Yeh Y, Hughes WT. Surfactant phospholipids and lavage phospholipase A_2 in experimental *Pneumocystis carinii* pneumonia. Am Rev Respir Dis 1986; 134:526–531.
27. Peglow SL, Smulian AG, Linke MJ, Pogue CL, Nurre S, Crisler J, Phair J, Gold JWM, Armstrong D, Walzer PD. Serologic responses to *Pneumocystis carinii* antigens in health and disease. J Infect Dis 1990; 161:296–306.
28. DiPrima MA, Sorice M, Vullo V, Mastroianni CM, Amendolea MA, Masala C. Anticardiolipin antibody in the acquired immunodeficiency syndrome: a marker of *Pneumocystis carinii* infection? J Infect 1989; 18:100–101.
29. Masala C, Sorice M, DiPrima MA, Lenti L, Misasi R, Mojow M, Contini C, Vullo V. Evidence for shared epitopes between cardiolipin and *Pneumocystis carinii*. J Infect Dis 1989; 160:736–737.
30. Lundgren B, Kovacs JA, Nelson NN, Stock F, Martinez A, Gill VJ. *Pneumocystis carinii* and specific fungi have a common epitope, identified by a monoclonal antibody. J Clin Microbiol 1992; 30:391–395.
31. Hassl A, Muller WA, Aspock H. An identical epitope in *Pneumocystis carinii* and *Toxoplasma gondii* causing serological cross reactions. Parasitol Res 1991; 77:351–352.
32. Smulian AG, Stringer JR, Linke MJ, Walzer PD. Isolation and characterization of a recombinant antigen of *Pneumocystis carinii*. Infect Immun 1992; 60:907–915.
33. Haidaris PJ, Wright TW, Gigliotti F, Haidaris CG. Expression and characterization of a cDNA clone encoding an immunodominant surface glycoprotein of *Pneumocystis carinii*. J Infect Dis 1992; 116:1113–1123.
34. Wakefield AE, Pixley FJ, Banerji S, Sinclaire K, Miller RF, Moxon ER, Hopkin JM. Detection of *Pneumocystis carinii* with DNA amplication. Lancet 1990; 336:451–453.

Part Two

EPIDEMIOLOGY

7

Transmission and Epidemiology

MELANIE T. CUSHION

University of Cincinnati College of Medicine
Cincinnati, Ohio

I. Introduction

Knowledge of the life cycle of *Pneumocystis carinii* remains quite rudimentary, limiting understanding of the mode of transmission of infection, identification of the transmissive agent, and reservoirs of infection. Developmental forms within the mammalian lung have been identified and several life cycles have been postulated incorporating these forms (1–6) (discussed in Chapter 2). Because a suitable in vitro system does not exist for the organism that would permit direct observation of the progression of development, all existing life cycles are based on static images supplied by microscopy and educated guesses as to the modes of replication. It appears likely that trophic forms replicate asexually and a sexual mode of reproduction results in at least one type of cyst form (3). Our information therein ends. The method of entry into the mammalian host and the events that follow have not been described. It is not known whether infected individuals can transmit the disease or if there is an environmental cycle that produces the infective agent. Understanding of the life cycle is necessary for control of the infection. If patients are able to transmit the infection, then barrier isolation may be required for these individuals, since many AIDS patients often reside on the same floor in a hospital. Strict hygienic control and sanitation, including filtered air, may be indicated if an environmental cycle is shown to produce the infective form.

II. Evidence for an Airborne Mode of Transmission

Animal experiments have been used to help delineate the mode of transmission of *P. carinii* infection. Exploiting the immunosuppressed rodent animal model of *P. carinii* pneumonia, a series of studies showed that the infection was likely transmitted by airborne contact with an infectious agent (7–12). All studies followed a basic design in which *P. carinii*–free (naïve) rats were exposed in varying ways to immunosuppressed, infected rats. After chronic immunosuppression, the once-naïve rats developed *P. carinii* pneumonia. In 1971 Hendley and Weller showed both close and distant contact between these two groups resulted in infection of the naïve animals (7). Walzer et al. extended these studies to include the use of *P. carinii*–infected nude mice as the distant contact source of infection for uninfected nude mice (8). Walzer et al. also had limited success in establishing the infection by intrapulmonary injection; in contrast, intranasal instillation of organisms did not cause infection. Studies by Hughes (9–11) explored several potential methods of transmission, including exposure of noninfected rats to unsterile water, air, food, and administration of infected lungs as a food source. As in previous studies, the infection was shown to be transmitted only by an airborne route. In a more recent study, Soulez et al. exposed *P. carinii*–free SCID (severe combined immune deficiency) mice to non-SCID mice (NSM) that had corticosteroid-induced *P. carinii* infection (12). The naïve SCID animals were exposed to the infected NSM for 1, 7, 26, 46, 60, or 120 days by housing the mice in the same cage, or in a separate cage but under the same filter bonnet. Control SCID mice isolated under a separate barrier did not develop the infection, showing that these mice were not latently infected with *P. carinii* organisms. Infection was shown to occur in SCID mice exposed to an infected mouse for as little as 1 day. During the first month of exposure, the time of exposure could be directly correlated with organism burden in the newly infected mice. Results from this experiment again supported an airborne mode of infection, since infected mice could transmit the infection to naïve mice housed in separate cages.

To address questions concerning reactivation of latent infection and airborne transmission, we conducted similar studies to those outlined above with the added dimension of characterization of the *P. carinii* isolates by electrophoretic karyotyping (13). The chromosomes of *P. carinii* and other lower eukaryotes can be separated by size, using techniques of pulsed field gel electrophoresis (PFGE) resulting in distinct and reproducible patterns of ethidium bromide–visualized DNA bands. These electrophoretic karyotypes were used as epidemiological markers, to identify the *P. carinii* isolates. In this study, we placed corticosteroid-immunosuppressed, *P. carinii*–infected rats in the same room, but on different cage racks, with corticosteroid-treated, *P. carinii*–free rats. The ability to identify a *P. carinii* isolate by its karyotypic pattern permitted us to show that the *P. carinii* harbored within the infected rat lungs was the same organism that caused infection in the naïve rats. Like the previous studies, these experiments supported an airborne mode of transmission, since the animals were at opposite ends of the room. In addition, it was shown that a specific type of *P. carinii* could be traced from one group of rats to another, illustrating the potential of electrophoretic karyotyping as an epidemiological tool. Primary exposure of the immunosuppressed naïve rats to an infected source resulted in fulminant pneumonia, expanding the concept of the origin of *P. carinii* pneumonia in immunosuppressed hosts to include newly acquired organisms as well as reactivation of latent infection.

In the second part of the same study, latently infected rats housed under barrier conditions and immunosuppressed produced fulminant *P. carinii* pneumonia with the same organism burden as their immunosuppressed littermates housed in cages open to the environment. These studies provide experimental evidence that reactivation of latent organisms leads to fulminant pneumocystosis, since the rats kept under the barrier were not exposed to any source of infection. They also suggest that organisms may be harbored in the immune competent host for at least a short while, since the barrier-isolated rats were permitted to acclimate for 10 days prior to initiation of immunosuppressive therapy. Studies have not been undertaken to assess the length of time the organism can persist in the lungs of immune competent hosts or if they can exist for any period of time ex vivo. Little evidence for colonization or a carrier state can be found in the literature, although one recent report detected *P. carinii* in an apparently healthy 20-year-old adult (14). Detection of *P. carinii* product in immune depressed individuals without apparent clinical disease suggests that transitory colonization may occur in selected populations (15,16) (discussed below).

From these studies, it seems clear that the agent of infection is contacted through the air, yet the focus or reservoir of infection remains unknown. If one considers the dissemination of the tubercle bacillus as a possible model for the transmission of *P. carinii*, then the infected hosts would serve to discharge the infective particle through a process of coughing or wheezing. Like droplet nuclei, this infective particle would be able to remain suspended in the air for extended periods of time and take advantage of air or thermal currents for dispersion to susceptible individuals. Alternatively, an environmental cycle may be an intermediate step required for the production of vast numbers of infective forms (e.g., spores).

III. Origin of Infection

A. Residence Within the Mammalian Host

Several seroepidemiological studies have shown that the vast majority of the human population becomes seropositive to *P. carinii* by the age of 4 years (17,18), attesting to the suspected ubiquitous distribution of the organism. Thus far, no definitive clinical manifestations of primary exposure to *P. carinii* have been described and the primary infection is thought to be asymptomatic in the immunecompetent host. The origin of the fulminant infection manifested by immunocompromised individuals has been thought to result from an activation of organisms acquired early in life, a "reactivation of latent organisms." Such an event would imply some mechanism for circumventing the host immune surveillance system, as well as raise questions as to the place of residence of the latent organisms or consequences of environmental exposure to a new source of infection by an immunocompromised individual.

If *P. carinii* is ubiquitous in the environment and if organisms are harbored in the human lung, one might expect to frequently encounter organisms in the lung during postmortem examination or as a result of antemortem diagnostic procedures. Within the past 3 decades, five studies have addressed the prevalence of *P. carinii* at autopsy using histological staining methods of detection (19–23). The detection of *P. carinii* in these varied populations ranged between 0 and 8%. In all cases, the presence of *P. carinii* was associated with an underlying state of immune depression due to malignancy or chronic disease. Healthy adults did not appear to harbor latent organisms. These postmortem studies were limited by a variety of factors, including selection of certain subpopulations of patients with underlying disease, retrospective review of medical records for diagnosis, and most important, method of detection. Histological staining of random lung samples for organisms that may be in low numbers is an insensitive method at best.

More recently, the technology of molecular biology was used to evaluate postmortem tissue and antemortem samples for the presence of *P. carinii*. Autopsy material from 15 cases and 10 bronchoalveolar lavage fluids (BALF) were analyzed by the polymerase chain reaction (PCR) (24,25). PCR technology permits very small amounts of DNA (theoretically as low as a single DNA molecule) to be amplified to levels that can be analyzed for size and sequence composition. In the studies cited, primers designed to amplify a portion of the mitochondrial ribosomal RNA of human-derived *P. carinii* were used. Products were detected in BALF from patients with clinical *P. carinii* infection. When BALF from nonimmunocompromised patients were analyzed, no products of the expected size were produced. In the second study, one entire lobe of lung from each of 15 individuals examined at autopsy was homogenized and portions were then used for analysis. The right and left upper and lower lobes were sampled in rotation from each of the 15 cases. PCR of these homogenates did not yield a positive result. By seeding normal human lung with organisms, these investigators determined the sensitivity of the reaction to be minimally 100 organisms. Although the ability of bronchoalveolar lavage to recover organisms in healthy adults may be questionable, homogenization of entire lobes of lungs should provide a suitable sample for these analyses. These studies imply that *P. carinii* are not harbored for any significant length of time in the healthy individual. Yet the possibility of a carrier state or transitory colonization cannot be totally excluded. Conflicting data, such as the recent report of the recovery of *P. carinii* cysts from a healthy adult by bronchoalveolar lavage, suggest that *P. carinii* may reside in immunologically intact individuals (14). PCR studies with larger sample sizes and perhaps a survey of other organ systems may provide more definitive information.

In another study, PCR was compared with immunofluorescence for the detection of *P. carinii* in sputum samples from asymptomatic patients, immunosuppressed patients, and renal and heart/lung transplant patients (15). The PCR reaction was directed to the same mitochondrial RNA sequences as in the previous studies (24,25). Of these three groups of 10 patients, all 30 were negative by immunofluorescence, but three renal and two heart/lung patients were positive by PCR amplification. One of these five patients went on to develop symptomatic pneumocystosis 6 weeks after sampling. The authors hypothesized that the organ transplant patients rendered immune incompetent by antirejection therapy were colonized by the organism and that this apparent colonization does not necessarily result in fulminant infection since 4/5 cases did not result in clinical disease.

Lipschik et al. used two PCR methods for the detection of *P. carinii* in induced sputum and BALF of humans and in blood of humans and rats (16). One PCR method used the same single primer pair directed to mitochondrial rRNA gene sequence of human-derived *P. carinii* reported by Wakefield et al. (24). In the second technique, two primer pairs based on nuclear rRNA sequences of rat-derived *P. carinii* were used in a nested PCR procedure (16). Nested PCR involves two rounds of amplification with two sets of primers, resulting in enhanced sensitivity and specificity. Of 71 sputum samples analyzed, 17 patients with confirmed *P. carinii* pneumonia were all correctly identified by nested PCR reaction, while 50 of the 54 microbiologically negative samples were found negative by the nested reaction. In contrast, PCR with a single primer pair detected the presence of organisms in 12 of the 17 diagnosed cases and was negative in 51 of the 54 of the apparently noninfected samples. Results from 113 BALF evaluated showed there were no significant differences in sensitivity between either PCR method.

Detection of the presence of organisms in blood was not as successful as with BALF or sputum samples. Blood samples from 14 patients with documented *P. carinii* pneumonia produced three positive results with nested PCR only. Of the three infections detected by nested PCR, two of three patients with disseminated pneumocystosis were positive, but only 1/11 cases restricted to the lung were correctly identified. None of the seven control blood samples from patients without the infection were positive by either PCR method.

Analyses of blood from infected and noninfected rats were more promising; 11 of 14 samples of rats with documented infection were positive by both PCR techniques, and all three uninfected rats were negative by both PCR techniques.

Like Leigh et al. (15), these investigators found PCR products in samples without histologically documented infection. They also concluded that these findings indicated the presence of low numbers of organisms present in these patients, since most of the "false-positive" samples were positive by both PCR methods (7/11). Since the PCR methods were based on unrelated gene sequences and controls remained negative, it seems unlikely that these reactions are spurious. Most of the patients apparently colonized were patients treated with immunosuppressive drugs or were HIV-positive, with CD4 counts below 0.2×10^9/L. Only 1 in 10 of these patients progressed to fulminant infection during a 6-month period, suggesting, again, that this low level of organism burden rarely proceeds to clinical pneumonia.

Although PCR technology needs improvement before it gains widespread use as a diagnostic tool, the studies by Leigh et al. (15) and Lipschik et al. (16) are striking for their detection of low levels of organisms in immunosuppressed patient populations [e.g., HIV(+), transplant recipients]. These reports also provide evidence for the presence of *P. carinii* in other locations beside the lung and suggest a hematogenous spread of the organism in disseminated cases.

Some other evidence supportive of transitory colonization was recently reported. *P. carinii* cysts were recovered from a 20-year-old female college student who underwent BAL as a control subject (14). She appeared to be in good health, except that cysts were found in her BALF by staining procedures. Laboratory findings showed an increase in both the total number of lymphocytes and the proportions of lymphocyte classes in the BALF, but not in the peripheral blood. Serological evaluation revealed an increase in antibody titer to Epstein-Barr virus, consistent with a reactivation or resolution of infection. Her CD4+/CD8+ ratio was within the normal range. Twenty-six weeks later another BAL was performed and no organisms were found. The BALF did not show the lymphocytosis associated with the organisms in the first BALF. The authors suggested that the small numbers of organisms and the associated lymphocytosis may have represented subclinical infection with *P. carinii*. It is of interest that this individual was employed as a research technician and frequently exposed to bronchoscopy specimens from both immunosuppressed patients and those with AIDS. She had no respiratory complaints and her chest X-ray was clear. Four years later she remains free of pneumonia.

B. Residence Outside the Mammalian Host?

The previous discussion considered the location(s) of *P. carinii* within the infected or colonized individual and provided evidence that *P. carinii* may be somewhat mobile within the mammalian host. However, the origin of the organisms that initiate infection has yet to be identified. The issue of the natural place of residence of *P. carinii* is clouded by several factors. First is the problem of taxonomy.

Consideration of *P. carinii* as a protozoon or a fungus is important in elucidating its natural history. Protozoons such as *Trypanosoma* often have insect vectors or intermediate hosts that are required for the completion of their life cycle. Many protozoan parasites of humans do not require the human for replication, but end up there accidentally and cause disease as a result. Generally, protozoan parasites do not have environmental amplification cycles; rather they require animals (vertebrates and invertebrates, insects and other protists) for continuation of the species. Fungi, in contrast, often have complex cycles involving plants or materials in the environment such as soil or decaying organic matter. Among the medically important fungi, the ability to temperature-shift permits them access to the human being. Again, humans are rarely required for completion of a fungal life cycle, although some fungi like *Candida* exist on humans without causing significant harm. Obligate parasitism is yet another mode of existence that cannot be ruled out; members of both the Fungi and Protozoa are known to follow this life-style.

The taxonomic association of *Pneumocystis* has been controversial since it was first identified by Chagas in the early 1900s (27). At one time *P. carinii* was considered a protozoan parasite, but did not fit neatly into any existing class of parasites. A collection of molecular genetic evidence, including nuclear small ribosomal subunit sequence, gene sequences, and mitochondrial ribosomal sequences, as well as other supportive biochemical evidence, now points to the organism's fungal identity (26,28–31). Some investigators place *P. carinii* with the smuts and rusts (red yeasts) based on comparison of partial mitochondrial RNA sequences (32). Yet, *P. carinii* cannot be grown on the simple artificial medium that many of the red yeasts readily grow on; indeed, *P. carinii* cannot be grown on or in any in vitro system. It is likely not a "typical" yeast and unlikely a protozoon.

The second factor that has confounded understanding of the life cycle of *P. carinii* is a lack of in vitro culture system. The development of the organism cannot be directly observed, and potential environmental reservoirs cannot be inoculated onto artificial media to test the hypothesis.

The third confounding factor has been the availability of technology that would permit investigators to approach an organism that was refractory to in vitro propagation. The tools with which to approach the characterization and identification of organism isolates have only recently become available. Codon usage, intron structure, repetitive elements, chromosome number, strain/species variation, and taxonomic affiliation have been revealed by molecular biological approaches. It is likely the agent of transmission will be identified by use of tools such as PCR.

Related to the question of the focus or reservoir of infection is the method by which the transmissible agent is contacted. Is the airborne "spore" generated from an environmental source or from an infected individual? A person-to-person spread is supported by the clusters of outbreaks reported in various population groups as well as by the organism's apparent thermotropism. That the organism can be found in polar, temperate, or tropical climates may be a function of direct contact among mammals without a separate environmental cycle. Molecular genetic and antigenic data recently have provided evidence for species-level differences among *P. carinii* isolates from humans, rats, mice, and ferrets (28,33–38), which would argue against the organism as a zoonosis and support transmission by direct contact. At least in wild rodents, there is some evidence that the infection can be carried at low levels in apparently immune-competent animals (e.g., 22% in 150 wild brown rats in Denmark) (39). In contrast, the organism does not seem to reside in the lungs of healthy adults in even low levels, although some immunosuppressed patients may harbor organisms, as reported by investigators using PCR as a detection tool (15,16). Congenitally acquired human infection has been reported in a few cases (40–42). Although animal experiments designed to detect transplacental transmission suggested that it was possible (43), this mode of transmission is probably not a major form of transmission.

It is difficult to imagine that sufficient numbers of organisms (i.e., transmissive forms) can be produced by either infected individuals or carriers. The ubiquitous distribution of *P. carinii* almost begs for an amplification cycle as a means to explain the apparent abundance of the organism in the environment and our immediate contact with it early in life. Faced with these incongruities, we cannot yet reach a conclusion as to the focus or reservoir of the infective particle. Resolution of this question will likely involve the use of molecular biological approaches, such as PCR, in combination with various environmental and biological sampling methods.

IV. Epidemiology

A. Influence of Climate or Geography on Occurrence of Infection

Hughes recently reviewed the global and climatological distribution of *P. carinii* (9a) and concluded that the organism did not exhibit regional tropism, as in the case of *Histoplasma capsulatum*, and had little preference as to climate or geography, since countries in temperate and tropical zones, as well as those in polar regions, have reported cases of pneumocystosis. Likewise, there did not appear to be a specific geoclimate favored by the organism, as coastal regions, arid climates, and rain forests all appear to sustain *P. carinii*.

P. carinii seems to reside only in mammals. Although exhaustive studies have not been undertaken to sample all reptile species or other invertebrates, data from the few reports available indicate that the poikilotherms are not conducive to the existence of *P. carinii*. A thorough study to evaluate the presence of the organism in birds was undertaken in Holland and no evidence of the organism was detected (44). The body temperature of birds is approximately 41°C. It is interesting to note that in a series of studies designed to identify the optimal temperature for maintenance of *P. carinii* in vitro, 41°C was found to be inhibitory for *P. carinii* in either of the cell lines evaluated, whereas 35–37°C supported replication in both lines (45). The absence of the organism in animals with body temperature below 35°C and above 41°C suggests that *P. carinii* may have very specific temperature requirements for growth. This requirement could explain its predilection for mammalian species.

The seasonal occurrence of *P. carinii* pneumonia has been evaluated in only a few studies. In 1974, Walzer and colleagues analyzed 194 confirmed *P. carinii* cases in the United States over a 3-year period (46). When the cases were broken down on a month-by-month basis (Fig. 1), no real pattern of temporal distribution emerged. Likewise, in a study conducted at the University of Cincinnati AIDS Treatment Center (ATC) from 1986 to 1989, a total of 118 confirmed cases of *P. carinii* pneumonia evaluated did not display any seasonal predilection (Tables 1 and 2) (47).

An epidemiological pattern of upper respiratory illness and *P. carinii* in homosexual men was thought to occur in a Multicenter AIDS Cohort study designed to address the transmission of infection (48). Almost 5000 homosexual men in four cities (Baltimore, Chicago, Los Angeles, and Pittsburgh) participated in the study from 1986 through 1988. The incidence of upper respiratory infections

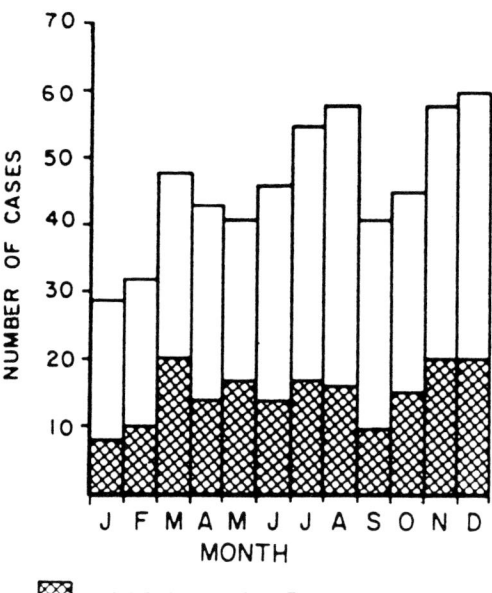

Figure 1 Cases of *Pneumocystis* pneumonia, by month, in the United States, 1968–1970. (From Ref. 46 and unpublished data, Peter D. Walzer.)

Table 1 Distribution of *Pneumocystis* Pneumonia Cases by Month of Diagnosis, Cincinnati AIDS Treatment Center, 1986–1989

Month	1986	1987	1988	1989	Number of cases/months
January	2	6	2	7	17
February		2	3	4	9
March			3	2	5
April		6	4	2	12
May	1		2	3	6
June	1	2	1	2	6
July	1			6	7
August		3	5	3	11
September		3	2	3	8
October	2	1	5	6	14
November	1	3	4	2	10
December	1	3	3	6	13
Total	9	29	34	46	118

Source: Adapted from Ref. 47.

(URI) peaked midwinter to late winter and was at the lowest point during late summer. Conversely, the peak of *P. carinii* cases occurred 4 months after the peak in URI, during May to June, and the nadir of *P. carinii* cases lagged 4 months behind the trough of URI, from November to December. It does not seem likely that the URI represented a *P. carinii* pneumonia prodrome since the upper airways do not appear to harbor *P. carinii* organisms. Rather, the authors of this study proposed that the association of *P. carinii* with the respiratory viruses may have been due to similar modes of transmission. A geographic association seemed to be suggested by the data. Pittsburgh and Chicago had the highest reported rates of URI coincident with the highest proportion of AIDS cases with *P. carinii* pneumonia as the initial diagnosis. Since no temporal or geographic associations were observed for non–*P. carinii* pneumonia or other HIV-related symptoms, it was thought these associations were real and specific for *P. carinii*. The apparent geographic and seasonal association would have been strengthened by presentation of the data by site and year, to evaluate whether the seasonal pattern was consistent across these four geographic locations. The presentation of the data in this manner would have added significant weight to a temporal trend in disease occurrence. As the authors point out, these findings suggest a person-to-person spread of *P. carinii* pneumonia among immunosuppressed individuals, but may also indicate a spurious finding.

Table 2 Calculated Rate of *Pneumocystis* Pneumonia Among Cincinnati AIDS Treatment Center Populations 1986–1989

Month	P. carinii pneumonia cases	At risk	Rate[a]	Month	P. carinii pneumonia cases	At risk	Rate[a]
1	2	35	0.057143	25	2	352	0.005682
2	0	43	0.000000	26	3	367	0.008174
3	0	49	0.000000	27	3	378	0.007937
4	0	53	0.000000	28	4	393	0.010178
5	1	64	0.015625	29	2	411	0.004866
6	1	73	0.013699	30	1	431	0.002320
7	1	85	0.011765	31	0	446	0.000000
8	0	96	0.000000	32	5	476	0.010504
9	0	107	0.000000	33	2	491	0.004073
10	2	126	0.015873	34	5	502	0.009960
11	1	132	0.007576	35	4	508	0.007874
12	1	147	0.006803	36	3	518	0.005792
13	6	163	0.036810	37	7	560	0.012500
14	2	176	0.011364	38	4	572	0.006993
15	0	188	0.000000	39	2	596	0.003356
16	6	235	0.025532	40	2	606	0.003300
17	0	215	0.000000	41	3	615	0.004878
18	2	223	0.008969	42	2	625	0.003200
19	0	242	0.000000	43	6	637	0.009419
20	3	250	0.012000	44	3	659	0.004552
21	3	262	0.011450	45	3	677	0.004431
22	1	284	0.003521	46	6	706	0.008499
23	3	304	0.009868	47	2	739	0.002706
24	3	319	0.009404	48	6	762	0.007874

[a]Rate = number of *P. carinii* pneumonia cases divided by ATC population at risk.
The hypothesis that a seasonal variation of increase in rates occurs in November, December, and January was investigated. For each month, the rate of *P. carinii* pneumonia was calculated as the number of cases per number of AIDS Treatment Center population. The denominator included the total number of patients enrolled, adjusted for deaths from the previous month. Patients who had previously been diagnosed with *P. carinii* pneumonia were excluded from the denominator at risk population. Multiple regression models failed to identify a significant pattern in rates.
Source: Adapted from Ref. 47.

Two brief reports claimed a seasonal variation among *P. carinii* cases in England and Switzerland (49,50). These reports are difficult to interpret since no distinction was made between recurrent pneumonia or primary cases; the numbers of patients were not reported and rates of infection could not be calculated; and the data were shown graphically with number of cases by month combined with plots of rainfall and temperature. No statistical analyses of these relationships were presented and there appears to be no correlation between the peak of *P. carinii* pneumonia cases and temperature or humidity based on the information contained in these reports.

Until more information is available in terms of defined populations and means of assessing recurrent or primary infection, it is difficult to declare a temporal occurrence of *P. carinii* pneumonitis at this time.

B. Clusters of Human *P. carinii* Pneumonitis

Although the organism seems to be common in the environment, several reports of clusters of human *P. carinii* pneumonitis suggest direct or close contact as important means of transmission.

In 1965 Watanabe et al. reported a case of what appeared to be familial transmission (51). After presenting with acute lymphocytic leukemia, the father was treated and went into remission. Two months after his initial diagnosis, his 7-year-old daughter experienced respiratory symptoms that lasted 3 months. During her daughter's respiratory illness, the mother developed a dry cough and dyspnea and other symptoms characteristic of *P. carinii* pneumonia, including extensive pulmonary infiltrates on chest X-ray. Less than 1 week after presentation, she died. Postmortem exam revealed organisms consistent with *P. carinii*. Two days later, the father was admitted to the hospital with symptoms similar to those experienced by his wife; 8 days later, he succumbed to *P. carinii* pneumonia, established by identification of organisms at autopsy. This outbreak was curious for a number reasons. The mother and daughter were immunologically intact, and the father, although diagnosed with leukemia, was experiencing a remission and was in good health until presenting with the symptoms of *P. carinii* pneumonia. Both the mother and father had histologically documented pneumocystosis. The daughter survived and had not undergone any diagnostic procedure to recover organisms, so her diagnosis of *P. carinii* pneumonia was presumptive, but likely; she also had diffuse bilateral pulmonary infiltrates on chest X-ray. The virulence of the disease in this setting and its apparently highly contagious presentation mark this outbreak as unusual, since pneumocystosis is usually confined to severely immunocompromised hosts. Another unusual feature of this outbreak is the likelihood that the daughter introduced the infection into the family, yet was not immunologically compromised herself.

Reports of unusual clusters involving several patients have been reported in sufficient frequency to suggest that direct transmission among susceptible individuals is a significant way to contract the infection. Eleven cases of *P. carinii* pneumonia occurred within a 3-month period in 1975 at Memorial Hospital in New York in patients with leukemia, lymphoma, or other cancers (52). This rise in cases was found to differ at a significant level from other 3-month increments, but information on other infections was not reported nor was the chemotherapeutic regimen, which may have increased the susceptibility to opportunistic infections. The lack of an epidemiological marker made it impossible to trace the source of the outbreak.

The intensity of chemotherapy was linked to the incidence of pneumocystosis in two studies. In the first study, 10 cases were reported in children with acute lymphoblastic leukemia at the James Whitcomb Riley Hospital for Children in Indianapolis (53). Cases were distributed throughout the year with no more than three reported cases per month. The rate of infection was higher among children receiving more intensive chemotherapy. It is interesting to note that physicians in close contact with the patients had higher antibody titers to the organism than other staff members or family members. At St. Jude's Children's Research Hospital in Memphis, postmortem examination of 827 children revealed 19 cases of *P. carinii* pneumonia (2.3%), 17 of which were diagnosed between 1968–1969 (54). More intensive chemotherapy was associated with the incidence of pneumonia. In 1978 an outbreak of *P. carinii* pneumonia was reported at Milwaukee Children's Hospital (55). There, 11 cases were diagnosed in children with underlying malignancies between January 1974 and April 1977, without a significant clustering of cases in any one month. Adoption of more intensive chemotherapy modeled after regimens used by St. Jude's was thought to be coincident with *P. carinii* pneumonia.

In a more recent study, the incidence of pneumocystosis was associated with the type and intensity of chemotherapy. In 1986, Browne et al. reported a higher incidence of the infection in patients receiving ProMACE-CytaBOM (3/37), which includes cytarabine and bleomycin, as compared to those receiving ProMACE-MOPP (0/37) (56). As in the other studies discussed, the source of infection could not be determined as exogenous or as a reactivation of latent infection.

Direct transmission of *P. carinii* has been suggested by a few reported cases. In 1990, Goesch et al. (57) described an apparent transfer of the infection from one leukemic patient with clinical infection to another in a hospital in Hamburg, Germany. The first individual displayed few characteristic symptoms of *P. carinii* pneumonia, except that a chest X-ray showed diffuse bilateral infiltrations. Bronchoalveolar lavage produced no *P. carinii*. Fifty-eight days after hospitalization and chemotherapy, patient 1 expired. Autopsy findings revealed *P. carinii* pneumonia. Patient 2 had shared a room with patient 1 for 14 days. After chemotherapy, patient 2 went into remission, but 50 days after the first patient's death, he developed pneumonia concurrent with marrow aplasia. Bronchoalveolar lavage produced *P. carinii* organisms and he recovered after treatment with intravenous pentamidine treatment.

Similar to the case reported by Goesch et al., Brazinsky and Phillips reported the potential transmission of *P. carinii* from one lymphoma patient to his hospital roommate (58). The first patient had pulmonary symptoms on admission and *P. carinii* organisms were found at autopsy. Patient 1 share the room for 5 weeks with the second patient, who had received radiation therapy. The second patient developed pneumonia and *P. carinii* were found in the lung tissue at autopsy. Since both patients shared the same room and experienced the infection within the same relatively short time period, transmission was suggested, but reactivation of latent organisms could not be ruled out.

Persuasive evidence for the transmission of *P. carinii* in a susceptible population is provided in a report of five cases of *P. carinii* pneumonia among renal transplant recipients (59). The cases occurred within a 22-month period in the transplant patients undergoing treatment for acute graft rejection. The renal transplant patients shared a common outpatient room with AIDS patients, which was thought to have been the site of transmission. This concept was supported by a case-control study that implied that the infected renal cases had more contact with AIDS patients with *P. carinii* than the uninfected renal transplant recipients.

Unlike the outbreaks of pneumocystosis in the populations of susceptible, immunosuppressed patients, Jacobs et al. describe the occurrence of *P. carinii* in individuals without identifiable risk factors or severely depressed immune states (60). No underlying malignancies were detected in any of five elderly hospitalized patients at the New York Hospital–Cornell Medical Center who developed *P. carinii* pneumonia during their stay. Although numbers of T and B lymphocytes as well as T-cell subsets were normal or slightly below normal, all three of the patients tested did have decreased ability to respond to T-cell lectin, phytohemagglutinin, and T-cell-dependent B-cell mitogen, pokeweed mitogen. Therefore, most patients had a slight immune deficiency and were not totally immunologically intact. Of note is the small number of organisms recovered in the BALF. Prior to AIDS, the presence of low numbers of organisms in respiratory secretions was considered diagnostic for the pneumonia, and the presentation of *P. carinii* pneumonia in this cluster may be more like the pre-AIDS pneumocystosis than that form seen in AIDS patients. There has been one report of histopathologically detectable *P. carinii* in respiratory secretions of an apparently healthy adult (14), but recent studies employing the exquisitely sensitive technique of PCR did not find any evidence of the organism in healthy adults. However, Leigh et al. could detect PCR product in some patients who had received antirejection therapy for organ transplants (15), and Lipschik et al. (16) found that some HIV-positive patients produced PCR products without apparent infection. When 5/6 and 9/10 of these patients, in the respective studies, did not go on to develop fulminant infection, they hypothesized that immunosuppressed individuals could be colonized with the organism. Thus, this colonization only rarely progressed to clinical infection. In keeping with this hypothesis, perhaps the decreased immune function of the elderly patients permitted a pseudoinfection of *P. carinii* analogous to the apparent colonization of the transplant patients.

Interpretation of transmission of infection suggested by the clustering of cases described above and the evidence for transitory colonization is flawed by a lack of epidemiological markers. Without such tools it is impossible to document transmission patterns: acquired infection versus reactivation of latent organisms. Complicating our understanding of these apparent outbreaks is insufficient information in the many cases that have been reported. All too frequently, data are presented without case controls or denominator populations at risk, leading to speculation or inaccurate conclusions.

As we enter the second decade of AIDS, it is imperative that we begin to focus on the characterization of *P. carinii* isolates. The occurrence of the infection in the elderly patients as well as the increase of disseminated infections may herald a change in the genetic makeup of some organisms (61). The strong suggestion of person-to-person transmission among susceptible populations from infected sources suggests that a reconsideration of hospital policy for control of this infection may be warranted (62). Currently, isolation is not recommended for patients with *P. carinii* infection although there have been recommendations for such action (61,62). Some hope for isolate characterization lies in basic research presently being conducted (15,16,24,25,28,38). Using the rat infection as a paradigm, it appears likely that human *P. carinii* will have strain variation detectable by electrophoretic karyotyping (28,63) and further sequence differences will be revealed by application of PCR technology (28,38). With these tools, we can then begin to address the questions of transmission and epidemiology.

References

1. Barton EG Jr, Campbell G. *Pneumocystis carinii* in lungs of rats treated with cortisone acetate. Ultrastructural observations relating to the life cycle. Am J Pathol 1969; 54:209.
2. Campbell WG Jr. Ultrastructure of *Pneumocystis* in human lung: life cycle of human pneumocystosis. Arch Pathol 1972; 93:312.
3. Matsumoto Y, Yoshida Y. Sporogony in *Pneumocystis carinii*: synaptonemal complexes and meiotic nuclear divisions observed in precysts. J Protozool 1984; 31:420.
4. Matsumoto Y, Yoshida Y. Advances in *Pneumocystis* biology. Parasitol Today 1986; 5:137.
5. Vossen MEMH, Beckers PJA, Meuwissen JHE, Stadhouders AM. Developmental biology of *Pneumocystis carinii* and alternative view on the life cycle of the parasite. Z Parasitenkd 1978; 55:101.
6. Cushion MT, Ruffolo JJ, Walzer PD. Analysis of the developmental stages of *Pneumocystis carinii*, in vitro. Lab Invest 1988; 58:324.
7. Hendley JO, Weller TH. Activation and transmission in rats of infection with *Pneumocystis*. Proc Soc Exp Biol Med 1971; 137:1401–1404.
8. Walzer PD, Schnelle V, Armstrong, D, Rosen PP. Nude mouse: a new experimental model for *Pneumocystis carinii* infection. Science 1977; 197:177–179.

9. Hughes WT. Natural habitat and mode of transmission in: *Pneumocystis carinii* pneumonitis, Vol I. Boca Raton, FL: CRC Press, 1987:97–105.
9a. Hughes WT. Geographic distribution. In: *Pneumocystis carinii* Pneumonitis, Vol I. Boca Raton, FL: CRC Press, 1987:33–57.
10. Hughes, WT. Natural mode of acquisition for de novo infection with *Pneumocystis carinii*. J Infect Dis 1982; 145:842–848.
11. Hughes WT, Bartley DL, Smith BM. A natural source of infection due to *Pneumocystis carinii*. J Infect Dis 1983; 147:595.
12. Soulez B, Palluault F, Cesbron J-Y, Dei-Cas E, Capron A, Camus D. Introduction of *Pneumocystis carinii* in a colony of SCID mice. J Protozool 1991; 38:123S–125S.
13. Cushion MT, Stringer JR, Walzer PD. Cellular and molecular biology of *Pneumocystis carinii*. Int Rev Cytol 1991; 131:59–107.
14. Stiller RA, Paradis IL, Dauber JH. Subclinical pneumonitis due to *Pneumocystis carinii* in a young adult with elevated antibody titons to Epstein-Barr virus. J Infect Dis 1992; 166:926–930.
15. Leigh TR, Wakefield AE, Peters SE, Hopkin JM, Collins JV. Comparisons of DNA amplification and immunofluorescence for detecting *Pneumocystis carinii* in patients receiving immunosuppressive therapy. Transplantation 1992; 54:468–470.
16. Lipschik GY, Gill VJ, Lundgren JD, Andrawis VA, Nelson NA, Nielsen JO, Ognibene FP, Kovacs JA. Improved diagnosis of *Pneumocystis carinii* infection by polymerase chain reaction on induced sputum and blood. Lancet 1992; 340:203–206.
17. Meuwissen JHETh, Tauber I, Leeuwenberg ADEM, Beckers PJA, Sieben M. Parasitologic and serologic observations of infection—*Pneumocystis* in humans. J Infect Dis 177; 136:43–49.
18. Pifer LL, Hughes WT, Stagno S, Woods D. *Pneumocystis carinii* infection: evidence for high prevalence in normal and immunosuppressed children. Pediatrics 1978; 61: 35–41.
19. Robinson JJ. Two cases of pneumocystosis. Observation in 203 adult autopsies. Arch Pathol 1961; 50:156–159.
20. Easterly, JA. *Pneumocystis carinii* in lungs of adults at autopsy. Am Rev Respir Dis 1968; 97:935–937.
21. Meuwissen JHE. Infections with *Pneumocystis carinii*. Natl Cancer Inst Monogr 1976; 43:133–136.
22. Sedaghatian MR, Singer DB. *Pneumocystis carinii* in children with malignant disease. Cancer 1972; 29:772–777.
23. Settnes OP, Genner J. *Pneumocystis carinii* in human lungs at autopsy. Scand J Infect Dis 1986; 18:489–496.
24. Wakefield AS, Pixley FJ, Banerji S, Sinclair K, Miller RF, Hopkin JM. Detection of *Pneumocystis carinii* with DNA amplification. Lancet 1990; 336:451–453.
25. Peters SE, Wakefield AE, Sinclair K, Millard PR, Hopkin JM. A search for *Pneumocystis carinii* in post mortem lungs by DNA amplification. J Pathol 1992; 166: 195–198.
26. Edman JC, Kovacs JA, Masur H, Santi DV, Elwood HJ, Sogin ML. Ribosomal RNA sequence shows *Pneumocystis carinii* to be a member of the fungi. Nature 1988; 334: 519–522.

27. Chagas C. Nova tripanomia zaea humana. Ueber eine neve trypano somiasis de menschen. Mem Inst Oswaldo Cruz 1909; 1:159–218.
28. Stringer JR, Stringer SL, Zhang J, Baughman R, Smulian AG, Cushion MT. Molecular genetic evidence that *Pneumocystis* from rats and humans are different species. 1992 (submitted).
29. Zhang J, Stringer JR. Cloning and characterization of an α-tubulin gene from *Pneumocystis carinii* derived from laboratory rats. GENE (in press).
30. Matsumoto Y, Yamada M, Amagai T. Yeast glucan of *Pneumocystis carinii* cyst wall: an excellent target for chemotherapy. J Protozool 1991; 38:6S–7S.
31. Pixley FJ, Wakefield AE, Banerji S, Hopkin JM. Mitochondrial gene sequences show fungal homology for *Pneumocystis carinii* pneumonia. Mol Microbiol 1991; 5:1347–1351.
32. Wakefield AE, Peters SE, Banerji S, Bridge PD, Hall GS, Hawksworth DL, Guiver LA, Allen AG, Hopkin JM. *Pneumocystis carinii* shows DNA homology with the ustomycetous red yeast fungi. Mol Microbiol 1992; 6(14):1903–1911.
33. Gigliotti F. Host species-specific antigenic variation of a mannosylated surface glycoprotein of *Pneumocystis carinii*. J Infect Dis 1992; 165:329–336.
34. Graves DC, McNabb SJ, Ivey MH, Worley MA. Development and characterization of monoclonal antibodies to *Pneumocystis carinii*. Infect Immun 1986; 51:125–133.
35. Kovacs JA, Halpern JL, Swann JC, Moss J, Parrillo JE, Masur H. Identification of antigens and antibodies specific for *Pneumocystis carinii*. J Immunol 1988; 140: 2023–2031.
36. Walzer PD, Linke MJ. A comparison of the antigenic characteristics of rat and human *Pneumocystis carinii* by immunoblotting. J Immunol 1987; 138:2257–2265.
37. Gigliotti F, Ballou LR, Hughes WT, Mosley BD. Purification and initial characterization of a ferret *Pneumocystis carinii* surface antigen. J Infect Dis 1988; 158:848–854.
38. Sinclair K, Wakefield AE, Banerji S, Hopkin JM. *Pneumocystis carinii* organisms derived from rat and human hosts are genetically distinct. Mol Biochem Parasit 1991; 45:183–184.
39. Settnes DP, Lodal J. Prevalence of *Pneumocystis carinii*. Delanoe & Delanoe, 1912, in rodents in Denmark. Nord Vet Med 1980; 32:17–27.
40. Bazaz GR, Manfredi OL, Howard RG, Claps AA. *Pneumocystis carinii* pneumonia in three full-term siblings. J Pediatr 1970; 76:767–769.
41. Pavlica F. The first observation of congenital *Pneumocystis* pneumonia in a fully developed stillborn child. Ann Paediatr 1967; 198:177–184.
42. Dutz W, Post C, Vessal K, Kohout E. Endemic infantile *Pneumocystis carinii* infection: the Shiraz Study. Nat Cancer Inst Monogr 1976; 43:31–40.
43. Pifer LL, Latuada CP, Edwards CC, Woods DR, Owens DR. *Pneumocystis carinii* infection in germ-free rats: implications for human patients. Diagn Microbiol Infect Dis 1984; 2:23–36.
44. Poelma FG. *Pneumocystis carinii* infections in zoo animals. Ztschr Parasitenkrankh 1975; 46:61–68.
45. Cushion MT, Ruffolo JJ, Linke MJ, Walzer PD. *Pneumocystis carinii*: growth variables and estimates in the A549 and WI-38 VA13 human cell lines. Exp Parasitol 1985; 60:43–54.

46. Walzer PD, Perl DP, Krogstad DJ, Rawson PG, Schultz MG. *Pneumocystis carinii* pneumonia in the United States. Epidemiologic, diagnostic, and clinical features. Ann Intern Med 1974; 80:83–93.
47. Vigdorth EM. Epidemiology of *Pneumocystis carinii* pneumonia at the University of Cincinnati AIDS Treatment Center 1986–1989. Doctoral dissertation, University of Cincinnati College of Medicine, Department of Environmental Health, 1992.
48. Hoover DR, Graham NMH, Bacellar H, Schrager LK, Kaslow R, Visscher B, Murphy R, Anderson R, Saah A. Epidemiologic patterns of upper respiratory illness and *Pneumocystis carinii* pneumonia in homosexual men. Am Rev Respir Dis 1991; 144:756–759.
49. Miller RF, Grant AD, Foley NM. Seasonal variation in presentation of *Pneumocystis carinii* pneumonia. Lancet 1992; 339:747–748.
50. Vanhems P, Hirschel B, Morabia A. Seasonal incidence of *Pneumocystis carinii* pneumonia. Lancet 1992; 339:1182.
51. Watanabe JM, Chinchinian H, Weitz C, McIlvanie SK. *Pneumocystis carinii* pneumonia in a family. JAMA 1965; 193:685–686.
52. Singer C, Armstrong D, Rosen PP, Schottenfeld D. *Pneumocystis carinii* pneumonia: a cluster of eleven cases. Ann Intern Med 1975; 82:772–777.
53. Ruebush TK, Weinstein RA, Baehner RL, Wolff D, Barlett M, Gonzales-Crussi F, Sulzer A, Schultz MG. An outbreak of *Pneumocystis* pneumonia in children with acute lymphocytic leukemia. Am J Dis Child 1978; 132:143–148.
54. Perera DR, Western KA, Johnson HD, Johnson WW, Schultz MG, Ahers PV. *Pneumocystis carinii* pneumonia in a hospital for children. JAMA 1970; 214:1074–1078.
55. Chusid MJ, Heyrman KA. An outbreak of *Pneumocystis carinii* at a pediatric hospital. Pediatrics 1978; 62:1031–1035.
56. Browne MJ, Hubbard SM, Longo DL, Fisher R, Wesley R, Ihde DC, Young RC, Pizzo PA. Excess prevalence of *Pneumocystis carinii* pneumonia in patients treated for lymphoma with combination chemotherapy. Ann Intern Med 1986; 104:338–344.
57. Goesch TR, Gotz G, Stellbrinck KH, Albrecht H, Weh HJ, Hossfeld DK. Possible transfer of *Pneumocystis carinii* between immunodeficient patients. Lancet 1990; 336:627.
58. Brazinsky JH, Phillips JE. *Pneumocystis* pneumonia transmission between patients with lymphoma. JAMA 1969; 209:1527.
59. Chave J, David S, Wauters J, Mille G, Franciolo P. Transmission of *Pneumocystis carinii* from AIDS patients to other immunosuppressed patients: a cluster of *Pneumocystis carinii* pneumonia in renal transplant recipients. AIDS 1991; 5:927–932.
60. Jacobs JL, Libby DM, Winters RA, Gelmont DM, Fried ED, Hartman BJ, Laurence J. A cluster of *Pneumocystis carinii* pneumonia in adults without predisposing illnesses. N Engl J Med 1991; 324:246–250.
61. Walzer PD. *Pneumocystis carinii*—new clinical spectrum? N Engl J Med 1991; 324: 263–265.
62. Giron JA, Martinez S, Walzer PD. Should inpatients with *Pneumocystis carinii* be isolated? Lancet 1982; 2:46.
63. Cushion MT, Zhang J, Kaselis M, Stringer SL, Stringer JR. Evidence for two species of *Pneumocystis* coinfecting laboratory rats. J Clin Microbiol (in press).

8

Serological Studies of *Pneumocystis carinii* Infection

A. GEORGE SMULIAN and PETER D. WALZER

Cincinnati Veterans Affairs Medical Center
and University of Cincinnati College of Medicine
Cincinnati, Ohio

I. Introduction

Serology has been used in various infectious diseases for epidemiological and diagnostic purposes. Over the past three decades, the serological investigation of *Pneumocystis carinii* infection has evoked much interest, although it has been unable to fulfill such diagnostic or epidemiological roles. Studies have demonstrated a high prevalence of antibodies in normal populations. Thus far, workers have been unable to identify antibody responses of predictive, diagnostic, or pathogenetic importance. It is difficult to compare many of the studies because of differences in the techniques and antigen preparations used. These problems should be resolved as purified antigens become available from biochemical purification and molecular cloning of recombinant antigens. Consequently, serological investigation as an epidemiological tool should see significant progress in the future. This review will present the published results according to the technique used, to allow most appropriate comparison (Table 1).

Table 1 Serological Studies on *P. carinii* Infection

Ref.	Antigen	Subjects		Seropositivity		Comments
		Cases	Controls	Cases (%)	Controls (%)	
Complement fixation test						
Barta, 1969 (1)		119	120	90	3	Immunocompetent children
Indirect immunofluorescent antibody assay						
Nowoslawski and Brzosko, 1964 (2)	Human lung section (HLS)	6	50	100	16.7	Infants (epidemic type)
Brzosko et al., 1967 (3)	HLS	37		100		IgM antibodies in younger infants, IgG in older
Norman and Kagan, 1972 (4)	huPc cysts	89	85 contacts 50 controls	46	14 contacts 0 controls	United States, immunosuppressed children and adults
Norman and Kagan, 1973 (5)	huPc and rPc cysts, soluble Pc Ags	191	109 contacts 74 controls	44.5	7.3 contacts 1.4 controls	Titer > 1:8 positive; Similar results with huPc and rPc
Merwissen et al., 1977 (7)	huPc cysts	29	594	71	71.5 controls	43.2% of children antibody positive by age 2 years
Pifer et al., 1978 (6)	rPc cysts from tissue culture	31	120 children	71	64 controls	97% of patients seropositive during disease or convalescence
Sheperd et al., 1977 (9)	HLS	23	31 contacts 60 controls	86.9	55 contacts 57 controls	Antibody titers of patients elevated or rising
Maddison et al., 1984 (14)	rPc cysts	32	36 AIDS controls 135 non-AIDS	31	41 AIDS controls 25.9 non-AIDS	AIDS patients; ELISA also performed

Ref.	Antigen	Cases	Controls	% Cases	% Controls	Comments
Tamabe et al., 1985 (27)	rPc cysts	13	100 controls, 25 non-Pc pneumonia, 145 children	100 (≥ 1:40)	100, 84	Mean titers higher in patients with Pc pneumonia
Gerrard et al., 1987 (10)	HLS (parafin sections)				48	Older children had higher titers
Hofmann et al., 1988 (8)	huPc cysts	15	21 AIDS controls, 31 non AIDS	80	57 AIDS controls, 37.5 non-AIDS	IgM antibodies also detected
Chatterton et al., 1989 (11)	rPc cysts	24	148 controls, 464 patients with clinical symptoms	58.3	8.8 normal controls, 13.4 clinically ill	IgM not detected in confirmed cases
Burns et al., 1990 (12)	Rat lung sections (frozen)	38 AIDS, 37 non-AIDS	40 normal	63.2 AIDS, 70.2 non-AIDS	80	Serial testing performed on some patients.

ELISA

Ref.	Antigen	Cases	Controls	Comments
Maddison et al., 1982 (13)	Urea solubilized rPc	88 proved, 38 suspected	153 contacts, 105 controls, 49 pneumonia	High prevalence of antibodies; patients and controls similar
Maddison et al., 1984 (14)	rPc cysts	32	135 controls, 36 AIDS pts	
Nielsen et al., 1988 (15)	huPc sonicate	90		Good correlation of IFA and ELISA; ELISA more sensitive
Pifer et al., 1988 (16)	rPc	47 pediatric AIDS cases	25 children	No diagnostic value; mean titer higher in cases than controls
Wakefield et al., 1990 (17)	rPc sonicate		150 Britons (3 mo–40 yrs), 150 Gambians (6 mo–40 yrs)	70% seropositivity in both groups; no detectable IgM or IgA

Table 1 (Continued)

		Subjects		
Ref.	Antigen	Cases	Controls	Comments
Lundgren et al., 1991 (18)	huPc—purified gp95 antigen	30	27 infants 8 adults controls 16 AIDS controls	33% of cases positive, 23% indeterminate; 2% positive, 2 % indeterminate among controls
Lundgren et al., 1992 (19)	huPc—purified gp95 antigen	76	53 HIV-infected 20 HIV-negative	66% positivity in HIV-infected cases with Pc pneumonia vs 34% in HIV-infected cases without Pc pneumonia
Western blot				
Kovacs et al., 1988 (20)	huPc and rPc	10 non-AIDS 9 AIDS	8 children 8 adults 6 AIDS controls	12.5% positivity in children; 97% positive among adult controls and cases
Peglow et al., 1990 (21)	huPc	77	95 children 10 adult controls 44 non-AIDS (high-risk) 137 HIV	
Smulian et al., 1992 (22)	huPc		948 individuals	76.7% seropositivity overall in five geographic regions

Pc, *Pneumocystis carinii*; hu, human; r, rat; Ags, antigens.

II. Complement Fixation Assays

Barta reviewed the results of complement fixation assays performed on 1300 sera collected between 1952 and 1965 (1). These samples were from 119 histologically proved fatal cases and 120 control cases with pneumonitis from other causes among immunocompetent children. Complement-fixing antibodies were found in 90% of the 119 children with histologically proved *P. carinii* pneumonitis and in only 3% of the control cases of pneumonitis from other causes. Among children with clinical suspected disease, a seropositivity rate of between 75 and 85% was reported.

III. Indirect Immunofluorescent Assay

Indirect immunofluorescent antibody (IFA) assays have been used in most studies on humoral responses to *P. carinii*. This technique, which is dependent on the expertise of the operator in recognizing *P. carinii* organisms, has good specificity if fluorescence is recorded to cyst forms only. An initial study by Nowoslawski and Brzosko used formalin-fixed sections of infected lung, as the antigen, in studies of children with the epidemic form of pneumocystosis (2). This, and later studies by the same authors, concluded that IFA was as reliable as complement fixation (3). Later work demonstrated that IFA was superior in immunocompromised individuals, since complement-fixing antibodies were often not detectable. In the Polish studies, all 43 infants with documented or clinically suspected pneumocystosis demonstrated antibodies to *P. carinii*. When these cases were segregated by age, IgM antibodies alone were found in those under 8 weeks, combinations of IgM and IgG antibodies in some children 3–6 months old, and only IgG responses were detected those children older than 6 months of age. Antibodies to *P. carinii* were detected in only 2 of 37 asymptomatic controls younger than 2 years and 3 of 13 infants with mild respiratory symptoms.

Numerous studies of antibodies to *P. carinii* measured by IFA have been reported from the United States. With rat- or human-derived *P. carinii* prepared from homogenized infected lungs, Norman and Kagan detected anti-*P. carinii* antibodies in 44% of confirmed and clinically suspected cases of *P. carinii* pneumonia, whereas such antibodies were detected in only 7.3% of healthy contacts and 1.4% of healthy noncontacts (4,5). Antibody titers were lower among controls ($<$1:20) than among confirmed cases of *P. carinii* pneumonia ($>$1:20). A further study by this group found 61.1% of patients without *P. carinii* pneumonia had titers of anti-*P. carinii* antibodies higher than 1:8. This study failed to confirm their prior association of titers of 1:20 or higher and active disease. The antibodies detected in the healthy controls and patients with sporadic *P. carinii* infections were of the IgG class.

With use of rat-derived *P. carinii* cysts propagated in tissue culture as antigen, Pifer detected anti-*P. carinii* antibodies in 19% of infants younger than 1 year of age (6). The proportion demonstrating antibodies at a titer of 1:16 or higher, had increased to 83% by 4 years of age. This suggests that *P. carinii* is an ubiquitous organism, and exposure occurs in early childhood.

In the Netherlands, Merwissen, using a pronase-treated cyst suspension from infected human lung, demonstrated that most children (>75%) developed antibodies (≥1:40) to *P. carinii* within the first 2 years of life (7). In Denmark, Hofmann detected anti-*Pneumocystis* antibodies (IgM or IgG) in 72% of healthy volunteers and in 13% of acquired immunodeficiency syndrome (AIDS) patients with *P. carinii* pneumonia (8).

In the United Kingdom, Sheperd studied 23 cases of proved or clinically suspected pneumocystosis among patients of an oncology unit (9). In the group, 10 patients demonstrated titers higher than 1:32, 5 patients showed a fivefold rise in antibody titer, 3 converted from negative to a 1:8 titer, and 1 proved case remained negative. Among 91 controls, 56% demonstrated antibodies, with the highest titer being 1:32. A subsequent British study, using the same infected human lung sections as antigen, detected antibodies at a titer of 1:8 or higher in 48% in nonimmunosuppressed children (10). A trend for more of the older children to have higher levels of antibody was noted.

Two further IFA studies, reported from Scotland, used rat-derived *P. carinii* an antigen. Chatterton detected antibodies at a titer of 1:8 or higher in 58.3% of 24 immunosuppressed patients with histologically proved or strongly suspected cases of *P. carinii* pneumonia (11). They detected antibodies in only 8.8% of normal controls and 13.4% of 464 patients symptomatic with pulmonary symptoms or fever. No IgM antibodies were detected in the sera from the case or control groups. Burns studied immunosuppressed patients (AIDS, lymphoid and myeloid malignancies) and controls by IFA to frozen sections of *P. carinii*-infected rat lung (12). They detected antibodies in 63.2% of AIDS patients, 70.2% of non-AIDS patients, and 80% of controls.

IV. Enzyme Immunoassay

Numerous enzyme immunoassays (EIA) have been developed to detect and quantitate anti-*P. carinii* antibodies. As opposed to IFA, for which fluorescence is visualized on the *P. carinii* organisms, the specificity of an EIA is dependent on the purity of the antigen preparation used to coat the well. Most published reports have used intact organisms or extracts (sonicates or urea extracts) of organisms derived from lung homogenates. These preparations almost certainly contain non-*P. carinii* antigens in addition to specific *P. carinii* antigens. The validity of results, therefore, are predicated on the use of rigorous and extensive controls. This problem will be overcome with the availability of purified native antigens and recombinant antigens.

Similar antibody levels were detected in serum from patients and normal controls in an initial study performed by Maddison, who used an urea extract of rat-derived *P. carinii* extract as antigen (13). The assay confirmed the high prevalence of antibodies to *P. carinii*, but demonstrated no diagnostic value of such an assay. A subsequent study, by the same group of investigators, detected antibodies in 47% of AIDS patients with *P. carinii* pneumonia (14). Positive ELISA reactions were observed in 56% of AIDS patients without clinical evidence of *P. carinii* pneumonia and in 48 and 50% of healthy homosexual and heterosexual controls, respectively.

A comparison of IFA and EIA was performed by Nielsen on 90 specimens, using human-derived *P. carinii* organisms (15). Results from the EIA correlated well with IFA results, and the EIA was noted to be more sensitive. Pifer studied 47 pediatric AIDS patients and 25 control children and demonstrated no difference in the titer of antibodies to *P. carinii*, although patients with documented *P. carinii* pneumonia had higher antibody titers (16). With a sonicate of rat-derived organisms as antigen, Wakefield detected IgG antibodies in 70% of individuals from Britain and Gambia (17). No IgM or IgA responses were observed in either group.

In an attempt to overcome the problem of using crude antigen preparations or whole *P. carinii* organisms, Lundgren used purified gp95 antigen, a major surface antigen of human-derived *P. carinii*, in an ELISA assay (18). Among their control group, 98% demonstrated no antibodies to *P. carinii*, whereas 2% had indeterminate antibody levels. In AIDS and non-AIDS patients with a history of *P. carinii* pneumonia, 33% had antibody levels deemed positive, 44% were antibody-negative, and in a further 23% antibodies were of an indeterminate level. This study was the first to use a purified *P. carinii* antigen preparation. Subsequently, these authors have examined responses to this purified antigen in AIDS patients with pneumonia (19). Rising titers of antibodies were detected in 43% of patients with *P. carinii* pneumonia, but in only 3% of the patients in whom another etiological agent was identified.

V. Immunoblotting

Many workers have used Western blotting to identify and characterize the major antigens of rat- and human-derived *P. carinii*. Similar techniques have also been used to identify serological responses to specific *P. carinii* antigens. Because only responses to specific *P. carinii* antigens are reported, the purity of the antigen preparation used is not as critical as with other methods. Kovacs found specific anti-*P. carinii* antibodies in 97% of cases and adult controls (20); among children, only 12.5% had detectable antibodies.

Peglow studied the serum of children and adults, in both low- and high-risk groups, for *P. carinii* pneumonia by both IFA and immunoblotting (21). Antibodies to the 40-kDa antigen were the most common antibody response detected in all groups. Antibodies to any *P. carinii* antigen were found in 94% of children by 30 months of age. Antibody to *P. carinii* were found in 74% of adults, but were detected more frequently in healthy controls than in immunosuppressed patients (71 vs 48%, $p < 0.05$).

In a study of 948 individuals from five geographic regions, Smulian et al. detected antibodies to any major *P. carinii* antigen in 76.7% of individuals (Fig. 1) (22). The prevalence of antibodies was similar in all regions, confirming the ubiquitous nature of the organism. Antibodies to the 30–40-kDa antigen were the most commonly detected antibody response.

Different antibody responses were noted in different regions of the world. The most notable differences were in antibody responses to the high molecular mass antigens, suggesting exposure to antigenically different strains of *P. carinii* in different regions.

A 55-kDa antigen of rat-derived *P. carinii* has been cloned and shown to share epitopes with the 30–40-kDa antigen of human-derived *P. carinii* (23). With this antigen, antibodies were detected in 6 of 20 normal individuals and 5 of 20 human immunodeficiency virus (HIV)-infected patients. In patients with multiple episodes of *P. carinii* pneumonia, the presence of antibodies varied over time. This variation included the development of antibodies to the recombinant antigen with a

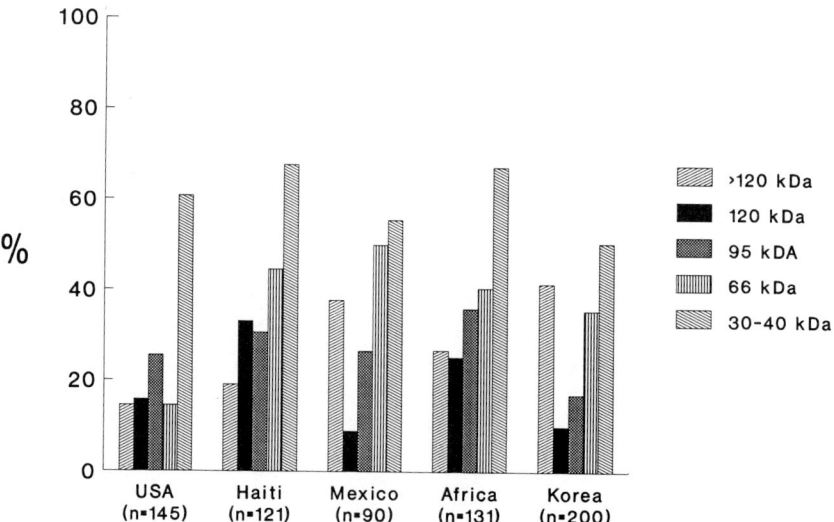

Figure 1 Responses to specific *P. carinii* antigens among HIV-negative samples from different geographic regions. Prevalence of antibodies to the major *P. carinii* antigens is shown among HIV-negative specimens from each geographic region. Regional differences in antibody prevalence was most marked to high molecular mass antigens. (From Ref. 22.)

second episode of *P. carinii* pneumonia or a gradual decrease in the antibody response.

VI. Serology of *Pneumocystis carinii* Outbreaks

During outbreaks of interstitial plasma cell pneumonia in Central Europe, Barta et al. studied antibody responses among patients and hospital personnel by the complement fixation test (1). Complement-fixing antibodies were detected in 75–95% of infected infants, 15% of hospital personnel in the institutions where outbreaks occurred, and only 0–3% of the general healthy population. Similar findings were reported by Ruebush et al. following a cluster of cases of *P. carinii* pneumonia among children with acute lymphocytic leukemia (24). Antibody titers by IFA were higher in children with *P. carinii* pneumonia than in the other individuals studied. Significantly more physicians and nurses directly exposed to the patients were seropositive than other nurses and physicians in the hospital. In a cluster of cases among oncology cases in New York, Singer et al. detected significantly higher titers of antibody to *P. carinii* in two physicians closely associated with the cases than in other hospital personnel (25). Antibody titers in a group of exposed hospital workers rose progressively over time to develop significantly higher levels than other hospital workers in a study performed in New York by Giron et al. (26).

VII. Conclusion

These studies have determined that *P. carinii* is a ubiquitous organism to which most of the population is exposed in early childhood. As a result, the mere presence of anti-*P. carinii* antibodies is of little diagnostic or epidemiological value. Changes in humoral responses do, however, appear to occur in the setting of clinical disease. By using purified or recombinant antigens, it is hoped that subsets of antibodies involved in the humoral response will be identified. These may serve to enhance our understanding of the pathogenesis of the disease and may be of diagnostic or prognostic value.

References

1. Barta K. Ann Int Med 1969; 70–235.
2. Nowoslawski A, Brzosko WJ. Indirect immunofluorescence test for serodiagnosis of *Pneumocystis carinii* infection. Bull Acad Pol Sci 1964; 12:143–147.
3. Brzosko WJ, Madalinski K, Nowoslawski A. Fluorescent antibody and immunoelectrophoretic evaluation of the immune reaction in children with pneumonia induced by *Pneumocystis carinii*. Exp Med Microbiol 1967; 19:397–405.

4. Norman L, Kagan IA. A preliminary report of an indirect fluorescent antibody test for detecting antibodies to cysts of *Pneumocystis carinii* in human sera. Am J Clin Pathol 1972; 58:170–176.
5. Norman L, Kagan IA. Some observations on the serology of *Pneumocystis carinii* infections in the United States. Infect Immun 1973; 8:317–321.
6. Pifer LL, Hughes WT, Stago S, Woods D. *Pneumocystis carinii* infection: evidence for high prevalence in normal and immunosuppressed children. Pediatrics 1978; 61:35–41.
7. Meuwissen JHE, Tauber I, Leeuwenberg ADE, Beckers PJA, Sieben M. Parasitologic and serologic observations of infection with *Pneumocystis* in humans. J Infect Dis 1977; 136:43–49.
8. Hofmann B., Nielsen PB, Odum N, Gerstoft J, Platz P, Ryder LP, Poulsen AG, Mathiesen L, Dickmeiss E, Norrild B, Andersen HK, Westergaard BF, Nielsen CM, Holten-Andersen W, Mojon M, Nielsen JO, Svejgaard A. Humoral and cellular responses to *Pneumocystis carinii*, CMV, and herpes simplex in patients with AIDS and in controls. Scand J Infect Dis 1988; 20:389–394.
9. Sheperd V, Jameson B, Knowles GK. *Pneumocystis carinii* pneumonitis: a serological study. J Clin Pathol 1979; 32:773–777.
10. Gerrard MP, Eden OB, Jameson B, Craft AW. Serological study of *Pneumocystis carinii* infection in the absence of immunosuppression. Arch Dis Child 1988; 62:177–179.
11. Chatterton JM, Joss AW, Williams H, Ho-Yen DO. *Pneumocystis carinii* antibody testing. J Clin Pathol 1989; 42:865–868.
12. Burns SM, Read JA, Yap PL, Brettle RP. Reduced concentrations of IgG antibodies to *Pneumocystis carinii* in HIV-infected patients during active *Pneumocystis carinii* infection and the possibility of passive immunisation. J Infect 1990; 20:33–39.
13. Maddison SE, Walls KW, Haverkos HW, Juranek DD. Evaluation of serologic tests for *Pneumocystis carinii* antibody and antigenemia in patients with acquired immunodeficiency syndrome. Diagn Microbiol Infect Dis 1984; 2:69–73.
14. Maddison SE, Hayes GV, Slemenda SB, Norman LG, Ivey MH. Detection of specific antibody by enzyme-linked immunosorbent assay and antigenemia by counterimmunoelectrophoresis in humans infected with *Pneumocystis carinii*. J Clin Microbiol 1982; 15:1036–1043.
15. Nielsen PB, Mojon M. Enzyme-linked immunosorbent assay compared with indirect immunofluorescence test for detection of *Pneumocystis carinii* specific immunoglobulins G, M, and A. APMIS 1988; 96:649–654.
16. Pifer LL, Woods DR, Edwards CC, Joyner RE, Anderson FJ, Arheart K. *Pneumocystis carinii* serologic study in pediatric acquired immunodeficiency syndrome. Am J Dis Child 1988; 142:36–39.
17. Wakefield AE, Stewart TJ, Moxon ER, Marsh K, Hopkin JN. Infection with *Pneumocystis carinii* is prevalent in healthy Gambian children. Trans R Soc Trop Med Hyg 1990; 84:800–802.
18. Lundgren B, Lipschik GY, Kovacs JA. Purification and characterization of a major human *Pneumocystis carinii* surface antigen. J Clin Invest 1991; 87:163–170.
19. Lundgren B, Lundgren JD, Nielsen T, Mathiesen L, Nielsen JO, Kovacs JA. Antibody

responses to a major *Pneumocystis carinii* antigen in human immunodeficiency virus-infected patients with and without *P. carinii* pneumonia. J Infect Dis 1992; 165:1151–1155.
20. Kovacs JA, Halpern JL, Swan JC, Moss J, Parrillo JE, Masur H. Identification of antigens and antibodies specific for *Pneumocystis carinii*. J Immunol 1988; 140:2023–2031.
21. Peglow SL, Smulian GA, Linke MJ, Crisler J, Phair JWM, Gold J, Armstrong D, Walzer PD. Serologic responses to specific *Pneumocystis carinii* antigens in health and disease. J Infect Dis 1990; 161:296–306.
22. Smulian AG, Sullivan DW, Linke MJ, Halsey NH, Quinn TC, MacPhail AP, Hernandez-Avila MA, Hong ST, Walzer PD. Geographic variation in humoral responses to *Pneumocystis carinii*. J Infect Dis (in press).
23. Smulian AG, Stringer JR, Linke MJ, Walzer PD. Isolation and characterization of a recombinant antigen of *Pneumocystis carinii*. Infect Immun 1992; 60:907–915.
24. Ruebush TK, Weinstein RA, Baehner RL, Wolff D, Bartlett M, Gonzales-Crussi F, Sulzer AJ, Schultz MG. An outbreak of pneumocystis pneumonia in children with acute lymphocytic leukemia. Am J Dis Child 1978; 132:143–148.
25. Singer C, Armstrong D, Rosen PP, Schottenfeld D. *Pneumocystis carinii* pneumonia: a cluster of eleven cases. Ann Intern Med 1975; 82:772–777.
26. Giron JA, Martinez S, Walzer PD. Should in patients with *Pneumocystis carinii* be isolated? Lancet 1982; 2:46.
27. Tanabe K, Furuta T, Ueda K, Tanaka H, Shimada K. Serological observations of *Pneumocystis carinii* infection in humans. J Clin Microbiol 1985; 22:1058–1060.

Part Three

PATHOPHYSIOLOGY

9

Pathological Features

WILLIAM D. TRAVIS

National Cancer Institute
National Institutes of Health
Bethesda, Maryland
and Armed Forces Institute of Pathology
Washington, D.C.

I. Introduction

The existence of *Pneumocystis carinii* was recognized eight decades ago by Chaga, who thought it was a form of trypanosoma (1). Shortly thereafter, Delanoe and Delanoe proved that it was a distinct organism (1). In subsequent years, it was found to be an important opportunistic pneumonia in immunocompromised hosts. However, over the past decade, owing to the acquired immunodeficiency syndrome (AIDS) epidemic, there has been an explosion of interest and publications on the subject of *P. carinii* pneumonia (PCP). As a result, the body of information about the pathology of PCP has expanded enormously (2–12). Despite intensive laboratory efforts, *P. carinii* has not yet been grown in culture, and it remains uncertain whether it should be classified as a fungus or as a parasite (1,13). Understanding the pathology remains important, despite the decreased number of lung biopsies required for the diagnosis of *P. carinii* pneumonia, owing to the sensitivity of bronchoscopic (14–16) and cytological techniques (17–23) in the examination of bronchoalveolar lavage (BAL) (24–28), bronchial wash (29,30), and sputum specimens (31,32).

This review will discuss the fascinating spectrum of unusual pathological features of pneumocystosis with emphasis on those features observed during the

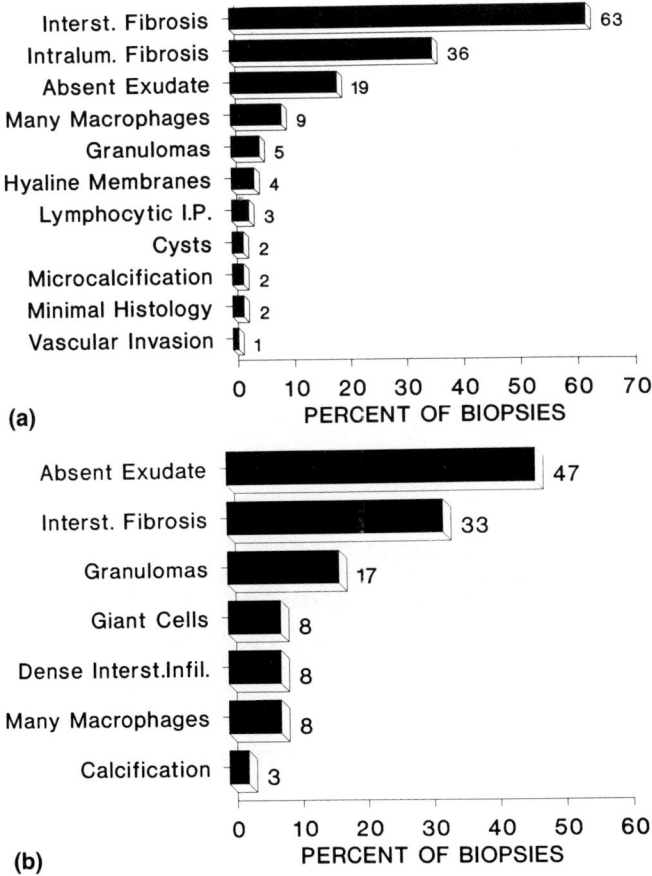

Figure 1 (a) Summary of unusual histological features of *P. carinii* pneumonia in patients with AIDS. Summarized from reference (3) (interst, interstitial; intralum, intraluminal; IP, interstitial pneumonitis). (b) Summary of unusual histological features of *P. carinii* pneumonia in patients without AIDS (33) (infil, infiltrate).

AIDS epidemic, including cysts, granulomas, vasculitis, and extrapulmonary dissemination. These features have been reviewed previously in patients with (Fig. 1a) (3) and without (Fig. 1b) (33) AIDS.

II. Classic Histopathology

The classic histopathological appearance of *P. carinii* pneumonia is characterized by a prominent eosinophilic foamy intra-alveolar exudate accompanied by a mild, interstitial pneumonitis (Fig. 2) (3,33). The pneumonitis is typically characterized by mild interstitial chronic inflammation and proliferation of type II pneumocytes.

The light microscopic diagnosis of *P. carinii* pneumonia requires identification of cysts of the organism within the alveolar exudate. The organisms are detected with special stains, such as the Gomori methenamine silver (GMS) or

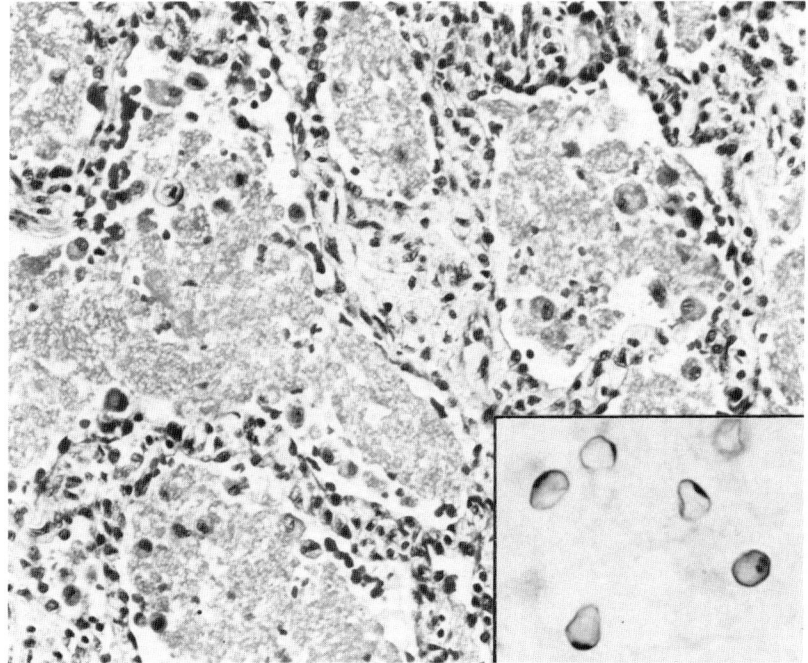

Figure 2 Typical histology of *P. carinii* pneumonia is characterized by prominent intra-alveolar, foamy, eosinophilic exudate (H&E ×250). (Insert) Multiple round to oval cysts of the organism with eccentrically located darkly stained foci are seen (Gomori methenamine silver ×1250).

toluidine blue. The cysts of *P. carinii* are uniform in size, measuring 5–7 μm. These structures easily collapse and may form curved shapes that have been compared to helmets, crescents, bananas, footballs, and gnome's hats (34). The cysts also frequently have darkly stained foci, which represent discoid thickenings of the capsule (35).

III. Unusual Histological Features

A. Diffuse Alveolar Damage

It is well recognized that diffuse alveolar damage occurs in pneumocystosis (3,36); however, the chronic organizing phase is more common than the acute exudative phase. The relative frequency of organizing diffuse alveolar damage is

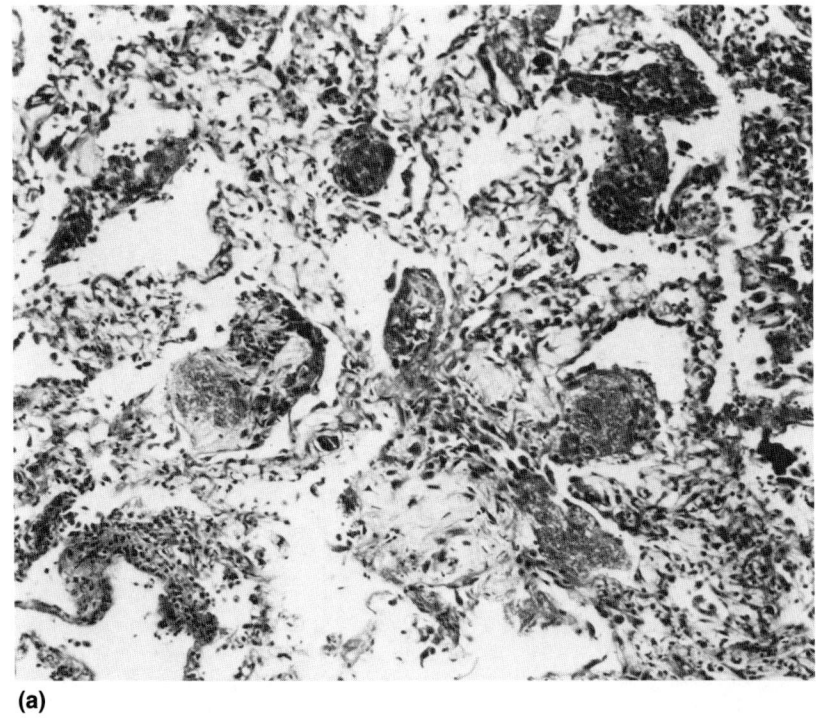

(a)

Figure 3 (a) The loose interstitial fibrosis in this biopsy reflects the organizing phase of diffuse alveolar damage. (b) This biopsy of resolving *P. carinii* pneumonia following therapy shows prominent intraluminal fibrosis with the pattern of organizing pneumonia similar to that seen in bronchiolitis obliterans with organizing pneumonia (BOOP) (a,b: H&E ×125). (From Ref. 3.)

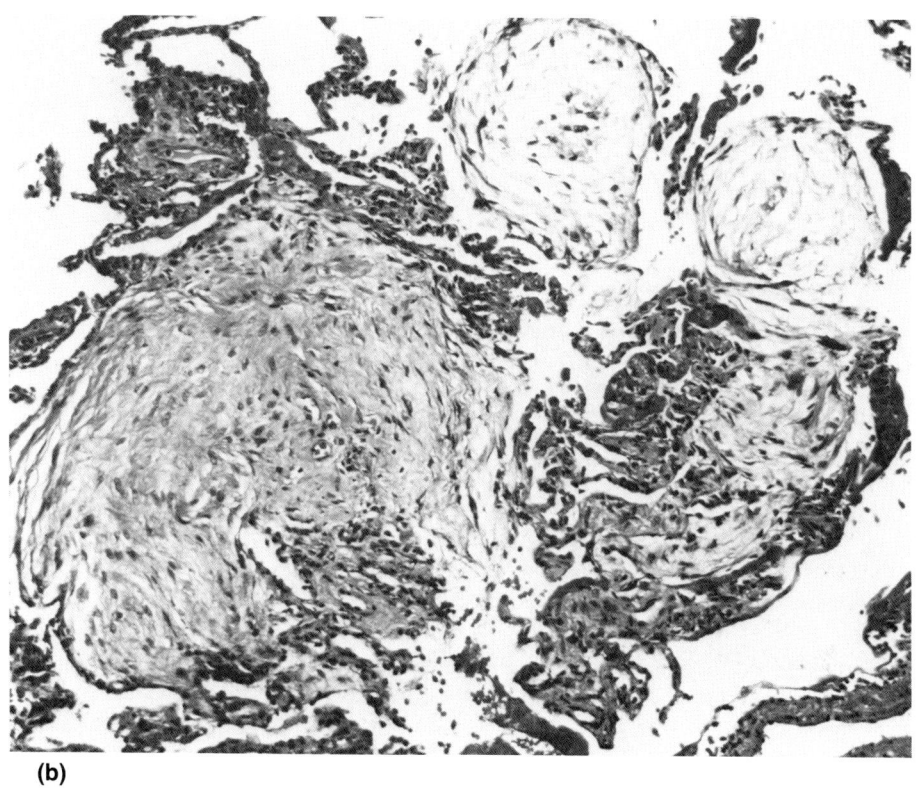
(b)

reflected by the finding of interstitial fibrosis in 63% (Fig. 3a) and intraluminal fibrosis in 36% (see Fig. 3b) of lung biopsies from AIDS patients with *P. carinii* pneumonia (3). This fibrosis was usually loose and organizing, similar to that seen in organizing diffuse alveolar damage (3). The relative infrequency of acute diffuse alveolar damage is reflected by the rarity of hyaline membranes, which were found in only 4% of lung biopsies from AIDS patients with *P. carinii* pneumonia (3). With severe acute diffuse alveolar damage, prominent hyaline membranes (Fig. 4a) may obscure the alveolar exudate of *P. carinii* pneumonia and cause difficulty in recognition of the diagnosis (3,36). This problem could also occur if the interstitial fibrosis of organizing diffuse alveolar damage is extensive (see Fig. 4b).

B. Absence of Alveolar Exudate

Since the eosinophilic alveolar exudate is a key histological clue to the diagnosis of pneumocystosis, it is important to be aware that this exudate may be absent in a

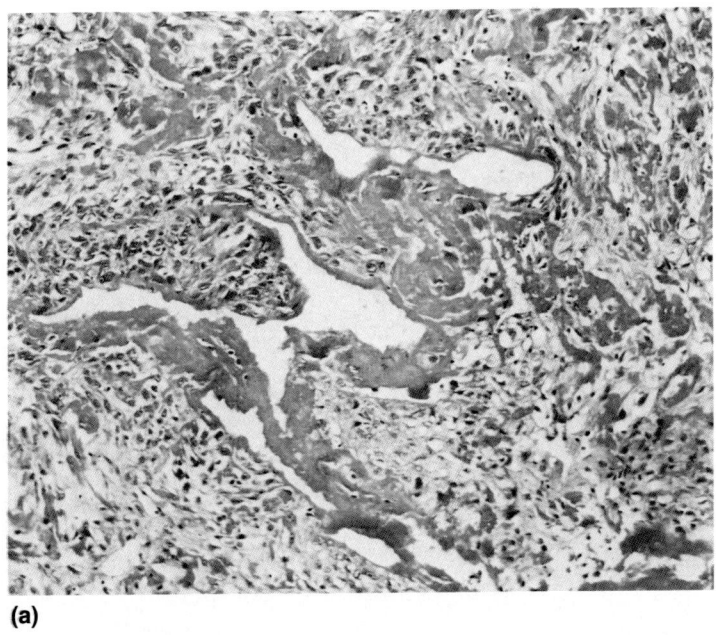

(a)

Figure 4 (a) Hyaline membranes, interstitial thickening, and inflammation in this biopsy specimen reflect manifestations of acute diffuse alveolar damage. (b) The nodular foci of fibrosis, prominent type II pneumocyte hyperplasia, and interstitial inflammation are features of organizing diffuse alveolar damage that obscured the intra-alveolar exudate here (a,b: H&E; a ×125, b ×62).

substantial percentage of cases. Absence of alveolar exudate has been described in up to 47% of cases of *P. carinii* pneumonia in patients without AIDS (see Fig. 1b) (33) and in up to 19% in AIDS patients (see Fig. 1a) (3). The alveolar exudate may be obscured by either intra-alveolar red blood cells (Fig. 5a), usually a result of artifactual, biopsy-induced hemorrhage, or by atelectasis (see Fig. 5b), or by prominent histological features, such as diffuse alveolar damage or lymphocytic interstitial pneumonia. Rarely, in *P. carinii* pneumonia there may be minimal histological reaction in addition to absence of exudate. In such cases, a few organisms may be seen along the edge of the alveolar septa (Fig. 6) (3).

C. Cystic and Cavitary Lesions

Although before the AIDS epidemic a few cases of pulmonary cysts or cavities were described in *P. carinii* pneumonia (37,38), the frequency of this complication increased dramatically in patients with AIDS (3,39–49). Pulmonary cysts in

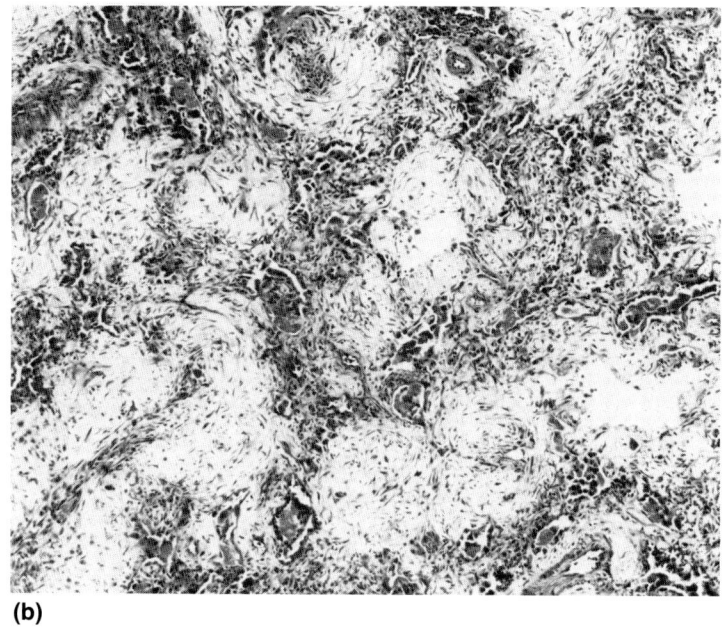
(b)

P. carinii pneumonia are found most often in the upper lobes and may present initially as cysts or as nodular lesions on chest radiographs that subsequently cavitate. Pneumocystosis has rarely been reported to present as a solitary pulmonary nodule, with or without cavitation (50–52). The cavities are typically multiple and bilateral; however, solitary cysts can occur. Spontaneous pneumothorax is a frequent complication, resulting from the rupture of cysts, and it may be the presenting clinical symptom of *P. carinii* pneumonia in human immunodeficiency virus (HIV)-infected patients (53–56). Hemoptysis may occur if blood vessels rupture within cavitary lesions (57). A cavitary lesion has presented in association with an endobronchial mass (52). Cavitary *P. carinii* pneumonia is often, but not always, associated with aerosolized pentamidine prophylaxis (58).

Cavitary pulmonary lesions may consist of either intraparenchymal cysts (Fig. 7) or subpleural bullous emphysematous blebs (Fig. 8). These correspond to the thin-walled cysts seen on chest radiographs and computed tomography (CT) scans (41,59). Most intraparenchymal cysts are located in the subpleural parenchyma (see Fig. 8), but they may also occur deep within the lung. Several types of histological features have been reported for intraparenchymal cavitary lesions in *P. carinii* pneumonia. They have been described as necrotic, infarct-like lesions (47,60) and necrotizing granulomas (61). More commonly, they consist of empty spaces (see Fig. 7) surrounded by walls that are lined by exudate or thin layers of

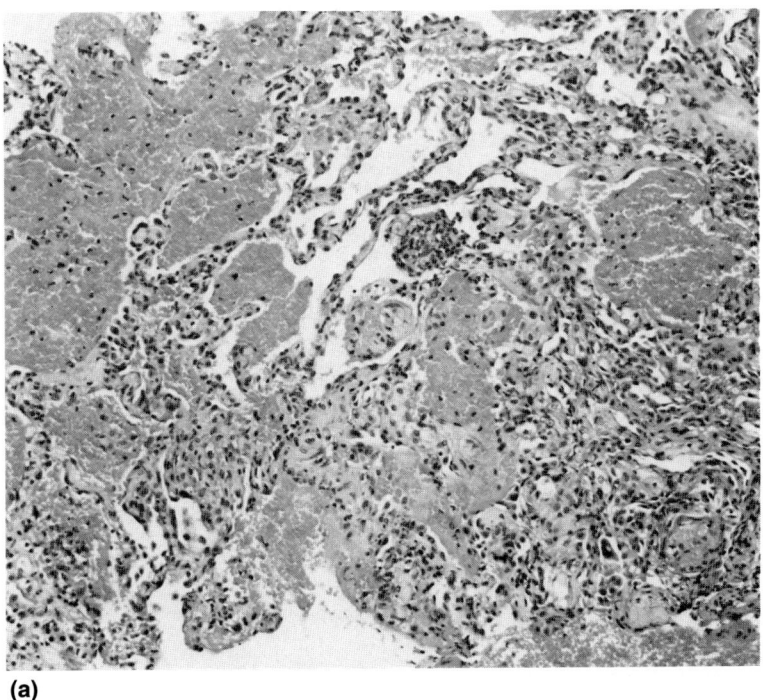

Figure 5 (a) The alveolar exudate in this specimen was obscured by the numerous red blood cells, which were an artifact of the biopsy procedure. (b) In this specimen, the atelectasis resulting from poor expansion of the alveolar walls during processing helped to obscure the alveolar exudate (a,b: H&E; a ×125, b ×30).

fibrous tissue and inflammatory cells (see Fig. 7). Subpleural emphysematous blebs have a fibrous wall (see Fig. 8) and the alveolar exudate or *P. carinii* organisms may be absent.

A variety of mechanisms have been proposed to explain the cyst formation in *P. carinii* pneumonia in HIV-infected patients, including interstitial emphysema, intravenous drug abuse (62), remodeling of the lung parenchyma associated with interstitial fibrosis, airway obstruction (63), necrotizing granulomas (61), infarction (47), proteolytic digestion of the lung induced by *P. carinii* pneumonia (64), and infection with HIV. Histological study of cavitary lesions of pneumocystosis suggests that the cystic destruction of lung parenchyma occurs within areas of active disease. This is consistent with the concept that *P. carinii* pneumonia causes necrosis and destruction of the lung parenchyma (64). Subpleural bullous emphysematous blebs may develop from rupture or confluence of intraparenchymal cysts

Pathological Features 163

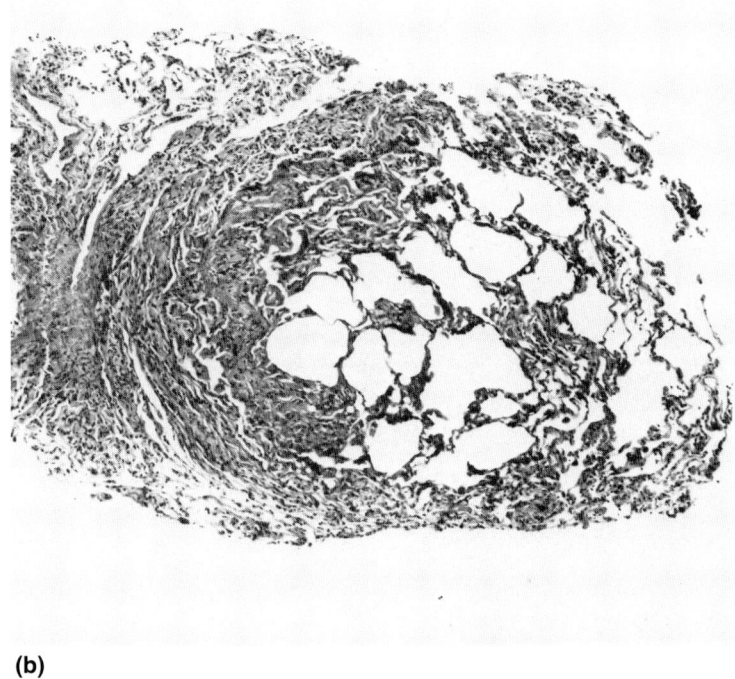

(b)

(3). Involvement of the pleura by *P. carinii* pneumonia has been described and may contribute to development of subpleural blebs (65).

Rupture of subpleural cavitary lesions may result in involvement of pleural fluid by *P. carinii* organisms (60), although pleural fluid involvement has also been reported without detectable cavitary lesions (66). Trophozoites may be especially prominent in pleural fluid, and these are well demonstrated with the Diff-Quik stain (67).

D. Granulomatous *Pneumocystis carinii* Pneumonia

Granulomatous inflammation in *P. carinii* pneumonia was a curiosity before the AIDS epidemic (51,68), although, in one study, it was described in up to 17% of lung biopsies (33). However, since the onset of the AIDS epidemic, there have been innumerable reports of granulomatous inflammation in *P. carinii* pneumonia (3,51,69–71). Granulomatous inflammation consisting of noncaseating granulomas (Fig. 9a) and scattered giant cells (see Fig. 9b) was described in 5% of lung biopsies of *P. carinii* pneumonia from a group of AIDS patients (3). Cavitating granulomas (61) and granulomas with central calcification (72) have also been

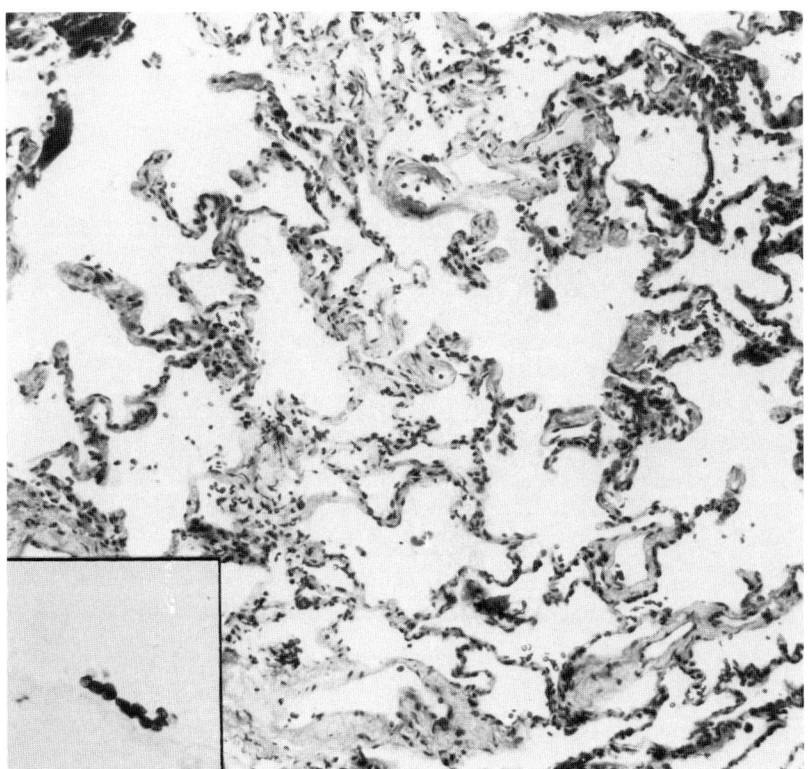

Figure 6 This biopsy shows little histological reaction to *P. carinii* with no visible alveolar exudate (H&E ×125) (Insert) Cysts of *P. carinii* are present lining the alveolar septa (Gomori methenamine silver ×500). (From Ref. 3.)

described; when these lesions are encountered, one must be careful to exclude other infectious agents commonly known to cause granulomatous inflammation, such as mycobacteria or fungi (3).

E. Lymphocytic–Plasmacellular Interstitial Pneumonitis

Early reports of *P. carinii* pneumonia in humans described an interstitial plasma cell pneumonia in 3 to 6-month-old marasmic institutionalized premature infants receiving artificial nutrition (1,73,74). The pulmonary interstitial plasma cell infiltrate in these infants was so striking that it has been suggested to be a distinctive manifestation of *P. carinii* pneumonia (1).

It is unusual to encounter such prominent lymphocytic or plasma cell infiltrates in adult patients with pneumocystosis. In one study of non–HIV-infected patients, dense interstitial infiltrates were described in 8% of lung

Pathological Features

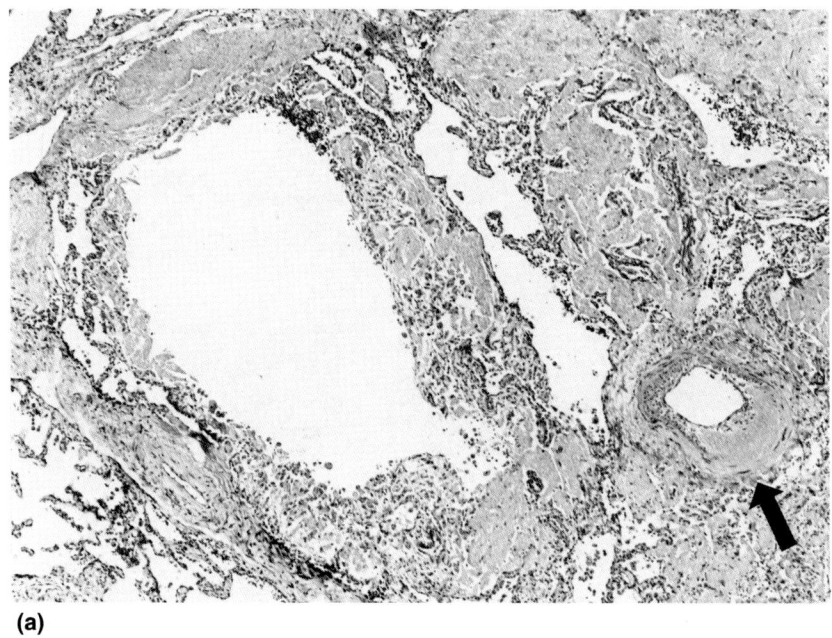

(a)

Figure 7 (a) Two unusual histological features of *P. carinii* pneumonia are present in this biopsy specimen: an intraparenchymal cyst and vascular permeation by *P. carinii* pneumonia. The parenchyma surrounding the cyst is involved by typical alveolar exudate of *P. carinii* pneumonia. (b) This intraparenchymal cyst is centered on a bronchiole. (c) High power of a cyst wall shows alveolar exudate of *P. carinii* pneumonia, macrophages, lymphocytes, and loose fibrous tissue (a–c: H&E; a ×50; b ×60, c ×125). (From Ref. 3.)

biopsies (see Fig. 1a) (33). Prominent lymphocytic infiltrates can occur in 3% of AIDS patients with *P. carinii* pneumonia (see Fig. 1b) (3). In rare cases, AIDS may present with *P. carinii* pneumonia associated with extensive lymphocytic interstitial pneumonia-like infiltrates that obscure the alveolar exudate and can delay recognition of the diagnosis (Fig. 10) (3,75). It is possible that the marked lymphoid proliferation in HIV patients may be due to the effects of *P. carinii*, HIV infection, or both (75,76).

F. Microcalcifications

Microcalcification has been described in lung biopsies of *P. carinii* pneumonia from 3% of non-AIDS patients (33) and from 2% of AIDS patients (3). In one recent study, microcalcifications were divided into four types: bubbly, plate-like, elongate, and conchoidal (77). Cysts of *P. carinii* were found with the GMS stain in all types of calcifications. In some cases, calcification was the only

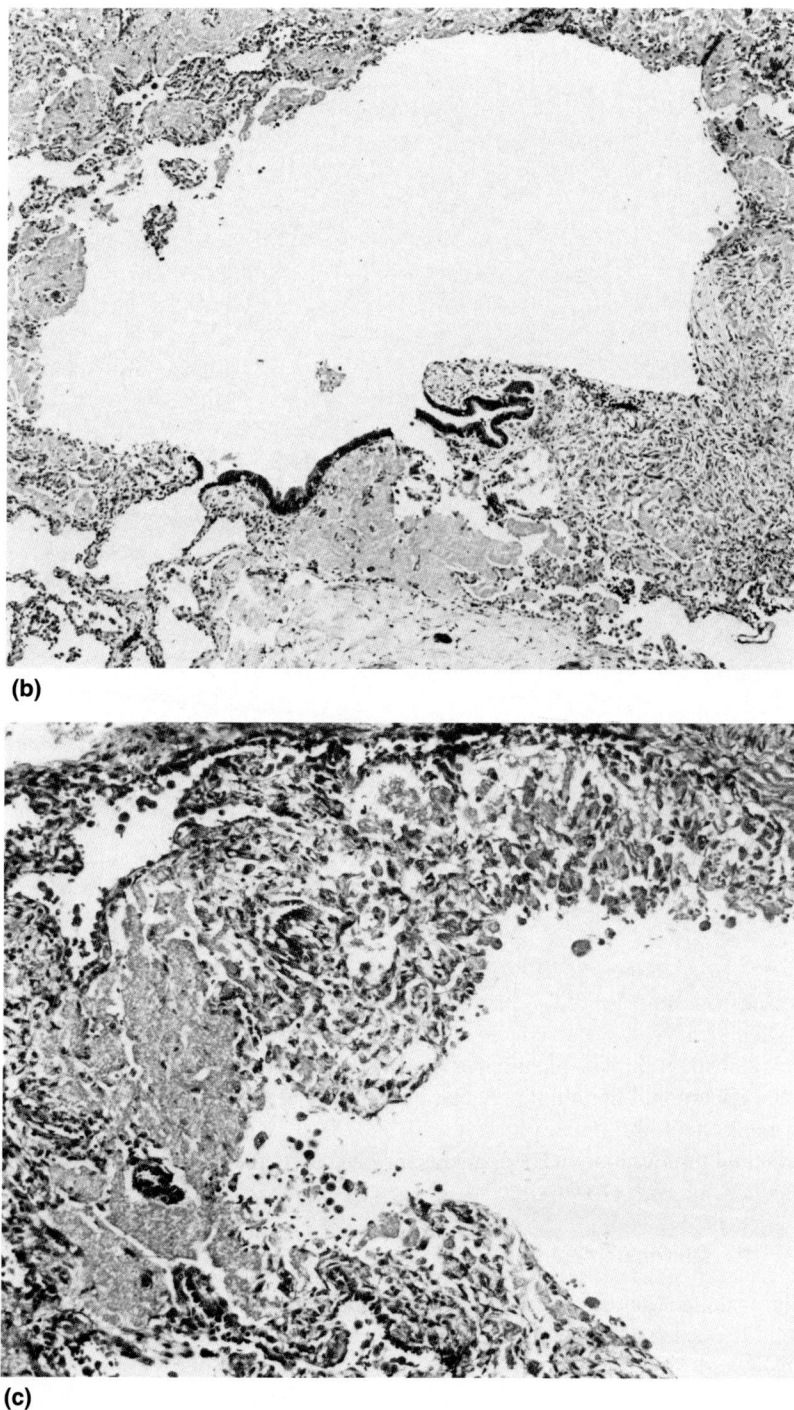

Figure 7 (Continued)

Pathological Features 167

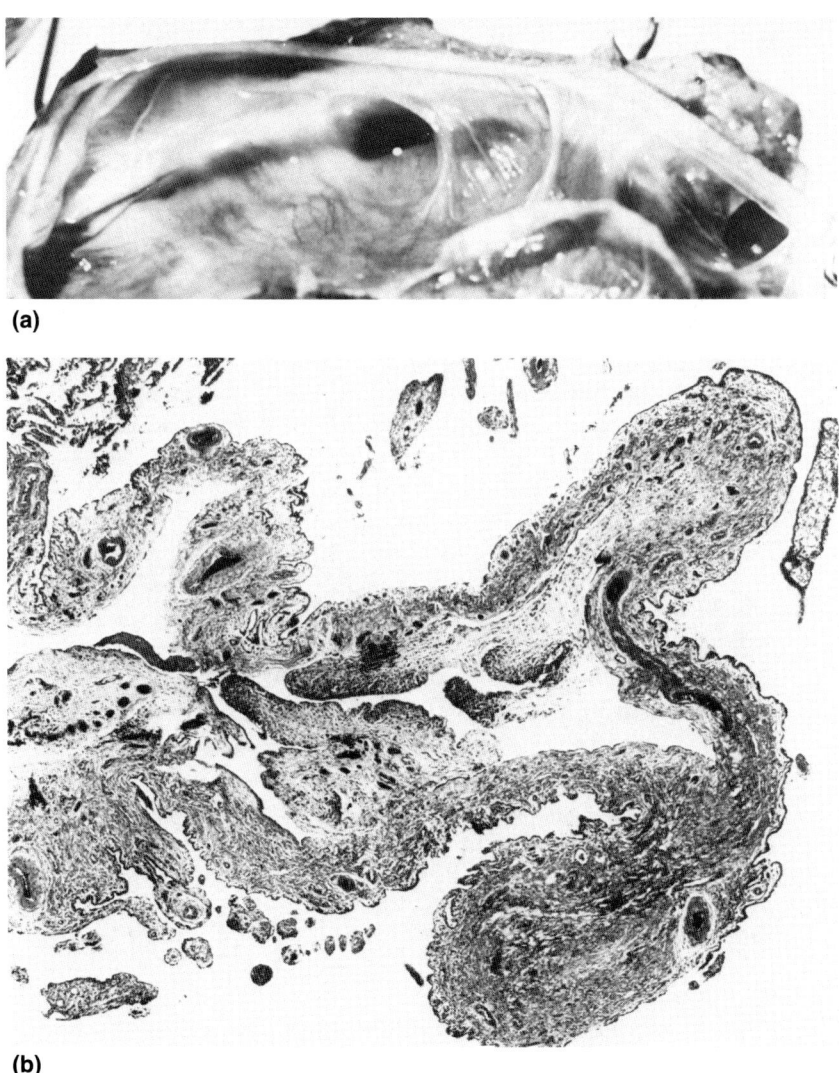

Figure 8 (a) This autopsy gross photograph shows marked subpleural cystic changes with the appearance of subpleural emphysematous blebs. This AIDS patient had numerous recurrent episodes of *P. carinii* pneumonia. (b) The tissue from this subpleural emphysematous bleb demonstrates tortuous folding of the fibrotic, thickened pleura. There is minimal inflammation in the fibrotic tissue (H&E ×30). (From Ref. 3.)

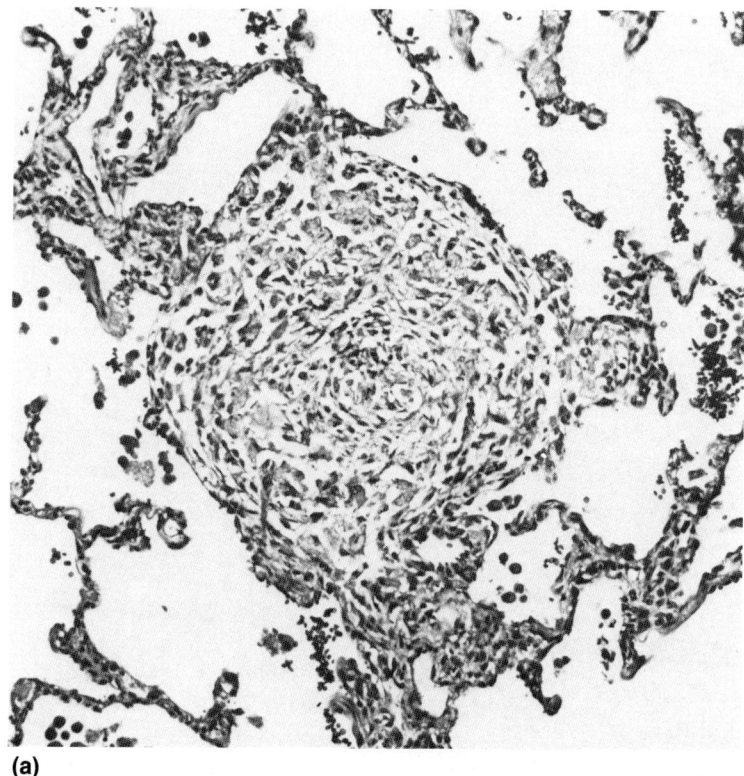

(a)

Figure 9 (a) This noncaseating granuloma consists of a nodular collection of epithelioid histiocytes intermixed with small foci of *P. carinii* pneumonia exudate. (b) This multinucleated giant cell was scattered within the background of organizing diffuse alveolar damage (a,b: H&E; a ×125, b ×250). (a, From Ref. 3.)

morphological clue on review of hematoxylin–eosin (H&E) stained-sections that *P. carinii* was present, since alveolar exudate was absent. Calcifications were also found in patients without prior diagnosis of *P. carinii* pneumonia or therapy. Therefore, it was felt that calcification is a potential reaction of the lung to dying *P. carinii*, regardless of therapy (77).

Calcification can occur in other tissues as well, and may be a marker for dissemination of *P. carinii* infection (78).

G. Marked Alveolar Macrophage Accumulation

Marked alveolar macrophage accumulation may be seen in a few cases of *P. carinii* pneumonia, and rarely, this may resemble the pattern seen in desquamative inter-

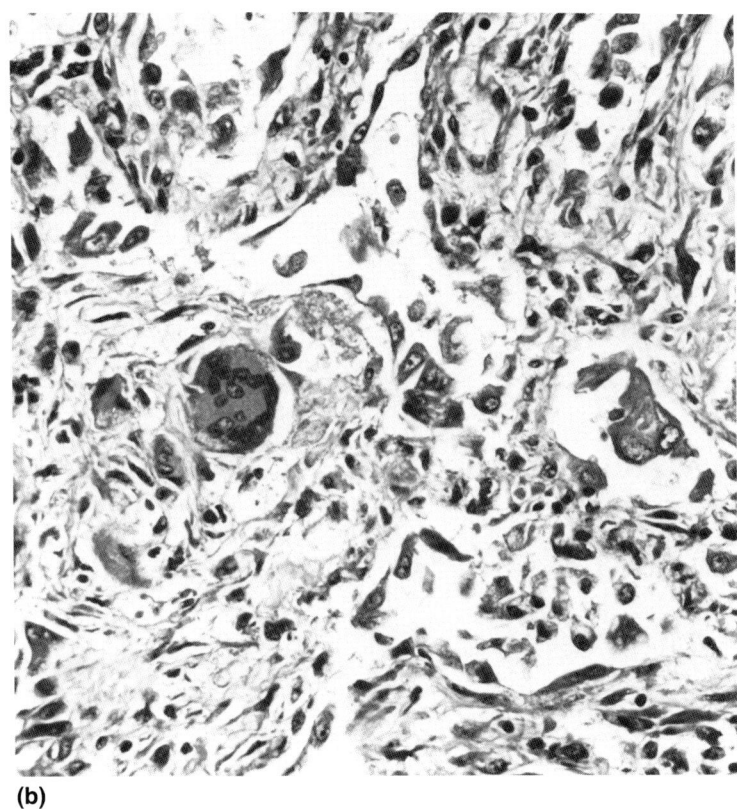
(b)

stitial pneumonia (DIP). Prominent alveolar macrophage accumulation was observed in 8% of *P. carinii* pneumonia lung biopsies from a series of non–HIV-infected patients (33) and in 9% of biopsies from AIDS patients (3).

H. Vascular Permeation and Vasculitis

Striking vascular permeation and vasculitis can rarely occur (3,47) (Fig. 11), and it may be associated with necrotizing or cavitary lung lesions (3,45,47,60). Given this association, it has been suggested that cavities are caused by ischemic necrosis. When identified, it may be a marker for widespread extrapulmonary dissemination (3,58).

I. Alveolar Proteinosis

Rare cases of alveolar proteinosis have been reported with *P. carinii* pneumonia (79–81); however, since the exudate of pneumocystosis may resemble the protein-

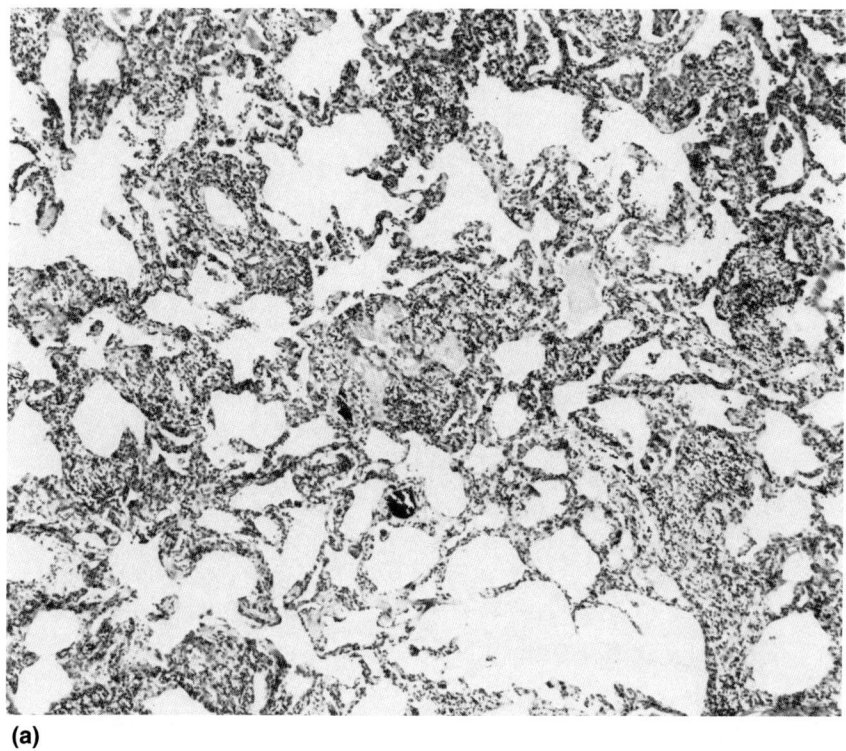

Figure 10 (a) In this case the prominent lymphocytic interstitial pneumonia delayed recognition of the *P. carinii* pneumonia exudate. (b) At higher power the alveolar exudate is more readily apparent (a,b: H&E; a ×60, B ×125). (From Ref. 3.)

aceous alveolar material of alveolar proteinosis, *P. carinii* pneumonia can be mistaken for alveolar proteinosis. The intra-alveolar material in *P. carinii* pneumonia is foamy and vacuolated; this is in contrast with alveolar proteinosis in which the alveolar material is finely granular, with occasional coarse clumps and cholesterol clefts. The *P. carinii* organisms should be sought rigorously with special stains in cases of suspected alveolar proteinosis, especially in HIV-infected patients. It should be kept in mind that the intra-alveolar exudate stains positively for periodic-acid-Schiff (PAS), with and without diastase digestion, in both *P. carinii* pneumonia and alveolar proteinosis. Other methods that have been used to detect alveolar proteinosis in cases of *P. carinii* pneumonia include immunohistochemical, which may show positive staining for surfactant apoprotein (79,80), and electron microscopy, which may show lipoproteinaceous material with myelin-like bodies (79).

Pathological Features 171

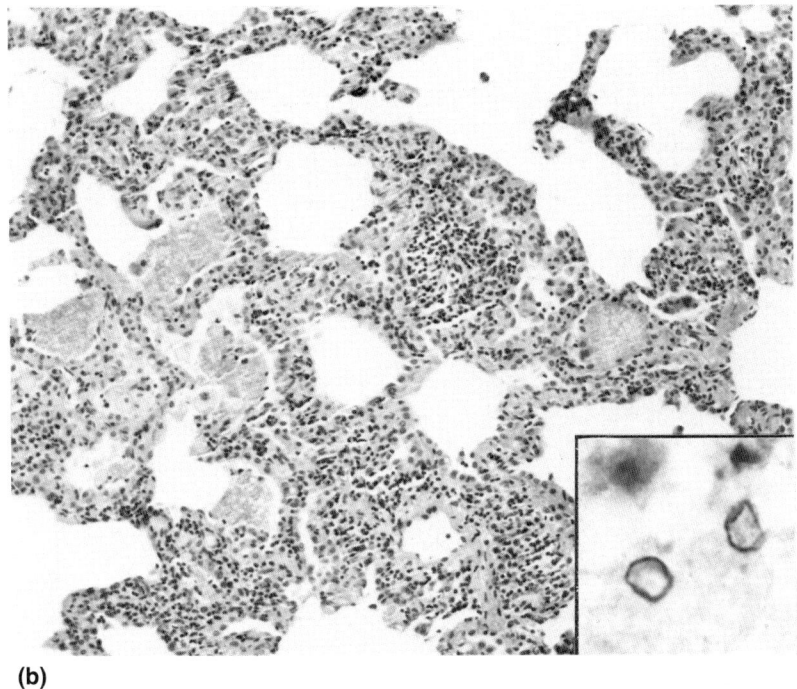

(b)

IV. Concomitant Processes

Since patients who contract *P. carinii* pneumonia are immunosuppressed, additional lesions, such as other opportunistic infections or neoplasms, may also be found in the lung. The most commonly associated infection is cytomegalovirus (CMV) (12), but a wide variety of other infectious agents may be found, including bacterial pneumonia, *Cryptococcus neoformans*, and *Mycobacterium intracellular* (3,82). In HIV-infected patients, both Kaposi's sarcoma and malignant lymphoma have been found in the lungs in patients with pneumocystosis (3,82).

V. Treated *Pneumocystis carinii* Pneumonia

There are few studies on the pathology of *P. carinii* pneumonia following therapy. In one study, serial lung biopsies 4–6 weeks after therapy showed persistent inflammation, but failed to show any detectable change in the number of *P. carinii* organisms or in the appearance of the alveolar exudate, regardless of how well patients responded to pentamidine or to trimethoprim–sulfamethoxasole (83).

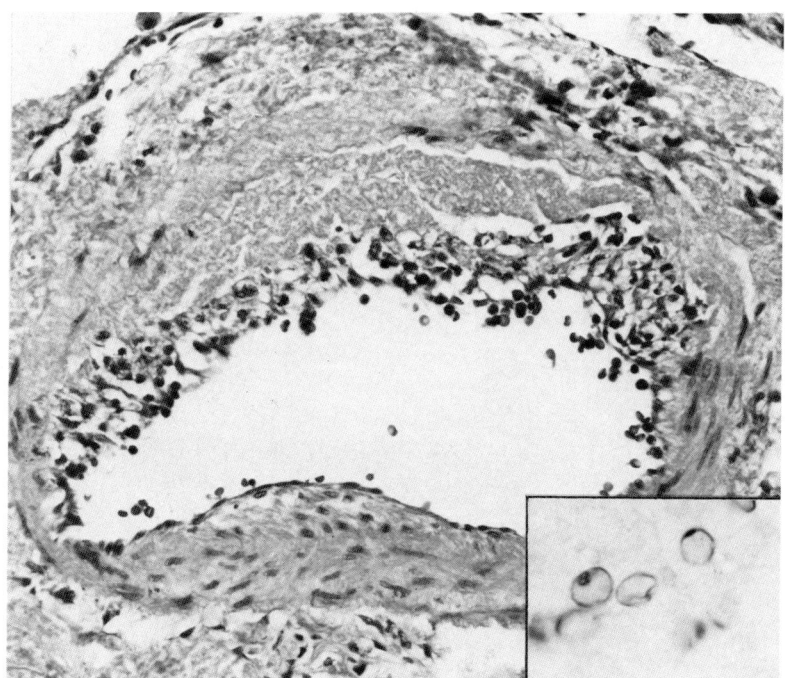

Figure 11 This blood vessel shows destruction of the smooth-muscle wall by eosinophilic *P. carinii* pneumonia exudate and associated inflammation or vasculitis. The patient subsequently developed widespread dissemination (58) (H&E ×250). (Insert) Immunohistochemistry for the 2G2 antigen shows positive staining of the cyst wall. (From Ref. 3.)

These results suggested that resolution of *P. carinii* pneumonia was slower in AIDS patients than in patients without AIDS (83). After successful therapy, trophozoites may also be detected by electron microscopy in lung biopsies from AIDS patients (84).

In another study, follow-up lung biopsies an average of 25.2 days after initial diagnosis, revealed persistent *P. carinii* cysts in 38% of patients who improved on therapy for *P. carinii* pneumonia (85). On the basis of a group of clinical parameters, it was not possible to distinguish patients whose lung biopsies showed persistent organisms from those whose biopsies were negative (85).

In an autopsy study, Saldana et al. found that the lungs of most patients who die with fulminant *P. carinii* pneumonia have abundant alveolar exudate with numerous organisms and show histological features of the exudative or early organizing phases of diffuse alveolar damage (82). Following therapy, in these patients, the alveolar exudate became partly or totally compacted and showed fewer cysts on GMS stains (82). In cases of unresolved *P. carinii* pneumonia, the major histological feature was that of the organizing phase of diffuse alveolar damage, and exudates became incorporated into intra-alveolar fibroblastic proliferation (82). Extensive fibrosis was found in patients with "cured" *P. carinii* pneumonia; in such cases it was difficult to identify the organisms, and it was difficult to exclude other causes of interstitial fibrosis, such as oxygen or drug toxicity and other infections (82).

VI. Disseminated (Extrapulmonary) *Pneumocystis carinii* Infection

Before the AIDS epidemic, extrapulmonary *P. carinii* infection was extraordinarily rare (68), but the number of reported cases has exploded over the past 10 years (56,68,78,86–92). Virtually all organs can be affected, including the skin (58), spleen (93,94), liver (55,93), kidney (93), myocardium (93), thoracic (56,93) or abdominal lymph nodes (93–95), thymus (93), parathyroid glands (93), pancreas (93), adrenal glands (93,94), choroid (44,96,97), gastrointestinal mucosa (93,95), thyroid (87,95), brain (98), diaphragm (95), and bone marrow (91,93,94). Many cases appear to be associated with lymphatic or vascular invasion. Extensive involvement by *P. carinii* can lead to organ failure and result in fatal complications (90). Visceral calcification detected by computed tomography may be a marker for extrapulmonary *P. carinii* infection (78).

VII. Immunohistochemistry

The development of monoclonal antibodies to *P. carinii* has led to attempts to apply this tool as a diagnostic technique in paraffin-embedded tissue sections (3,90,99,100). Several different antibodies have been described including 2G2, R13/3G4-6, 5E12, 2E3, 3F6, 7D7, and 6B8 (see Fig. 10b) (99,100). However, these provide little advantage over routine silver stains for diagnosis, since the latter are cheaper and more rapid. Monoclonal antibody staining may be of use in cases of disseminated *P. carinii* infection or if the differential diagnosis with other organisms, such as *Histoplasma capsulatum*, is raised.

VIII. Conclusion

In summary, the pathology of *P. carinii* pneumonia includes several typical and atypical histological features. The AIDS epidemic has drawn attention to several interesting atypical histological features, including absence of alveolar exudate, cystic or cavitary lesions, granulomatous inflammation, lymphocytic interstitial pneumonitis, microcalcifications, alveolar proteinosis, and vascular permeation or vasculitis. In addition, numerous reports of extrapulmonary *P. carinii* infection have documented involvement of virtually every organ. Use of immunohistochemical methods in formalin-fixed, paraffin-embedded tissue sections may be useful for documentation of disseminated infection or in cases where the differential diagnosis with other organisms, such as *Histoplasma capsulatum*, is raised; however, immunohistochemistry does not appear to be superior to GMS staining for routine diagnosis in lung biopsy specimens.

References

1. Dutz W. *Pneumocystis carinii* pneumonia. Pathol Annu 1970; 5:309–341.
2. Travis WD, Lack EE, Ognibene FP, Suffredini AF, Shelhamer J. Lung biopsy interpretation in the acquired immunodeficiency syndrome: experience of the National Institutes of Health with literature review. Prog AIDS Pathol 1989; 1:51–84.
3. Travis WD, Pittaluga S, Lipschik GY, et al. Atypical pathologic manifestations of *Pneumocystis carinii* pneumonia in the acquired immune deficiency syndrome. Review of 123 lung biopsies from 76 patients with emphasis on cysts, vascular invasion, vasculitis, and granulomas. Am J Surg Pathol 1990; 14:615–625.
4. Watts JC, Chandler FW. Evolving concepts of infection by *Pneumocystis carinii*. Pathol Annu 1991; 26(pt 1):93–138.
5. Genner J, Settnes OP. Pathological characteristics for the diagnosis of *Pneumocystis carinii* pneumonia. A retrospective autopsy study. APMIS 1990; 98:1098–1104.
6. Marchevsky A, Rosen MJ, Chrystal G, Kleinerman J. Pulmonary complications of the acquired immunodeficiency syndrome: a clinicopathologic study of 70 cases. Hum Pathol 1985; 16:659–670.
7. Hui AN, Koss MN, Meyer PR. Necropsy findings in acquired immunodeficiency syndrome: a comparison of premortem diagnoses with postmortem findings. Hum Pathol 1984; 15:670–676.
8. Guarda LA, Luna MA, Smith JL Jr, Mansell PW, Gyorkey F, Roca AN. Acquired immune deficiency syndrome: postmortem findings. Am J Clin Pathol 1984; 81: 549–557.
9. Nash G, Fligiel S. Pathologic features of the lung in the acquired immune deficiency syndrome (AIDS): an autopsy study of seventeen homosexual males. Am J Clin Pathol 1984; 81:6–12.
10. Rosen P, Armstrong D, Ramos C. *Pneumocystis carinii* pneumonia. A clinicopathologic study of twenty patients with neoplastic diseases. Am J Med 1972; 53: 428–436.
11. Travis WD, Roth, DB. Histopathologic evaluation of lung biopsy specimens. In: Shelhamer J, Pizzo PA, Parrillo JE, Masur H, eds. Respiratory Disease in the Immunosuppressed Host. Philadelphia: JB Lippincott, 1991:182–217.
12. McKenzie R, Travis WD, Dolan SA, et al. The causes of death in patients with human immunodeficiency virus infection: a clinical and pathologic study with emphasis on the role of pulmonary diseases. Medicine 1991; 70:326–343.

13. Edman JC, Kovacs JA, Masur H, Santi DV, Elwood HJ, Sogin ML. Ribosomal RNA sequence shows *Pneumocystis carinii* to be a member of the fungi. Nature 1988; 334:519–522.
14. Chuang MT, Rosen MJ, Teirstein AS, Brown LK, Padilla ML, Tow TW. Flexible bronchoscopy in the diagnosis of *Pneumocystis carinii* pneumonia in patients with acquired immune deficiency syndrome. South Med J 1986; 79:1363–1365.
15. Mones JM, Saldana MJ, Oldham SA. Diagnosis of *Pneumocystis carinii* pneumonia. Roentgenographic–pathologic correlates based on fiberoptic bronchoscopy specimens from patients with the acquired immunodeficiency syndrome. Chest 1986; 89: 522–526.
16. Harcup C, Baier HJ, Pitchenik AE. Evaluation of patients with the acquired immunodeficiency syndrome (AIDS) by fiberoptic bronchoscopy. Endoscopy 1985; 17:217–220.
17. Flint A, Beckwith AL, Naylor B. *Pneumocystis carinii* pneumonia. Cytologic manifestations and rapid diagnosis in routinely prepared Papanicolaou-stained preparations. Am J Med 1986; 81:1009–1011.
18. Francis ND, Goldin RD, Forster SM, et al. Diagnosis of lung disease in acquired immune deficiency syndrome: biopsy or cytology and implications for management. J Clin Pathol 1987; 40:1269–1273.
19. Duggan MA, Pomponi C, Robboy SJ. Pulmonary cytology of the acquired immune deficiency syndrome: an analysis of 36 cases. Diagn Cytopathol 1986; 2:181–186.
20. Orenstein M, Webber CA, Heurich AE. Cytologic diagnosis of *Pneumocystis carinii* infection by bronchoalveolar lavage in acquired immune deficiency syndrome. Acta Cytol 1985; 29:727–731.
21. Greaves TS, Strigle SM. The recognition of *Pneumocystis carinii* in routine Papanicolaou-stained smears. Acta Cytol 1985; 29:714–720.
22. Selvaggi SM, Gerber M. Pulmonary cytology in patients with the acquired immunodeficiency syndrome (AIDS). Diagn Cytopathol 1986; 2:187–193.
23. Guarner J, Robey SS, Gupta PK. Cytologic detection of *Pneumocystis carinii*: a comparison of Papanicolaou and other histochemical stains. Diagn Cytopathol 1986; 2:133–137.
24. Griffiths MH, Kocjan G, Miller RF, Godfrey-Faussett P. Diagnosis of pulmonary disease in human immunodeficiency virus infection: role of transbronchial biopsy and bronchoalveolar lavage. Thorax 1989; 44:554–558.
25. McKenna RJ Jr, Campbell A, McMurtrey MJ, Mountain CF. Diagnosis for interstitial lung disease in patients with acquired immunodeficiency syndrome (AIDS): a prospective comparison of bronchial washing, alveolar lavage, transbronchial lung biopsy, and open-lung biopsy. Ann Thorac Surg 1986; 41:318–321.
26. Caughey G, Wong H, Gamsu G, Golden J. Nonbronchoscopic bronchoalveolar lavage for the diagnosis for *Pneumocystis carinii* pneumonia in the acquired immunodeficiency syndrome. Chest 1985; 88:659–662.
27. Hartman B, Koss MN, Hui A, Baumann W, Athos L, Boylen T. *Pneumocystis carinii* pneumonia in the acquired immunodeficiency syndrome (AIDS). Diagnosis with bronchial brushings, biopsy, and bronchoalveolar lavage. Chest 1985; 87: 603–607.

28. Stover DE, White DA, Romano PA, Gellene RA. Diagnosis of pulmonary disease in acquired immune deficiency syndrome (AIDS). Role of bronchoscopy and bronchoalveolar lavage. Am Rev Respir Dis 1984; 130:659–662.
29. Chandra P, Delaney MD, Tuazon CU. Role of special stains in the diagnosis of *Pneumocystis carinii* infection from bronchial washing specimens in patients with the acquired immune deficiency syndrome. Acta Cytol 1988; 32:105–108.
30. Rorat E, Garcia RL, Skolom J. Diagnosis of *Pneumocystis carinii* pneumonia by cytologic examination of bronchial washings. JAMA 1985; 254:1950–1951.
31. Pitchenik AE, Ganjei P, Torres A, Evans DA, Rubin E, Baier H. Sputum examination for the diagnosis of *Pneumocystis carinii* pneumonia in the acquired immunodeficiency syndrome. Am Rev Respir Dis 1986; 133:226–229.
32. Bigby TD, Margolskee D, Curtis JL, et al. The usefulness of induced sputum in the diagnosis of *Pneumocystis carinii* pneumonia in patients with the acquired immunodeficiency syndrome. Am Rev Respir Dis 1986; 133:515–518.
33. Weber WR, Askin FB, Dehner LP. Lung biopsy in *Pneumocystis carinii* pneumonia: a histopathologic study of typical and atypical features. Am J Clin Pathol 1977; 67: 11–19.
34. Bedrossian CW. Ultrastructure of *Pneumocystis carinii*: a review of internal and surface characteristics. Semin Diagn Pathol 1989; 6:212–237.
35. Watts JC, Chandler FW. *Pneumocystis carinii* pneumonitis. The nature and diagnostic significance of the methenamine silver-positive "intracystic bodies. Am J Surg Pathol 1985; 9:744–751.
36. Askin FB, Katzenstein AL. Pneumocystic infection masquerading as diffuse alveolar damage: a potential source of diagnostic error. Chest 1981; 79:420–422.
37. Doppman JL, Geelhoed GW, De Vita VT. Atypical radiographic features in *Pneumocystis carinii* pneumonia. Radiology 1975; 114:39–44.
38. Luddy RE, Champion LAA, Schwartz AD. *Pneumocystis carinii* pneumonia with pneumatocele formation [letter]. Am J Dis Child 1977; 131:470.
39. Praz JO, Lorenzi P, Chevrolet JC. *Pneumocystis carinii* pneumonia and acquired immunodeficiency syndrome: an atypical presentation with lung cavitations. Eur Respir J 1990; 3:1221–1223.
40. Judson MA, Postic B, Weiman DS. *Pneumocystis carinii* pneumonia manifested as a hilar mass and cavitary lesion: an atypical presentation in a patient receiving aerosolized pentamidine prophylaxis. South Med J 1990; 83:1309–1312.
41. Moskovic E, Miller R, Pearson M. High resolution computed tomography of *Pneumocystis carinii* pneumonia in AIDS. Clin Radiol 1990; 42:239–243.
42. Summers QA, Helprin GA, Tarala RA, French MA. Multiple pneumatocoeles and bilateral tension pneumothoraces complicating pneumocystis pneumonia in AIDS. Aust NZ J Med 1990; 20:257–260.
43. Gurney JW, Bates FT. Pulmonary cystic disease: comparison of *Pneumocystis carinii* pneumatoceles and bullous emphysema due to intravenous drug abuse. Radiology 1989; 173:27–31.
44. Rao NA, Zimmerman PL, Boyer D, et al. A clinical, histopathologic, and electron microscopic study of *Pneumocystis carinii* choroiditis. Am J Ophthalmol 1989; 107: 218–228.

45. Case records of the Massachusetts General Hospital. Weekly clinicopathological exercises. Case 9-1989. A 32-year-old man with AIDS and a cavitary pulmonary lesion. N Engl J Med 1989; 320:582–587.
46. Pincus PS, Sandler MA, Naude GE, Kallenbach JM, Isaacson C, Zwi S. Multiple pulmonary cavities—an unusual complication of *Pneumocystis carinii* pneumonia. S Afr Med J 1987; 72:871–872.
47. Liu YC, Tomashefski JF Jr, Tomford JW, Green H. Necrotizing *Pneumocystis carinii* vasculitis associated with lung necrosis. Arch Pathol Lab Med 1989; 113:494–497.
48. Barrio JL, Suarez M, Rodriguez JL, Saldana MJ, Pitchenik AE. *Pneumocystis carinii* pneumonia presenting as cavitating and noncavitating solitary pulmonary nodules in patients with the acquired immunodeficiency syndrome. Am Rev Respir Dis 1986; 134:1094–1096.
49. Gronbeck C. *Pneumocystis carinii* pneumonia presenting as cavitary lung disease. Milit Med 1988; 153:314–316.
50. Bier S, Halton K, Krivisky B, Leonidas J. *Pneumocystis carinii* pneumonia presenting as a single pulmonary nodule. Pediatr Radiol 1986; 16:59–60.
51. Hartz JW, Geisinger KR, Scharyj M, Muss HB. Granulomatous pneumocystosis presenting as a solitary pulmonary nodule. Arch Pathol Lab Med 1985; 109:466–469.
52. Gagliardi AJ, Stover DE, Zaman MK. Endobronchial *Pneumocystis carinii* infection in a patient with the acquired immune deficiency syndrome. Chest 1987; 91:463–464.
53. McGarry TM. Pneumatoceles and pneumothorax in *Pneumocystis carinii* pneumonia. NY State J Med 1991; 91:287–288.
54. Beers MF, Sohn M, Swartz M. Recurrent pneumothorax in AIDS patients with pneumocystis pneumonia. A clinicopathologic report of three cases and review of the literature. Chest 1990; 98:266–270.
55. Saldana MJ, Mones JM. Cavitation and other atypical manifestations of *Pneumocystis carinii* pneumonia. Semin Diagn Pathol 1989; 6:273–286.
56. Afessa B, Green WR, Williams WA, et al. *Pneumocystis carinii* pneumonia complicated by lymphadenopathy and pneumothorax. Arch Intern Med 1988; 148:2651–2654.
57. Mascarenhas DA, Vasudevan VP, Vaidya KP. *Pneumocystis carinii* pneumonia. Rare cause of hemoptysis. Chest 1991; 99:251–253.
58. Davey RT Jr, Margolis D, Kleiner D, Deyton L, Travis WD. Digital necrosis and disseminated *Pneumocystis carinii* infection after aerosolized pentamidine prophylaxis. Ann Intern Med 1989; 111:681–682.
59. Feuerstein IM, Archer A, Pluda JM, et al. Thin-walled cavities, cysts, and pneumothorax in *Pneumocystis carinii* pneumonia: further observations with histopathologic correlation. Radiology 1990; 174:697–702.
60. Balachandran I, Jones DB, Humphrey DM. A case of *Pneumocystis carinii* in pleural fluid with cytologic, histologic and ultrastructural documentation. Acta Cytol 1990; 34:486–490.
61. Klein JS, Warnock M, Webb WR, Gamsu G. Cavitating and noncavitating granulomas in AIDS patients with pneumocystis pneumonitis. AJR 1989; 152:753–754.

62. Goldstein DS, Karpel JP, Appel D, Williams MH Jr. Bullous pulmonary damage in users of intravenous drugs. Chest 1986; 89:266–269.
63. Quigley MJ, Fraser RS. Pulmonary pneumatocele: pathology and pathogenesis. AJR 1988; 150:1275–1277.
64. Eng RH, Bishburg E, Smith SM. Evidence for destruction of lung tissues during *Pneumocystis carinii* infection. Arch Intern med 1987; 147:746–749.
65. Dyner TS, Lang W, Busch DF, Gordon PR. Intravascular and pleural involvement by *Pneumocystis carinii* in a patient with AIDS [letter]. Ann Intern Med 1989; 111:94.
66. Mariuz P, Raviglione MC, Gould IA, Mullen MP. Pleural *Pneumocystis carinii* infection. Chest 1991; 99:774–776.
67. Elwood LJ, Dobrzanski D, Feuerstein IM, Solomon D. *Pneumocystis carinii* in pleural fluid. The cytologic appearance. Acta Cytol 1991; 35:761–764.
68. LeGolvan DP, Heidelberger KP. Disseminated, granulomatous *Pneumocystis carinii* pneumonia. Arch Pathol 1973; 95:344–348.
69. Cupples JB, Blackie SP, Road JD. Granulomatous *Pneumocystis carinii* pneumonia mimicking tuberculosis. Arch Pathol Lab Med 1989; 113:1281–1284.
70. Blumenfeld W, Basgoz N, Owen WF Jr, Schmidt DM. Granulomatous pulmonary lesions in patients with the acquired immunodeficiency syndrome (AIDS) and *Pneumocystis carinii* infection. Ann Intern Med 1988; 109:505–507.
71. Bleiweiss IJ, Jagirdar JS, Klein MJ, et al. Granulomatous *Pneumocystis carinii* pneumonia in three patients with the acquired immune deficiency syndrome. Chest 1988; 94:580–583.
72. Gal AA, Koss MN, Strigle S, Angritt P. *Pneumocystis carinii* infection in the acquired immune deficiency syndrome. Semin Diagn Pathol 1989; 6:287–299.
73. Dutz W. *Pneumocystis carinii* infection and interstitial plasma cell pneumonia: what does history teach? Semin Diagn Pathol 1989; 6:195–202.
74. Thomas SF, Dutz W, Khodadad EJ. *Pneumocystis carinii* pneumonia (plasma cell pneumonia); roentgenographic, pathologic and clinical correlation. Am J Roentgenol Radium Ther Nucl Med 1966; 98:318–322.
75. Murphy PM, Fox C, Travis WD, Koenig S, Fauci AS. Acquired immunodeficiency syndrome may present as severe restrictive lung disease. Am J Med 1989; 86:237–240.
76. Kassel SH, Echevarria RA, Guzzo FP. Midline malignant reticulosis (so-called lethal midline granuloma). Cancer 1969; 23:920–935.
77. Lee MM, Schinella RA. Pulmonary calcification caused by *Pneumocystis carinii* pneumonia. A clinicopathological study of 13 cases in acquired immune deficiency syndrome patients. Am J Surg Pathol 1991; 15:376–380.
78. Feuerstein IM, Francis P, Raffeld M, Pluda J. Widespread visceral calcifications in disseminated *Pneumocystis carinii* infection: CT characteristics. J Comput Assist Tomogr 1990; 14:149–151.
79. Tran Van Nhieu J, Vojtek AM, Bernaudin JF, Escudier E, Fleury-Feith J. Pulmonary alveolar proteinosis associated with *Pneumocystis carinii*. Ultrastructural identification in bronchoalveolar lavage in AIDS and immunocompromised non-AIDS patients. Chest 1990; 98:801–805.
80. Ruben FL, Talamo TS. Secondary pulmonary alveolar proteinosis occurring in two

patients with acquired immune deficiency syndrome. Am J Med 1986; 80:1187–1190.
81. Prakash UB, Barham SS, Carpenter HA, Dines DE, Marsh HM. Pulmonary alveolar phospholipoproteinosis: experience with 34 cases and a review. Mayo Clin Proc 1987; 62:499–518.
82. Saldana MJ, Mones JM, Martinez GR. The pathology of treated *Pneumocystis carinii* pneumonia. Semin Diagn Pathol 1989; 6:300–312.
83. Shelhamer JH, Ognibene FP, Macher AM, et al. Persistence of *Pneumocystis carinii* in lung tissue of acquired immunodeficiency syndrome patients treated for pneumocystis pneumonia. Am Rev Respir Dis 1984; 130:1161–1165.
84. el-Sadr W, Sidhu G. Persistence of trophozoites after successful treatment of *Pneumocystis carinii* pneumonia. Ann Intern Med 1986; 105:889–890.
85. DeLorenzo LJ, Maguire GP, Wormser GP, Davidian MM, Stone DJ. Persistence of *Pneumocystis carinii* pneumonia in the acquired immunodeficiency syndrome. Evaluation of therapy by follow-up transbronchial lung biopsy. Chest 1985; 88:79–83.
86. Dembinski AS, Smith DM, Goldsmith JC, Woods GL. Widespread dissemination of *Pneumocystis carinii* infection in a patient with acquired immune deficiency syndrome receiving long-term treatment with aerosolized pentamidine. Am J Clin Pathol 1991; 95:96–100.
87. Drucker DJ, Bailey D, Rotstein L. Thyroiditis as the presenting manifestation of disseminated extrapulmonary *Pneumocystis carinii* infection. J Clin Endocrinol Metab 1990; 71:1663–1665.
88. Berman SM, Shah B, Wyle FA, Dacosta-Iyer M, McRae DM. Disseminated *Pneumocystis carinii* in a patient receiving aerosolized pentamidine prophylaxis. West J Med 1990; 153:82–86.
89. Ravalli S, Garcia RL, Vincent RA, Shein R. Disseminated *Pneumocystis carinii* infection in the acquired immunodeficiency syndrome. NY State J Med 1990; 90:155–157.
90. Cote RJ, Rosenblum M, Telzak EE, May M, Unger PD, Cartun RW. Disseminated *Pneumocystis carinii* infection causing extrapulmonary organ failure: clinical, pathologic, and immunohistochemical analysis. Mod Pathol 1990; 3:25–30.
91. Batra P, Wallace JM, Ovenfors CO, Heyman MR, Rasmussen P. Efficacy and complications of transthoracic needle biopsy of lung in patients with *Pneumocystis carinii* pneumonia and AIDS *Pneumocystis carinii* involvement of the bone marrow in acquired immunodeficiency syndrome. Am J Clin Pathol 1987; 87:780–783.
92. Cohen OJ, Stoeckle MY. Extrapulmonary *Pneumocystis carinii* infections in the acquired immunodeficiency syndrome. Arch Intern Med 1991; 151:1205–1214.
93. Amin MB, Abrash MP, Mezger E, Sekerak GF. Systemic dissemination of *Pneumocystis carinii* in a patient with acquired immunodeficiency syndrome. Henry Ford Hosp Med J 1990; 38:68–71.
94. Unger PD, Rosenblum M, Krown SE. Disseminated *Pneumocystis carinii* infection in a patient with acquired immunodeficiency syndrome. Hum Pathol 1988; 19:113–116.
95. Matsuda S, Urata Y, Shiota T, et al. Disseminated infection of *Pneumocystis carinii*

in a patient with the acquired immunodeficiency syndrome. Virchows Arch [A] 1989; 414:523–527.
96. Rosenblatt MA, Cunningham C, Teich S, Friedman AH. Choroidal lesions in patients with AIDS. Br J Ophthalmol 1990; 74:610–614.
97. Freeman WR, Gross JG, Labelle J, Oteken K, Katz K, Wiley CA. *Pneumocystis carinii* choroidopathy. A new clinical entity. Arch Ophthalmol 1989; 107:863–867.
98. Mayayo E, Vidal F, Alvira R, Gonzalez J, Richart C. Cerebral *Pneumocystis carinii* infection in AIDS [letter]. Lancet 1990; 336:1592.
99. Radio SJ, Hansen S, Goldsmith J, Linder J. Immunohistochemistry of *Pneumocystis carinii* infection. Mod Pathol 1990; 3:462–469.
100. Linder J, Radio SJ. Immunohistochemistry of *Pneumocystis carinii*. Semin Diagn Pathol 1989; 6:238–244.

10

Animal Models

MARTINE Y. K. ARMSTRONG

Yale University School of Medicine
New Haven, Connecticut

MELANIE T. CUSHION

University of Cincinnati College of Medicine
Cincinnati, Ohio

I. Introduction*

Animal models of *Pneumocystis carinii* pneumonia have played and continue to play a central role in research on this organism. Observations made in the 1950s and 1960s that pneumocystis pneumonia could be provoked in rats and rabbits by cortisone treatment alone (1–4) led to the realization that latent *P. carinii* infection was widespread among these animals. Over the past 25 years, the most widely used animal model of pneumocystis pneumonia has been the latently infected rat in which *P. carinii* infection is reactivated by prolonged corticosteroid administration. Increasingly, however, this classic model is plagued by significant variability in the severity of the induced *P. carinii* pneumonia. This chapter will consider the rat model in some detail and will focus on the possible causes of its variability. The use and development of alternative animal models of pneumocystosis will also be

---

*This chapter is based in part on presentations and discussions in the session "Pneumocystosis: Animal Models" at the Second International Workshop on *Pneumocystis, Cryptosporidium*, and Microsporidia held in Bozeman, Montana, June 28–July 2, 1991. The authors cochaired the session.

reviewed and their advantages and disadvantages discussed. The final section discusses molecular genetic evidence that supports the existence of strain and species variations among *P. carinii* organisms isolated from different mammalian hosts.

II. The Classic Corticosteroid-Treated Rat Model of *Pneumocystis carinii* Pneumonia

Frenkel and his colleagues established the parameters of the rat model in experiments designed to study agents effective against *P. carinii* pneumonia (5). They demonstrated that (1) *P. carinii* pneumonia could be produced in 200-g Sprague–Dawley rats by twice weekly subcutaneous injections of 25 mg cortisone acetate for 6–8 weeks; (2) many rats treated with such high doses of corticosteroids died of intercurrent infections before pneumocystis pneumonia could develop; (3) the most common cause of such deaths, *Corynebacterium kutscheri* bronchopneumonia, could be prevented by the addition of chlortetracycline to the drinking water, at a dose of at least 50 mg/100 mL; (4) suppression of intercurrent infections permitted the development of fatal *P. carinii* pneumonia; (5) cessation of corticosteroid administration allowed resolution of the *P. carinii* pneumonia; (6) the corticosteroid-induced rat model of pneumocystosis could be treated effectively in the continuing presence of corticosteroids with a combination of sulfadiazine–pyrimethamine, as well as with pentamidine.

Although reactivation of rat pneumocystosis has been provoked by other agents that affect the immune system, such as cyclophosphamide (5) and cyclosporine (6), corticosteroid administration remains the most efficacious method of *P. carinii* pneumonia induction (7). The specific corticosteroid preparation used and the route of administration appear to reflect investigators' personal experience. Thus, in some studies, cortisone acetate or methyl prednisolone acetate are injected subcutaneously, twice weekly or once weekly, respectively (8,9). In other studies, dexamethasone is added to the drinking water (8,10). Although oral medication cuts down on the amount of animal manipulation, the dose that each animal actually receives is more variable. Since severe protein malnutrition alone has been associated with *P. carinii* infection in both humans and rats (11), a low-protein (8%) diet is frequently included as part of the immunosuppressive regimen, for its enhancing effect on the *P. carinii* pneumonia induced by corticosteroid administration (12). Addition of antibiotics (e.g., tetracycline, ampicillin) to the drinking water remains the standard approach to the control of secondary bacterial infection. There is some evidence, however, that hyperchlorinated water may have a comparable effect (13). The routine use of antifungal drugs, such as amphotericin B, injected subcutaneously three times weekly at a dose of 1 mg (14) or nystatin added to the drinking water at a dose of 200,000 U/mL (15), has not been widely adopted, probably because their effectiveness in preventing fungal infections has yet to be proved, and also because of their relative toxicity. In addition, nystatin is poorly soluble.

Although reactivation of latent pneumocystosis has been observed in several rat strains that include Sprague–Dawley, Wistar, Lewis, Fisher, Holtzman, and Long–Evans (5,8,12,14), Sprague–Dawley rats are the most commonly used in the latently infected, corticosteroid-treated rat model, and these are usually male rats. From a small study designed to compare the susceptibility to, and survival from, *P. carinii* infection in male and female Sprague–Dawley rats, Hughes (8) concluded that both sexes are equally susceptible to reactivation of *P. carinii* infection by corticosteroids, but that the male rat survives the infection longer. With male and female Wistar rats, Settnes also found each sex to be equally susceptible to pneumocystis infection, but the females survived on average 12 days longer (16).

A. The Role of the Rat Model in *Pneumocystis carinii* Research

The corticosteroid-treated rat model of pneumocystosis has been the mainstay of *P. carinii* research since it was first established in 1966 by Frenkel et al. (5) because it mirrors so faithfully the disease in humans and because its response to preventive and therapeutic measures predicts so accurately that of the human disease. Thus, this rat model has provided much of our current information on the pathogenesis, immunology, diagnosis, and therapy of pneumocystis pneumonia, as well as on the morphology, life cycle, and transmission of the organism itself (17).

The rat model was developed specifically to evaluate the therapeutic potential of drugs in the treatment and prevention of *P. carinii* pneumonia. In their landmark study (5), Frenkel et al. confirmed that pentamidine, previously shown to be effective in the treatment of human pneumocystis pneumonia (18), was also effective in clearing the reactivated rat infection. The study also demonstrated, for the first time, that the combined use of pyrimethamine and sulfadiazine, two drugs with antiprotozoal activity, prevented *P. carinii* reactivation when given concurrently with the corticosteroids, and significantly reduced the incidence and severity of the pneumocystosis when given after 30 days of corticosteroids.

In the absence of standardized, readily reproducible *P. carinii* culture methods, the classic corticosteroid-treated rat has, until recently, been the principal tool of drug development (19) and continues as a major source of the organism for basic biological studies.

B. Understanding the Rat Model

The standard immunosuppressive regimen used to reactivate latent *P. carinii* infection in rats is associated with increasing debility, wasting, and marked involution of all lymphoid tissues (12,20). The latter results in a profound lymphocyte depletion. Analysis of lymphocyte subsets at different body sites revealed that the lymphopenia in the peripheral blood was characterized by a greater fall in T-helper than in T-suppressor cells, resulting in reversal of the T-helper/T-suppressor cell ratio (20). Although the T-helper/T-suppressor cell ratio was also reversed in the lungs, this was associated with an actual increase in number of T-suppressor cells, a phenomenon that is also seen in patients with the acquired immunodeficiency syndrome (AIDS) who develop *P. carinii* pneumonia (21).

The critical role of corticosteroids in the standard immunosuppressive regimen was confirmed by Walzer and colleagues, who compared the effects of tetracycline and a low-protein diet with and without corticosteroids on the growth, nutrition, and lymphoid systems of rats (12). Rats receiving either tetracycline or a low-protein (8%) diet alone for 7 weeks developed few abnormalities. Rats receiving both tetracycline and the low-protein diet developed lower body and lymphoid organ weights, lower serum albumin levels, and fewer circulating lymphocytes. However, only when corticosteroids were given did the characteristic reversal of T-helper/T-suppressor cell ratio occur. Whereas long-term tetracycline administration by itself does not promote the development of *P. carinii* pneumonia (12), tetracyclines have a variety of effects that could potentiate the immunosuppressive action of corticosteroids. Tetracyclines have been shown to inhibit certain lymphocyte functions in rats (22), to affect leukocyte chemotaxis and phagocytosis (23), and to induce changes in alveolar epithelial cells (24). Protein–caloric restriction may also enhance critical aspects of corticosteroid immune suppression. Severe protein–calorie malnutrition in rats depresses not only cell-mediated immune responses, but also impairs recruitment of macrophages to the lungs (25).

Corticosteroids also inhibit circulating antibody production in rats and, in addition to their striking effects on lymphoid tissues and cells, they influence a wide variety of processes involved in inflammation, immunological responses, and the handling of infectious agents (26). It has been suggested that suppression of polymorphonuclear leukocytic inflammatory response may underlie corticosteroid-induced activation of *P. carinii* infection (27). This is based on the observation that rats receiving intratracheal injections of *Pseudomonas aeruginosa*, resulting in a striking polymorphonuclear leukocytosis in bronchoalveolar lavage fluid, were significantly less likely to develop detectable pneumocystosis following corticosteroid treatment than rats injected with *Staphylococcus aureus*, which does not induce a polymorphonuclear leukocytic alveolar exudate (27).

C. Variability in the Rat Model

At the time that Frenkel and his colleagues developed the classic rat model in the 1960s, laboratory animals were infected not only with *P. carinii*, but also with a host of other microbial agents (28,29). Over the past decade, a growing awareness that adventitious infectious agents represent an uncontrolled variable in animal research has resulted in an increased demand for the production of pathogen-free rats and mice. Improvements in laboratory animal science and husbandry have enabled animal producers to establish animal colonies that are free of specific pathogens (29). As a result, it has been the common experience among *P. carinii* investigators that whereas the incidence of serious intercurrent infection among corticosteroid-treated rats has dropped significantly, the provocation of *P. carinii* pneumonia has become more problematic (30). As documented by Walzer and colleagues, over a decade ago, rats placed on a standard immunosuppressive regimen of corticosteroids and a low-protein diet developed a pneumocystis infection that intensified fairly predictably over time, culminating in a severe *P. carinii* pneumonia after 7–8 weeks (31). Assessment of the severity of the induced pneumocystis infection, using a semiquantitative scoring system, established that rats characteristically developed infections involving over 75% of the alveoli, with cyst counts in lung homogenates reaching up to 10^9/g of lung (31).

Many cesarian-rederived and barrier-raised colonies of rats and mice are now free of latent pneumocytosis, so that *P. carinii* pneumonia may no longer be inducible by corticosteroid treatment alone. In practice, most certified virus-free laboratory rodent colonies are also free of *P. carinii*, whereas latent pneumocystosis may still present among colonies that continue to harbor viral agents (30). Of all the possible viruses that naturally infect laboratory mice and rats (Table 1), and that are still widely prevalent, those identified in the table in bold italics could have a decisive effect on the induction of *P. carinii* pneumonia (28). In the rat, these include several parvovirus strains, the coronavirus sialodacryoadenitis virus, and two paramyxoviruses: Sendai virus and pneumonia virus of mice. An active infection with sialodacryoadenitis virus, Sendai virus, or pneumonia virus of mice may cause pneumonia in immunocompromised animals, whereas both Sendai virus and parvovirus infections may themselves be immunosuppressive. Parvoviruses are generally believed to cause persistent infections and, hence, can be potentially activated upon immunosuppression (28).

It is quite possible that the effects of such viruses on the host could contribute to the increasing variability in corticosteroid inducibility of *P. carinii* pneumonia and its severity among rat colonies in which latent pneumocystosis is still present. Two recent studies have sought to examine factors that might influence pneumocystis infection in the immunocompromised rat (10,32). In one of the studies (10), the intensity of the induced *P. carinii* pneumonia was assessed in five groups of rats acquired sequentially over a two-year period from the same colony of a particular vendor and placed on the same immunosuppressive regimen. The rats were barrier-raised, but were not certified to be virus-free. Upon receipt from the vendor, they were housed singly in unprotected cages in a room dedicated to these specific rats. Serum was obtained when the rats were euthanized after 9–12 weeks of immunosuppression and was tested for the presence of

Table 1 Viruses Known to Naturally Infect Laboratory Mice and Rats

Virus group	Mice	Rats
DNA		
Adenovirus	Mouse adenovirus K87, FL	Rat adenovirus
Herpesvirus	Mouse cytomegalovirus	Rat cytomegalovirus
	Mouse thymic necrosis virus	
Papovavirus	Polyoma virus	Polyoma-like virus
	K virus	
Parvovirus	*__Minute virus of mice__*	*__Kilham's rat virus__*
		__Toolan's H-1 virus__
	__Mouse orphan parvovirus__	*__Rat orphan parvovirus__*
Poxvirus	Ectromelia virus	Cowpox virus
RNA		
Arenavirus	Lymphocytic choriomeningitis virus	
Coronavirus	*__Mouse hepatitis virus__*	*__Sialodacryoadenitis virus__*
Hantavirus		Hemorrhagic fever virus
Paramyxovirus	*__Pneumonia virus of mice__*	*__Pneumonia virus of mice__*
	__Sendai virus__	*__Sendai virus__*
Picornavirus	Mouse encephalomyelitis virus	MHG virus
Reovirus	Epizootic diarrhea of infant mice virus	Infectious diarrhea of infant rats virus
	Reovirus 3	Reovirus 3
Togavirus	Lactate dehydrogenase-elevating virus (LDHE-V)	

Viruses in italic, bold print could have an effect on *P. carinii* pneumonia development, as discussed in the text.
Source: Modified from Ref. 28.

antibodies to rat corona- and parvoviruses, Sendai virus, pneumonia virus of mice, and *Mycoplasma pulmonis*. Although antibodies were detected to parvovirus in 22% of the total 60 rats examined, to pneumonia virus of mice in 48%, and to Sendai virus in 78%, there was no apparent correlation between the presence or absence of antibodies to these agents and the severity of the *P. carinii* pneumonia, assessed in part by the total number of organisms extracted from the lungs (10). Although the presence of specific antibody detected at death indicates past infection, it provides little information about when such infection occurred. Thus, these findings do not preclude the possibility that an active infection with such agents at a critical period during the course of immunosuppression could influence *P. carinii* reactivation and the intensity of the resultant pneumocystis pneumonia. In the other study (32), virus-free rats, shown to be free of latent pneumocystosis, developed *P. carinii* pneumonia when immunosuppressed with corticosteroids and placed in unprotected cages in an open room housing *P. carinii* infected rats. In this setting, these initially virus-free rats also became infected with rat coronavirus, Sendai virus, and pneumonia virus of mice. Even though the role of concomitant viral infection in the development of pneumocystosis could not be determined in this study, it is of interest that the rats were able to mount an antibody response to the viral agents, despite the immunosuppressive effects of corticosteroid administration, but that they did not develop antibodies to *P. carinii*.

Other possible causes of variability now inherent in the classic corticosteroid-treated rat model are further discussed in the section on inoculated rodent models (see Sect. IV). It is also possible that different strains of *P. carinii* vary in their pathogenicity and that variability in reactivated pneumocystis infection reflects *P. carinii* strain variation (see Sect. VII).

III. *Pneumocystis carinii* Infection in Mice

Mice, like rats, may be latently infected with *P. carinii*. Their potential for use as an animal model of pneumocystis infection was explored in the late 1970s and early 1980s by Walzer and colleagues (33–36). A comprehensive study of *P. carinii* pneumonia in different strains of cortisonized mice established that pneumocystis infection was present among mice of all eight strains examined (33). Seven of these were inbred strains, namely, C3H/HeN, BALB/cAnN, C57BL/6N, B10.A(2R), AKR/J, DBA/2N, DBA/1J; one was the outbred Swiss Webster strain. The intensity of pneumocystis infection in the lungs was assessed using the scoring system already referred to, based on the number of *P. carinii* cysts detected in lung sections by the methenamine silver stain (33). The corticosteroid-induced *P. carinii* infection varied in intensity among the different strains, with C3H/HeN mice consistently developing the heaviest degree of infection and DBA/2N and DBA/1J the lowest frequency and lightest intensity (Table 2). The optimal immunosuppressive regimen consisted of twice-weekly subcutaneous injections of 1 mg cortisone acetate, a low-protein (8%) diet, and tap water with 1 mg/mL tetracycline added (33,36). A corticosteroid dose of 1mg cortisone acetate in a 20 g mouse represents less than half the 25 mg dose in a 200 g rat. This may account for the generally less intense infection induced in mice, compared with that in the corticosteroid-treated rat model; few mice developed infection involving more than 75% of the alveoli (see Table 2). Raising the cortisone acetate dose to 2.5 mg resulted in greatly increased early mortality from intercurrent fungal and bacterial infections (33). Mouse *P. carinii* stained with methenamine silver or Giemsa were morphologically indistinguishable from rat *P. carinii*. The histopathology of the infected lungs was similar among the different strains of mice and resembled that of the corticosteroid-treated rat, although the infection was generally less severe in mice than in rats in terms of organism burden.

Table 2 *Pneumocystis carinii* Infection in Different Strains of Normal Mice

Mouse strain	No. infected/total	Mean *P. carinii* score[a]
Steroid treated		
C3H/HeN	27/30	1.9
BALB/cAnN	31/38	1.5
AKR/J	17/17	1.3
C57BL/6N	15/20	1.2
B10.A (2R)	10/14	1.1
Swiss Webster	13/16	1.1
DBA/2N	5/14	0.8
DBA/1J	4/17	0.8
Controls		
C3H/HeN	2/12	0.5
BALB/cAnN	4/19	0.5
AKR/J	2/6	0.5
C57BL/6N	1/6	0.5
B10.A (2R)	1/6	0.5
Swiss Webster	1/9	0.5
DBA/2N	0/6	0.0
DBA/1J	0/3	0.0

[a]A standardized procedure was established for grading the intensity of *P. carinii* infection (33). At least three pieces of lung were removed, one each from the upper and lower portions of the right lung, and one from the midportion of the left lung. The lung sections were stained with methenamine silver, coded, and read blindly. The following scoring system for infection was used: 0 = no *P. carinii* found; 0.5+ = minimal infection, <1% alveoli involved; 1+ = light, 1–25% alveoli involved; 2+ = moderate, 25–50% alveoli involved; 3+ = heavy, 50–75% alveoli involved; 4+ = very heavy infection, >75% alveoli involved. For comparison, the mean score of the group was calculated only from those members in which *P. carinii* was demonstrated (i.e., with a score ≥0.5+).
Source: Ref. 35.

In a second study (36), Walzer and colleagues compared the *P. carinii* pneumonia induced by corticosteroid treatment and an 8%-protein diet in C3H/HeJ mice with that induced in C3Heb/FeJ mice. C3H/HeJ mice, shown in their previous study (33) to develop the heaviest degree of *P. carinii* infection of all eight strains tested, are unresponsive to bacterial lipopolysaccharide (LPS), have defects in macrophage function, and have increased antibody responses to orally administered T-dependent antigens, all by virtue of a single autosomal gene mutation (37). C3Heb/FeJ mice are immunologically normal. Although pneumocystosis was present in all corticosteroid-treated mice, the intensity of the infection was significantly greater among C3H/HeJ mice.

Both these studies (33,36) established the validity of using the corticosteroid-treated mouse as an experimental model for *P. carinii* pneumonia, but also highlighted some of the disadvantages of the model. The hope that well-defined genetic differences among inbred strains of mice might reveal important factors in host susceptibility to *P. carinii* has not been realized. This, in part, is due to the confounding effect of corticosteroids on the host immune system and the possibility that genetic differences in susceptibility to corticosteroids, rather than to *P. carinii*, may determine the course of the reactivated *P. carinii* infection. In the mouse, as in the rat, corticosteroid administration results in severe lymphopenia and impaired lymphocyte function (26). In addition, corticosteroids render normal macrophages unresponsive to lymphokines (38). It is not known, for example, if the increased susceptibility to *P. carinii* infection in C3H/HeJ mice is due to their inherent immune deficit, or if it results from an altered corticosteroid response.

The studies of Walzer and colleagues on *P. carinii* infection in steroid-treated normal mice (33,36) also illustrated the difficulty of titrating the immunosuppressive regimen to maximize the relatively slow development of pneumocystis pneumonia, without a substantial increase in early death from intercurrent infections. The frequency of the latter may well reflect that, at the time these studies were conducted, laboratory rodents characteristically harbored many more infective agents than they do now.

A recent report documents the transmission of *P. carinii* infection in viral antigen-free inbred mice raised under barrier conditions (39). C3HeB/FeJ mice obtained from Jackson Laboratories were identified as having a latent pneumocystis infection following the induction of *P. carinii* pneumonia by a 6-week regimen of 8 mg dexamethasone per liter in the drinking water, together with an 8%-protein diet. The viral status of these "seed" mice was not given. Preliminary experiments showed that optimal *P. carinii* infection could be achieved in seed mice with 4 mg dexamethasone per liter given for 8–10 weeks and that substitution of a normal (23%)-protein diet for the low-protein diet did not reduce the intensity of the infection. No premature mortality was observed in mice on this latter regimen. After 5–8 weeks of such immunosuppression, seed C3HeB/FeJ mice were placed for 2 weeks in microisolator cages that contained viral antigen-free "recipient" mice. All the cage residents received the immunosuppressive regimen, which was continued for a further 6 weeks after the seed mice were removed. Several recipient mouse strains were used, including C3HeN, DBA/2N, BALB/c and BALB/c nu/nu. All recipient immunosuppressed mice developed *P. carinii* infection; immunosuppressed littermates not exposed to seed mice did not have detectable pneumocystis infection. The total number of *P. carinii* cysts present in the homogenized preparation of excised lungs was used as an index of the level of pneumocystis infection produced. Table 3 shows that the level of

Table 3 Transmission of *P. carinii* to Various Mouse Strains by Short-Term Exposure to C3HeB/FeJ Mice with Acute *P. carinii* Pneumonia

Recipient[a]	Dexamethasone (mg/L)	Seed period (wk)	Incubation postseeding (wk)	Mean no. of cysts (± SEM)[b] in mice that were	
				Seeded	Not seeded
C3HeN	8	1	6	5.41 ± 0.15	0
DBA/2N	4	2	5	5.71 ± 0.04	0
BALB/c	4	2	5	5.55 ± 0.05	0
nu/nu	0	2	6	5.63 ± 0.06	0

[a]There were six to ten animals per group, except for the nu/nu group, which had two animals. All animals were fed 23% protein rodent chow, except for the C3HeN mice, which were on an 8%-protein diet.
[b]Numbers are the geometric mean numbers of cysts per lung. Detection limit is 3.36 cysts per lung ($\log_{10}$).
Source: Ref. 39.

infection was comparable among mice of different strains and that dexamethasone was not necessary to establish infection in athymic BALB/c nu/nu mice. The mean cyst counts were also similar to those of seed mice sampled at a comparable time during immunosuppression. The cyst loads were slightly lower than those in the larger lungs of the corticosteroid-treated rat (31).

These recent experiments (39) raise several intriguing possibilities. Short-term cohabitation with infected seed mice appears to produce a much more uniform and intense *P. carinii* infection in immunosuppressed recipient mice, irrespective of strain, than reactivation of a latent pneumocystis infection by immune suppression. It may be that the variation in intensity of the reactivated latent infection among different mouse strains reflects host strain differences in response to the primary *P. carinii* infection, or a dose effect, or differences in host susceptibility to various *P. carinii* strains. Unfortunately, the original source of the *P. carinii* organisms in the C3Heb/FeJ seed mice is unknown. The success of this mode of transmission offers the prospect that the method can be used to achieve continuous propagation of pneumocystis infection within a colony of immunosuppressed, otherwise pathogen-free, mice. It would be interesting to know if the infected, recipient mice described in this study (39) were free of specific viral agents.

IV. Development of Inoculated Rodent Models

There have been conflicting reports throughout the past four decades on the success of establishing *P. carinii* infection in animal models by inoculation or injection (1–4,34,35,40–42). Two general approaches were used: (1) inoculation of frozen or fresh organisms into rodents rendered immune incompetent by steroid administration, or (2) inoculation of such preparations into congenitally athymic rodents, the so-called nude mouse or rat, the genetic defect of which produces profound immunosuppression. Most investigators used a same-species inoculation scheme (e.g., rat organisms into rat host), although heterologous transfer has been sporadically attempted. Successful propagation of human organisms in nude mice was reported in the late 1970s and also in a more recent study (69). However, no one inoculation method reliably established *P. carinii* infection, and the corticosteroid-provoked reactivation model of infection became the most widely used of animal models.

In recent years, significant progress has been made toward establishing a reproducible inoculated rodent model of *P. carinii* infection. After identifying sources of rats that were free of latent *P. carinii*, Bartlett and colleagues (43) used these animals as recipients of organism-containing lung homogenates by transtracheal introduction (44). All of the rats inoculated were reported as manifesting the infection. Later studies designed to assess the usefulness of this model for the purpose of drug evaluation confirmed the consistent production of infection (45). This procedure and its application are discussed in greater detail in Chapter 24.

A variation of the intratracheal inoculation technique was reported by Boylan and Current (13) who used noninvasive intratracheal intubation to inoculate the *P. carinii* organisms. These investigators detected no difference in the intensity of the induced infection in the three rat strains evaluated, Sprague–Dawley, Fischer 344, and Lewis. Hyperchlorination of water was used to control secondary microbial infections. The kinetics of infection were evaluated by enumeration of all developmental forms of the organisms. Other characteristics that were also considered included body weight, cause of death, and the effect of single-, double-, and triple-organism doses (of approximately 10^6 organisms per dose) on the parasite burden of the ensuing infection. Mortality caused by *P. carinii* pneumonia, and greater body weight loss, were associated with double- and triple-organism inoculations, compared with the single-inoculation regimen.

Bartlett et al. have recently reported successful infection of steroid-immunosuppressed BALB/c mice with *P. carinii* from scid mice, using the same surgical tracheal instillation technique described for the rat model (46). Only BALB/c mice, but not C_3H/HeJ, NIH Swiss, non-Swiss albino, ND4 Swiss Webster, nor ICR mice were found to be suitable for the inoculation-induced *P. carinii* infection. The C_3H/HeJ mice already had latent infection, and the other strains never developed the infection, although they were profoundly immunosuppressed.

The inoculated rodent model of pneumocystosis offers some distinct advantages over the standard model of steroid-provoked infection. Since the organism cannot be continuously cultured in vitro, the task of providing the investigator with a steady supply of parasites falls to the animal model of infection. It is well-known that rats received from the same vendor, in the same shipment, from the same room, will not all develop infections with an equivalent organism burden when administered steroids. Some immunosuppressed rats never develop a fulminant infection, even if they are caged with other infected rats. The pneumonitis in the standard model of infection is generally thought to be initiated by a reactivation of latent organisms acquired at some point in the rat's life. Whether these organisms colonize the lung or other organs of the immune competent mammal for extended periods, or exist for only a short time before the immune system eradicates them, is unknown. Likewise, the minimum number required to initiate the infection has not been determined. Thus, the exposure to and dosage of *P. carinii* are not controlled in the naturally acquired infection. The ability to somewhat control these factors in the inoculated model produces a more consistent infection among rats in a given colony, and the time required for a fulminant infection to develop is also reduced from 8–12 weeks for the natural infection to 5–7 weeks with the inoculated model. Because viral antibody-negative rats seem to be necessary for the success of the inoculated model, their use is associated with a reduction in the incidence of secondary microbial infections. Since they have been raised under barrier conditions, exposure to environmental pathogens has been minimized. They are not, however, pathogen-free, and their normal flora can cause intercurrent infections. The loss of animals from secondary infections, once a serious problem with the model of naturally acquired reactivated infection, has been minimized by the use of barrier-housing systems, such as microisolators, laminar flow rooms, and high-efficiency particulate air (HEPA)-filtered bubbles (47).

The disadvantages of the inoculated model revolve around the artificiality of the infection and questions of reproducibility. Investigators in the field of *P. carinii* have questioned if the induced infection is reflective of the natural pneumonitis in terms of life cycle stages represented, pathogenesis, and progress of disease (Second International Workshop on *Pneumocystis*, *Cryptosporidia*, and Microsporidia, Bozeman, Montana, July 1991, Session on *Pneumocystis*: Animal Models). Induction of the pneumonia using either of the inoculated models has not been successful in several laboratories that have attempted to establish these techniques. One of us (MTC) has been successful in infecting one group of rats using the technique of Boylan and Current (13), but encountered problems in subsequent attempts using a different preparation of frozen organisms. It is apparent from the collective mixed results that the technique of administration, the viability, and life cycle stages in the inocula may be important factors that determine the success or failure of the inoculated model.

Perhaps more important to the understanding of the infection is the loss of the diversity associated with exclusive use of the inoculated model. Genetic variations among *P. carinii* isolates that suggest strain or species differences, as well as coinfection with two *P. carinii* variants in individual rats, have been identified by differences in electrophoretic karyotypes, DNA sequences, and hybridization profiles (48–50) (discussed later). The very existence of strain variation and coinfection could have been detected only by use of the naturally acquired rat model of infection. Indeed, one of the dangers of using the inoculated model as the sole model of infection is the loss of the wild-type strains of *P. carinii*. The extent of the variation among *P. carinii* isolates is just beginning to be realized by electrophoretic karyotyping surveys of the various viral antibody-positive rats still available (50). The biological significance of these various strains is unknown, but current technology has the potential to identify strains that vary in virulence or antibiotic resistance.

It is clear that each model has its own advantages and disadvantages, depending on the scope of the research proposed. An investigator does not have to choose one over the other, but could employ each model as a complement to the other. For example, the inoculated model currently provides the only means by which to amplify the various isolates of *P. carinii* until a suitable culture method can be identified. It is conceivable that the drug assays could be performed with these isolates in the inoculated rat model to identify sensitive or resistant strains.

Previous attempts by investigators to induce *P. carinii* infection by inoculation in various animal recipients met with little success. It is important to reflect on the differences between present-day techniques used by Bartlett et al. (44–46) and Boylan and Current (13) and those used in previous unsuccessful attempts. The major difference appears to be the mode of inoculation. Whereas most of the earlier studies used intranasal inoculation (presumably because the transmission of infection is thought to be by an airborne particle), the more recent studies directly instill the organisms into the trachea, with little doubt about the final destination of the parasites. The germ-free status of animals in previous experiments was likely more variable than that of rodents today, since surveillance and isolation techniques currently used by vendors are more stringent than those used in the past. There is some reported evidence that animals already harboring latent organisms do not "take" the inoculated infection (46). In our own unpublished experience, attempts to produce infection by inoculation in rats harboring latent *P. carinii* were unsuccessful. The inability to establish infection in latently infected animals may have been due to an immune response mounted by the host since the rats received only one or two doses of steroids prior to inoculation. This limited immunosuppressive regimen may have left the host with an immune response sufficient to prevent the organisms from establishing the infection.

V. *Pneumocystis carinii* Infection in Immunodeficient Mice and Rats

Spontaneous outbreaks of *P. carinii* pneumonia have occurred in colonies of nude mice and mice with severe combined immunodeficiency (51–53). Spontaneous pneumocystosis has also been reported in a breeding colony of nude rats (54).

A. *Pneumocystis carinii* Infection in Immunodeficient Mice

Walzer and colleagues investigated large outbreaks of *P. carinii* pneumonia in colonies of immunodeficient mice at four different institutions (53). Of the five outbreaks described, three were among mice homozygous for the nu (nude) mutation, and two involved mice homozygous for the scid (severe combined immunodeficiency) mutation. Outbred Crl: CD1(ICR)nu/nu mice from the same commercial breeder were involved not only in two of these outbreaks, which occurred in different institutions, but also in a *P. carinii* pneumonia cluster reported previously from a third institution (52). A common source also appeared to link the development of pneumocystosis among C.B-17/Icr scid/scid mice bred and housed in two separate institutions, one of which also maintained a BALB/c nu/nu mouse colony known to have been infected with *P. carinii* for several years (53). It is of interest to note that the first documented spontaneous outbreak of *P. carinii* pneumonia among immunodeficient mice, reported by Ueda and colleagues in Japan, also occurred among BALB/c nu/nu mice (51).

In all the reports, the spontaneous development of *P. carinii* pneumonia in immunodeficient mice was associated with wasting, cyanosis, and dyspnea (51–53). Although the severity of the infection varied among individual mice, in general, it was more severe in scid/scid mice than in nu/nu mice (53), in older mice (51,53), and in mice housed together in microisolator cages or in cages on positive-pressure laminar flow racks (52,53). Lung homogenates from *P. carinii*-infected immunodeficient mice were analyzed in immunofluorescence and immunoblotting studies using mouse antiserum to mouse *P. carinii*, rabbit antiserum to rat *P. carinii*, and rabbit antiserum to human *P. carinii* (53). The results of these studies were consistent with *P. carinii* infection of mouse origin.

The Nude Mouse Model of Pneumocystis carinii Pneumonia

Whereas natural transmission among nude mice may result in severe and fatal *P. carinii* pneumonia, attempts to experimentally transmit human, rat, or mouse *P. carinii* to nude mice, or to reactive latent *P. carinii* infection in nude mice by exogenous immunosuppression, have often failed (35,53). When *P. carinii* infection has been experimentally induced, infection is typically mild, with a light to moderate organism burden (34,51). On the other hand, Furuta and colleagues have described in their studies (55,56) the sequential passage of *P. carinii* in BALB/c nu/nu mice through the intranasal inoculation of organisms in infected lung homogenate preparations. The original source of the *P. carinii* organisms was a naturally infected BALB/c nu/nu mouse. Although nude mice, by virtue of their congenital athymic defect, have greatly reduced numbers of mature functional T cells, they are capable of mounting a number of protective responses (37). It has been speculated that such responses, provoked by a variety of endogenous microbial flora, might determine relative susceptibility or resistance to *P. carinii* infection (53). At any rate, variability in the nude mouse response to *P. carinii* infection has limited its usefulness as a model.

The scid Mouse Model of Pneumocystis carinii Pneumonia

The scid mouse holds considerably more promise than the nude mouse for studies of *P. carinii* pneumonia. The autosomal recessive scid mutation was first identified in the BALB/c congenic inbred mouse strain C.B-17 (BALB/c.C57BL/Ka-lgh-l^{b}/lcr) at the Institute for Cancer Research, Fox Chase Cancer Center, Philadelphia, Pennsylvania (57). The scid mutation has been maintained in the C.B-17 congenic strain and has also been transferred to several other inbred mouse strains (58).

Homozygous scid/scid mice, commonly referred to as scid mice, have greatly reduced numbers of T cells and B cells and lack detectable levels of circulating immunoglobulins (37). They have a rudimentary thymic medulla without cortex, relatively empty splenic follicles and lymph nodes, and underdeveloped bronchial and intestinal lymphocytic foci (59). The scid mutation is associated with a defect in the rearrangement of genes that code for antigenic-specific receptors on B cells and T cells, resulting in defective lymphoid differentiation (37). The mutation does not appear to seriously impair the hematopoietic microenvironment necessary for lymphoid differentiation because reconstitution of lymphoid tissues with functional T cells and B cells can be achieved by transplantation of bone marrow cells from normal syngeneic mice. Cells of the myeloid lineage and natural killer cells appear to be normal in scid mice (37).

The scid mouse presents an ideal model system for studying lymphoid deficiency and for elucidating the differentiation of the lymphoid system after reconstitution with appropriate normal murine precursor cells (60). The characteristics of the scid defect have been further exploited to reconstruct the human immune system within mice with the scid mutation (61). The potential power of the scid mouse system has generated intense interest in its use (62). The spontaneous occurrence of pneumocystosis in research colonies of scid mice offers, on the one hand, a promising new animal model of *P. carinii* pneumonia, on the other, a threat to experimentation unrelated to *P. carinii* research (53).

A recent study from the Jackson Laboratory documents the occurrence and pathobiology of pneumocystosis in populations of scid breeders and offspring mice specifically held for life span analysis and pathology (58). These populations were established from C.B-17/lcr scid mice originally obtained from the breeding colony of the Institute for Cancer Research, Philadelphia, where the scid mutation was identified (57), and where an outbreak of *P. carinii* pneumonia was first recognized in 1984 among a colony of approximately 900 scid/scid mice (53). A total of 535 C.B-17 scid mice were followed at the Jackson Laboratory: 89 male and 121 female mice housed in a barrier facility and 149 male and 176 female mice conventionally housed. Mice in both these animal facilities developed profound *P.*

carinii pneumonia and died within the first year of life. The cumulative percentage survival of C.B-17 scid mice maintained in a conventional room was compared with that of C.B-17 scid mice maintained in a barrier room (Fig. 1). The scid mice from conventional quarters had a dramatic reduction in median life span (expressed as survival age at which 50% of the mice were still alive) compared with mice housed in the barrier facility; male mice from both barrier and conventional rooms died earlier than corresponding female mice. Although scid mice housed in a conventional animal room developed severe *P. carinii* pneumonia earlier than barrier-housed scid mice, very few mice in either facility survived beyond a year. Twenty ill scid mice underwent comprehensive necropsy. All showed evidence of moderate to severe interstitial pneumonitis characteristic of pneumocystis infection. Numerous *P. carinii* cysts and trophozoites were identified in lung sections stained with Grocott's methenamine silver and Giemsa, respectively. By far the most obvious sign of morbidity was loss of body weight. Female and male scid mice weighed 40% and 30% less, respectively, than similarly aged congenic normal controls. By contrast, the lungs of clinically ill mice with 30% or more reduction in body weight were strikingly enlarged, with a grayish, often mottled appearance, and weighed 2.5 times more than those of similarly aged congenic normal controls. The pulmonary histopathological appearance in scid mice with *P. carinii* pneumonia was quite similar to that in humans and rats with pneumocystosis and included the typical foamy, eosinophilic alveolar exudate containing massed *P. carinii* trophozoites and cysts, as well as alveolar macrophages. The authors speculate that the presence of other opportunistic pathogens in the conventional animal facility may have accelerated the course of the pneumocystosis. This hypothesis is supported by two studies in which pneumocystosis in scid mice was exacerbated by inoculation with pneumonia virus of mice (PVM), a virus that is relatively nonpathogenic in normal mice (63,64). In the first study, C3H/HeSnJ scid mice naturally infected with *P. carinii* became ill and died of pneumocystis pneumonia within 28 days of PVM inoculation. No morbidity or mortality occurred in control noninoculated scid mice nor in inoculated normal congenic C3H mice. A second study extended these findings to BALB/c scid mice and confirmed that PVM inoculation of scid mice free of infection with *P. carinii* caused little morbidity and no mortality, although widespread lesions typical of PVM infection were noted in the lungs (64).

Two studies helped to elucidate the immune mechanisms involved in host resistance to *P. carinii* (58,65). In the first study, spontaneous *P. carinii* pneumonia in scid mice was used to analyze the effect on *P. carinii* infection of reconstitution of scid mice with bone marrow cells from normal congenic mice (58). Surprisingly, some two-thirds of the recipient mice died about 1 month after reconstitution, whereas none of 15 scid mice receiving scid bone marrow cells died at a comparable time. The deaths were attributed to a striking pulmonary inflammatory response, presumably caused by the preexisting *P. carinii* infection.

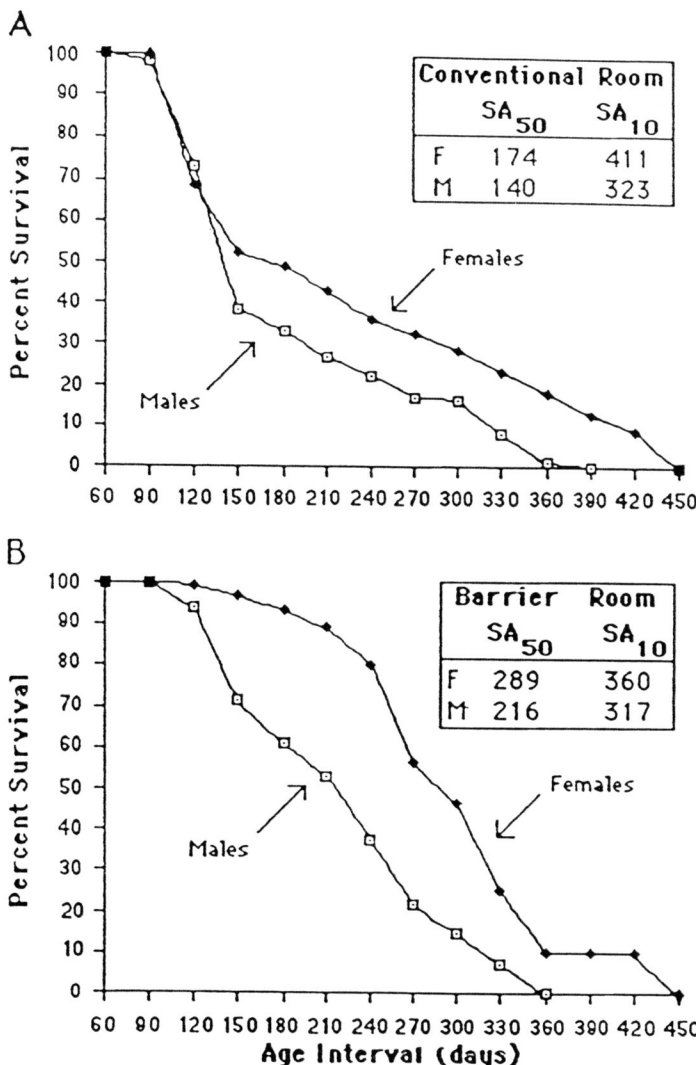

Figure 1 Cumulative percentage of survival of C.B-17-scid mice maintained in either (A) conventional or (B) barrier mouse room. The survival age (SA) at which 50% and 10% of the female and male mice remained alive is indicated. (From Ref. 58.)

Most alveoli contained massive numbers of macrophages, whereas others were filled with edema fluid, and there was prominent perivascular and peribronchial infiltration by well-differentiated lymphocytes. Essentially complete resolution of the pneumocystosis occurred among those marrow-treated scid mice that survived the period of hyperinflammation. Among scid mice receiving scid bone marrow, however, the pneumocystis infection intensified with time, and overt *P. carinii* pneumonia developed.

In the second study, the scid mice carrying the *P. carinii* infection eliminated almost all cysts 4 weeks after transfer of either 5 million sensitized or nonsensitized lymph node cells (LNC) (65). Transfer of 500,000 sensitized LNC resulted in a decrease of cyst load by 68%, but the same number of nonsensitized LNC did not cause a significant reduction. Transfer of 5×10^4 of sensitized or nonsensitized LNC had no effect on the number of cysts. Similar to the bone marrow recipients in the previous study, a hyperinflammatory reaction was observed along with mortality, especially in mice receiving 5×10^5 LNC. The LNC-supplemented mice also mounted a humoral response, as evidenced by near-normal levels of IgM levels in the lung. However, increases in specific anti-*P. carinii* antibody (both IgM and IgG2a) were observed only in scid mice that received 5 million LNC from *P. carinii*-immunized donors.

In the same study, adoptive transfer of lymphocyte subsets and passive hyperimmune serum therapy were evaluated for antipneumocystis response. Fluorescence-activated cell sorter (FACS)-sorted $CD4^+$ T cells reduced cyst numbers to 5% of the untreated controls, whereas transferred $CD8^+$ T cells were ineffective in decreasing organism load. Again, mice receiving the $CD4^+$ cells experienced increased lung mass attributable to a hyperinflammatory response. These studies demonstrate the importance of $CD4^+$ cells for resistance to *P. carinii* and also underscores the potentially lethal hyperinfla/mmatory response associated with transfer. The specific humoral immune response initiated by transfer of $CD4^+$ cells offers a second line of resistance to *P. carinii* infection.

Other reconstitution experiments using scid mice have established the essential role of $CD4^+$ T cells in resistance to *P. carinii* infection (66). Harmsen and Stankiewicz treated *P. carinii*-infected scid mice with infusions of spleen cells from immunocompetent mice and demonstrated a striking reduction in the *P. carinii* lung burden within 3–4 weeks of reconstitution (66). No mortality was reported, although lung lavage fluids contained numerous lymphoblasts, lymphocytes, neutrophils, and macrophages. When such reconstituted scid mice were depleted of $CD4^+$ T cells with injections of anti-CD4 monoclonal antibody, their acquired ability to resolve their pneumocystis infection was eliminated (66). A subsequent report by these same investigators suggested that B cells are also necessary (67). This conclusion was based on the finding that there was no resolution of the *P. carinii* infection when scid mice were reconstituted with cell populations that contained T cells, but that were depleted of B cells. The *P. carinii*-infected scid mouse model reconstituted with immunocompetent mouse spleen cells was further used to investigate the role of cytokines in host resistance to *P. carinii* (68). Such reconstituted mice were given intraperitoneal injections of either anti–tumor necrosis factor-alpha IgG or anti–interferon gamma IgG. Clearance of the *P. carinii* infection was inhibited by anti–tumor necrosis factor-alpha IgG, but not by anti–interferon gamma IgG.

The scid mice have also been reported to propagate human *P. carinii* in vivo. Sethi inoculated *P. carinii* organisms obtained by bronchoalveolar lavage from an AIDS patient with pneumocystis pneumonia into the trachea of scid mice (69). Since these mice were known to be infected with mouse *P. carinii*, monoclonal antibodies to human and to mouse *P. carinii* were used in a double-immuno-fluorescence staining procedure to distinguish human from mouse organisms in impression smears of lungs from mice sampled at intervals following inoculation. From the results of this procedure, it was determined that the lungs of recipient mice were colonized by the human *P. carinii*, the number of which increased substantially within 10 days of inoculation. After 20 days, the number of mouse *P. carinii* in inoculated mice also increased markedly, compared with control uninoculated scid mice. It is clearly desirable to exploit this potential for growth of human *P. carinii* in scid mice that are free of endogenous mouse *P. carinii*. Colonies of scid mice free of *P. carinii* have been successfully established by cesarian rederivation and maintenance under strict specific pathogen-free (SPF) conditions (e.g., Taconic Farms, Germantown, New York; Harlan Sprague-Dawley, Inc., Indianapolis, Indiana).

The T-cell–Depleted Mouse Model of Pneumocystis carinii Pneumonia

Shellito and colleagues have developed a new mouse model of *P. carinii* infection by selective depletion of helper T lymphocytes in virus-free, *P. carinii*-free BALB/c mice that are given intratracheal inoculations of *P. carinii* derived from the lungs of chronically infected athymic mice (70). Helper T-cell depletion was achieved by weekly injections of anti-CD4 monoclonal antibody. Two intratracheal inoculations were made a week apart after two anti-CD4 antibody injections had been given, and consisted of an inoculum of at least 2×10^4–2×10^5 *P. carinii* cysts obtained from two separate pools of infected lungs. The intensity of the resultant infection was graded by histological examination of lung tissue, using a modification of existing semiquantitative scoring methods. The induced infection was stable and persisted for 3 months with continued antibody treatment, but cleared spontaneously when antibody treatment was stopped (Fig. 2).

This model is being used to examine the components of the host defense against *P. carinii*. A recent study sought to test the hypothesis that *P. carinii* pneumonia in AIDS may result from impaired local release of interferon gamma in the lungs and subsequent failure of macrophage activation (71). Mice rendered immunodeficient by selective depletion of $CD4^+$ lymphocytes and infected by intratracheal *P. carinii* inoculation were exposed 4 weeks thereafter to daily

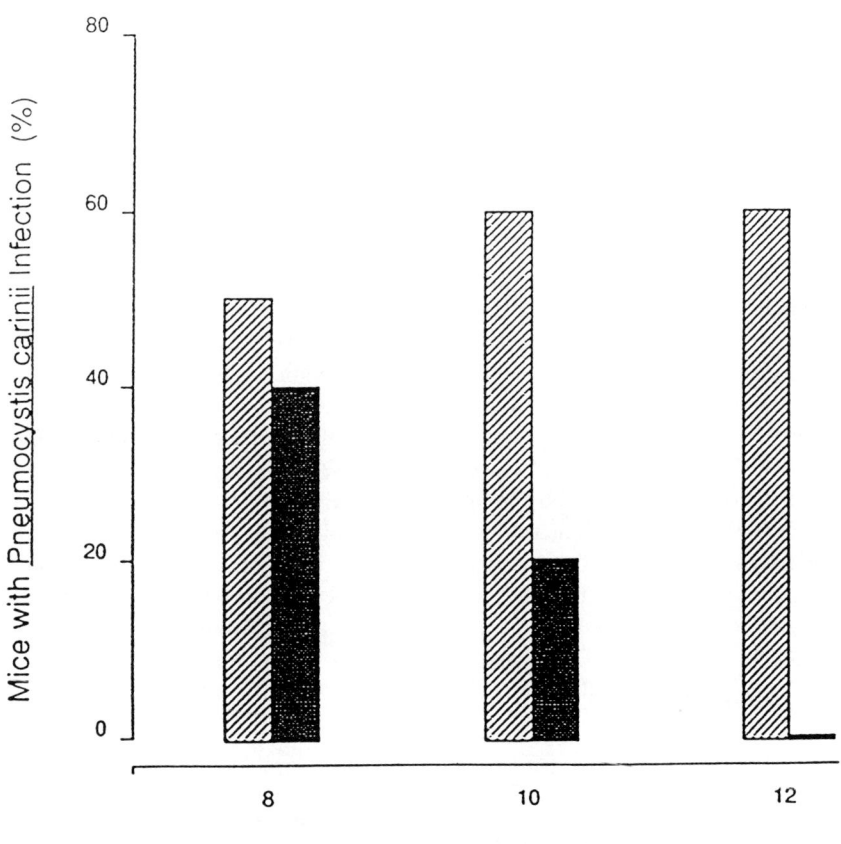

Figure 2 Percentage of mice with *P. carinii* infection. Data at each time point represent the results for at least five mice. Hatched bars, mice given two intratracheal inoculations of *P. carinii* organisms and weekly anti-CD4 antibody; shaded bars, mice given two intratracheal inoculations of *P. carinii* and anti-CD4 treatment stopped 2 weeks after the second intratracheal injection. (Reproduced from J Clin Invest 1990; 85:1686–1693 by copyright permission of the Am Soc Clin Invest.)

aerosolized recombinant murine interferon gamma for 2 weeks. This resulted in significant reduction in the intensity of the *P. carinii* infection.

The inflammatory lung responses to *P. carinii* in T-cell–depleted mice are characterized by perivascular infiltration with mononuclear cells, increase in cell number in bronchoalveolar lavage (particularly $CD8^+$ lymphocytes) and activation of alveolar macrophages (72). Although recruitment and activation of inflammatory cells in the lung still occurs even when CD4+ cells are depleted, such responses are insufficient to prevent pneumocystis infection.

B. *Pneumocystis carinii* Infection in Immunodeficient Rats

Although it is clear that *P. carinii* pneumonia may develop spontaneously in rats homozygous for the nude (rnu) mutation (54,73), there have been no reported outbreaks of pneumocystosis among nude rat colonies in the United States.

Japanese workers at the University of Tokyo have made extensive use of nude rats as a source of *P. carinii* organisms. Infection among these rats was initiated in the following way. Outbred Rowett hooded rats, homozygous for the rnu mutation (74), were inoculated intranasally with *P. carinii*-infected lung homogenates prepared from a cortisone-treated Wistar rat (75). The inoculum contained 10^5 *P. carinii* cysts. The rats were then injected with 25 mg of cortisone acetate subcutaneously twice weekly for 8 weeks. When emaciation became obvious, at 2–3 months after intranasal inoculation, rats were sacrificed and their lungs used for the next passage. It is not possible from this report to determine whether the induced *P. carinii* pneumonia was due to reactivation of a latent infection or to successful transmission of the inoculated *P. carinii* organisms. However, whatever the mechanism, there seems little doubt from the published data that the combined use of intranasal inoculation of *P. carinii* organisms and corticosteroid administration in nude rats at Tokyo University resulted in severe pneumocystosis after 4–8 weeks, allowing a significant harvest of trophozoites from bronchoalveolar lavage performed after emaciated and cyanotic rats were killed (76). Investigators in the United States, on the other hand, have had little success in reproducing the Japanese experience with nude rats. Several limited attempts to establish *P. carinii* infection in nude rats have failed (Walzer PD, Armstrong MYK, unpublished observations). In one of these attempts Rowett nude rats supplied by the NCI Animal Program received intranasal instillation of *P. carinii* organisms and were placed for 10 weeks on an immunosuppressive regimen consisting of dexamethasone added to the drinking water in a dose of 0.25–0.5 mg/liter and a low (8%)-protein diet (Armstrong MYK, unpublished data). The *P. carinii* organisms inoculated were isolated from the heavily infected lungs of corticosteroid-treated Sprague–Dawley rats that were barrier-raised, but not certified virus-free. No *P. carinii* were detected in the lungs in any of the 11 recipient nude mice, 2 of which were killed at 6 weeks, 2 at 9 weeks, and the remainder at 10 weeks. Failure to induce *P. carinii* pneumonia under these conditions could reflect resistance to the particular strain of *P. carinii* instilled, absence of latent *P. carinii* infection in the recipients, or insufficient immunosuppression. However, the fact that the Japanese nude rats are given the full immunosuppressive dose of corticosteroids, namely cortisone acetate 25 mg subcutaneously twice weekly for up to 8 weeks, suggests that the nude rats used do not have an immune defect that readily permits the growth of *P. carinii* and that the induced *P. carinii* pneumonia observed by the

Japanese workers could well reflect reactivation of widespread latent pneumocystis infection with a particularly virulent strain of the organism.

VI. *Pneumocystis carinii* Infection in Other Mammals

In his monograph on *P. carinii* pneumonitis, Hughes details the worldwide occurrence of pneumocystis infection in various mammalian species (77). By using histological stains, such as Giemsa or Grocott's methanamine silver, impression smears of the lungs from multiple animal species were examined for the presence of the cyst form, considered an irrefutable diagnostic feature of infection or colonization. *Pneumocystis carinii* was detected in many wild animals worldwide, including rats, mice, hares, rabbits, dogs, goats, swine, horses, marmosets, monkeys, chimpanzees, and cats. A survey of zoo animals in the Netherlands revealed the presence of the organism in exotic animal species, such as the sloth, kangaroo, red panda, fennec fox, and hyrax, as well as in several primate species (78). The organism has not been found outside the mammalian kingdom. The most extensive studies have been conducted in birds (78), but sporadic surveys of reptiles, amphibians, or fish have not produced any organisms resembling those recognized as *P. carinii*. The absence of the organism in these animals may be due to suboptimal body temperatures, or to a lack of suitable transmission environment, as in fish. It is perhaps important to note that within the mammalian species assayed, the golden hamster was found to be refractory to attempts to induce the infection by inoculation (5) and provocation by immunosuppressive agents (79). Analysis of this animal's immune function and components may provide clues to the immune factors needed for resistance to *P. carinii* infection.

Although the infection can be induced in almost any mammalian species, the immunosuppressed rodent model has served as the standard model of infection because of its low maintenance, abundant supply from commercial vendors, and relative sensitivity to the immunosuppressive actions of corticosteroids, while maintaining some resistance to the resultant cachexia. However, several investigators have turned to alternative models of infection for a variety of reasons.

A. The Ferret Model of *Pneumocystis carinii* Infection

Having been used previously as a suitable model for the study of other respiratory infections, the ferret (*Mustela pulorius furo*) was developed as an alternative, larger animal model of pneumocystis pneumonia by Stokes et al. (80). Infections appeared after about 10 weeks of corticosteroid immunosuppression (cortisone acetate 20 mg/kg), a time period equivalent to development of infection in the rodent model. Postmortem examination of the ferret lungs by light microscopic and ultrastructural techniques revealed organisms with morphology identical with those from rat and human sources. Likewise, the histological assessment of the lungs showed the characteristic interstitial pneumonitis and alveolitis previously reported in other mammalian hosts. However, unlike rats, ferrets were steroid-insensitive. Steroid administration in sensitive animal species, like rats and mice, results in dramatic loss in body weight and regression of lymphoid tissue, whereas in insensitive species, like humans, these changes are less dramatic, while sustaining similar immune system depression. Because of the ferret's steroid insensitivity, it is healthier in appearance and is able to sustain more experimental manipulations. One such manipulation in bronchoalveolar lavage, a technique that permits serial sampling of the infected lungs, rather than a terminal evaluation at death. Bronchoalveolar lavage is quite difficult to perform on a live rat or mouse. The size of the ferret lungs is 8–12 g, as compared with 1–2 g of the rat, which also facilitates the lavage technique and recovery of significant numbers of organisms. The ferret model has been used to develop innovative treatment modalities such as the administration of monoclonal antibodies targeted at major antigens of ferret *P. carinii* (81).

B. The Newborn and Adult Rabbit Model of *Pneumocystis carinii* Infection

Experimental induction of *P. carinii* pneumonia in rabbits was first reported by Sheldon in 1959 (3). The infection developed in young or old rabbits that were intranasally inoculated with human- and rabbit-derived *P. carinii* organisms and subsequently immunosuppressed with cortisone acetate (5–10 mg/kg). The infection was also observed to develop in the control groups of immunosuppressed rabbits that received no inocula or boiled inocula. Sheldon concluded that his inoculations were not the origin of infection in these animals, since the uninoculated, immunosuppressed control groups were equally infected. The pulmonary lesions of the pneumonia in the rabbits were reported to resemble a subclinical form of pneumonitis in human patients, compared with a widespread pneumonia that occurred in infected infants at that time (3). Since the rabbits were at most immunosuppressed for 44 days, perhaps continued immunosuppression would have produced more involvement of the rabbit lung.

In a more recent study, Soulez et al. reported induction of *P. carinii* infection in white rabbits of various ages (82). The parasite density was higher in younger, rather than older, rabbits and in those younger rabbits immunosuppressed with orally administered prednisolone, as compared with those injected subcutaneously with hydrocortisone. Sufficient numbers of organisms were obtained for immunological, ultrastructural, and in vitro experiments. After making the observation that 80–100% of untreated young rabbits obtained from two vendors in France were heavily infected with *P. carinii*, the same group went on to use this nonimmunosuppressed model for ultrastructural and in vitro studies (83–85). Numbers of organisms per lung decreased from $68 \pm 50 \times 10^6$ cysts at 4 days postweaning to $23 \pm 9 \times 10^6$ cysts after 8 days (84). When the neonate rabbits were administered steroids for 2–3 weeks after weaning, cyst counts averaged

$55 \pm 50 \times 10^6$. Although the young or weanling rabbit model of infection has advantages, such as the ability to study the infection without the confounding factor of steroid administration, this model has limitations in terms of organism yield or in drug evaluations because of the self-limiting nature of the infection.

C. Pneumocystis carinii Infection in the Hairless Athymic Guinea Pig

The occurrence of *P. carinii* infection in hairless athymic guinea pigs was first described during the Third International Workshop on Nude Mice held in Bozeman, Montana, 1979 (86). In 1975, a colony of hairless athymic Hartley guinea pigs was established after a mutation in this breed appeared (86). Similar to nude mice and rats, the hairless guinea pigs were smaller than their unaffected littermates, had wrinkled skin, and little to no hair. Normal thymic tissue was absent, and the T-cell regions in the spleen and lymph nodes were cell-depleted. The animals were hypogammaglobulinemic and were susceptible to microbial infections. The mode of inheritance of the defect is not well understood and has not been proved to behave as an autosomal recessive, as in the nude rat or mouse. Hairless guinea pigs were able to survive for up to 6 months, as long as they were separated from their mothers and littermates at birth and placed in HEPA-filtered chambers.

Pneumocystis carinii infection was cited as a frequent cause of death of these animals (86) along with other infectious agents such as cytomegalovirus, viral and fungal infections, and systemic balantidiasis, an infection caused by *Balantidium caviae*, a ciliated protozoan found naturally in the intestinal tract of guinea pigs. The number of animals surveyed was not reported, but two cases of *P. carinii* pneumonia were discussed (86). Histological sections of the lung showed large areas of the alveolar fields to be filled with pink foamy material when stained with hematoxylin–eosin, and with cysts when stained with methenamine silver.

Although athymic hairless guinea pig colonies chronically infected with *P. carinii* have not yet been established, it would appear that this model could serve a function similar to that of other immunodeficient rodent models.

D. The Porcine Model of Pneumocystis carinii Infection

Commercial producers of pigs are well aware of the predisposition of these animals to respiratory infections. The etiologic agents responsible for the coughing observed in many of these herds historically have been identified as bacterial and viral in origin (87). Recent studies from Denmark have identified *P. carinii* as another causative agent of pneumonia in commercially raised piglets (88,89). In one study, pneumonia associated with *P. carinii* was found in almost 40% of piglets aged 4–10 weeks (89). The condition in sick piglets was characterized by growth retardation, dyspnea, and dry coughing before and after weaning, with some cases of diarrhea observed among the herd. The infection was refractory to antibiotic therapy. Postmortem findings included enlarged lungs, with diffuse consolidation. Histopathological findings were typical of pneumocystis pneumonia in other animals; interstitial pneumonia, foamy, acidophilic honeycomb material in the alveoli, and crescent-shaped cysts stained by the Grocott methenamine silver method. As these piglets had not received any immunosuppressive agents, it was hypothesized that the piglets' exposure to stress factors, such as overcrowding, early weaning, or malnutrition resulting from frequent bouts of diarrhea, may have resulted in a depressed immune system (89). The spontaneous infection in piglets without the administration of exogenous steroids holds promise as an alternative animal model of *P. carinii* pneumonia. The size of the piglet should facilitate bronchoalveolar lavage as well as the administration of treatment protocols involving aerosolization of compounds. The very large size of the lungs relative to the rodent or ferret should permit large numbers of organisms or host cells to be harvested for experimental purposes. The major disadvantages of the porcine model are also associated with its size; pigs are expensive to purchase and house when compared with smaller animals, even when kept as piglets or when "minipigs" are used. Another disadvantage is the transitory nature of the *P. carinii* pneumonia. The infections reportedly disappear from the herds as spontaneously as they appear (89).

E. *Pneumocystis carinii* Infection in Cats and Dogs

Surveys of cats in the United States (90), Mexico (91,92), and Denmark (93) reported the detection of *P. carinii* cysts in the lungs at frequencies of 0% (0 of 36), 4% (4 of 100), and 4% (3 of 75), respectively. The study conducted in the United States retrospectively analyzed 36 paraffin blocks from cats with documented feline leukemia virus in Ohio (90), in contrast with the other studies that examined domestic populations of stray animals (91–93). No evidence of *P. carinii* was found in this subpopulation of cats that had marked immunodeficiencies associated with their viral infection. It may be that the cat has some intrinsic factors in its immune system, differences in viral or microbial flora, or metabolism that impart some resistance to *P. carinii*, since corticosteroid immunosuppression of even young animals does not produce a fulminant infection (discussed in the following).

Yoshida and Ikai found cysts in 15% (2 of 13) dogs that were trapped and examined in Kyoto, Japan (94), whereas Davalos (91) reported that cysts were found in 2.7% (3 of 108) dogs in Mexico City, 1963. Ten years later, Zavala and Rosado found *P. carinii* organisms in 6.3% (4 of 63) dogs and in 12.6% (10 of 79) cats of Merida, Yucatan (92). In 1984, Settnes and Hasselager (93) found the organism in 1 of 106 dogs examined in Denmark.

Cases of naturally occurring pneumonia caused by organisms identified as *P.*

carinii by the usual staining procedures (e.g., methenamine silver) have been reported in dogs (95–99), but not in cats. In 1960, van den Akker and Goedbloed reported the occurrence of *P. carinii* pneumonia in a 1-year-old dog (of unknown breed) in Utrecht (95). The dog had a history of coughing for months, was short of breath, and tired easily. After increasing dyspnea, the dog died. The lungs were found to be gray and consolidated at necropsy. There also appeared to be involvement of other organs, as fluid was found in the thoracic and abdominal cavities, the liver was congested, and the right chamber of the heart was dilated. Microscopic examination of lung tissue revealed alveoli filled with periodic acid–Schiff (PAS)–positive-staining foamy material, interstitial pneumonia with a small number of plasma cell present, and varying degrees of cellular infiltration. Many cysts were identified within the honeycomb matrix.

Subsequent reports of canine pneumocystosis usually involved several dogs, especially younger animals and those of the dachshund breed (96–99). In 1972, Farrow et al. (96) described the occurrence of *P. carinii* pneumonia in six male miniature dachshunds with ages ranging from 9 to 12 months, over a 3-year period. The symptoms were identical with those just described, except that two dogs experienced diarrhea, and all animals were reported to lose weight, despite an unaltered appetite. Chest x-rays showed diffuse infiltrates. Hematological evaluation of the six dogs showed all to have increased numbers of white blood cells concomitant with granulocytosis, and evidence of lymphopenia. Five of the six dogs exhibited polycythemia. *Pneumocystis carinii* organisms were found in all three dogs that underwent percutaneous lung biopsy. The dogs were administered pentamidine isethionate and appeared to improve, despite poor weight gain. The dogs were euthanized after 2 months and underwent postmortem evaluation. Although the severity of the infection was variable, all had foamy amorphous material within the alveoli and many *P. carinii* organisms. The authors noted that five of the six dogs were closely related, which raises the possibility of an immune defect responsible for the predisposition to pneumocystis infection.

Copland also reported pneumonia in pedigree miniature dachshunds, with subsequent infection of their two puppies (97). The dog and bitch were imported into Papua New Guinea from Australia and mated. After 18 months of residence, the bitch developed dyspnea, fatigue, failed to gain weight, and died of respiratory distress. No postmortem was performed. The dog developed similar symptoms and also died. The puppies developed a respiratory illness, but recovered without treatment.

Postmortem findings on the dog were characteristic of canine *P. carinii* pneumonia. The lungs were gray and solid, with frothy material exuding from the cut surface. Large numbers of organisms were detected by silver and Giemsa staining. Two cases of the infection were subsequently reported in dachshunds in South Africa in 1979 (98,99). The symptoms and postmortem findings were in keeping with the foregoing cases.

From these case reports of pneumocystosis in dogs, it seems evident that the infection has an affinity for the dachshund breed, which may suggest a congenital immune defect in at least some pedigreed lines.

Although naturally occurring pneumonia in cats has not been observed, the infection could be detected in cats rendered immune incompetent by administration of exogenous steroids (100). Shiota et al. injected cats of both sexes that ranged in age from 2 to 5 months and adult cats of 12 months. Corticosteroids were delivered in two dose regimens: twice weekly intramuscular injections of 2 mg of betamethasone sodium phosphate for 97–141 days, or 10–25 mg of prednisolone acetate for 11–168 days. Lung imprint smears from each lower lung lobe stained with Giemsa and Gomori's methenamine silver nitrate were used to assess the infections. Twelve of the 17 cats treated with corticosteroids produced light *P. carinii* infection, 1 cat treated with the 25 mg prednisolone regimen for 90 days had no evidence of infection, whereas 4 cats that were immunosuppressed with betamethasone for longer than 100 days did not develop infection. Of the 12 cats that did have light *P. carinii* infection, 1 cat had been immunosuppressed for only 11 days. None of the cats developed moderate or heavy infection, even with increased corticosteroid dose or extended time periods. Organisms were not found in 6 untreated cats used as controls and sacrificed at the start of the experiment, indicating that latent organisms may not be harbored by this animal, or the organisms do not remain for any extended periods in their lungs. The immunosuppressed cats lost weight owing to the catabolic effects of the steroids, but other symptoms, such as dyspnea or cyanosis, were not noted. Microscopic examination of the lightly infected lungs did not show the characteristic foamy exudate, and the inflammatory changes were noted as insignificant. Ultrastructural analysis revealed that the host tissue was unaffected by the infection.

The apparent paucity of latent organisms harbored by the cat and the failure to induce the infection even with extended administration would indicate that the cat is not a suitable model for *P. carinii* infection.

F. *Pneumocystis carinii* Infection in Arabian Foals with Combined Immunodeficiency

Pneumocystis carinii infection in horses was first reported in two Arabian foals in 1973, in Ithaca, New York (101). Two 3-month-old colts underwent evaluation because of apparent weakness, lethargy, loss of weight, and labored breathing. Chest x-ray films revealed diffuse bilateral infiltrates. The colts did not respond to therapy, including triple sulfonamides or sulfamethazine. Coughs in both colts grew progressively worse and the animals died. Microscopic examination of the lungs of the one foal showed diffuse proliferation of the alveolar epithelium, thickened alveolar septae, and honeycomb exudate that filled the alveolar lumens. Organisms were detected throughout the alveoli, but not in any other organ.

Microscopic evaluation of the other set of lungs did not exhibit the involvement shown by the first, although many alveoli contained the honeycomb exudate and some *P. carinii* cysts were detected. *Corynebacterium equi* was cultured from the nasopharynx and it was thought that *P. carinii* contributed to, but was not the sole cause of death in the second foal.

The severe combined immunodeficiency (SCID) disorder in foals was first described by McGuire and Poppie in 1973 (102). The SCID is a genetic disorder inherited as an autosomal recessive trait and has only been found in Arabian horses to date. A herd of SCID horses is maintained at Washington State University where adult horses are heterozygous for the gene (103,104). Affected foals do not live past 4–5 months of age, exhibit lymphopenia (<1000 lymphocytes per cubic millimeter) at birth, and are unable to synthesize immunoglobulins. These animals are susceptible to a wide variety of viral, bacterial, and fungal infections, including *P. carinii* pneumonia (105). Perryman et al. reported *P. carinii* pneumonia in 30% (22 of 66) of SCID foals examined at autopsy (105).

The SCID horse model has been used to evaluate immunotherapy of cryptosporidiosis (103) and holds promise as a model for selected studies of *P. carinii* infection requiring larger animals, such as bronchoalveolar lavage.

G. *Pneumocystis carinii* Infection in Nonhuman Primates

Reports of the detection of *P. carinii* organisms in various monkeys can be found in the literature, with descriptions of some cases that may have clinical import. These studies predate the emergence of simian models of the acquired immune deficiency syndrome currently being developed. It will be interesting to see the incidence of this opportunistic pathogen in animals infected with SIV, the simian equivalent of human immunodeficiency virus (HIV).

One early study described the frequency of pulmonary infection with *P. carinii* in a colony of marmoset monkeys (106). The study was undertaken as a retrospective evaluation of necropsies done between the years 1966 and 1975. Of the 441 lung specimens available for study, 50 animals (11.3%) were found to harbor the organism by histological staining methods. Most infections were slight or moderate, although two monkeys had enough organisms to be considered of clinical significance. The younger animals and those residing in the colony for the longest periods had a higher prevalence rate.

Pulmonary pneumocystosis was detected in two aged male owl monkeys (*Aotus trivirgatus*) and two chimpanzees (*Pan troglodytes*) held for 5 years at the Centers for Disease Control, Atlanta, Georgia (107). One owl monkey had received 1 million *Treponema pallidum* organisms to induce experimental syphilis in 1965, the other was uninoculated. In 1969, both monkeys became ill and exhibited weight loss and anorexia and died later in the same year. Necropsy of the owl monkeys showed patchy areas of alveolar involvement, with groups of alveoli filled with an eosinophilic, vacuolated, granular material, proteinaceous fluid, and organisms detected by methenamine silver staining. Extrapulmonary *P. carinii* were not observed.

Both chimpanzees had an underlying immunosuppressive state caused by myeloproliferative malignant neoplasms (107). The chimpanzees developed anorexia, had elevated white blood cell counts, showed extensive infiltrates on chest x-ray films, and exhibited cyanosis. After showing clinical improvement with antibiotic, corticosteroid, or pentamidine therapy, the therapy was discontinued and the animals subsequently relapsed and died of *P. carinii* infection. In one case, the lungs were diffusely consolidated; in the other, areas of discrete consolidation were scattered. Histologically, the alveoli contained the honeycomb exudate as well as large numbers of the organisms.

In six splenectomized owl monkeys maintained at Ft. Detrick, Maryland, interstitial pneumonia caused by *P. carinii* was found in two of the monkeys (108). Both monkeys were emaciated at death, and numerous organisms were found in the alveoli, accompanied by the frothy exudate typical of *P. carinii* pneumonia. However, the authors concluded that only in one monkey was pneumocystis pneumonia of clinical significance (108).

An extensive study of macaque monkeys in Japan was undertaken by Matsumoto et al. in 1987 (109). Lung samples of 128 monkeys were retrospectively examined for the presence of *P. carinii* by silver staining of the paraffin blocks. Cysts were found in 5 of the 128 monkeys examined (4%). The 5 monkeys that were positive were found in two species of the genus, *Macaca*; 4 of 52 *M. fuscata fuscata* and 1 of 13 *M. fasicularis*. Three of the 5 *P. carinii*-positive monkeys were debilitated, with influenza-like symptoms, diarrhea, and emaciation. One of these was diagnosed with pneumonia. Two of the cases were infants younger than 1 year old, and 3 were young monkeys younger than 3 years old. Three were debilitated at the time of death. Necropsy revealed only minor infection with *P. carinii* and lack of findings characteristic of pneumocystosis (e.g., foamy exudate). It was concluded that pneumocystis infection was not the cause of death in any of the 5 cases.

Evaluation of the collective presentations of pneumocystosis described in the foregoing indicate that fulminant pneumocystosis is not a common form of pneumonia among nonhuman primates.

VII. *Pneumocystis carinii* Strain and Species Variations

The organism known as *P. carinii* has been identified in a multitude of mammalian species, usually in animals with some underlying condition that decreases immunocompetence. One question that remains unanswered and that is crucial to our understanding of the epidemiology and transmission of human *P. carinii* infection is that of the identity of the organism. Is *P. carinii* a zoonosis, infecting man and animals indiscriminately, or are there organism species that are capable of infecting only a given mammalian species? Previous studies offer some data that indicate species-level differences. Early serological studies suggested that there were both shared and distinct antigenic epitopes on organisms from different hosts (5,110). Later, studies of rat-, human-, mouse-, and ferret-derived organisms reached similar conclusions with the more sensitive technique of immunoblotting (111–115).

On the other hand, numerous studies of the various developmental forms of *P. carinii* at the light microscopic or ultrastructural levels have not identified any morphological differences among isolates of different animal origin (116–120).

Differences among *P. carinii* isolates at the genotypic level have been identified recently using a variety of techniques. Pulsed field gel electrophoresis (PFGE) gave the first indication of the heterogeneity among organisms isolated from rats. At least three laboratories have published electrophoretic karyotypes of *P. carinii* obtained from different rat strains (121–123). Although the studies used different PFGE techniques, clear differences among the numbers and sizes of the ethidium bromide-stained chromosome bands of organisms were evident. Most of the rat-derived isolates separated within a 250- to 750-kb range and contained 13–15 bands. In a recent study over 100 *P. carinii* isolates from viral-positive rats were analyzed by pulsed field electrophoresis techniques (124). Several rat strains from different commercial vendors were sampled during the study, including Lewis, Fischer 344, Wistar, Long-Evans, and Sprague–Dawley rats. Examples of electrophoretic karyotypes of *P. carinii* from several different rat strains produced by contour-clamped homogeneous electrical field (CHEF) are shown in Figure 3. Generally, the same karyotype was produced by isolates from the same breeding colony, but different rat colonies contained different types of

---

Figure 3 Separation of rat-derived *P. carinii* by contour-clamped homogeneous electrical field (CHEF). Organisms were isolated from the infected lungs of various rat strains and embedded in low-melt agarose according to previous protocols (122). One percent agarose gels prepared in 45 mM Tris HCl–0.125 M EDTA–45 mM boric acid (0.5× TBE) were loaded with organism plugs and run at 14°C at 6.4 V/cm, 60–100 sec continuous ramp for 120 hr. Isolates in the lanes shown are identified by the vendor and rat strain; isolate/rat number; and time of immunosuppression by corticosteroids (pi). Lambda ladder size markers are in the first lane and single isolates of *P. carinii* from the following rat strains and vendors are in adjacent lanes: (HH) Harlan, Inc. (Indianapolis, Indiana) Holtzman rat; (SH) Sasco, Inc. (Omaha, Nebraska) Holtzman; (ZM-SD) Zivic-Miller Sprague–Dawley (Zelienople, Pennsylvania); (HF) Hilltop (Scottdale, Pennsylvania) Fischer 344; (HW) Hilltop Wistar; (CRL) Charles River Laboratories (Wilmington, Massachusetts) Lewis; (CRLE) Charles River Long Evans; (CRBN) Charles River Brown Norway.

Animal Models 211

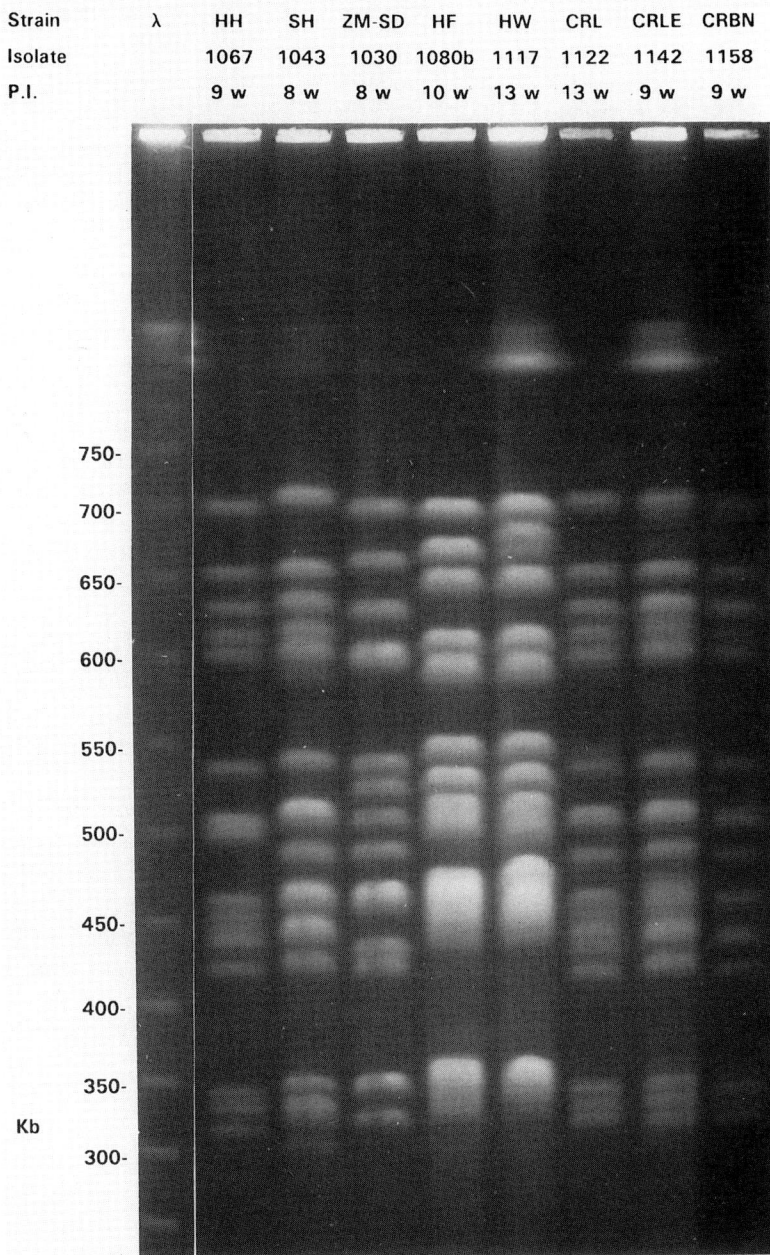

P. carinii. For example, all Sprague–Dawley rats from Zivic-Miller (Zelionople, Pennsylvania) produced a 13-banded karyotype (see Fig. 3, lane 4, ZM–SD), but this was distinct from the karyotype produced by *P. carinii* isolated from Hilltop (Scottdale, Pennsylvania) Fischer rats (see Fig.3 , lane 5, HF). However, some rat colonies produced a few isolates that did not contain the typical 13- to 15-band karyotype, but instead contained 22 bands (<10% frequency). By using a combination of DNA hybridization, the polymerase chain reaction (PCR), and DNA sequencing, it was determined that the 22-band patterns resulted from coinfection with two types of *P. carinii* that were genetically distinct (48).

The identification of two entities within the infected lung raises exciting possibilities for understanding the mechanism of recurrent episodes of pneumocystosis. It is conceivable that strains resistant to current therapies may coexist with sensitive strains, producing what initially appears to be a clinical response (eradication of the sensitive organism), with a subsequent lag phase, followed by replication of the resistant strain. With these molecular biological techniques to characterize *P. carinii* isolates, it is now possible to approach this question as well as other epidemiological and taxonomic questions. Such tools are essential for determining the origin of disseminated *P. carinii* infection, as well as for the characterization of those organisms capable of causing pneumonitis in patient populations without underlying immunosuppression (125). If there are gradations of virulence among *P. carinii* strains, these techniques should provide a means of identifying them. The existence of *P. carinii* variants and coinfection in the immunosuppressed rat predicts that a similar situation likely exists in humans, since in almost every aspect evaluated, the rat model mirrors the infection in humans.

Few karyotypic separations have been performed on *P. carinii* isolates from sources other than immunosuppressed rats. Electrophoretic karyotypes produced from ferret-derived organisms and presented at the Second International Workshop on *Pneumocystis*, *Cryptosporidia*, and Microsporidia appeared to contain eight bands, although some bands could have been obscured by the host DNA present in the lanes or not resolved by the conditions used (126). Evaluable karyotypes have not been obtained from porcine-derived *P. carinii* owing to the poor condition of the shipped organisms (Cushion M, Settnes OP, unpublished data). Hong et al. produced electrophoretic karyotypes from organisms derived from human postmortem and bronchoalveolar lavage fluids (122). Ten to twelve bands were visible in the human-derived patterns, but the low numbers of organisms present in the samples produced a faint image that was somewhat difficult to interpret. From studies of rat-derived organisms, it is apparent that at least 5×10^7 organism nuclei are needed to produce a visible ethidium bromide-stained pattern on these gels, an amount not always available from bronchoalveolar lavage fluid. Recent studies by Stringer et al. (49) show a clear electrophoretic pattern from human organisms derived from postmortem lung tissue. The human-derived pattern is clearly distinct from that of the rat (Fig. 4; compare with Fig. 3). Although the bands separated within the same size range (250–750 kb) as those of the rat *P. carinii*, the sizes of the bands larger than 550 kb differ from the rat's as well as bands between 400 and 500 kb. The human karyotype has only one small band below 300 kb, whereas the rat organisms typically display a triplet in this size range. Other dramatic differences at the genetic level were found between the human and rat isolates. DNA sequences known to be repeated in rat-derived organisms were not detected by hybridization techniques in human isolates; total DNA from rat-derived organisms failed to hybridize to *P. carinii* DNA from the human; and the sequences at two genetic loci were slightly more divergent than were sequences from the corresponding regions of *Candida albicans* and *C. tropicalis*. The base composition of the α-tubulin gene from rat-derived organisms was rich in adenine and thymine, whereas the base composition of this gene from human-derived *P. carinii* was rich in guanine and cytosine. These data help to explain the lack of hybridization observed when total rat-derived *P. carinii* DNA was used to probe the human *P. carinii* karyotypes (50). Collectively, these data suggest clear differences between the rat- and human-derived organisms.

One mouse *P. carinii* karyotype was successfully produced from the combined lungs of four scid mice obtained from Charles Sidman, University of Cincinnati College of Medicine (124). DNA hybridization techniques showed that the ribosomal locus of the mouse and rat *P. carinii* were on different-sized chromosomes and that the repeated DNAs isolated from the rat-derived organisms were not present in the *P. carinii* of the mouse. Sequencing studies are underway to determine the extent of the differences.

VIII. Conclusion

The corticosteroid-treated rat model of *P. carinii* pneumonia has been the mainstay of *P. carinii* research. This model has been involved in virtually all phases of investigative work on the organism and is still a critical source of *P. carinii* for molecular and biochemical studies. Increasingly, however, its reliability and very existence are jeopardized by the general trend to use cleaner animals for biomedical research and, specifically, by the demand for laboratory rodents that are free of major rodent viruses and other pathogens. Commercial vendors have responded with an ongoing elimination of virus-positive animals (i.e., rats and mice that may still be latently infected with *P. carinii* as well as with a variety of rodent viruses). In addition, some laboratory animal resource programs now prohibit the introduction of virus-positive rodents into their animals facilities. Improvements in animal husbandry practices have also led to a decreased prevalence of pneumocystis infection among rats and mice in colonies where *P. carinii* is still present. The resultant unpredictability of *P. carinii* pneumonia induction by corticosteroids

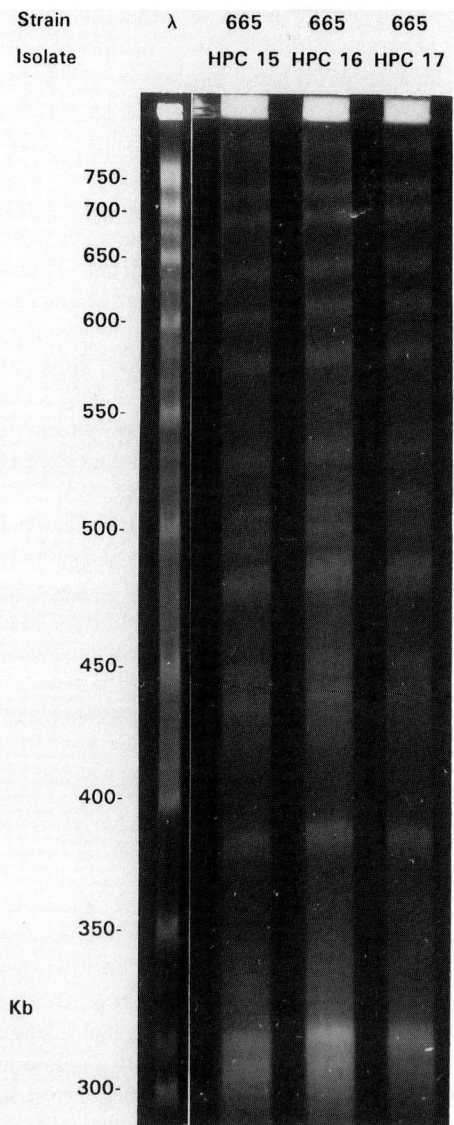

Figure 4 Separation of human-derived *P. carinii* by field inversion gel electrophoresis (FIGE). Organisms were isolated from human postmortem lung tissue according to previous protocols (122). Low-melt agarose-embedded organisms were electrophoresed through 1% agarose gels in 0.5× TBE (as described in Fig. 3, with 0.1 M glycine added) at 6.5 V/cm for 48 hr, followed by 4.9 V/cm for 96 hr, with a 50sec:25sec forward to backward pulse. The first lane contains lambda size markers. The next three lanes contain agarose-embedded organisms sequentially prepared from the infected human lung.

and the overall decrease in intensity of the reactivated infection have driven the development of alternative animal models.

The *P. carinii*-inoculated virus-negative rat models developed by Bartlett and colleagues (44,45) and by Boylan and Current (13) have provided reproducible models for the testing of new potential anti-*P. carinii* drugs in a setting in which the risk of intercurrent infection has been minimized. The natural transmission mouse model of Powles and colleagues (39) also provides a predictable pneumocystis pneumonia of uniform intensity, as well as a small-animal model for the testing of those potential anti-*P. carinii* drugs that are available in only small quantities. The naturally occurring *P. carinii* infection of scid mice and the induced infection in T-cell–depleted mice offer exciting new opportunities for sophisticated immunological studies of host resistance to *P. carinii*, without the confounding effects of corticosteroids.

The current status of animal models in *P. carinii* research was the subject of an entire session at the Second International Workshop on *Pneumocystis, Cryptosporidium*, and Microsporidia held in Bozeman, Montana, in 1991, and provoked intense discussion. Rats are still the most widely used animals in pneumocystis research. There was general consensus among the participants that, although the inoculated virus-negative rat model has much to offer, the continued availability of latently infected virus-positive rats needs to be safeguarded. There are several compelling arguments for the continued production of such rats. They more closely mimic conditions in the human lung that is exposed to a variety of organisms from the environment and, thus, they provide opportunities to study the role of associated lung microbial flora as cofactors in the pathogenesis of *P. carinii* pneumonia. In addition, as recent work has shown, there is significant diversity among *P. carinii* organisms isolated from various rat strains in different colonies. This new area of investigation should yield important information concerning the organism's transmission, virulence, and response to drugs, and would be lost with the elimination of virus-positive rats.

In the absence of sustained and substantial *P. carinii* growth in culture, a reliable animal source of organisms sufficient for basic studies remains a top priority. The National Institutes of Health workshop in future directions in discovery and development of therapeutic agents for opportunistic infections associated with AIDS (127) recommended federal support for a central animal source to guarantee the continued availability of animals naturally infected with *P. carinii*. Such a resource would provide a major boost for *P. carinii* research.

References

1. Weller R. Zur erzeugung von Pneumocystosen im tierversuch. Z Kinderheilk 1955; 76:366–378.
2. Weller R. Weitere untersuchungen über experimentele rattenpneumocystose in

hinblick auf die interstitielle pneumonie der frühgeborenen. Z Kinderheilk 1956; 78: 166–176.
3. Sheldon WH. Experimental pulmonary *Pneumocystis carinii* infection in rabbits. J Exp Med 1959; 110:147–160.
4. Frenkel JK, Havenhill MA. The corticoid sensitivity of golden hamsters, rats, and mice. Lab Invest 1963; 12:1204–1220.
5. Frenkel JK, Good JT, Shultz JA. Latent pneumocystic infection of rats, relapse and chemotherapy. Lab Invest 1966; 15:1559–1577.
6. Hughes WT, Smith B. Provocation of infection due to *Pneumocystis carinii* by cyclosporin A. J Infect Dis 1982; 145:767.
7. Hughes WT. Animal models for *Pneumocystis carinii* pneumonia. J Protozool 1989; 36:41–45.
8. Hughes WT. Experimental animal models. In: *Pneumocystis carinii* Pneumonitis. Vol 1. Boca Raton: CRC Press, 1987:71–95.
9. DeStefano JA, Trinkle LS, Walzer PD, Cushion MT. Flow cytometric analysis of lectin binding to *Pneumocystis carinii* surface carbohydrates. J Parasitol 1992; 78: 271–280.
10. Armstrong MYK, Smith AL, Richards FF. Common viral infections may modify the development of *Pneumocystis carinii* in the rat model. J Protozool 1991; 38:136S–137S.
11. Hughes WT, Price RA, Sisko F, Havron S, Kafatos AG, Schonland M, Smythe PM. Protein–calorie malnutrition. A host determinant for *Pneumocystis carinii* infection. Am J Dis Chid 1974; 128:44–52.
12. Walzer PD, LaBine M, Redington TJ, Cushion MT. Predisposing factors in *Pneumocystis carinii* pneumonia: effects of tetracycline, protein malnutrition, and corticosteroids on hosts. Infect Immun 1984; 46:747–753.
13. Boylan CJ, Current WL. Improved rat model of *Pneumocystis carinii* pneumonia: induced laboratory infections in pneumocystis-free animals. Infect Immun 1992; 60: 1589–1597.
14. Chandler FW, Frenkel JK, Campbell WG. Animal model: *Pneumocystis carinii* pneumonia in the immunosuppressed rat. Am J Pathol 1979; 95:571–574.
15. Pottratz ST, Martin WJ II. Role of fibronectin in *Pneumocystis carinii* attachment to cultured lung cells. J Clin Invest 1990; 85:351–356.
16. Settnes OP, Genner J. Survival periods in male and female Wistar rats with steroid-induced *Pneumocystis carinii* pneumonia. APMIS 1989; 97:556–558.
17. Walzer PD, Kim CK, Cushion MT. *Pneumocystis carinii*. In: Walzer PD, Genta RM, eds. Parasitic Infections in the Compromised Host. New York: Marcel Dekker, 1989: 83–178.
18. Rogers TS, Haggie MHK. *Pneumocystis carinii* pneumonia associated with hypogammaglobulinemia responding to pentamidine. Lancet 1964; 1:1042.
19. Walzer PD. Experimental *Pneumocystis carinii* infection. In: Zak O, Sande MA, eds. Experimental Models in Antimicrobial Chemotherapy. Vol. 3. Orlando: Academic Press, 1986:185–201.
20. Walzer PD, LaBine, M, Redington TJ, Cushion MT. Lymphocyte changes during chronic administration of and withdrawal from corticosteroids: relation to *Pneumocystis carinii* pneumonia. J Immunol 1984; 133:2502–2508.

21. Young KR, Rankin JA, Naegel GP, Paul ES, Reynolds HY. Bronchoalveolar lavage cells and proteins in patients with the acquired immunodeficiency syndrome. Ann Intern Med 1985; 103:522–533.
22. Van den Bogert C, Kroon MA. Effects of oxytetracycline on in vivo proliferation and differentiation of erythroid and lymphoid cells in the rat. Clin Exp Immunol 1982; 50:327–335.
23. Belshem J, Gnarpe H, Persson S. Tetracyclines and host defense mechanisms: interference with leukocyte chemotaxis. Scand J Infect Dis 1979; 11:141–145.
24. Gottschall JI, Walzer PD, Yoneda K. Morphological changes in the rat type II pneumocytes induced by oxytetracycline. Lab Invest 1979; 41:5–12.
25. Martin TR, Altman LC, Alvares OF. The effects of severe protein–calorie malnutrition on antibacterial defense mechanisms in the rat lung. Annu Rev Respir Dis 1983; 128:1013–1019.
26. Claman HN. Corticosteroids and lymphoid cells. N Engl J Med 1972; 287:388–397.
27. Pesanti EL. Effects of bacterial pneumonitis on development of pneumocystosis in rats. Annu Rev Respir Dis 1982; 125:723–726.
28. Barthold SW. A review of common infectious disease agents of laboratory mice and rats: potential influence on *Pneumocystis carinii*. J Protozool 1991; 38:131S–133S.
29. Russell RJ, McGinley JR. *Pneumocystis carinii*—animal production perspective. J Protozool 1991; 38:128S–129S.
30. Walzer PD. Overview of animal models of *Pneumocystis carinii* pneumonia. J Protozool 1991; 38:122S–123S.
31. Walzer D, Powell RD, Yoneda K, Rutledge ME, Milder JE. Growth characteristics and pathogenesis of experimental *Pneumocystis carinii* pneumonia. Infect Immun 1980; 27:928–937.
32. Cushion MT, Linke MJ. Factors in influencing pneumocystis infection in the immunocompromised rat. J Protozool 1991; 38:133S–135S.
33. Walzer PD, Powell RD Jr, Yoneda K. Experimental *Pneumocystis carinii* pneumonia in different strains of cortisonized mice. Infect Immun 1979; 24:939–947.
34. Walzer PD, Schnelle V, Armstrong D, Rosen PP. Nude mouse: a new experimental model for *Pneumocystis carinii* infection. Science 1977; 197:177–179.
35. Walzer PD, Powell RD Jr. Experimental *Pneumocystis carinii* infection in nude and steroid-treated normal mice. In: Reed ND, ed. Proceedings of the Third International Workshop on Nude Mice. New York: Gustav Fisher Verlag, 1982:123–132.
36. Walzer PD, Rutledge ME, Yoneda K. Experimental *Pneumocystis carinii* in C3H/HeJ and C3HeB/FeJ mice. J Reticuloendothel Soc 1983; 33:1–9.
37. Shultz LD, Sidman CL. Genetically determined murine models of immunodeficiency. Annu Rev Immunol 1987; 5:367–403.
38. Masur H, Murray HW, Jones TC. Effect of hydrocortisone on macrophage response to lymphokine. Infect Immun 1982; 35:709–714.
39. Powles MA, McFadden DC, Pittarelli LA, Schmatz DM. Mouse model for *Pneumocystis carinii* pneumonia that uses natural transmission to initiate infection. Infect Immun 1992; 60:1397–1400.
40. Linhartova A. Experimentelle pneumocystose bei ratten. Zentralbl Bakteriol Abt I Orig 1956; 167:178–186.
41. Csillag A, Brandstein L. The role of *Blastomyces* species in the etiology of

interstitial plasmocytic pneumonia of the premature infant. Acta Microbiol Hung 1954; 1:179–190.
42. Armstrong D, Walzer PD. Experimental infections in the nude mouse. In: Fogh J, Giovanella BC, eds. The Nude Mouse in Experimental and Clinical Research. New York: Academic Press, 1978:477–489.
43. Bartlett MS, Durkin MM, Jay MA, Queener SF, Smith JW. Sources of rats free of latent *Pneumocystis carinii*. J Clin Microbiol 1987; 25:1794–1795.
44. Bartlett MS, Fishman JA, Queener SF, Durkin MM, Jay MA, Smith JW. New rat model of *Pneumocystis carinii* infection. J Clin Microbiol 1988; 26:1100–1102.
45. Bartlett MS, Fishman JA, Durkin MM, Queener SF, Smith JW. *Pneumocystis carinii*: improved models to study efficacy of drugs for treatment of prophylaxis of pneumocystis pneumonia in the rat (*Rattus* spp.). Exp Parasitol 1990; 70:100–106.
46. Bartlett MS, Queener SF, Durkin MM, Shaw MM, Smith JW. Inoculated mouse model of *Pneumocystis carinii* pneumonia. J Protozool 1991; 38:130S–131S.
47. Walzer PD, Foy J, Steele P, Kim CK, White M, Klein RS, Otter BA, Allegra C. Activities of antifolate, antiviral, and other drugs in an immunosuppressed rat model of *Pneumocystis carinii* pneumonia. Antimicrob Agents Chemother 1992; 36:1935–1942.
48. Cushion MT, Zhang J, Kaselis M, Stringer SL, Stringer JR. Evidence for two types of *Pneumocystis* co-infecting laboratory rats. J Clin Microbiol (in press).
49. Stringer JR, Stringer SL, Zhang J, Baughman R, Smulian AG, Cushion MT. Molecular genetic evidence that *Pneumocystis* from rats and humans are different species. (submitted).
50. Cushion MT, Kaselis MT, Zhang J, Stringer JR. Variation among rodent and human *Pneumocystis* detected by electrophoretic karyotyping (submitted).
51. Ueda K, Goto Y, Yamazaki S, Fujiwara K. Chronic fatal pneumocystosis in nude mice. Jpn J Exp Med 1977; 47:475–482.
52. Weir EC, Brownstein DG, Barthold SW. Spontaneous wasting disease in nude mice associated with *Pneumocystis carinii* infection. Lab Anim Sci 1986; 36:140–144.
53. Walzer PD, Kim CK, Linke MJ, Pogue SL, Huerkamp MJ, Chrisp CE, Lerro AV, Wixson SK, Hall E, Shultz LD. Outbreaks of *Pneumocystis carinii* pneumonia in colonies of immunodeficient mice. Infect Immun 1989; 57:62–70.
54. van Hooft JIM, van Zwieter MJ, Solleveld HA. Spontaneous pneumocystosis in the athymic nude rat (abstr). Lab Anim Sci 1986; 36:P33.
55. Furuta T, Ueda K, Fujiwara K, Yamanoughi K. Cellular and humoral immune responses of mice subclinically infected with *Pneumocystis carinii*. Infect Immun 1985; 47:544–548.
56. Furuta T, Ueda K, Kyuwa S, Fujiwara K. Effect of T-cell transfer on *Pneumocystis carinii* infection in nude mice. Jpn J Exp Med 1984; 54:57–64.
57. Bosma GL, Custer RP, Bosma MJ. A severe combined immunodeficiency mutation in the mouse. Nature 1983; 301:527–530.
58. Roths JB, Marshall JD, Allen RD, Carlson GA, Sidman CL. Spontaneous *Pneumocystis carinii* pneumonia in immunodeficient mutant scid mice. Am J Pathol 1990; 136:1173–1186.
59. Custer RP, Bosma GC, Bosma MJ. Severe combined immunodeficiency (SCID) in the mouse. Pathology, reconstitution, neoplasms. Am J Pathol 1985; 120:464–477.

60. Yancopoulos GD, Alt FW. Reconstruction of an immune system. Science 1988; 241: 1581–1583.
61. McCune JM, Namikawa R, Kaneshima H, Schultx LD, Lieberman M, Weissman IL. The SCID-hu mouse: murine model for the analysis of human hematolymphoid differentiation and function. Science 1988; 241:1632–1639.
62. The SCID Mouse in Biomedical and Agricultural Research. Conference held at Ontario: The University of Guelph, August 5–7, 1992.
63. Roths JB, Smith AL, Sidman CL. Lethal exacerbation of *Pneumocystis carinii* pneumonia (PCP) in scid mice after infection by pneumonia virus of mice (PVM). J Exp Med (in press).
64. Bray MV, Barthold SW, Sidman CL, Roths JB, Smith AL. Exacerbation of *Pneumocystis carinii* pneumonia in immunodeficient (scid) mice by concurrent infection with a pneumovirus. Infect Immun (in press).
65. Roths JB, Sidman CL. Both immunity and hyperresponsiveness to *Pneumocystis carinii* result from transfer of CD4$^+$ T cells into severe combined immunodeficiency mice. J Clin Invest 1992; 90:673–678.
66. Harmsen AG, Stankiewicz M. Requirement for CD4$^+$ cells in resistance to *Pneumocystis carinii* pneumonia in mice. J Exp Med 1990; 172:937–945.
67. Harmsen AG, Stankiewicz M. T cells are not sufficient for resistance to *Pneumocystis carinii* pneumonia in mice. J Protozool 1991; 38:44S–45S.
68. Chen W, Havell EA, Harmsen AG. Importance of endogenous tumor necrosis factor alpha and gamma interferon in host resistance against *Pneumocystis carinii* infection. Infect Immun 1992; 60:1279–1284.
69. Sethi KK. Multiplication of human-derived *Pneumocystis carinii* in severe combined immunodeficient (SCID) mice. Experientia 1992; 48:63–67.
70. Shellito J, Suzara VV, Blumenfeld W, Beck JM, Steger HJ, Ermak TH. A new model of *Pneumocystis carinii* infection in mice selectively depleted of helper T lymphocytes. J Clin Invest 1990; 85:1686–1693.
71. Beck JM, Liggitt HD, Brunette EN, Fuchs HJ, Shellito JE, Debs RJ. Reduction in intensity of *Pneumocystis carinii* pneumonia in mice by aerosol administration of gamma interferon. Infect Immun 1991; 59:3859–3862.
72. Beck JM, Warnock ML, Curtis JL, Sniezek MJ, Arraj-Peffer SM, Kaltreider HB, Shellito JE. Inflammatory responses to *Pneumocystis carinii* in mice selectively depleted of helper T lymphocytes. Am J Respir Cell Mol Biol 1991; 5:186–197.
73. Ziefer A, Jacobs T, Hedrich HJ, Seitz HM. *Pneumocystis carinii* infections in immunosuppressed and in thymus deficient rats (abstr). Zentralbl Bakteriol Hyg 1984; A258:387.
74. Festing MFW, May D, Connors TA, Lovell D, Sparrow S. An athymic nude mutation in the rat. Nature 1978; 274:365–366.
75. Furuta T, Ueda K, Fujiwara K. Experimental *Pneumocystis carinii* infection in nude rats. Jpn J Exp Med 1984; 54:65–72.
76. Watanabe J, Tanabe K, Shimada K. Separation of trophozoites of *Pneumocystis carinii* from lung of the inoculated nude rat. Jpn J Exp Med 1987; 57:295–297.
77. Hughes WT. Natural occurrences in animals. In: *Pneumocystis carinii* Pneumonitis. Vol. 1. Boca Raton: CRC Press. 1987:57–70.
78. Poelma FG. *Pneumocystis carinii* in zoo animals. Parasitenkunde 1975; 46:61.

79. Yoshida Y, Yamada M, Shiota T, et al. Provocation experiment: *Pneumocystis carinii* in several kinds of animals. Zentralbl Bakteriol Microbiol Hyg Abt I Orig 1981; A250:206–212.
80. Stokes DC, Gigliotti F, Rehg JE, Snellgrove RL, Hughes WT. Experimental *Pneumocystis carinii* pneumonia in the ferret. Br J Exp Pathol 1987; 68:267–276.
81. Gigliotti F, Hughes WT. Passive immunoprophylaxis with specific monoclonal antibody confers partial protection against *Pneumocystis carinii* pneumonitis in animal models. J Clin Invest 1988; 81:1666–1668.
82. Soulez B, Dei-Cas E, Camus D. Le lapin, hote experimental de *Pneumocystis carinii*. Ann Parasitol 1988; 63:5–15.
83. Dei-Cas E, Jackson H, Paulluault F, Aliouat EM, Hancock V, Soulez B, Camus D. Ultrastructural observations on the attachment of *Pneumocystis carinii* in vitro. J Protozool 1991; 38:205S–207S.
84. Soulez B, Dei-Cas E, Charet P, Mougeot G, Caillaux M, Camus D. The young rabbit: a nonimmunosuppressed model for *Pneumocystis carinii* pneumonia. J Infect Dis 1989; 160:355–356.
85. Dei-Cas E, Soulez B, Camus D. Ultrastructural study of *Pneumocystis carinii* in explant cultures of rabbit lung and in cultures with and without feeder cells. J Protozool 1989; 36:555–575.
86. Reed C, O'Donoghue JL. The hairless athymic guinea pig. In: Reed N, ed. Proceedings of the Third International Workshop on Nude Mice. Vol. 1. New York: Gustav Fischer, 1982:51–57.
87. Mugera GM. Some observations on the pathology of pneumonia of pigs in Kenya. Vet Rec 1967; Oct 7:372–376.
88. Settnes OP, Henriksen SA. *Pneumocystis carinii* in large domestic animals in Denmark. A preliminary report. Acta Vet Scand 1989; 30:437–440.
89. Bille-Hansen V, Jorsal SE, Henriksen SAa, Settnes OP. *Pneumocystis carinii* pneumonia in Danish piglets. Vet Rec 1990; 127:407–408.
90. Hagler DN, Kim CK, Walzer PD. Feline leukemia virus and *Pneumocystis carinii* infection. J Parasitol 1987; 73:1284–1286.
91. Davalos AM. Infeccion latente producida por *Pneumocystis carinii* en animales domesticos de la civdad de Mexico. Salud Publica Mex 1963; 5:975–977.
92. Zavala JV, Rosado R. *Pneumocystis carinii* en animales domesticas de la Ciudad de Merida, Yucatan. Salud Publica Mex 1972; 14:103–106.
93. Settnes OP, Hasselager E. Occurrence of *Pneumocystis carinii* Delanoe and Delanoe, 1912 in dogs and cats in Denmark. Nord Vet Med 1984; 36:179–181.
94. Yoshida Y, Ikai T. *Pneumocystis carinii* pneumonia: epidemiology in Japan, and cyst concentration method. Zentralbl Bakteriol Hyg Abt I Orig 1979; A244:405–410.
95. van den Akker S, Goedbloed E. Pneumonia caused by *Pneumocystis carinii* in a dog. Trop Geogr Med 1960; 12:54–58.
96. Farrow BRH, Waterson ADJ, Hartley WJ, Huxtable CRR. *Pneumocystis* pneumonia in the dog. J Comp Pathol 1972; 82:447–458.
97. Copland JW. Canine pneumonia caused by *Pneumocystis carinii*. Aust Vet J 1974; 50:515–518.
98. Botha WS, van Rensburg IB. Pneumocystosis: a chronic respiratory distress syndrome in dog. J S Afr Vet Assoc 1979; 50:173–179.

99. McCully RM, Lloyd J, Kuys D, Schneider DJ. Canine pneumocystis pneumonia. J S Afr Vet Assoc 1979; 50:207–209.
100. Shiota T, Shimada Y, Kurimoto H, Oikawa H. *Pneumocystis carinii* infection in corticosteroid-treated cats. J Parasitol 1990; 76:441–445.
101. Shively JN, Dellers RW, Buergelt CD, Hsu FS, Kabelac LP, Moe KK, Tennant B, Vaughn JT. *Pneumocystis carinii* pneumonia in two foals. J Am Vet Med Assoc 1973; 162:648–652.
102. McGuire TC, Poppie MJ, Banks KL. Combined (B- and T-lymphocyte) immunodeficiency: a fatal genetic disease in arabian foals. J Am Vet Med Assoc 1974; 164:70–76.
103. Perryman LE, Bjorneby JM. Immunotherapy of cryptosporidiosis in immunodeficient animal models. J Protozool 1991; 38:98S–100S.
104. Perryman LE, McGuire TC, Magnuson NS. Combined immunodeficiency (severe), Swiss-type agammaglobulinemia, Model No. 38, Supplement update, 1983. In: Capen CC, Hackel DB, Jones TC, Migaki G, eds. Handbook: Animal Models of Human Disease. Fasc. 12. Washington, DC: Registry of Comparative Pathology, Armed Forces Institute of Pathology, 1983.
105. Perryman LE, McGuire TC, Crawford TB. Maintenance of foals with combined immunodeficiency: cause and control of secondary infections. Am J Vet Res 1978; 39:1043.
106. Richter CB, Humason GL, Godbold JH Jr. Endemic *Pneumocystis carinii* in a marmoset colony. J Comp Pathol 1978; 88:171–180.
107. Chandler FW, McClure HM, Campbell WG. Pulmonary pneumocystosis in nonhuman primates. Arch Pathol Lab Med 1976; 100:163–167.
108. Long GG, White JD, Stookey JL. *Pneumocystis carinii* infection in splenectomized owl monkeys. J Am Vet Med Assoc 1975; 167:651–654.
109. Matsumoto Y, Yamada M, Tegoshi T, Yoshida Y, Gotoh S, Suzuki J, Matsubayashi K. *Pneumocystis* infection in macaque monkeys: *Macaca fuscata fuscata* and *Macaca fascicularis*. Parasitol Res 1987; 73:324–327.
110. Walzer PD, Rutledge ME. Comparison of rat, mouse, and human *Pneumocystis carinii* by immunofluorescence. J Infect Dis 1980; 142:449.
111. Graves DC, McNabb SJ, Ivey MH, Worley MA. Development and characterization of monoclonal antibodies to *Pneumocystis carinii*. Infect Immun 1986; 51:125–133.
112. Graves DC, McNabb SJ, Worley MA, Downs JD, Ivey MH. Analysis of rat *Pneumocystis carinii* antigens recognized using Western immunoblotting. Infect Immun 1986; 54:96–103.
113. Walzer PD, Kim CK, Linke MJ, Pogue CL, Huerkamp MJ, Chrisp CE, Lerro AV, Wixson SK, Hall E, Shultz LD. Outbreaks of *Pneumocystis carinii* pneumonia in colonies of immunodeficient mice. Infect Immun 1989; 57:62–70.
114. Walzer PD, Linke MJ. A comparison of the antigenic characteristics of rat and human *Pneumocystis carinii* by immunoblotting. J Immunol 1987; 138:2257–2265.
115. Gigliotti F, Ballou LR, Hughes WT, Mosley BD. Purification and initial characterization of a ferret *Pneumocystis carinii* surface antigen. J Infect Dis 1988; 158:848–854.
116. Campbell WG. Ultrastructure of *Pneumocystis* in human lungs: life cycle of human pneumocystosis. Arch Pathol 1972; 93:312–324.

117. Barton EG, Campbell WG. Further observations on the ultrastructure of pneumocystosis. Arch Pathol 1967; 83:527–534.
118. Shiveley JN, Moe KK, Dellers RW. Fine structure of spontaneous *Pneumocystis carinii* pulmonary infection in foals. Cornell Vet 1974; 64:72–88.
119. Settnes OP, Genner J. *Pneumocystis carinii* in human lungs at autopsy. Scand J Infect Dis 1986; 18:489–496.
120. Yoshida Y, Ogino K, Arizono N, Kondo K, Matsuno K. Studies on *Pneumocystis carinii* and pneumocystis pneumonia. (1) Appearance of this protozoa in cortisone treated rats. Jpn J Parasitol 1974; 23 (suppl 23; in Japanese).
121. Yoganathan T, Lin H, Buck GA. An electrophoretic karyotype and assignment of ribosomal genes to resolved chromosomes of *Pneumocystis carinii*. Mol Microbiol 1989; 3:1473–1480.
122. Hong ST, Steele PE, Cushion MT, Walzer PD, Stringer SL, Stringer JR. *Pneumocystis carinii* karyotypes. J Clin Microbiol 1990; 28:1785–1795.
123. Lundgren B, Cotton R, Lundgren JD, Edman JC, Kovacs JA. Identification of *Pneumocystis carinii* chromosomes and mapping of five genes. Infect Immun 1990; 58:1705–1710.
124. Zhang J, Cushion MT, Stringer JR. Molecular characterization of a novel repetitive element from *Pneumocystis carinii* from rats. J Clin Microbiol 1993; 31:244–248.
125. Jacobs JL, Libby DM, Winters RA, Gelmont DM, Fried ED, Hartman BJ, Laurence J. A cluster of *Pneumocystis carinii* pneumonia in adults without predisposing illnesses. N Engl J Med 1991; 324:246–250.
126. Weinberg GA, Bartlett MS. Comparison of pulsed field gel electrophoresis karyotypes of *Pneumocystis carinii* derived from rat lung, cell culture, and ferret lung. J Protozool 1991; 38:64S–65S.
127. Laughon BE, Allaudeen HS, Becker JM, Current WL, Feinberg J, Frenkel JK, Hafner R, Hughes WT, Laughlin CA, Meyers JD, Schrager LK, Young LS. Summary of the workshop on future directions in discovery and development of therapeutic agents for opportunistic infections associated with AIDS. J Infect Dis 1991; 164:244–251.

11

New Animal Models for *Pneumocystis carinii* Research: Immunodeficient Mice

CHARLES L. SIDMAN and JOHN B. ROTHS

University of Cincinnati College of Medicine
Cincinnati, Ohio

I. Introduction: Advantages of Mutant Mouse Models

Traditionally, most research on *Pneumocystis carinii* has been undertaken using deliberately (i.e., experimental) or nondeliberately (i.e., human patients) immunosuppressed mammals. In the past several years, however, increasing use has been made of mouse strains that are congenitally immunodeficient due to homozygosity for the mutant gene "severe combined immunodeficiency" (*scid*) (1). This chapter summarizes our laboratory's experience with these and other strains of immunodeficient mice and discusses their advantages plus the salient conclusions about *P. carinii* to which their use has led. At least six distinct aspects can be delineated that favor the use of these newer immunodeficient mouse strains in *P. carinii* research:

First, the development and natural history of pneumocystosis in such strains is highly reproducible and well defined (2,3). Our laboratory has maintained numerous stocks of *scid* and other immunodeficient mice for over 8 years and has observed a reasonably consistent course of pneumocystosis in each stock over that period. Thus, by maintaining long-term and stable colonies of immunodeficient mice, one can avoid the uncertainties and potential for nonreproducibility that have been experienced by investigators who rely on experimental activation of latent *P. carinii* infection in animals from external suppliers (who can and do alter their husbandry practices in the pursuit of "better and cleaner" animals). The state of immunodeficiency allowing active infection in these mutant mouse strains is also much simpler in origin and more manipulatable, being due to defined and Mendelian inherited genetic traits rather than a complex and interacting regimen of steroidal immunosuppression, antibiotic supplementation, and caloric deprivation (4).

A second major advantage of using genetically immunodeficient mice in *P. carinii* research is that these mice offer the opportunity to study a long-term and chronic infection comparable to human immunodeficiencies rather than the single acute episode that is provided by the steroid-based suppression model. As described previously (2,3), pneumocystosis regularly develops in three phases in our *scid* mouse colonies: an initial period of 1–2 months when *P. carinii* organisms are detectable but rare in the lungs, another interval of 1–2 months when *P. carinii* organisms rapidly increase to final plateau levels, and finally, a period of 2–6 months during which the disease state becomes steadily worse and the animal ultimately dies. This natural history suggests that factors separate from the induction of disease limit the extent of infection by *P. carinii*, and that host pathology becomes clinically evident only after extensive infection is achieved. Such insights may have substantial significance for the spontaneous pneumocystosis of human immunodeficiency patients.

A third opportunity for *P. carinii* research provided by genetically immunodeficient mice is that both spontaneous and deliberately induced infections can be investigated in the same species. While most of this chapter discusses the spontaneous course of infection as experienced in our and others' colonies, *scid* mice can be cleansed of their *P. carinii* by hysterectomy derivation and so maintained for extended periods in isolator systems. Alternatively, these animals can be rendered *P. carinii*–free by pharmacological treatment (see below). In both cases, intratracheal inoculation is a highly reproducible way of deliberately initiating *P. carinii* infection (5). Illustrative results of such experiments are presented in Section IV.

The above-described aspects of reproducibility, chronic nature, and possibilities for either spontaneous or induced infection together constitute a fourth and major opportunity for using immunodeficient mice in *P. carinii* research, namely, the ability to conduct either short- or long-term therapy studies, including investigation of potential relapse and reinfection. Such opportunities are being vigorously exploited in our and others' laboratories (see Section III).

A fifth practical advantage of using immunodeficient mice in *P. carinii* research is that their small size allows much cheaper and thus more feasible pharmacological studies of new compounds at a given dose per body weight ratio. This aspect will no doubt find great application in the development of new chemical therapies for *P. carinii* as well as other infectious agents.

New Animal Models

Finally, the sixth advantage of immunodeficient mice for *P. carinii*, as for much other biomedical research, is the extensive wealth of animal stocks, genetic tools and information, reagents, and so forth that are readily available in this species. In the following sections we discuss some of the progress already made, as well as future lines of development, using the unique capabilities of the mouse as an experimental system.

II. *scid* Mice and Mechanisms of Immunity to *P. carinii*

In the years since its discovery, our laboratory transferred the *scid* mutation from its original C.B-17 background (1) to multiple additional inbred mouse strains by at least 10 generations of backcrossing followed by intercrossing for homozygosity. This process was accomplished fairly rapidly by simultaneously test-mating males of each generation with C.B-17-*scid/scid* females and with additional females of the target strain; offspring of the first cross were typed for *scid* homozygosity by ELISA assays for serum Ig, and the corresponding backcross progeny of the *scid/+* males thus discovered were further mated for the next cycle. In our colony, all these homozygous congenic *scid* stocks have displayed roughly equivalent levels of *P. carinii* infection and lifespans (Fig. 1). The median

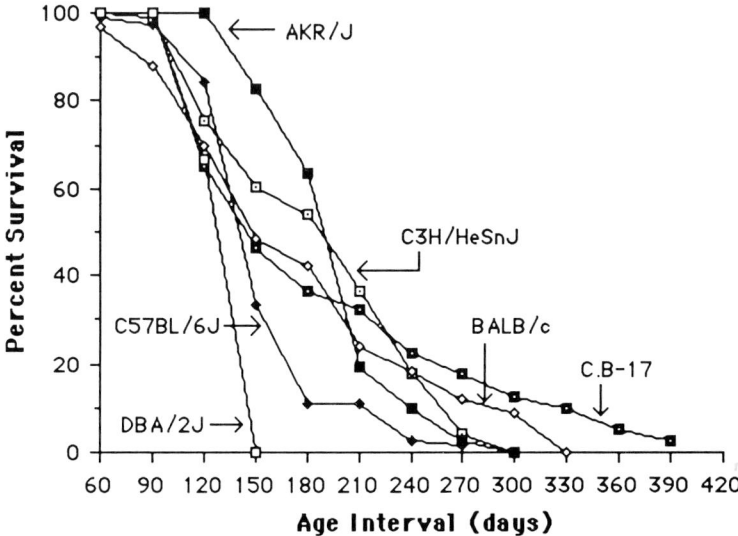

Figure 1 Survival curves for various congenic stocks of homozygous *scid* mice, calculated as per Ref. 2.

longevities of stocks of homozygous *scid* mice on different genetic backgrounds have ranged from a low of about 5 months (DBA/2-*scid*) to a high of about 7 months (BALB/c-*scid* and C.B-17-*scid*), periods that could reflect genetic background differences in cell subsets or cytokine levels that in turn affect the overall pathological process. All these stocks seem to die exclusively from equivalent *P. carinii* infections, except AKR-*scid* animals, which regularly die with *P. carinii* but apparently from a reproducible and early-onset form of T-lymphocyte lymphoma reminiscent of that characteristic of older AKR-+/+ animals (6). These homozygous *scid* congenic stocks may thus prove useful for other fields of investigation, such as tumor biology, in addition to infectious disease research.

Using several of these congenic *scid* strains, pharmacological as well as immunological modes of therapy for *P. carinii* have been explored; the salient features of some of these are presented in Table 1. The classic anti–*P. carinii* drug combination, trimethoprim-sulfamethoxazole (TMP-SMZ) (7), was found in our hands to be completely effective in clearing *scid* mice of their endogenous organism with a 2-week treatment regimen delivered through the drinking water. Such animals remained essentially free of *P. carinii* for the remainder of their lives but could be deliberately reinfected (see below) after cessation of treatment. Despite its efficacy, TMP-SMZ is noted as a therapeutic modality of moderate risk of complications because it is poorly tolerated in some AIDS patients (8). Moreover, we have had substantial difficulty in propagating TMP-SMZ–treated *scid* mice for successive generations, suggesting the possibility of an as yet poorly understood reproductive side effect in this species and with this dose level. It should be noted that continued prophylactic treatment of *scid* mice for 3 days per week and with the same dilution into the drinking water has not interfered with breeding performance (9), but the 2-week regimen that we have used for definitive treatment may not be as benign.

In contrast to pharmacological treatment, two modes of immunological resistance and therapy of *P. carinii* have been demonstrated (3,10). In one, a regimen of six weekly transfers of 0.25 ml of serum from congenic +/+ mice repeatedly immunized with *scid* mouse lung-derived *P. carinii* has proved ca-

Table 1 Comparison of Different Modes of *P. carinii* Therapy

Mode of therapy	Risk of complications	Duration of benefit	Possibility of reinfection
TMP-SMZ	Moderate	Long	High
Humoral	None	Temporary	Certain
Cellular	High	Permanent	None
Combined humoral and cellular	Low	Permanent	None

pable of reducing the *P. carinii* burden of *scid* mice by greater than 80% without detectable complications. Most impressively, this form of treatment is effective in *scid* mice at all ages up to and including near-moribund animals, essentially rescuing such mice from their figurative deathbeds! Nevertheless, such serotherapy merely temporarily checks, but does not cure, *scid* mice of their pneumocystosis, since disease returns with vigor once weekly serum transfers are stopped. However, continuing serum transfers have extended the lifespan of *scid* mice to over twice their untreated levels, thus proving the practical efficacy of this mode of therapy and indicating that resistance to *P. carinii* can be mediated by humoral factors.

A second mode of immunological resistance to and therapy for *P. carinii* lies in the transfer and action of helper T lymphocytes (10). After fractionation of immunocompetent lymphocytes from congenic normal animals using a fluorescence-activated cell sorter (FACS) and transfer of these into *scid* mice, CD8-bearing T cells were found to be without effect, while CD4-bearing T cells were intensely reactive to *P. carinii*. In the lungs of *scid* recipients, these helper T cells caused a vigorous inflammatory reaction that actually killed one-half to two-thirds of the recipient mice by about 1 month after transfer. However, the minority of mice that survived this hyperinflammatory episode were then permanently free of and protected from reinfection with *P. carinii*.

In summary, these transfer experiments showed that (presumably) antibodies and helper T cells constitute two independently effective immunological mechanisms of resistance to *P. carinii*. Each of these separate immunological mechanisms has advantages and disadvantages therapeutically, but the two can be combined to produce an optimal treatment regimen. Thus, after reducing their *P. carinii* burden by 6 weeks of hyperimmune serum transfers, *scid* mice given cellular reconstitution no longer experienced the fatal inflammatory reaction, but instead were rendered uniformly and permanently free of and resistant to *P. carinii*. Such a biphasic regimen of first reducing organism levels by pharmacological or humoral means, followed by permanent restoration of cellular immunity, may prove to be the optimal treatment protocol for *P. carinii* in humans.

III. Non-*scid* Mouse Models of *P. carinii*

Mice homozygous for the *scid* mutation are not the only immunodeficient strains suffering from *P. carinii* and thus useful for *P. carinii* research. Rather, a variety of immunologically mutant mice besides *scid* animals also show measurable cyst levels and provide important lessons about *P. carinii* biology (Table 2).

In light of the above-described transfer experiments into *scid* mice that demonstrated two essentially independent immunological mechanisms of resistance against *P. carinii* provided by B and helper T lymphocytes, it was of interest

Table 2 *P. carinii* Cyst Density in Immunoaberrant Mutant Strains of Mice

Strain background	+/−	bgJ/bgJ	gld/gld	lpr/lpr	mev/mev	μMT/μMT	nu/nu	scid/scid
AKR	0[a] [0/6][b] 202 ± 33[c]							436 ± 152 [9/9] 158 ± 28
BALB/cBy or C.B-17	0.2 ± 0.2 [1/9] 301 ± 60		69 ± 34 [10/19] 164 ± 5	0.1 ± 0.1 [1/28] 178 ± 6	3.3 ± 2.5 [3/17] 79 ± 12			231 ± 36 [27/27] 159 ± 10
C3H/He	0 [0/4] 210 ± 28		0 [0/5] 176 ± 5	1.3 ± 1.3 [1/6] 176 ± 1	3.6 ± 3.1 [3/13] 103 ± 14			367 ± 68 [14/14] 160 ± 9
C57BL/6	0 [0/4] 153 ± 22	0 [0/5] 141 ± 0	0 [0/7] 179 ± 8	0 [0/7] 233 ± 3	0.9 ± 0.9 [1/5] 80 ± 5	423 ± 79 [10/10] 102 ± 5	33 ± 33 [1/6] 221 ± 39	469 ± 143 [11/11] 141 ± 5
MRL/Mp	0 [0/6] 175 ± 10		63 ± 29 [6/14] 166 ± 7	170 ± 69 [8/9] 164 ± 5	4.2 ± 3.7 [2/7] 61 ± 7			
SJL	0 [0/3] 239 ± 65		21 ± 14 [3/14] 110 ± 5	1.2 ± 0.9 [2/6] 136 ± 12	0 [0/2] 36 ± 0			

[a]Mean ± S.E. cyst density (cysts/mm^2).
[b][No. of mice cyst-positive/total mice examined.]
[c]Mean ± S.E. age at necropsy (days).

to see the effect of genetically deleting one or the other of these arms of the immune system. Athymic and thus T-cell-deficient "nude" (*nu*) mice (11) and rats (12) have been used in the past as *P. carinii* models, but in our experience have shown only modest levels of infection in terms of either the percentage of animals showing detectable organisms or the number of those organisms. In contrast, a homologous-recombination "knockout" mouse strain that lacks B cells and humoral immune function ("μ*MT*" mice) (13) surprisingly shows consistency of infection and levels of *P. carinii* cyst density comparable to those of *scid* animals. The first of these results can be explained either that the still substantial antibody levels in *nu* mice provide considerable protection against *P. carinii*, or that their remaining T cells, mostly of the γ/δ receptor type (14), are able to perform this function. The μ*MT* result is more surprising because helper T cells were shown to be an effective mechanism of resistance to *P. carinii* even in the absence of B cells and antibody (10); these mice may represent the best evidence to date that antigen presentation to T cells in vivo is critically dependent on B cells rather than macrophages (15,16).

A third class of immunologically abnormal animals that are *P. carinii*–susceptible are certain autoimmune mouse strains. After finding anti–*P. carinii* antibodies in the sera of some mice congenic for the autoimmunity-causing mutations "generalized lymphoproliferative disease" (*gld*) (17), "lymphoproliferation" (*lpr*) (18), and "viable motheaten" (*me^v*) (19), we quantitated *P. carinii* cyst levels and found that certain of these congenic strain-mutation combinations exhibited substantial *P. carinii* infections. Prominent among these were MRL-*lpr*, MRL-*gld*, and BALB/c-*gld*. One important lesson that derives from these data is that the immunological dysregulations that underlie autoimmunity can also prevent normal immune protection against opportunistic infections such as *P. carinii*. Second, the overall immunoregulatory picture in such animals is a complex result of both the already defined single mutant genes and as-yet-unknown polymorphisms differing between the various genetic backgrounds. The *P. carinii* susceptibility of autoimmune mouse strains may thus provide a useful means for investigating immunologically important background genes. Finally, it is interesting that *me^v* mice did not show appreciable *P. carinii* cyst density even though they did contain substantial antibody to this organism. Their extremely high levels of spontaneously produced polyclonal immunoglobulin (20) thus may have protected them from actual *P. carinii* infection.

One of the salient opportunities of working with genetically defined, immunologically mutant mouse strains is that their mutant alleles can be rearranged by classical Mendelian genetics (i.e., controlled breeding) to provide additional insights into *P. carinii* biology. An example of this was the set of autoimmune congenic strains discussed above. Another was provided by the creation of mice doubly homozygous for *scid* and other mutations that affect nonspecific immune function. Table 3 shows comparative cyst densities and

Table 3 *P. carinii* Cyst Density in Double-Mutant C57BL/6 Mice

	Genotype		
	scid	*scid, bg*	*scid, Lps^d*
Cyst density	469 ± 143[a]	283 ± 48	857 ± 143
	[11][b]	[15]	[7]
	141 ± 5[c]	134 ± 4	188 ± 19
Longevity[d]	137 [75]	286 [29]	ND[e]

[a]Mean ± S.E. cyst density (cysts/mm^2).
[b][No. of mice.]
[c]Mean ± S.E. age at necropsy (days).
[d]Survival age (days) at which 50% of the mice remained alive (based on cumulative percent survival) and [*n*] number of mice at risk from weaning.
[e]Not done.

longevities for singly mutant *scid* and doubly mutant *scid, bg* and *scid, Lps^d* mice, all on the C57BL/6 background. The "beige" (*bg*) (21) mutation produces anomalous lysosomes resulting in defective function in several types of cells such as granulocytes and macrophages, while the "lipopolysaccharide-deficiency" (*Lps^d*) (22) allele prevents normal macrophage and other cell responses to microorganisms' cell-wall lipopolysaccharides. It is important to note that neither the *bg* mutation (Table 2) nor the *Lps^d* allele (carried by the C3H/He-+/+ strain shown in Table 2) by themselves lead to any appreciable spontaneous *P. carinii* density [although earlier work by others suggested that C3H/He mice carrying the *Lps^d* allele were more susceptible to *P. carinii* in the steroid suppression model (23)]. However, double mutants homozygous for both *scid* and either of these additional mutations show either substantially greater longevity (*scid,bg* for sure, and perhaps *scid,Lps^d* as well; studies in progress) or higher *P. carinii* cyst loads (*scid,Lps^d*) than their single-mutant *scid* counterpart. These models allow emphasis on the importance of the nonspecific immune system (macrophages, granulocytes, etc.) in controlling *P. carinii* infections in the absence of B and T lymphocytes and lead to the realization that a major component of the pathology of *P. carinii* infection may be the uncontrolled activity of non-antigen-specific cells in the alymphocytic and immunodeficient environment.

IV. *P. carinii* Derived from Mouse Versus Other Species

The ability to render normally *P. carinii*–infected *scid* mice permanently free of *P. carinii* by TMP-SMZ treatment (see above) has allowed studies involving deliberate inoculation and reinfection by exogenous organisms. In a series of experiments performed with Dr. W. Current (Lilly Research Labs, Indianapolis, IN), *P. carinii* organisms were isolated from the lungs of either nontreated, spontaneously infected *scid* mice or steroid-suppressed, *P. carinii*–infected rats (24). Then, both preparations were inoculated into the lungs of either TMP-SMZ–treated *scid* mice or steroid-suppressed rats from a supplier whose animals did not carry endogenous *P. carinii*. Control animals from both groups received no inoculation and did not develop significant pneumocystosis as judged by organism counts. In contrast, animals receiving the homologous *P. carinii* preparation did develop vigorous pneumocystosis within 2–3 months. These results proved the viability and infectivity of the *P. carinii* preparations. Most interestingly, animals given *P. carinii* isolated from the other species developed little or no pneumocystosis, demonstrating for the first time a functional host range specificity for *P. carinii* organisms. Combined with previous results concerning antigenic (25) and karyotypic differences (24,26) between *P. carinii* isolates within and between host species, it seems likely that the term "*Pneumocystis carinii*" actually encompasses a broad range of microorganisms of distinct functional, genetic, and antigenic properties. The potential cross-infectivity of animal-derived *P. carinii* for humans, and vice versa, is an interesting question that is currently under investigation.

V. Synergy Between *P. carinii* and Other Organisms

In addition to the foregoing, a second caveat regarding *P. carinii* is that pneumocystosis can represent a synergism between distinct organisms rather than a single homogeneous infection. The original impetus for a series of coinfection experiments was our experience that colonies of genetically identical *scid* mice housed in different mouse rooms had significantly different life expectancies (2). Both populations showed similar levels and time courses of development of *P. carinii* organisms in their lungs, and both died from severe pneumocystosis. We also knew that certain usually nonpathogenic microorganisms were regularly or intermittently present in one room but never in the other. Therefore, in collaboration with Dr. Abigail Smith (Yale University, New Haven, CT), *scid* mice carrying endogenous *P. carinii* were deliberately coinfected with a variety of pneumotropic microorganisms including those we had reason to suspect may have been present in the mouseroom where *scid* mice showed shorter longevities (27). Of the five microorganisms tested to date [pneumonia virus of mice (PVM), Sendai virus, murine hepatitis virus strain Y, respiratory syncytial virus (RSV), and *Pasturella pneumotropica*], only PVM significantly altered the course of *P. carinii* infection in *scid* mice, but it did so in a dramatic fashion. At almost a uniform 28 days after PVM infection, doubly infected *scid* mice died of terminal pneumocystosis with little evidence of the characteristic histopathology of solitary PVM infection. Importantly, PVM infection of normal immunocompetent mice or non–*P. carinii*-infected *scid* mice produced only slight histopathological responses and no mortality for at least 3 months postinfection; the immunocompetent animals rapidly cleared their inoculated PVM, while the *P. carinii*–free *scid* mice experienced a persistent, but nonfatal, course of PVM infection (28).

This finding of a functional interrelationship rather than merely an additive simultaneous infection by two microorganisms may have profound clinical importance, in that diagnosis and treatment of synergizing microorganisms may be as important and effective in the management of pneumocystosis as attention to the *P. carinii* organism itself. Interestingly, PVM is considered a relative of human RSV, another only mildly pathogenic pneumotropic microorganism. Efforts are continuing to search for additional microorganisms that functionally synergize with *P. carinii*.

At the fundamental level, one might ask about the mechanism underlying the significant interaction between *P. carinii* and PVM. The observation that in doubly infected *scid* mice the two microorganisms only rarely coincided microanatomically suggests that their interaction was indirect rather than contact-mediated (27). Some possibilities currently under consideration for this mechanism are (1) a reduction in the recruitment or activation of *P. carinii*–resisting macrophages by PVM, (2) a PVM-induced alteration in the production of specific cytokines or other polypeptides, and (3) changes in such biochemical parameters as pH, nutrients, and so forth. In any case, the opportunity for extensive genetic and microbiological manipulation makes *scid* and other immunodeficient mouse strains ideal systems for investigating the fascinating and important issues of microbial synergy and ecology.

VI. Considerations for Colony Maintenance

The discussion above of a variety of findings concerning the biology and therapy of *P. carinii* infections has significance for the management of colonies of these immunodeficient mice. In our laboratory, colonies of *scid* and other severely immunodeficient mice have been maintained for approximately 8 years. *P. carinii* has been endogenous in these mice for that entire period, but in the absence of synergizing coinfecting organisms, *P. carinii* alone has not interfered significantly with breeding and experimentation. Obviously, barrier isolation and strict control of material and animal traffic are critical to maintaining this performance, probably mostly by preventing the entry of synergizing coinfectious microorganisms.

If one requires more extended longevity than that provided by *P. carinii*–infected *scid* or other mice, several means of eliminating or controlling this organism are available. Most completely, several colonies of *scid* mice have been rendered apparently free of *P. carinii* by hysterectomy rederivation and fostering and have been so maintained for years. On the other hand, such a procedure is extremely laborious, and even with this effort, *P. carinii* has frequently returned to isolator-maintained colonies. One must wonder whether *P. carinii* is equally or more able than other organisms to survive autoclaving, and what is the immediate source of the newly reinfecting *P. carinii* in this case?

For laboratories not equipped to operate a complete isolator facility, several less laborious methods are available to temporarily eliminate or reduce the levels of *P. carinii* infection. Drugs such as TMP-SMZ have been used either briefly as an intensive treatment (24) or more mildly for ongoing prophylaxis (9) against *P. carinii*. Alternatively, mice can be laboriously maintained by continuing humoral immunotherapy, or more efficiently, immunologically reconstituted with functional lymphocytes for service as breeding stock. In the latter case, reduction of the *P. carinii* organism load by humoral or pharmacological treatment before cellular reconstitution reduces the vigor of the hyperinflammatory response and greatly improves the percentage of animals surviving. Finally, for colony maintenance, any of these immunodeficiency alleles can be bred through the immunocompetent heterozygous state to cleanse the stock of the bulk of its opportunistic infectious agents. In all instances, housing of the animals in microisolators, changing of cages in laminar flow cabinets with sterile technique, and feeding of autoclaved food and filtered water are recommended to maintain both *P. carinii* and other possibly synergizing microorganisms at minimum levels.

VII. Conclusions

This chapter has reviewed our laboratory's experience in the use of *scid* and other immunodeficient mouse strains in *P. carinii* research. These mice offer unique experimental opportunities that complement the more traditional systems reviewed elsewhere in this volume and, as discussed above, have led and continue to lead to insights about *P. carinii* that are fascinating from a fundamental perspective and perhaps may soon lead to clinical application.

References

1. Bosma GC, Custer RP, Bosma MJ. A severe combined immunodeficiency mutation in the mouse. Nature 1983; 301:527–530.
2. Roths JB, Marshall JD, Allen RD, Carlson GA, Sidman CL. Spontaneous *Pneumocystis carinii* pneumonia in immunodeficient mutant *scid* mice: natural history and pathobiology. Am J Pathol 1990; 136:1173–1186.
3. Roths JB, Sidman CL. Single and combined humoral and cell-mediated immune

therapy of *Pneumocystis carinii* pneumonia in immunodeficient *scid* mice. Infect Immun 1993 (in press).
4. Frenkel JK, Good JT, Shultz JA. Latent *Pneumocystis* infection of rats, relapse, and chemotherapy. Lab Invest 1966; 15:1559–1577.
5. Boylan CJ, Current WL. Improved rat models of *Pneumocystis carinii* pneumonia: induced laboratory infections in *Pneumocystis*-free animals. Infect Immun 1992; 69: 1589–1597.
6. Hoag, WG. Spontaneous cancer in mice. Ann NY Acad Sci 1963; 108:805–831.
7. Hughes WT, McNabb PC, Makres TD. Efficacy of trimethoprim and sulfamethoxazole in the prevention and treatment of *Pneumocystis carinii* pneumonitis. Antimicrob Agents Chemother 1974; 5:289–293.
8. Gordin FM, Simon GL, Wofsy CB, Mills J. Adverse reactions to trimethoprim-sulfamethoxazole in patients with the acquired immunodeficiency syndrome. Ann Intern Med 1984; 100:495–499.
9. Walzer PD, Kim CK, Linke MJ, Pogue CL, Huerkamp MJ, Chrisp CE, Lerro AV, Wixson SK, Hall E, Shultz LD. Outbreaks of *Pneumocystis carinii* pneumonia in colonies of immunodeficient mice. Infect Immun 1989; 57:62–70.
10. Roths JB, Sidman CL. Both immunity and hyper-responsiveness to *Pneumocystis carinii* result from transfer of $CD4^+$ but not $CD8^+$ T cells into "severe combined immunodeficiency" (*scid*) mice. J Clin Invest 1992; 90:673–678.
11. Walzer PD, Schnelle V, Armstrong D, Rosen PP. Nude mouse: a new experimental model for *Pneumocystis carinii* infection. Science 1977; 197:177–179.
12. Furata T, Ueda K, Fujiwara K. Experimental *Pneumocystis carinii* infection in nude rats. Jpn J Exp Med 1984; 54:65–72.
13. Kitamura D, Rajewsky K. Targeted disruption of μ chain membrane exon causes loss of heavy-chain allelic exclusion. Nature 1992; 356:154–156.
14. Yoshikai K, Matsuzaki G, Takeda Y, Ohga S, Kishihara K, Yuuki H, Nomoto K. Functional T cell receptor δ chain gene messages in athymic nude mice. Eur J Immunol 1988; 18:1039–1043.
15. Ron Y, DeBaetselier P, Gordon J, Feldman M, Segal S. Defective induction of antigen-reactive proliferating T-cells in B-cell-deprived mice. Eur J Immunol 1981; 11:964–968.
16. Chesnut RW, Grey HM. Antigen representation by B cells and its significance in T-B interactions. Adv Immunol 1986; 39:51–94.
17. Roths JB, Murphy ED, Eicher EM. A new mutation (*gld*) producing lymphoproliferation and autoimmunity in C3H/HeJ strain mice. J Exp Med 1984; 159:1–20.
18. Murphy ED, Roths JB. A single gene model for massive lymphoproliferation with immune complex disease in new mouse strain MRL. Proc 16th Internat Cong Hematol, Excerpta Medica, Amsterdam, 1978, pp 69–72.
19. Shultz LD, Coman DR, Bailey CL, Beamer WG, Sidman CL. "Viable motheaten," a new allele at the motheaten locus. I. Pathology. Am J Pathol 1984; 116:179–192.
20. Sidman CL, Shultz LD, Hardy RR, Hayakawa K, Herzenberg LA. Production of immunoglobulin isotypes by Ly-1(+) B cells in viable motheaten and normal mice. Science 1986; 232:1423–1425.
21. Gallin JI, Bujak JS, Patten E, Wolff SM. Granulocyte function in the Chediak-Higashi syndrome of mice. Blood 1974; 43:201–206.

22. Glode LM, Rosenstreich DL. Genetic control of B cell activation by bacterial lipopolysaccharide is mediated by multiple distinct genes or alleles. J Immunol 1976; 117:2061–2066.
23. Walzer PD, Rutledge ME, Kokichi Y. Experimental *Pneumocystis carinii* pneumonia in C3H/HeJ and C3HeB/FeJ mice. J Reticulendothel Soc 1983; 33:1–9.
24. Current WL, Boylan CJ, Keely S, Roths JB, Sidman CL. (in preparation).
25. Walzer PD, Linke MJ. A comparison of the antigenic characteristics of rat and human *Pneumocystis carinii* by immunoblotting. J Immunol 1987; 138:2257–2265.
26. Hong S-T, Steele PE, Cushion MT, Walzer PD, Stringer SL, Stringer JR. *Pneumocystis carinii* karyotypes. J Clin Microbiol 1990; 28:1785–1795.
27. Roths JB, Smith AL, Sidman CL. Lethal exacerbation of *Pneumocystis carinii* pneumonia (PCP) in *scid* mice after infection by pneumonia virus of mice (PVM). J Exp Med 1993 (in press).
28. Bray MV, Barthold SW, Sidman CL, Roths JB, Smith AS. Exacerbation of *Pneumocystis carinii* pneumonia in immunodeficient *scid* mice by concurrent infection with a pneumovirus. Infect Immun 1993 (in press).

12

Mechanisms of *Pneumocystis carinii* Attachment to Lung Cells

SCOTT T. POTTRATZ and WILLIAM J. MARTIN II

Indiana University Medical Center
Indianapolis, Indiana

I. Introduction

Attachment of pathogenic organisms to host cells has been demonstrated to be an essential initial event in the pathogenesis of many infections (1,2). The same is thought to be true for the pathogenesis of *Pneumocystis carinii* infection. This hypothesis has been supported by pathological specimens that have demonstrated the close apposition between *P. carinii* and host cell membranes. Recent advances in the quantitative assessment of pneumocystis-binding to target lung cells (3) has led to studies that have improved our understanding of the mechanisms involved in *P. carinii* attachment to host cells. This review will outline concepts gained from both ultrastructural data on *P. carinii* attachment, with recently published data examining cellular constituents thought to mediate this attachment.

II. Pathogen Attachment Mechanisms

Pathogen attachment is important in the initiation and propagation of host infection for numerous pathogens, including *Escherichia coli* (4), *Staphylococcus aureus* (5), streptococci (6), *Candida albicans* (7), *Leishmania* sp. (8), *Plasmodium* sp. (9), *Entamoeba histolytica* (10), and *Trypanosoma* sp. (11). The cellular mechanisms involved in pathogen attachment are quite variable within this group. Two major classes of pathogen adherence will be further discussed, as they seem to bear the most relevance for *P. carinii* attachment to host cells: (1) attachment mediated by adhesive proteins and (2) attachment mediated by lectins.

A wide variety of cell adhesive glycoproteins have been isolated and characterized. The most abundant and best studied of these is the extracellular matrix protein fibronectin (Fn). Fibronectin is a 500-kDa glycosylated molecule present throughout the body in both cell-associated and soluble forms. It binds to cells by specific transmembrane receptors present on a wide variety of cells, including epithelial cells (12), endothelial cells (13), macrophages (14), lymphocytes (15), and neutrophils (16). The Fn receptors are members of the large group of cell surface receptors known as integrins (17). This family of receptors is composed of at least 15 different receptor molecules, all of which are heterodimers containing distinct α- and β-subunits (18). The integrins function to provide a link between extracellular adhesion molecules and the cell cytoskeleton. Integrins are essential components for optimal cell–cell and cell–matrix attachment. The major integrin-binding site on Fn has been termed the classic Fn cell-binding domain and is made up of the tetrapeptide sequence Arg-Gly-Asp-Ser (RGDS). The RGD sequence is common to many other cell adhesion glycoproteins that bind to integrins (17,18). The wide distribution of both Fn and Fn receptors makes it an optimal target for use in pathogen adherence mechanisms.

Early studies of Fn-mediated adherence of bacteria focused on *S. aureus* because of its ability to bind to endothelial cells, which are laden with surface Fn. Initial studies demonstrated that Fn binding to *S. aureus* was both saturable and specific (19). Further studies showed that *S. aureus* attachment to host cells in vitro could be inhibited by blocking the function of Fn. An Fn-binding protein has recently been isolated from *S. aureus* (20), and this may provide a novel target for the development of new antistaphylococcal therapies.

Similar studies have been performed with streptococci, and Fn has been noted to bind to the lipoteichoic acid moiety present on the surface of many streptococcal strains (21). These same strains appear to show enhanced binding to oropharyngeal epithelial cells, which have an abundance of Fn on their surface (22).

A role for Fn in mediating fungal attachment has been demonstrated for *C. albicans* (23). This organism also demonstrates specific binding to Fn that appears to be mediated by the RGD cell-binding domain of Fn (24). A specific Fn receptor has not yet been isolated from *C. albicans*, but of interest is that a study by Marcantonio and Hynes (25) showed that an antibody to the highly conserved cytoplasmic domain of the β_1-integrin subunit reacts with a candidal protein by Western blot.

Protozoans also appear to use Fn for their adherence to host cells. *T. cruzi* organisms have been demonstrated to bind to Fn in a specific and reversible manner (26). Trypanosomal infection of cultured cells is inhibited by the addition of RGD-containing peptides that mimic the active site of the Fn cell-binding sequence (27). In addition, *Leishmania* sp. bind to Fn (8) and attachment of leishmanial promastigotes to cultured macrophages is inhibited by RGD-containing peptides (28).

Thus, there are examples of Fn-dependent pathogen attachment for a wide variety of organisms, including bacteria, fungi, and protozoans. The ubiquitous distribution of Fn and Fn receptors has made it a natural target for pathogenic organisms.

The second attachment mechanism that is pertinent to *P. carinii* is lectin-mediated attachment. Lectins are proteins that recognize and bind to specific saccharide components of other molecules (29). Therefore, lectin-mediated attachment involves either recognition of saccharide subunits on the surface of host cells by pathogens or the binding of pathogen surface saccharides to host cell lectins. Most previous studies have investigated the functions of specific surface lectins present on bacteria.

Many different bacterial lectins have been identified. These most commonly occur in the form of fimbriae, which are specialized filamentous structures present on many pathogenic bacteria. The best characterized of these are the type I (mannose-specific) fimbriae present on *E. coli* and many other pathogenic enteric gram-negative organisms (30). Type I fimbriae bind to short oligomannose chains of N-linked glycoproteins, which are common constituents of eukaryotic cell surfaces. Bacteria with type I fimbriae bind to uroepithelium (31), respiratory epithelium (32), and intestinal epithelial cells (33).

Several other bacterial lectins have been defined by inhibition studies using various saccharides. These include P fimbriae (galactose binding) (34), S fimbriae (sialyl galactoside binding) (35), and type 2 fimbriae (β-galactosyl binding) (36). In addition, more recent studies have demonstrated bacterial adherence to specific saccharide subunits present on cell surface glycolipids (37), leading to further investigations into the possible role of cell surface glycolipids in pathogen attachment.

Lectin-mediated attachment in eukaryotic pathogens has been demonstrated for the fungi *C. albicans*, *Cryptococcus neoformans*, and *Saccharomyces cerevisiae* (38), as well as for the protozoan *Entamoeba histolytica* (39). Lectin-mediated adherence has been best defined for *E. histolytica* in a series of studies by Ravdin and co-workers. These studies demonstrated that *E. histolytica* binding is inhibited by galactose-containing saccharides. Furthermore, inhibition of attachment also blocked the cytotoxic effects of the organism on cultured intestinal epithelial cells (39). Additional studies led to the isolation of galactose-specific cell surface lectin from *E. histolytica* (40). It is anticipated that the development of new therapies directed against this surface lectin would be highly specific and efficacious in the treatment of amebic infection.

Host immune cells also use lectin-mediated attachment to induce nonopsonic phagocytosis of pathogens. Mannose-specific lectins have been characterized on the surface of peritoneal (41) and alveolar macrophages (42). These surface lectins may aid in early host defense against organisms containing an abundance of cell surface mannose, such as fungi.

III. *Pneumocystis carinii* Attachment

Initial descriptions of the relation between *P. carinii* and alveolar epithelial cells by light microscopy emphasized clumping of the *P. carinii* organisms within a large conglomeration of amorphous eosinophilic material. The intimate relation between *P. carinii* and host cells was not well appreciated until electron microscopic (EM) studies were performed to examine infected lung tissue. Electron micrographs demonstrated the tight binding of *P. carinii* to alveolar epithelial cells in both rat (43) and human (44) lung tissue. The *P. carinii* cell membranes interdigitate with the host cell membranes, but there is no evidence of membrane fusion or intracellular uptake of the organisms by the alveolar epithelial cells (45).

Further ultrastructural studies have demonstrated the existence of filopodia on *P. carinii* (46). Initially, these were thought to be involved in organism attachment; however, further study has shown that the *P. carinii* filopodia are generally directed away from the host cell surface and, therefore, are not likely to be involved in attachment (47).

The most detailed EM studies of *P. carinii*–host cell interaction (48,49) illustrated the complex nature of *P. carinii* binding. The cell membranes of both the *P. carinii* and host cell are involved. The *P. carinii* outer membrane invaginates into the host cell membrane and, in this way, "grabs on" to the host cell, enabling the organism to maintain its position on the host cell and avoid alveolar clearance mechanisms.

The first investigation to go beyond a purely descriptive study of *P. carinii* attachment was performed by Limper and Martin (3). In this study, the investigators developed an assay to quantify *P. carinii* attachment to A549 cells, a lung epithelial cell line. In brief, the *P. carinii* were labeled with a radionuclide, and attachment was quantified by measuring radionuclide activity associated with the cell monolayer. With this assay, *P. carinii* attachment was reproducibly quantified and was shown to be dependent on intact cytoskeletal function. This finding was consistent with the ultrastructural studies demonstrating the intricate interposition of *P. carinii* and host cell membranes; an event likely to require *P. carinii* cellular motility and intact cytoskeletal function.

Furthermore, this study demonstrated that *P. carinii* attachment to host cells was necessary to produce a cytopathological effect on the host cells. Attachment of *P. carinii* inhibited proliferation of A549 cells. This effect was reversed by blocking *P. carinii* attachment through inhibition of cytoskeletal function. The cause of *P. carinii*-induced growth inhibition of the target cells was not specifically addressed, although there was no evidence of either direct cellular injury to the A549 cells or of depletion of nutrients in the culture medium. Thus, the precise mechanisms of the growth inhibitory effects of *P. carinii* remain open to speculation.

IV. Fibronectin-Mediated *Pneumocystis carinii* Attachment

Additional investigations into the cellular components of *P. carinii* attachment led to the elucidation of the role of the extracellular matrix protein fibronectin (Fn) as a mediator in *P. carinii* binding. Fibronectin binds to many pathogenic microorganisms and aids in their attachment to host cells. It is a known constituent of both the normal and inflamed alveolus. It has also been demonstrated to bind to type I alveolar epithelial cells (50), making it an ideal candidate to act as a mediator of *P. carinii* attachment in vivo (Fig. 1a).

Initial studies demonstrated that ^{125}I-Fn binding to *P. carinii* organisms in suspension was both a saturable and a specific process, with approximately 6.4×10^5 binding sites per organism and a K_d of 1.2×10^{-8} (51). These values correspond with those previously reported for Fn binding to *S. aureus* and *C. albicans* (19,24). More recent studies have shown that *P. carinii* organisms bind specifically to Fn-coated tissue culture plates, but not to either laminin- or albumin-coated plates (52).

Fibronectin is a large molecule, made up of multiple subunits that contain several different binding sites, including those for heparin, collagen, fibrinogen, *S. aureus*, and a eukaryotic cell-binding domain (53). The latter has been well studied, and its active site has been determined to involve the tetrapeptide sequence Arg-Gly-Asp-Ser (RGDS). Further studies were performed to determine the *P. carinii*-binding site on the Fn molecule. Addition of excess RGDS effectively blocked binding of ^{125}I-Fn to *P. carinii* organisms in suspension (51). Similarly, addition of RGDS inhibited attachment of *P. carinii* to Fn-coated culture plates (52). Therefore, *P. carinii* binding to Fn appears to be mediated by the known eukaryotic cell-binding site on the Fn molecule.

Further studies examined the possible role of Fn in *P. carinii* attachment to alveolar epithelial cells (51). Initial studies demonstrated that *P. carinii* binding to cultured lung epithelial cells could be inhibited by addition of polyclonal anti-Fn antibodies. Furthermore, a direct role for the RGD cell-binding domain in *P. carinii* binding to Fn was obtained by addition of synthetic peptides that mimic the active site of the cell-binding domain. Addition of the tetrapeptide RGDS completely abolished *P. carinii* binding to either alveolar epithelial cells or to immobilized Fn, whereas the nonfunctional peptide RGES had no effect on *P. carinii*

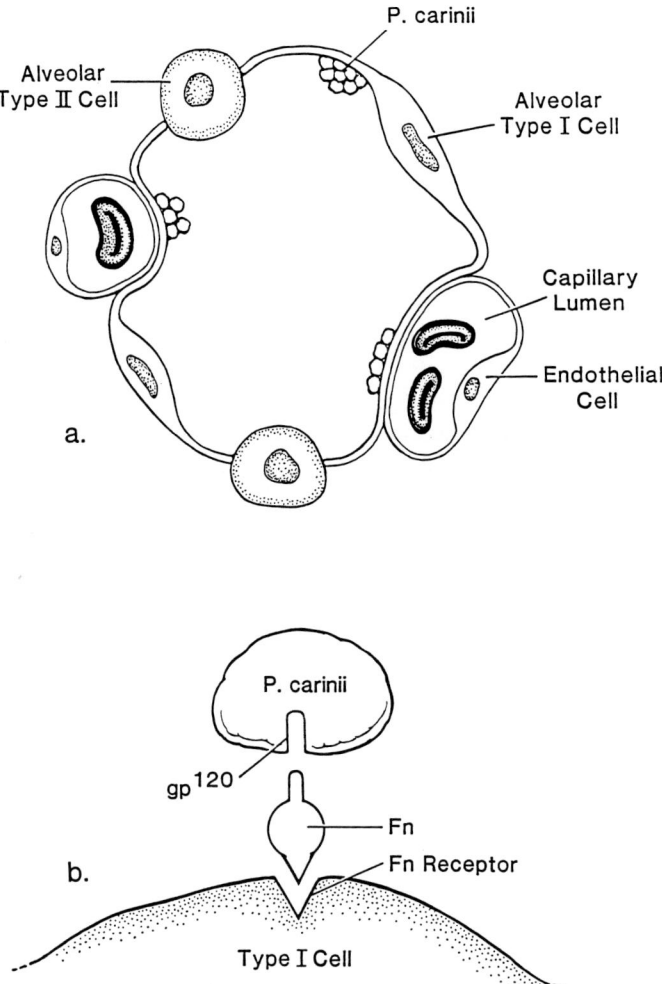

Figure 1 The role of fibronectin in *P. carinii* attachment to alveolar epithelial cells. (a) Attachment of *P. carinii* within the alveolus appears to occur predominantly to type I alveolar epithelial cells. (b) Proposed mechanism of Fn-mediated attachment of *P. carinii* organisms to type I alveolar epithelial cells. Fn acts as a "bridge" binding to gp120 on the *P. carinii* and to Fn receptors present on the alveolar epithelial cell.

attachment (52). Together these data indicate that *P. carinii* binding to Fn is mediated, at least in part, by the RGD cell-binding domain of Fn.

Additional investigation into the interaction between *P. carinii* and Fn involved determination of the *P. carinii* cell surface antigen that interacted with Fn. The most abundant surface component of *P. carinii* is a 110- to 120-kDa mannose-containing glycoprotein, which has been termed gp120 (54). The relative abundance of gp120, coupled with the essential role of *P. carinii* attachment in growth and replication of the organism, made gp120 a good candidate for a *P. carinii*-specific attachment factor.

Initial studies of gp120 demonstrated that in very low concentrations it inhibited *P. carinii* attachment to cultured lung epithelial cells (55). Additionally, gp120 caused a concentration-dependent decrease in specific binding of ^{125}I-Fn to *P. carinii* organisms. To clarify the interaction between gp120 and Fn, *P. carinii* antigen preparations were separated by sodium dodecyl sulfate–polyacrylamide gel electrophoresis (SDS–PAGE) and blotted with ^{125}I-Fn. This resulted in specific binding of the ^{125}I-Fn to gp120 (55). Moreover, this binding was inhibited by addition of excess unlabeled RGDS. This provided further evidence that gp120 acts as a surface receptor on *P. carinii* for the binding of Fn (see Fig. 1b).

Previous work had determined that the β_1-integrin seemed to be the most evolutionarily conserved of the integrin subunits. In particular, the cytosolic domain of this membrane-spanning molecule was very similar to that in drosophila and in humans. Marcantonio and Hynes (25) demonstrated that specific antibodies to this site on the β_1-integrin reacted with a cell surface molecule on candida. Use of this same antibody in Western blots of *P. carinii* cell preparations showed that the antibody also found specifically to gp120 (55). Thus, it appears that gp120 has a shared antigenic domain with the β_1-integrins.

These studies were extended to evaluate the possible role of Fn in *P. carinii* binding to alveolar macrophages. Previous studies had shown that *P. carinii* organisms bind to alveolar macrophages in vitro, but that phagocytosis is induced only in the presence of opsonizing antipneumocystis antibodies (56,57). Clearly, antipneumocystis IgG provides a possible mechanism for *P. carinii* binding to alveolar macrophages through Fc receptors present on the surface of the macrophage (Fig. 2c). More recently, investigators have demonstrated the presence of IgG molecules bound to the surface of *P. carinii* isolated from human lungs (58). However, the role of opsonizing antibodies in the clearance of the organism from the alveolar space has not been thoroughly investigated.

To investigate the possible role of Fn in *P. carinii* binding to alveolar macrophages, experiments were performed using normal alveolar macrophages obtained by lung lavage of healthy rats, and *P. carinii* attachment to these cells was quantified. The binding of *P. carinii* to alveolar macrophages was markedly inhibited by the addition of anti-Fn antibodies or by the addition of RGDS (59). *Pneumocystis carinii* binding to alveolar macrophages was dependent on the

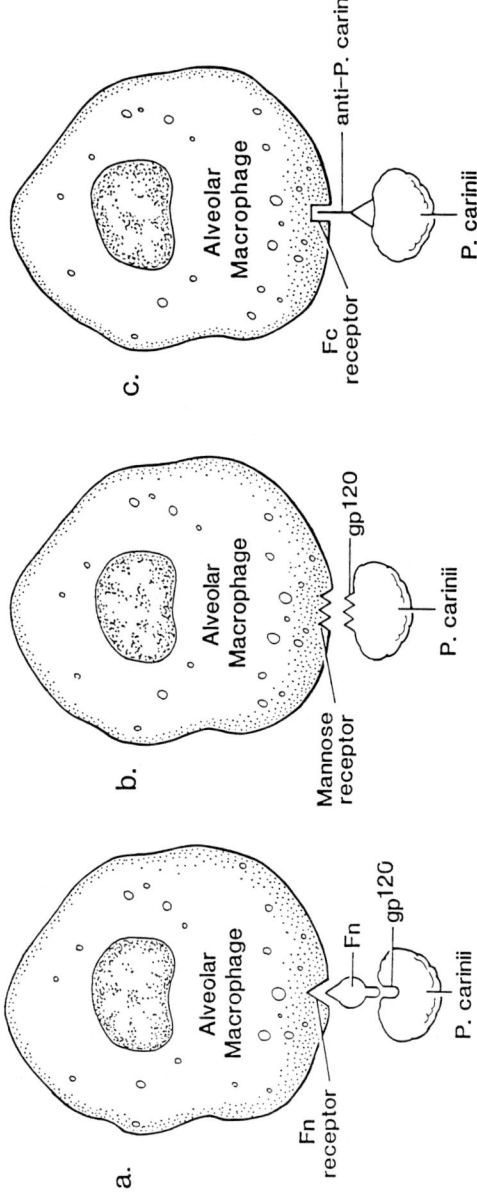

Figure 2 Proposed mechanisms of *P. carinii* binding to alveolar macrophages. (a) Fn-mediated binding of *P. carinii* to alveolar macrophages, which does not initiate activation of the macrophage. (b) Binding of mannose residues present on *P. carinii* gp120 to mannose receptors on the macrophage. This causes activation of the macrophage and phagocytosis of the *P. carinii* organisms. (c) antibody-mediated attachment via Fc receptors on the macrophage, which also activates the macrophage, as in (b).

presence of extracellular divalent cations. Furthermore, Fn-mediated *P. carinii* binding to the alveolar macrophages did not result in activation of the macrophages or in injury to the organisms (see Fig. 2a).

Thus, *P. carinii* organisms can bind in vitro to either alveolar epithelial cells or to alveolar macrophages by a mechanism that appears to be dependent on adhesive proteins, such as Fn, which serve as a bridge between the organism and the target cell. However, it is likely that microorganisms can successfully use more than one mechanism to attach to specific target cells. This redundancy increases the chances of survival for the organism in the otherwise hostile environment of the alveolar space.

V. Lectin-Mediated *Pneumocystis carinii* Attachment

Pneumocystis carinii organisms contain an abundance of cell surface mannose and *N*-acetylglucosamine by lectin-biding studies (60). The major cellular constituent of *P. carinii*, gp120, binds lectins in a similar manner (61), suggesting that it is the major cell surface glycoprotein of *P. carinii*.

Recent interest in the cellular mechanisms of *P. carinii* attachment to host cells has led to investigation into the possible role for lectin-mediated adherence in *P. carinii* binding. A recent report (62) indicates the presence of β-D-galactoside- and D-mannoside-binding activity on the surface of the organism. The investigators did not address whether this activity was endogenous to *P. carinii* or was due to the presence of soluble host lectins bound to the surface of the organism. Further investigation is required to determine the identity of the cellular components responsible for the endogenous *P. carinii* lectin activity noted in this study. In contrast, two recent studies have examined the possible role of cell surface mannose residues on *P. carinii* acting as mediators of attachment by binding to host cell surface lectins. A study by Ezekowitz et al. (63) demonstrated that *P. carinii* binding to alveolar macrophages can be mediated through the mannose-binding lectin present on the surface of the macrophage. In contrast to the previous study on Fn-mediated *P. carinii* binding to alveolar macrophages, mannose-mediated binding caused activation of the macrophage, with production of oxidants and phagocytosis of the organisms (see Fig. 2b). Thus, it appears mannose-mediated attachment of *P. carinii* to alveolar macrophages is likely a host defense mechanisms similar to nonopsonic binding of fungi by macrophages.

The second study to address the role of *P. carinii* surface mannose in *P. carinii* binding to host cells demonstrated modulation of *P. carinii* attachment to lung epithelial cells by addition of the mannose-binding lectin concanavalin A (Con A) (64). Preincubation of *P. carinii* with Con A inhibited *P. carinii* binding to the lung epithelial cell line A549. In contrast, preincubation of the target cells with Con A caused an increase in *P. carinii* binding. The explanation for this apparent paradox is the presence of multiple mannose-binding sites on Con A. Therefore, when Con A is preincubated with the *P. carinii* organisms in suspension, it is likely that all the Con A-binding sites are saturated by the mannose residues present in great abundance on the *P. carinii* organisms. Concanavalin A may inhibit binding of the *P. carinii* to target cell either by a specific blockade of mannose-mediated attachment or by a nonspecific steric inhibition of *P. carinii* gp120-mediated adherence. When the target epithelial cells are preincubated with Con A, it is possible that the Con A binds to the cells in such a way that there are multiple mannose-binding sites "sticking up" from the cell monolayer surface. This may effectively increase the number of *P. carinii*-binding sites on the monolayer, leading to the observed increase in *P. carinii* binding.

VI. Conclusion

Studies of *P. carinii* attachment to host cells have only recently advanced from ultrastructural electron microscopic studies to biochemical studies of the cellular mechanisms of attachment. The data presented thus far have not clearly established the roles of Fn- or lectin-mediated binding of *P. carinii* organisms. It is quite possible that multiple mechanisms of attachment may ultimately be defined for *P. carinii*. Further advances in the isolation and cloning of *P. carinii* surface antigens will be an immense aid in more clearly defining the mechanisms of organism attachment.

The insights gained for attachment mechanisms of *P. carinii* may provide important clues to the development of novel therapeutic strategies for *P. carinii* pneumonia. From a therapeutic viewpoint, the attachment of *P. carinii* to the alveolar epithelium is a vulnerable aspect of *P. carinii* survival in the alveolar environment. Targeting specific therapy to disrupt the mechanism of *P. carinii* attachment might provide an effective and safe means to stop the propagation of these organisms within the lung.

References

1. Keusch GT. The role of bacterial adherence in infection. Monogr Pathol 1982; 23:93–113.
2. Manocha MS, Chen Y. Specificity of attachment of fungal parasites to their hosts. Can J Microb 1990; 36:69–76.
3. Limper AH, Martin WJ. *Pneumocystis carinii*: inhibition of lung cell growth mediated by parasite attachment. J Clin Invest 1990; 85:391–397.
4. Svanborg-Eden C, Hanssen HA. *Escherichia coli* pili as possible mediators of attachment to human urinary tract epithelial cells. Infect Immun 1979; 21:229–237.

5. Aly R, Levit S. Adherence of *Staphylococcus aureus* to squamous epithelium: role of fibronectin and teichoic acid. Rev Infect Dis 1987; 9:S341–S350.
6. Beachey EH, Courtney HS. Bacterial adherence: the attachment of group A streptococci to mucosal surfaces. Rev Infect Dis 1987; 9:S475–S481.
7. King RD, Lee JC, Morris AL. Adherence of *Candida albicans* and other *Candida* species to mucosal epithelial cells. Infect Immun 19890; 27:667–674.
8. Wyler DJ, Sypek JP, McDonald JA. In vitro parasite–monocyte interactions in human leishmaniasis: possible role of fibronectin in parasite attachment. Infect Immun 1985; 49:305–311.
9. Roberts DD, Sherwood JA, Spitalnik SL, Panton LJ, Howard RJ, Dixit VM, Frazier WA, Miller LH, Ginsburg V. Thrombospondin binds falciparum malaria parasitized erythrocytes and may mediate cytoadherence. Nature 1985; 318:64–66.
10. Ravdin JI. Pathogenesis of disease caused by *Entamoeba histolytica*: studies of adherence, secreted toxins, and contact-dependent cytolysis. Rev Infect Dis 1986; 8: 247–260.
11. Ouaissi MA, Cornette J, Capron A. *Trypanosoma cruzi*: modulation of parasite–cell interaction by plasma fibronectin. Eur J Immunol 1985; 15:1096–1101.
12. Chen LB, Maitland N, Gallimore PH, McDougall JK. Detection of the large external transformation sensitive protein (fibronectin) on some epithelial cells. Exp Cell Res 1977; 106:39–46.
13. Conforti C, Zanetti A, Colella S, Abbadini M, Marchisio PC, Pytela R, Giancotti F, Tarone G, Languino LR, Dejana E. Interaction of fibronectin with cultured human endothelial cells: characterization of the specific receptor. Blood 1989; 73:1576–1585.
14. Wright SD, Meyer BC. Fibronectin receptor of human macrophages recognizes the sequence Arg-Gly-Asp-Ser. J Exp Med 1985; 162:762–767.
15. Hemler ME, Huang C, Schwarz L. The VLA protein family: characterization of five distinct cell surface heterodimers each with a common 130,000 molecular weight β-subunit. J Biol Chem 1987; 262:3300–3309.
16. Nathan C, Srimal S, Farber C, Sanchez E, Kabbash L, Asch A, Gailit J, Wright SD. Cytokine-induced respiratory burst of human neutrophils: dependence on extracellular matrix proteins and CD11/CD18 integrins. J Cell Biol 1989; 109:1341–1349.
17. Ruoslahti E, Pieschbacher MD. New perspectives in cell adhesion: RGD and integrins. Science 1987; 238:491–497.
18. Albelda SM, Buck CA. Integrins and other cell adhesion molecules. FASEB J 1990; 4:2868–2880.
19. Proctor RA, Mosher DF, Olbrantz PJ. Fibronectin binding to *Staphylococcus aureus*. J Biol Chem 1982; 257:14788–14794.
20. Froman G, Switalski LM, Speziale P, Hook M. Isolation and characterization of a fibronectin receptor from *Staphylococcus aureus*. J Biol Chem 9187; 262:6564–6571.
21. Courtney HS, Stanislawski L, Ofek I, Simpson WA, Hasty DL, Beachey EH. Localization of a lipoteichoic acid binding site to a 24-kilodalton NH_2-terminal fragment of fibronectin. Rev Infect Dis 1988; 10:S360–S362.
22. Simpson WA, Beachey EH. Adherence of group A streptococci to fibronectin on oral epithelial cells. Infect Immun 1983; 39:275–279.

23. Kalo A, Segal E, Sahar E, Dayan D. Interaction of *Candida albicans* with genital mucosal surfaces: involvement of fibronectin in adherence. J Infect Dis 1988; 157: 1253–1256.
24. Klotz SA, Smith RL. A fibronectin receptor on *Candida albicans* mediates adherence of the fungus to extracellular matrix. J Infect Dis 1991; 163:604–610.
25. Marcantonio EE, Hynes RO. Antibodies to conserved cytoplasmic domains of the integrin β_1 subunit react with proteins in vertebrates, invertebrates and fungi. J Cell Biol 1988; 106:1765–1772.
26. Ouaissi MA, Afchain D, Capron A, Grimaud JA. Fibronectin receptors on *Trypanosoma cruzi* trypomastigotes and their biological function. Nature 1984; 308:380–382.
27. Ouaissi MA, Cornette J, Afchain D, Capron A, Grasmasse H, Tartar A. *Trypanosoma cruzi* infection inhibited by peptides modeled from fibronectin cell attachment domain. Science 1986; 221:603–607.
28. Rizvi FS, Ouaissi MA, Marty B, Santoro F, Capron A. The major surface protein of *Leishmania* promastigotes is a fibronectin-like molecule. Eur J Immunol 1988; 18: 473–476.
29. Nicholson GL. The interactions of lectins with animal cells. Int Rev Cytol 1974; 39: 89–190.
30. Eshdat Y, Silverblatt F, Sharon N. Dissociation and reassembly of *Escherichia coli* type I pili. J Bacteriol 1981; 148:308–314.
31. Hultgren S, Porter T, Schaeffer A, Duncan J. Role of type I pili and effects of phase variation on lower urinary tract infections produced by *Escherichia coli*. Infect Immun 1985; 50:370–377.
32. Dal Nogare AR. Type I pili mediate gram-negative bacterial adherence to intact tracheal epithelium. Am J Respir Cell Mol Biol 1990; 2:433–440.
33. Knutton S, Lloyd DR, Candy DA, McNeish A. Adhesion of enterotoxigenic *Escherichia coli* to human small intestinal enterocytes. Infect Immun 1985; 48:824–831.
34. Wold A, Thorssen M, Hull S, Svanborg-Eden C. Attachment of *Escherichia coli* via mannose or Galα1-4Gal containing receptors to human colonic epithelial cells. Infect Immun 1988; 56:2531–2537.
35. Parkinnen J, Rogers GN, Korhonen T, Dahr W, Finne J. Identification of the *O*-linked sialyloligosaccharides of glycophorin A as the erythrocyte receptors for S-fimbriated *Escherichia coli*. Infect Immun 1986; 54:37–42.
36. Heeb MJ, Costello AH, Gabriel O. Characterization of a galactose-specific lectin from *Actinomyces viscosus* by a model aggregation system. Infect Immun 1982; 38:993–1002.
37. Karlsson KA. Animal glycosphingolipids as membrane attachment sites for bacteria. Annu Rev Biochem 1989; 58:309–350.
38. Jimenez-Lucho V, Ginsburg V, Krivan HC. *Cryptococcus neoformans*, *Candida albicans*, and other fungi bind specifically to the glycosphingolipid lactosylceramide (Galβ1- 4Glcβ1-1Cer), a possible adhesion receptor for yeasts. Infect Immun 1990; 58:2085–2090.
39. Ravdin JI, Guerrant RL. Role of adherence in cytopathologic mechanisms of *Entamoeba histolytica*. Study with mammalian tissue culture cells and human erythrocytes. J Clin Invest 1981; 68:1305–1313.

40. Petri WA, Smith RD, Shlesinger PH, Murphy CF, Ravdin JI. Isolation of the galactose-binding lectin that mediates the in vitro adherence of *Entamoeba histolytica*. J Clin Invest 1987; 80:1238–1244.
41. Inber MS, Pizzo SV, Johnson WS, Adams DO. Selective diminution of the binding of mannose by murine macrophages in the late stages of activation. J Biol Chem 1982; 257:5129–5135.
42. Stahl PD, Rodman JS, Miller MJ, Schlesinger PH. Evidence for receptor mediated binding of glycoproteins, glycoconjugates, and lysosomal glycosidases by alveolar macrophages. Proc Natl Acad Sci USA 1978; 78:1019–1022.
43. Yoneda K, Walzer PD. Attachment of *Pneumocystis carinii* to type I alveolar cells studied by freeze-fracture electron microscopy. Infect Immun 1983; 40:812–815.
44. Sueishi K, Hisano S, Sumiyoshi A, Tanaka K. Scanning and transmission electron microscopic study of human pulmonary pneumocystosis. Chest 1977; 72:213–215.
45. Millard PR, Wakefield AE, Hopkins JM. A sequential ultrastructural study of rat lungs infected with *Pneumocystis carinii* to investigate the appearances of the organism, its relationships and its effects on pneumocytes. Int J Exp Pathol 1990; 71:895–904.
46. Ham EK, Greenberg SD, Reynolds RC, Singer DB. Ultrastructure of *Pneumocystis carinii*. Exp Mol Pathol 1971; 14:362–372.
47. Henshaw NG, Carson JL, Culler AM. Ultrastructural observations of *Pneumocystis carinii* attachment to rat lung. J Infect Dis 1985; 151:181–186.
48. Long EG, Smith JS, Meier JL. Attachment of *Pneumocystis carinii* to rat pneumocytes. Lab Invest 1984; 54:609–615.
49. Itatani CA, Marshall GJ. Ultrastructural morphology and staining characteristics of *Pneumocystis carinii* in situ and from bronchoalveolar lavage. J Parasitol 1988; 74:700–712.
50. Rosenkrans WA, Albright JT, Hausman RE, Penny DP. Ultrastructural immunocytochemical localization of fibronectin in developing rat lung. Cell Tissue Res 1983; 234:165–177.
51. Pottratz ST, Martin WJ. Role of fibronectin in *Pneumocystis carinii* attachment to cultured lung cells. J Clin Invest 1990; 85:351–356.
52. Pottratz ST, Martin WJ. In vitro attachment of *Pneumocystis carinii* to fibronectin: a new model for pneumocystis adherence [abstract]. Clin Res 1991; 39:217A.
53. Ruoslahti E. Fibronectin and its receptors. Annu Rev Biochem 1988; 57:375–413.
54. Radding JA, Armstrong MYK, Ullu E, Richards FF. Identification and isolation of a major cell surface glycoprotein of *Pneumocystis carinii*. Infect Immun 1989; 57:2149–2157.
55. Pottratz ST, Paulsrud J, Smith JS, Martin WJ. *Pneumocystis carinii* attachment to cultured lung cells by pneumocystis gp120, a fibronectin binding protein. J Clin Invest 1991; 88:403–407.
56. Masur H, Jones TC. The interaction in vitro of *Pneumocystis carinii* with macrophages and L-cells. J Exp Med 1978; 147:157–170.
57. Von Behren LA, Pesanti EL. Uptake and degradation of *Pneumocystis carinii* by macrophages in vitro. Am Rev Respir Dis 1978; 118:1051–1059.
58. Blumenfeld W, Mandrell RE, Jarvis GA, Griffis JM. Localization of host immuno-

globulin G to the surface of *Pneumocystis carinii*. Infect Immun 1990; 58:456–463.
59. Pottratz ST, Martin WJ. Mechanism of *Pneumocystis carinii* attachment to cultured rat alveolar macrophages. J Clin Invest 1990; 86:1678–1683.
60. Cushion MT, Destefano JA, Walzer PD. *Pneumocystis carinii*: surface reactive carbohydrates detected by lectin probes. Exp Parasitol 1988; 67:137–147.
61. Linke MJ, Cushion MT, Walzer PD. Properties of the major antigens of rat and human *Pneumocystis carinii*. Infect Immun 1989; 57:1547–1555.
62. Vierbuchen M, Ortmann M, Uhlenbruck G. Endogenous carbohydrate-binding proteins in *Pneumocystis carinii*. Infect Immun 1990; 58:3143–3146.
63. Ezekowitz RAB, Williams DJ, Koziel H, Armstrong MYK, Warner A, Richards FF, Rose RM. Uptake of *Pneumocystis carinii* mediated by the macrophage mannose receptor. Nature 1991; 351:155–158.
64. Limper AH, Pottratz ST, Martin WJ. Modulation of *Pneumocystis carinii* adherence to cultured lung cells by a mannose-dependent mechanism. J Lab Clin Med 1991; 118:492–499.

13

Pathogenic Mechanisms

PETER D. WALZER

Cincinnati Veterans Affairs Medical Center
and University of Cincinnati College of Medicine
Cincinnati, Ohio

I. Introduction

As in any infectious disease, the pathogenesis of *Pneumocystis carinii* pneumonia involves a complex interaction between the organism and its mammalian host. The specific processes involved are poorly understood, and analysis of these factors inevitably leads to some overlap with other chapters in this book. The present chapter will focus on the pathophysiological changes in pneumocystosis and the current concepts of the underlying mechanisms.

The pathogenesis of *Pneumocystis carinii* pneumonia can be divided into four stages: establishment of the infection, organism proliferation, changes within the alveolar microenvironment, host inflammatory or immune response.

II. Establishment of the Infection

The portal of entry for *P. carinii* is the respiratory tract. Experimental studies have shown that *P. carinii* can be transmitted from one animal to another by the airborne route; however, there is little information about the infective stage or environmental source of the organism (1,2). *Pneumocystis carinii* can also be transmitted by intratracheal inoculation of infected lung homogenates (3). Airborne transmission is the presumed method of naturally acquired *P. carinii* infections in humans. Exposure to the organism occurs early in life and several epidemiological studies have shown that by age 2 or 3 years, about 80% of persons have developed serum antibodies to *P. carinii* (4–6).

Once inhaled, *P. carinii* does not appear to colonize the upper airways, but is deposited within the alveoli. The precise steps in initiation of infection are unknown. With many microbes, the first stage in this process is attachment to a specific host cell (see Chap. 12). *Pneumocystis carinii* also appears to follow this pattern, as judged by ultrastructural studies that have shown adherence of the trophic stage of the organism to the alveolar type I cell (7–11). The organism interdigitates tightly with the type I cell, but there is no fusion of the cell membranes. It has been difficult to analyze this interaction directly in vitro because the type I cell does not proliferate. Nevertheless, recent studies using other cell lines have begun to provide insights into the mechanisms involved. One line of investigation has suggested that fibronectin facilitates attachment by serving as a bridge between gp120, the principal surface antigen of *P. carinii*, and receptors on host cells (12–14). Other studies examining the interaction of *P. carinii* with alveolar macrophages have suggested role for mannose and Fc receptors (15–17). It is likely that other attachment mechanisms (e.g., lectin-mediated binding) exist, but definitive studies have not yet been published.

It is unclear what *P. carinii* inoculum size is needed to establish the infection, or after the infection has been established, how long the organism remains in the host. One school of thought holds that *P. carinii* remains quiescent in the host for long periods, perhaps for life (18). In essence, *P. carinii* become part of the normal microbial flora. With immunosuppression, the organisms would begin to proliferate and cause pneumonia by reactivation of this latent infection (19,20). Such a process has been thought to be the underlying mechanism for most cases of pneumocystosis, and has served as the rationale for not isolating *P. carinii* patients while in the hospital.

An alternative theory holds that *P. carinii* may remain in the host for only short periods, but that the host may be frequently exposed to sources of the organism during his or her lifetime (18). This hypothesis supports the idea of different strains of *P. carinii* and the possibility that the host may be infected with more than one strain of the organism at the same time. In addition, this theory emphasizes the communicability of *P. carinii* and the need to isolate patients with pneumocystosis from direct contact with other susceptible hosts. According to such a scenario, an immunosuppressed patient would provide fertile ground for the propagation of *P. carinii* if he or she were exposed to an exogenous source of the organism.

III. Organism Proliferation

The specific host immune defects that permit proliferation of *P. carinii* in the lung have not been elucidated. Its low virulence and the lack of a reliable in vitro cultivation system have hindered direct organism challenge experiments or cytotoxicity assays. Impaired cellular immunity is generally considered to be the major predisposing factor, based on the following lines of evidence: the underlying disease in *P. carinii* patients [e.g., acquired immunodeficiency syndrome (AIDS), cancer, protein malnutrition); type of immunosuppressive therapy (corticosteroids); and CD4 T-helper cell depletion and reconstitution studies in immunodeficient mice (21–25). A role for impaired humoral immunity has been suggested by the occurrence of pneumocystosis in patients with B-cell defects, the benefit of passive antibody administration in experimental animals, and the enhancement of phagocytosis by serum opsonins (17,21,25,26).

The proliferation of *P. carinii* in the host has been best studied in animal models. Rats raised in a conventional colony acquire latent *P. carinii* infection naturally from the environment; when administered corticosteroids for about 8 weeks, these animals develop *P. carinii* pneumonia spontaneously with histopathological features indistinguishable from those of the disease in humans (19,27). This system, which has been used for almost 40 years in *P. carinii* research, has been particularly valuable in studies of pathogenesis and therapy.

Propagation of *P. carinii* in the rat model has been studied at the light microscopic level by histological examination and by quantitation of the developmental stages of the organism in lung homogenates (27,28). A semiquantitative scoring system of lung sections stained with methenamine silver has been established to judge the severity of pneumocystosis based on the degree of alveolar involvement; the scale ranges from 0+ or negative (no alveoli), to 2+ or moderate (25–50% alveoli), to 4+ or very heavy (>75% alveoli). Reagents (e.g., toluidine blue O, cresyl echt violet) that selectively stain the cell wall of *P. carinii* cysts are used to enumerate this stage; the Giemsa stain or one of its more rapid variants (e.g., Diff-Quik) is used to count the nuclei of all life cycle stages. The lower limit of detection by these stains is about 10^5 organisms per lung. A high degree of correlation has been found among the quantitative and histological techniques.

Studies of rats administered corticosteroids for 8–10 weeks and sacrificed at regular intervals provide a good picture of the sequential development of pneumocystosis (Fig. 1). Animals examined before beginning the immunosuppressive regimen may have either undetectable *P. carinii* infection or rare organisms in their lungs. After receiving corticosteroids for 1–2 weeks, small clusters of *P. carinii* along alveolar septa can be found in widely scattered locations of the lungs, suggesting the infection is multifocal in origin. Over the next several weeks, the organisms continue to multiply and gradually fill the alveolar lumens. Thus,

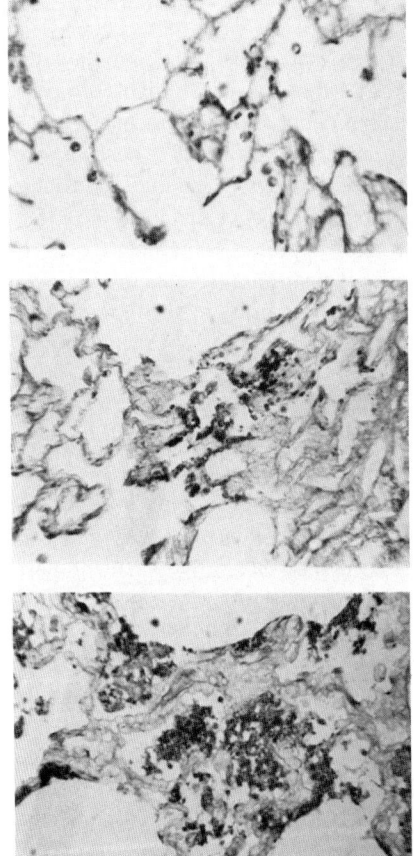

Figure 1 Sequential histological changes in experimental pneumocystosis in rats. Top, light infection; note scattered organisms in normal alveoli. Middle, moderate infection; note small clusters of organisms. Bottom, heavy infection; note alveolar filling with masses of organisms (methenamine silver stain, ×500).

P. carinii organisms in lung homogenates increase from $\leq 10^5$ per lung at the beginning of immunosuppression to 10^8–10^9 cysts and 10^9–10^{10} nuclei per lung, respectively, at peak intensity of the infection. These data indicate that *P. carinii* replicates slowly, but reaches high numbers in the lung.

Although studies of *P. carinii* proliferation in the rat model have been quite consistent, investigators have found that there may be variation in the peak organism burden and the time required to reach this level among rats. Factors influencing the development of pneumocystosis in a given experiment can be related to the rat that is used, method of establishing the infection, corticosteroid preparation, diet, associated microbial flora, and housing conditions.

Electron microscopic studies of *P. carinii* replication have focused on analyzing the organism's developmental stages and have formed the basis for most of our concepts about its life cycle (see Chap. 2). Although investigators have differed somewhat in their findings and terminology, they have identified three principal developmental stages: the trophic form or trophozoite, which is small, pleomorphic, and constitutes the most numerous stage; the cyst, which is characterized by its large size, thick cell wall, and the presence of up to eight intracystic bodies; the precyst, which is less well characterized, constitutes an intermediate stage.

Pneumocystis carinii proliferation in immunosuppressed rats appears to involve asexual and sexual phases of the life cycle (see Chap. 2). Trophic forms multiply by binary fission, whereas cyst development involves the fusion of gametes and a series of stages that culminate in the formation of the intracystic bodies; when these bodies were released from the cyst, they develop into trophic forms. Little is known about the factors that influence encystation or excystation.

Information about the *P. carinii* life cycle has also been derived from analyzing the effects of antimicrobial drugs. Agents such as trimethoprim–sulfamethoxazole (TMP–SMX) or pentamidine isethionate administered to rats to treat or prevent pneumocystosis lower both cyst and nuclei counts (29,30). These compounds have been thought to act mainly on the trophic form because the prominent cell wall of the cyst interfered with drug transport. The effects of these drugs on the cyst have been interpreted as indirect (i.e., through their effects on the trophic form, which is needed for the formation of the cyst).

Recent studies of drugs (e.g., echinocandins, papulocandins) which inhibit β-glucan synthesis challenge these concepts. These agents were originally developed as antifungal compounds; when ribosomal analysis pointed to the fungal nature of *P. carinii* and glucan (probably in the form of β-glucan) was found in the cell wall of the cyst stage (31), these drugs were investigated for their anti-*P. carinii* activity. β-Glucan inhibitors administered to immunosuppressed rats to treat pneumocystosis selectively lowered the cyst counts; the results were interpreted as indicating that these compounds acted only on the cyst form of the organism (32). However, when the β-glucan inhibitors were used as prophylactic agents, they lowered both the cyst and nuclei counts (33). These data suggested that formation of the cyst is essential to the general life cycle of *P. carinii*.

It is apparent from the foregoing that our understanding of the *P. carinii* life cycle is at a rudimentary level. Nevertheless, most workers have felt that it is legitimate to extrapolate about the life cycle of the organism in rats to other mammalian hosts. Available data suggest that human and mouse *P. carinii* closely resemble rat *P. carinii* in their developmental stages and response to antimicrobial drugs. Differences that have been found in these hosts appear to be more quantitative than qualitative. For example, the *P. carinii* burden achieved in normal mice with corticosteroid administration is not as great as that in rats (34). Pneumocystosis in immunodeficient mice is a more chronic illness and may have an even greater preponderance of trophic forms (24,35). Analysis about the frequency of specific *P. carinii* developmental stages in tissue specimens can be influenced by issues such as sampling technique or prior antimicrobial treatment; thus, we have found that the ratio of *P. carinii* trophic forms to cysts in rat or human lung homogenates or bronchoalveolar lavage fluids can vary from one subject to another (Cushion MT, Walzer PD, unpublished data).

Although the major site of *P. carinii* proliferation is the lung, the rising numbers of cases of disseminated pneumocystosis being reported in AIDS patients raise the intriguing possibility of parts of the organism's life cycle occurring at extrapulmonary sites (36). Investigation of this phenomenon might provide clues about *P. carinii* growth characteristics.

IV. Changes in the Alveolar Microenvironment

The development of pneumocystosis is accompanied by anatomical and physiological or biochemical changes in the host, but it has been difficult to establish a definite cause-and-effect relation. There is little evidence that *P. carinii* is invasive, has an intracellular phase in its developmental cycle, or secretes cytotoxic factors. The underlying conditions that predispose to pneumocystosis may produce broad changes in the host, and other opportunistic infections may also be present. However, with the use of animal models and careful controls, alterations in the host attributable to *P. carinii* have been delineated.

A. Anatomical Changes

The principal finding on hematoxylin–eosin (H&E)-stained lung sections is the foamy, vacuolated alveolar exudate. In corticosteroid-treated rats, this exudate develops with progressive *P. carinii* replication and consists of organisms, degenerative cell membranes, surfactant, and host proteins (9). Alveolar macrophages are present, but not conspicuous. The alveolar septa become thickened with hypertrophy and hyperplasia of the type II cells, interstitial edema, and a mild mononuclear cell infiltrate.

More detailed observations have been made by electron microscopy (9,37). During the early phase of corticosteroid administration, there are few alterations in the host other than attachment of *P. carinii* to the type I cell. The first change, that occurs when the organism burden nears or reaches its peak, consists of increased alveolar–capillary membrane permeability; this can be demonstrated by the leakage of an electron-dense marker (horseradish peroxidase) from the vascular space into the alveolar lumen. This is then followed by degenerative changes in the type I cell: subepithelial bleb formation, which represents fluid accumulation from the altered alveolar–capillary membrane permeability; denudation of the basement membrane, which appears to be the site of transport of serum fluid and proteins (e.g., fibrin) into the alveolar space to form the frothy exudate (Fig. 2).

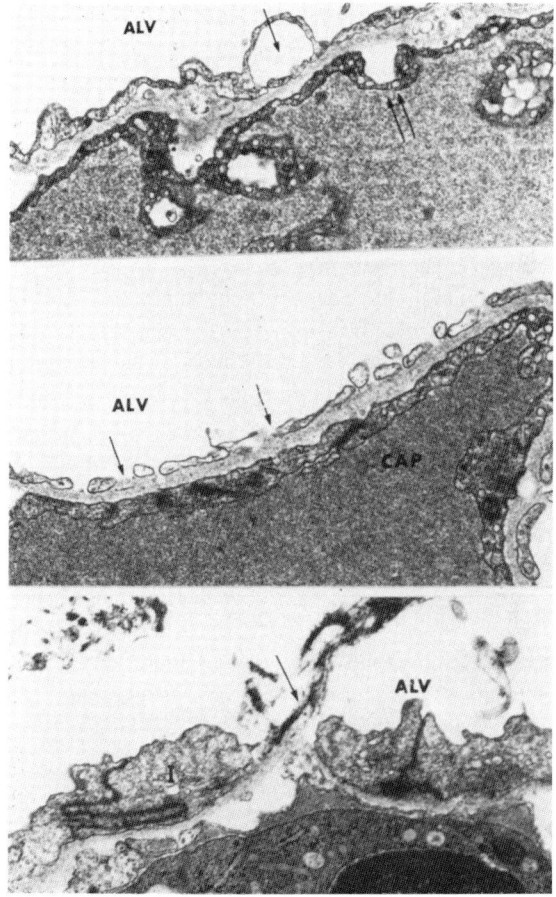

Figure 2 Sequential changes in the type I cell in experimental pneumocystosis. Top, subepithelial bleb formation (arrow). Middle, denudation of the basement membrane (arrow). Bottom, exudation of fibrin (arrow) and other serum proteins into the alveolar space (ALV) (×12,000).

Other morphological host changes require caution in interpretation. The hypertrophy of type II cells, which is seen on both light and electron microscopy, is a host reparative response to alveolar damage; under conditions that are poorly understood, the type II cells will differentiate into type I cells. However, type II cell hypertrophy can also result from administration of tetracyclines used in the immunosuppressive regimen to suppress bacterial infection (38). A decrease in the cell surface glycocalyx of the type I cell, as judged by histochemical stains (cationized ferritin, ruthenium red), has also been reported (Fig. 3) (39). This change, which owing to the effects of corticosteroids, may possibly alter the adhesive properties of the type I cell.

Overall, the changes described in the immunosuppressed rat model suggest diffuse alveolar injury. This histological picture is not specific for *P. carinii*, since it can be produced by a variety of other agents. However, the changes associated with pneumocystosis are distinctive in that they are slow to evolve, selectively involve the type I cell, and are related to organism attachment.

Studies using anatomical lung changes to investigate the pathogenesis of pneumocystosis in humans have been difficult to perform. Problems have included the need for an invasive procedure (e.g., transbronchial biopsy), the small amounts of tissue available for analysis, and the effects of agents used to treat *P. carinii* or the underlying disease on the pulmonary architecture. One report has demonstrated that *P. carinii* attaches to human type I cells in a manner similar to that in rats (40). Another study has found a correlation between the histological assessment of the severity of alveolar damage (as defined by the degree of interstitial edema) and long-term survival (41). Interstitial fibrosis can also be found on lung biopsy and autopsy specimens as a residual marker of lung injury (42).

B. Physiological and Biochemical Changes

Studies of the physiological and biochemical alterations in the lung that accompany pneumocystosis in the rat model have suggested a major role for the surfactant system in the disease pathogenesis (43–49). As in the anatomical

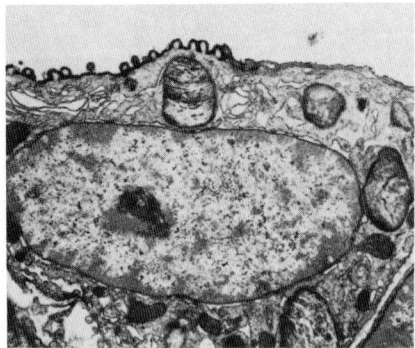 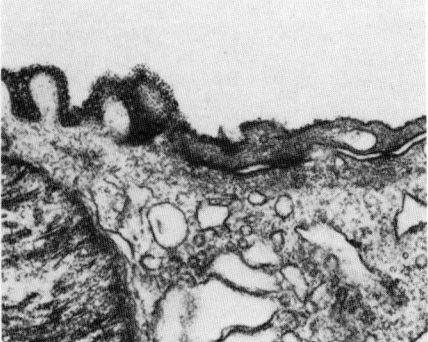

Figure 3 Deposition of the glycocalyx stain, cationized ferritin, in the alveolus of an immunosuppressed rat. Left, note the rather thin deposits on the type II cell and the near absence on the type I cell ($\times 7200$). Right, detailed view of same area ($\times 60,000$). (Adapted from Ref. 39.)

studies, care must be taken to distinguish changes caused by *P. carinii* from those caused by components of the immunosuppressive regimen. Typical controls include corticosteroid administration to rats without latent *P. carinii* infection, the use of TMP–SMX to prevent the development of pneumocystosis, and examining for the presence of other microbes.

The major findings in these studies have been impaired gas exchange, altered lung compliance and mechanics, and a decline in surfactant phospholipids in bronchoalveolar lavage fluid (BALF). Among the phospholipid constituents, there appears to be a fall in phostatidylcholine and a rise in sphingomyelin (46,49). Several hypotheses have been offered for the fall in surfactant phospholipids: increased catabolism, as evidenced by high phospholipase A_2 levels (43); impaired surfactant secretion, based on in vitro studies and the disparity between tissue and BALF concentrations of phospholipids in rats (Rice W, Walzer PD, unpublished data; 46); and binding of surfactant to *P. carinii* (50).

Along with the changes in surfactant phospholipids, increased levels of one of the major surfactant-associated proteins, surfactant protein A (SP-A), have been found (48). It is unknown whether this increase is due to *P. carinii* or is a nonspecific response to lung injury or inflammation. Surfactant protein A has several important functions, including regulation of surfactant phospholipid secretion and uptake by alveolar type II cells, absorption of phospholipid to the alveolar air–liquid interface, and lectin activity (51–54). Surfactant protein binds to the mannose residues of *P. carinii* gp120, possibly enhancing interaction of the organism with the alveolar epithelium and surfactant (55). It also interferes with the binding and internalization of *P. carinii* by alveolar macrophages, possibly altering host defenses (56).

Further evidence supporting the importance of the surfactant system in the pathogenesis of pneumocystosis comes from treatment experiments (47). Intratracheal instillation of surfactant improved oxygenation and pulmonary architecture in immunosuppressed rats with *P. carinii* pneumonia. These data suggest that surfactant replacement might have clinical application.

The physiological and biochemical changes in humans with pneumocystosis are generally similar to those in the rat model, but the types of studies have been different. Emphasis in human studies has been placed on arterial blood gas measurements because they are easy to perform and have important clinical significance. Pneumocystosis patients exhibit hypoxemia, increased alveolar–arterial oxygen gradient, and respiratory alkalosis. Early in the course of the disease, these patients display worsening oxygenation with exercise; this procedure has been suggested as an early diagnostic test (57). The degree of hypoxemia has been the most widely used marker for disease severity and prognosis.

Studies based on inhalation of the radionuclide, diethylenetriamine pentaacetic acid (DPTA), have suggested that *P. carinii* patients have increased alveolar–capillary permeability (58). The principal abnormality on pulmonary function tests is reduced diffusing capacity (DL); this involves the membrane diffusing capacity (DM), with no change in pulmonary capillary blood (V_c) (a picture of "alveolar–capillary block") (40). Impaired total lung capacity and vital capacity have also been reported (59). Studies of the surfactant system performed so far have shown a fall in surfactant phospholipids and a rise in SP-A levels (60–62). The physiological changes are reversible with successful anti-*P. carinii* therapy, but are slow to resolve.

Although the studies of the pathogenesis of pneumocystosis in animals and humans are at an early stage, enough information has been accumulated to formulate some general concepts. The hallmarks of the disease are impaired gas exchange and the foamy alveolar exudate; without treatment, there is progressive respiratory insufficiency and death of severe lung injury. These features result from the following mechanisms: the slow propagation of *P. carinii*, which fills the alveoli with masses of organisms; attachment of *P. carinii* to type I cells, which increases alveolar–capillary permeability and, ultimately, leads to damage of these cells; deficiency of surfactant phospholipids, which results in changes in alveolar surface tension, lung distensibility, and ventilation–perfusion abnormalities.

V. Host Inflammatory or Immune Response

It had long been thought that the host inflammatory or immune response plays little or no role in the pathogenesis of *P. carinii* pneumonia. This assumption was based on the fact that immunosuppressive agents are used to induce pneumocystosis, and the host inflammatory changes on histological examination are inconspicuous. It was only after withdrawal of corticosteroids in experimental pneumocystosis that the rats developed a vigorous response and cleared the organism from the lung (21). The process included phagocytosis of *P. carinii* by alveolar macrophages; the development lymphocytic infiltrates in peribronchial and perivascular areas and systemic lymphocytosis; continued proliferation of type II cells; a rise in local and systemic antibodies to the organism. Interstitial fibrosis also developed, thereby supporting the findings in humans that recovery was accompanied by evidence of lung damage.

However, in recent years, the occurrence of pneumocystosis in AIDS patients has raised the possibility that the host inflammatory or immune response may be deleterious. This hypothesis is supported by the deterioration in blood oxygenation soon after starting anti-*P. carinii* drugs; the effectiveness of corticosteroids in preventing this deterioration and in improving survival when given with anti-*P. carinii* drugs; and the association of increased neutrophils in BALF of *P. carinii* patients with poor prognosis (63,64).

What are the underlying mechanisms? The leading theory is that this host reaction is in response to dying organisms or lung damage; perhaps proteolytic enzymes are released from *P. carinii* or host cells (63). Some support for such an occurrence comes from studies that showed that rats with pneumocystosis that improved with surfactant replacement displayed emphysematous changes in their pulmonary architecture (47).

Insights into the cells mediating this host response have been gained from studies of immunodeficient mice that develop *P. carinii* pneumonia without the need for corticosteroids. SCID mice with pneumocystosis, which were immunologically reconstituted by bone marrow transplantation or infusion of CD4 cells, experienced early deaths from a hyperinflammatory reaction and then cleared *P. carinii* from their lungs (24,25). Other investigators have found that CD4 cell-depleted mice could also mount an inflammatory response to *P. carinii* (65). The histological picture in these studies resembled that found in rats when steroids were withdrawn.

These data illustrate the harmful and helpful effects of the host inflammatory or immune response. CD4 cells and other as yet undefined cell types can mediate this response; that these cells tend to congregate at specific regions of the lungs (i.e., perivascular and peribronchial areas) suggests that they may exert their effects by cytokines. The practical application of this work is that immunomodulators, which have far more specific effects on the host than corticosteroids, may play an important role in the treatment of pneumocystosis.

VI. Conclusion

The clinical and pathological features of *P. carinii* pneumonia are familiar to most physicians, but knowledge of pathophysiology is limited. Pathogenic mechanisms important in the development of pneumocystosis can be divided into four stages: attachment of *P. carinii* to the type I cell; alveolar filling by slow organism proliferation; changes in the alveolar microenvironment, which result in diffuse lung injury; the host immune or inflammatory response. Elucidation of these mechanisms will not only improve our understanding of the disease, but may also lead to new forms of therapy.

References

1. Walzer PD, Schnelle V, Armstrong D, Rosen PP. The nude mouse: a new experimental model for *Pneumocystis carinii* infection. Science 1977; 197:177–179.
2. Hughes WT. Natural mode of acquisition for de novo infection with *Pneumocystis carinii*. J Infect Dis 1982; 145:842–848.
3. Bartlett MS, Fishman JA, Queener SF, Durkin MM, Jay MA, Smith JW. New rat model of *Pneumocystis carinii* pneumonia. J Clin Microbiol 1988; 26:1100–1102.

4. Meuwissen JHE, Tauber I, Leewenberg ADEM, Beckers PJA, Shiehen J. Parasitologic and serologic observations of infection with *Pneumocystis* in humans. J Infect Dis 1977; 136:43–49.
5. Pifer LL, Hughes WT, Stagno S, Woods D. *Pneumocystis carinii* infection: evidence for high prevalence in normal and immunosuppressed children. Pediatrics 1978; 62:35–41.
6. Peglow SL, Smulian GA, Linke MJ, et al. Serologic responses to specific *Pneumocystis carinii* antigens in health and disease. J Infect Dis 1990; 161:296–306.
7. Lanken PN, Minda M, Pietra GG, Fishman AP. Alveolar response to experimental *Pneumocystis carinii* pneumonia in the rat. Am J Pathol 1980; 99:561–578.
8. Yoneda K, Walzer PD. The interaction of *Pneumocystis carinii* with host cells: an ultrastructural study. Infect Immun 1980; 29:692–703.
9. Yoneda K, Walzer PD. Attachment of *Pneumocystis carinii* to type I alveolar cells: study by freeze fracture electron microscopy. Infect Immun 1983; 40:812–815.
10. Henshaw NG, Carson JL, Collier AM. Ultrastructural observations in *Pneumocystis carinii* attachment to rat lung. J Infect Dis 1985; 151:181–186.
11. Long EC, Smith JS, Meier JL. Attachment of *Pneumocystis carinii* to rat pneumocytes. Lab Invest 1986; 54:609–614.
12. Pottratz ST, Martin WJ. Role of fibronectin in *Pneumocystis carinii* attachment to cultured lung cells. J Clin Invest 1990 85:351–356.
13. Limper AH, Martin WJ. *Pneumocystis carinii*: inhibition of lung cell growth mediated by parasite attachment. J Clin Invest 1990; 85:391–396.
14. Pottratz ST, Paulsrud J, Smith JS, Martin WJ. *Pneumocystis carinii* attachment to cultured lung cells by pneumocystis gp120, a fibronectin binding protein. J Clin Invest 1991; 88:403–407.
15. Ezekowitz RAB, Williams DJ, Koziel H, Armstrong MYK, Warner A, Richards FF, Rose RM. Uptake of *Pneumocystis carinii* mediated by the macrophage mannose receptor. Nature 1991; 351:155–158.
16. Limper AH, Pottratz ST, Martin WJ. Modulation of *Pneumocystis carinii* adherence to cultured lung cell by a mannose-dependent mechanism. J Lab Clin Med 1991; 118:492–499.
17. Masur H, Jones TC. The interaction in vitro of *Pneumocystis carinii* with macrophages and L-cells. J Exp Med 1978; 147:157–170.
18. Walzer PD. *Pneumocystis carinii*—new clinical spectrum? N Engl J Med 1991; 324:263–265.
19. Frenkel JK, Good JT, Schultz JA. Latent *Pneumocystis* infection of rats, relapse, and chemotherapy. Lab Invest 1966; 15:1559–1577.
20. Perera DR, Western KA, Johnson HD, et al. *Pneumocystis carinii* pneumonia in a hospital for children. JAMA 1970; 214:1074–1078.
21. Walzer PD, Kim CK, Cushion MT. *Pneumocystis carinii*. In: Walzer PD, Genta RM, eds. Parasitic infections in the compromised host. New York: Marcel Dekker, 1989:83–178.
22. Shellito J, Suzara VV, Blumenfeld W, Beck JM, Steger HJ, Ermak TH. A new model of *Pneumocystis carinii* infection in mice selectively depleted of helper T lymphocytes. J Clin Invest 1990; 85:1686–1693.

23. Harmsen AG, Stankiewicz M. Requirement for CD4+ cells in resistance to *Pneumocystis carinii* pneumonia in mice. J Exp Med 1990; 172:937–945.
24. Roths JB, Marshall JD, Allen RD, Carlson GA, Sidman CL. Spontaneous *Pneumocystis carinii* pneumonia in immunodeficient mutant SCID mice. Am J Pathol 1990; 136:1173–1186.
25. Roths JB, Sidman CL. Both immunity and hyperresponsiveness to *Pneumocystis carinii* result from transfer of $CD4^+$ but not $CD8^+$ T cells into severe combined immunodeficiency mice. J Clin Invest 1992; 90:673–678.
26. Gigliotti F, Hughes WT. Passive immunoprophylaxis with specific monoclonal antibody confers partial protection against *Pneumocystis carinii* pneumonitis in animal models. J Clin Invest 1988; 81:1666–1668.
27. Walzer PD, Powell RD, Yoneda K, Rutledge ME, Milder JE. Growth characteristics and pathogenesis of experimental *Pneumocystis carinii* pneumonia. Infect Immun 1980; 27:929–937.
28. Kim CK, Foy JM, Cushion MT, Stanforth D, Linke MJ, Hendrix HL, Walzer PD. Comparison of histologic and quantitative techniques in the evaluation of experimental *Pneumocystis carinii*. Antimicrob Agents Chemother 1987; 31:197–201.
29. Walzer PD, Kim CK, Foy JM, Linke MJ, Cushion MT. Inhibitors of folic acid synthesis in the treatment of experimental *Pneumocystis carinii* pneumonia. Antimicrob Agents Chemother 1988; 32:96–103.
30. Walzer PD, Kim CK, Foy JM, Linke MJ, Cushion MT. Cationic antitrypanosomal and other antimicrobial agents in the treatment of experimental *Pneumocystis carinii* pneumonia. Antimicrob Agents Chemother 1988; 32:896–905.
31. Cushion MT, Stringer JR, Walzer PD. Cell and molecular biology of *Pneumocystis carinii*. Int Rev Cytol 1991; 131:59–107.
32. Schmatz DM, Romanchek MA, Pittarelli LA, et al. Treatment of *Pneumocystis carinii* pneumonia with 1,3-β-glucan synthesis inhibitors. Proc Natl Acad Sci USA 1990; 87:5950–5954.
33. Schmatz DM, Powles M, McFadden DC, Pittarelli LA, Liberator PA, Anderson JW. Treatment and prevention of *Pneumocystis carinii* pneumonia and further elucidation of the *P. carinii* life cycle with 1,3-β-glucan synthesis inhibitor L-671,329. J Protozool 1991; 38:151S–153S.
34. Walzer PD, Powell RD, Yoneda K. *Pneumocystis carinii* pneumonia in different strains of cortisonized mice. Infect Immun 1979; 24:939–947.
35. Matsumoto Y, Frenkel JK, Aikawa M, Yoshida Y. Proliferation of *Pneumocystis* trophozoites in human lymph nodes and in nude mice lungs. J Protozool 1989; 36:33S–34S.
36. Telzak EE, Cote RJ, Gold JWM, Campbell SW, Armstrong D. Extrapulmonary *Pneumocystis carinii* infections. Rev Infect Dis 1990; 12:380–386.
37. Yoneda K, Walzer PD. Mechanism of alveolar injury in experimental *Pneumocystis carinii* pneumonia in the rat. Br J Exp Pathol 1981; 62:339–346.
38. Gottschall JI, Walzer PD, Yoneda K. Morphological changes in the rat type II pneumocytes induced by oxytetracycline. Lab Invest 1979; 41:5–12.
39. Yoneda K, Walzer PD. The effect of corticosteroid treatment on the cell surface glycocalyx of the rat pulmonary alveolus: relevance to the host–parasite relationship in *Pneumocystis carinii* infection. Br J Exp Pathol 1984; 65:347–354.

40. Sankary RM, Turner J, Lipavsky A, Howes EL, Murray JF. Alveolar–capillary block in patients with AIDS and *Pneumocystis carinii* pneumonia. Am Rev Respir Dis 1988; 137:443–449.
41. Brenner M, Ognibene FP, Lack EE, Simmons JT, Suffredini AF, Lane HC, Fauci AS, Parrillo JE, Shelhamer JH, Masur H. Prognostic factors and life expectancy of patients with acquired immunodeficiency syndrome and *Pneumocystis carinii* pneumonia. Am Rev Respir Dis 1987; 136:1199–1206.
42. Travis WD, Pittaluga S, Lipschik GY, et al. Atypical pathologic manifestations of *Pneumocystis carinii* pneumonia in the acquired immune deficiency syndrome. Review of 123 lung biopsies from 76 patients with emphasis on cysts, vascular invasion, vasculitis, and granulomas. Am J Surg Pathol 1990; 14:615–625.
43. Kernbaum S, Masliah J, Alcindor LG, Bouton C, Christol D. Phospholipase activities of bronchoalveolar lavage fluid in rat *Pneumocystis carinii* pneumonia. Br J Exp Pathol 1983; 64:75–80.
44. Brun-Pascaud M, Pocidalo JJ, Kernbaum S. Respiratory and pulmonary alterations in experimental *Pneumocystis carinii* pneumonia in rats. Bull Eur Physiopathol Respir 1985; 21:37–41.
45. Stokes DC, Hughes WT, Alderson PO, King RE, Garfinkel DJ. Lung mechanisms, radiography and ^{67}Ga scintigraphy in experimental *Pneumocystis carinii* pneumonia. Br J Exp Pathol 1986; 67:383–393.
46. Sheehan PM, Stokes DC, Yeh Y, Hughes WT. Surfactant phospholipids and lavage phospholipase A_2 in experimental *Pneumocystis carinii* pneumonia. Am Rev Respir Dis 1986; 134:526–531.
47. Eijking EP, van Daal GJ, Tenbrink R, Luijendijk A, Sluiters JF, Hannappel E, Lachmann B. Effect of surfactant replacement on *Pneumocystis carinii* pneumonia in rats. Intensive Care Med 1991; 17:475–478.
48. Phelps DS, Fishman JA, Rose RM. Surfactant protein A levels in glucocorticoid-immunosuppressed rats infected with *Pneumocystis carinii*. Am Rev Respir Dis 1992; 145:A246.
49. Su TH, Natarajan V, Martin WJ. Pulmonary surfactant in *Pneumocystis carinii* pneumonia is associated with a marked increase in sphingomyelin. Am Rev Respir Dis 1992; 145:A246.
50. Pesanti EL. Phospholipid profile of *Pneumocystis carinii* and its interaction with alveolar type II epithelial cells. Infect Immun 1987; 55:736–774.
51. Dobbs GL, Wright JR, Hawgood S, Gonzalez R, Venstrom K, Nellenbogen J. Pulmonary surfactant and its components inhibit secretion of phosphatidylcholine from cultured rat alveolar type II cells. Proc Natl Acad Sci USA 1987; 84:1010–1014.
52. Wright JR, Wager RE, Hawgood S, Dobbs L, Clements JA. Surfactant apoprotein M_r=26,000–36,000 enhances uptake of liposomes by type II cells. J Biol Chem 1987; 262:2888–2894.
53. Hawgood S, Benson BJ, Schilling J, Damm D, Clements J, White RT. Nucleotide and amino acid sequences of pulmonary surfactant protein SP 18 and evidence for cooperation between SP 18 and SP 28–36 in surfactant lipid absorption. Proc Natl Acad Sci USA 1987; 84:66–70.
54. Haagsman HP, Hawgood S, Sargeant T, Buckley D, White T, Drickamer K, Benson BJ.

The major lung surfactant protein, SP 8–36, is a calcium-dependent, carbohydrate-binding protein. J Biol Chem 1987; 262:13877–13880.
55. Zimmerman PE, Voelker R, McCormack FX, Paulsrud JR, Martin WJ. 120-kD Surface glycoprotein of *Pneumocystis carinii* is a ligand for surfactant protein A. J Clin Invest 1992; 89:143–149.
56. Koziel H, O'Riordan D, Phelps D, Fishman JA, Armstrong MYK, Richards FF, Rose RM. Surfactant protein-A inhibits binding and internalization of *Pneumocystis carinii* by alveolar macrophages. Am Rev Respir Dis 1992; 145:A247.
57. Stover DE, Greeno RA, Gagliardi AJ. The use of a simple exercise test for the diagnosis of *Pneumocystis carinii* pneumonia in patients with AIDS. Am Rev Respir Dis 1989; 139:1343–1346.
58. Mason GR, Duane GB, Mena I, Effros RM. Accelerated solute clearance in *Pneumocystis carinii* pneumonia. Am Rev Respir Dis 1987; 135:864–868.
59. Coleman DL, Dodek PM, Golden JA, Luce JM, Golden E, Gold WM, Murray JF. Correlation between serial pulmonary function tests and fiberoptic bronchoscopy in patients with *Pneumocystis carinii* pneumonia and the acquired immune deficiency syndrome. Am Rev Respir Dis 1984; 129:491–493.
60. Hoffman AGD, Lipchik G, Lawrence M, Kovacs J, Ognibene F, Suffredini AF, Masur H, Shelhamer JH. Pulmonary surfactant abnormalities in AIDS patients with *Pneumocystis* pneumonia. FASEB J 1990; 4:A2147.
61. Baughman RP, Hull W, Whitsett JA. *Pneumocystis carinii* alters surfactant associated protein-A concentrations found in bronchoalveolar lavage fluid. Clin Res 1992; 40:412A.
62. Phelps DS, Rose RM. Increased recovery of surfactant protein A in AIDS-related pneumonia. Am Rev Respir Dir 1991; 143:1072–1075.
63. The National Institutes of Health–University of California expert panel for corticosteroids as adjunctive therapy for *Pneumocystis carinii* pneumonia. Consensus statement on the use of corticosteroids as adjunctive therapy for pneumocystis pneumonia in the acquired immunodeficiency syndrome. N Engl J Med 1990; 323:1500–1504.
64. Mason GR, Hashimoto CH, Dickman PS, Foutty LF, Cobb CJ. Prognostic implications of bronchoalveolar lavage neutrophilia in patients with *Pneumocystis carinii* pneumonia and AIDS. Am Rev Respir Dis 1989; 139:1336–1342.
65. Beck JM, Warnock ML, Curtis JL, Sniezek MJ, Arraj-Peffer SM, Kaltreider HB, Shellito JE. Inflammatory responses to *Pneumocystis carinii* in mice selectively depleted of helper T lymphocytes. Am J Respir Cell Mol Biol 1991; 5:186–197.

14

Humoral and Cellular Immunity

DON C. GRAVES

University of Oklahoma Health Sciences Center
Oklahoma City, Oklahoma

**A. GEORGE SMULIAN
and PETER D. WALZER**

Cincinnati Veterans Affairs Medical Center
and University of Cincinnati College of Medicine
Cincinnati, Ohio

I. Introduction

Pneumocystis carinii is a ubiquitous organism that resides in the lungs of humans and a variety of other animals. Under conditions during which there is impaired immune response in the host (Table 1), this opportunistic organism can begin to propagate, resulting in pneumonia. If one carefully examines the underlying conditions predisposing the host to *P. carinii* pneumonia, one will notice that most of the defects seen in these patients, at least to some extent, are associated with T-cell function. This probably holds true for premature infants, because at their young age, they may have abnormal T-cell functions (1–3). It is possible that a similar situation is true for the patients with hypogammaglobulinemia, since most of these patients were infants younger than 1 year of age (4–8). Furthermore, many of the cases of infantile *P. carinii* pneumonia have been associated with malnutrition, which has been shown to have a major influence on cell-mediated immunity (2,9), specifically, a T-cell depression (3).

Pneumocystis carinii pneumonia in individuals with malignant neoplasias or those undergoing organ transplants is usually a result of immunosuppressive therapy (10). Corticosteroids and cyclosporin are commonly used drugs for immunosuppressive therapy, both of which have inhibitory effects on the cellular

267

Table 1 Predisposing Conditions Associated with *Pneumocystis carinii* Pneumonia

Condition	Ref.
Premature infants with malnutrition	1–3
Congenital (primary) immunodeficiency disease	4–8
Severe combined immunodeficiency	
Immunodeficiency with hypogammaglobulinemia	
Others	
Immunosuppressive therapy	4,5,10–14,18,20
Malignancies	
Organ transplantation	
Miscellaneous diseases treated	
Acquired immune deficiency syndrome (AIDS)	18,20–22

immune system and, in most cases, T lymphocytes (11–15). Other agents, such as methotrexate, cyclophosphamide, cytarabine, mechlorethamine, procarbazine, and radiation, used alone or in combination for therapy appear to predispose the patient to pneumocystosis, but their relative importance is unclear (16–18).

Perhaps the most striking evidence of the importance of T cells in host defenses against *P. carinii* comes from patients with acquired immunodeficiency syndrome (AIDS). Pneumocystosis was one of the original AIDS-defining illnesses (19,20) and remains one of the leading opportunistic infections (21). Among human immunodeficiency virus (HIV)-infected patients, the risk of *P. carinii* pneumonia can be directly correlated with the number of circulating CD4 cells (22). Recent CD4 depletion and reconstitution studies in mice also indicate that T cells are essential for protection and recovery from pneumocystosis (23–25).

Studies in experimental animals, involving passive immunization and B-cell reconstitution experiments, indicate that the humoral branch of the immune system also appears to be important in the host's ability to resist and recover from *P. carinii* pneumonia (26–28). The development of serological responses to *P. carinii* in recurrent episodes of pneumocystosis in AIDS patients further implies a role for humoral immunity (29). Thus, evidence is accumulating suggesting that both the humoral and cellular branches of the immune system are important for containing or eliminating the organism, but the specific components of each system and the role(s) of each component are poorly understood.

Immunological studies involving the humoral and cellular response in humans, as well as in animal models, to *P. carinii* will be presented in this chapter. Emphasis will be placed on the studies that have occurred in the past decade. The reader is referred to other references pertaining to the immunobiology of *P. carinii* for additional information (21,30–33).

II. Humoral Immunity

A. Studies in Animal Models

The indirect fluorescent antibody (IFA) assay, the enzyme-linked immunosorbent assay (ELISA) and, to a smaller extent, complement-fixation assay, are the techniques that have been most often used to study the host's immune response (a rise in serum antibody titer) to *P. carinii* pneumonia and have been summarized (21,30–33). However, it appears that environmental exposure to *P. carinii* stimulates an immune response and that most healthy hosts develop serum antibodies to the organism (34–37). The high prevalence of serum antibodies to *P. carinii* in the normal human population has limited the usefulness of these techniques as tools for the diagnosis of *P. carinii* pneumonia in the immunocompromised host. Furthermore, since many patients with AIDS have variable antibody titers to *P. carinii*, these serological assays are of limited value for diagnosing *P. carinii* infections in these patients (29).

The IFA, ELISA and, more recently, the immunoblot assays have provided valuable information about the humoral response of the host to *P. carinii*. With use of the IFA, sequential changes in rat IgG serum antibody titers to *P. carinii* were studied in the following groups of rats (38): (1) control rats not immunosuppressed, but housed in a conventional colony room; (2) corticosteroid-treated group (*P. carinii* pneumonitis induced); (3) a group treated with corticosteroid for the first 4 weeks and then corticosteroid tapered for the next 3 weeks to zero; (4) young rats (3–6 weeks old); and (5) retired breeders (about 6 months old) (Fig. 1). The results of the control group of rats not receiving corticosteroids, but housed in the conventional colony room, are shown in Figure 1a. The IgG antibody titers remained less than 1:4 for the first 8 weeks, but by 10 weeks, the titers began to increase to 1:16 or greater with time. The serum IgG antibody titers were generally suppressed during steroid treatment, a time of greatest *P. carinii* burden (see Fig. 1b). An inverse relation between the severity of disease and the antibody titer was usually observed. In the group of rats for which the steroid was tapered, antibody titers rose progressively with time to 1:256, or higher, and often reached levels higher than the untreated controls (see Fig. 1b). The young healthy rats usually lacked serum antibody titers to *P. carinii*, whereas the retired breeders had titers of 1:16, or higher (see Fig. 1c). Similar data were obtained using the ELISA for detecting sequential changes in serum IgG antibody (39). An additional observation made in this latter study was that normal adult cesarian-obtained, barrier-sustained rats had negligible levels of antibody titers to *P. carinii*.

Studies examining the immune response of mice to *P. carinii* have yielded results similar to those reported in the rat model (40,41). These studies indicate that rats and mice develop serum IgG antibodies in response to subclinical as well overt *P. carinii* infection, which is a situation that is also observed in humans (29,34–37). Furthermore, it has been observed that nu/+ mice and nu/+ rats develop good serum antibody titers upon recovery from infection, but nu/nu mice

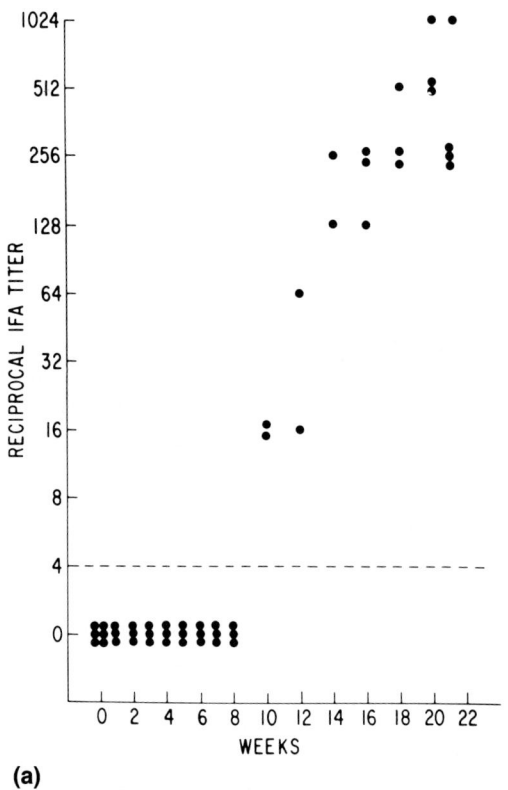

Figure 1 (a) Sequential changes in serum antibody titers to *P. carinii* among rats not receiving corticosteroids and housed in conventional colony room as measured by the IFA technique. (b) Sequential changes in rat serum antibody titers to *P. carinii* by IFA technique over time. ○, group A controls; ●, group B rats in the standard corticosteroid regimen; ▲, group C rats, the corticosteroid dose of which had been tapered after 4 weeks. (c) Serum antibody titers to *P. carinii* in rats from commercial breeders. ●, young adult rats; ○, retired breeder rats: A, ARS, Sprague-Dawley; B, Harlan; C, Charles River; D, Taconic; and E, Hilltop. (From Ref. 38.)

and nu/nu rats do not (40,42,43). Reconstitution of *P. carinii*-infected, severe combined immunodeficiency (SCID) mice, nu/nu mice, or nu/nu rats with spleen cells from immunocompetent donors also resulted in a serum antibody response to *P. carinii* as these animals recovered from *P. carinii* pneumonitis (23,43,44).

The host's IgM and IgA immune responses to *P. carinii* are not completely clear. One group of investigators, using the rat model, found that serum IgG and IgM antibodies developed at similar times in animals that recovered from induced pneumocystosis and in those with environmental exposure to *P. carinii*; the titers of each antibody varied in individual rats (45). In yet another study, using the rat

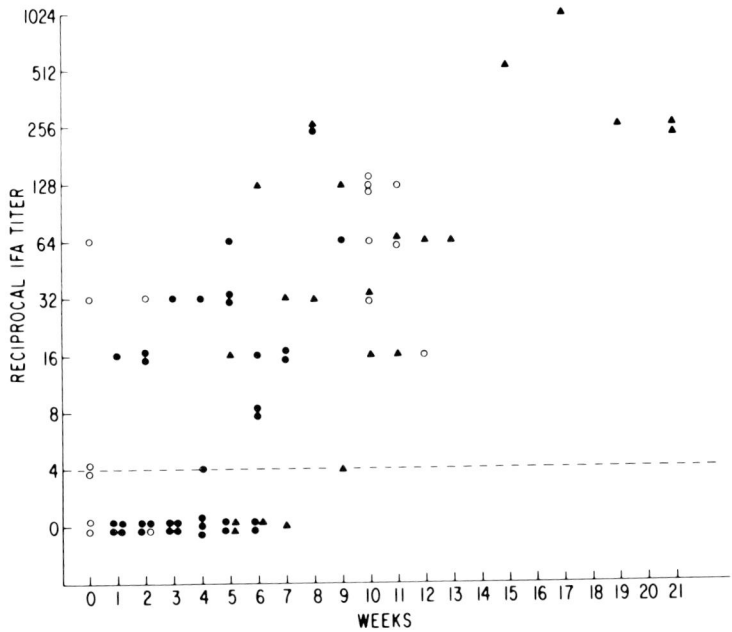

(b)

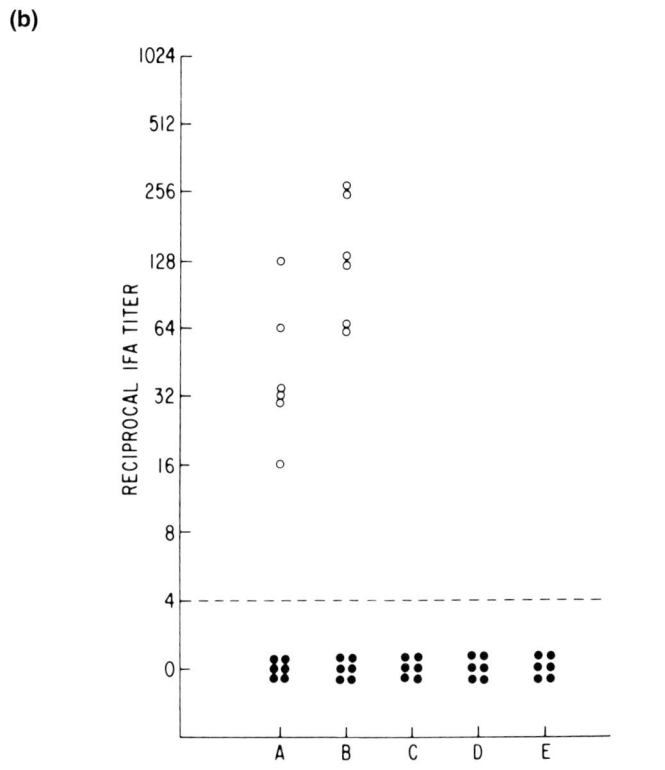

(c)

model, investigators found no IgM antibodies produced in response to *P. carinii* (42). When the mouse model was used, the IgM response was variable, depending on the strain of mouse studied and the serological technique used for the assays (40,46). With IFA, the IgM component of the immune response in mice (except C57 BL/6N strain) was low, whereas when the ELISA technique was used (46), the IgM antibodies assumed a more prominent role in the immune response to *P. carinii*.

The role of IgA in the immune response is poorly understood. Low levels of serum IgA antibodies were found in a small percentage of mice (both controls and those infected with *P. carinii*), but the titers were considerably lower than the IgG and IgM antibody titers to *P. carinii* in the same animals (40). Similar results have been observed in studies involving sera from humans (47–50). Variable results have been obtained in studies assaying for IgA antibodies to *P. carinii* in AIDS patients; however, AIDS patients, with and without *P. carinii* pneumonia, generally have IgA antibody titers similar to those of healthy controls (37,50). The fact that investigators have found IgA on the surface of *P. carinii* in bronchoalveolar lavage specimens suggests that IgA is involved in the host's local immune response to *P. carinii* infection (40,51,52). It has been implied that an IgA deficiency may be the predisposing factor in some patients with *P. carinii* pneumocystosis (53,54). However, patients with IgA deficiency, such as those with ataxia telangiectasia, are not prone to *P. carinii* pneumonia (4). Before any firm conclusions can be drawn on the role of IgA, more detailed studies need to be performed.

Until recently, there has been little experimental evidence indicating that antibodies to *P. carinii* play a role in the host's defense against *P. carinii*, even though they are frequently present. In one early study, rats immunized with *P. carinii* developed significant serum antibody titers (1:64–1:256 by IFA), but were not protected from fatal *P. carinii* pneumonia when subjected to immunosuppression by corticosteroids (55). In another study, in which mice were immunocompromised by cortisone and infected with *P. carinii* by intranasal inoculation, immune serum was not effective for recovery from *P. carinii* infection (43). These reports suggested that serum antibodies do not play a significant role as defense mechanisms against *P. carinii* infections. Recent studies, however, have provided information suggesting that antibodies to *P. carinii* are important components of the host's defense to this organism (26–28). In adoptive transfer experiments using SCID mice and functional T cells and spleen cells from immunocompetent donors, it was shown that B cells were necessary for the recipient mice to resolve their preexisting *P. carinii* pneumonia (26). Even though these studies did not show how B cells contributed to the resolution of *P. carinii* pneumonia, it was suggested that, with the help of T cells, B cells probably produce specific *P. carinii* antibodies that contributed to the process.

Further evidence supporting the importance of anti-*P. carinii* antibodies has come from immunoprophylaxis studies. Passive immunoprophylaxis, using a monoclonal antibody against a major antigenic component of ferret *P. carinii*, conferred partial protection to *P. carinii* pneumonia in steroid-induced immunosuppressed rats and ferrets (27). In a more recent immunotherapy study using SCID mice that have naturally acquired *P. carinii* pneumonia, administration of anti-*P. carinii* hyperimmune serum was successful in reducing the number of *P. carinii* in early, intermediate, and advanced stages of *P. carinii* pneumonia (28). In addition, administration of this hyperimmune serum on a continuing basis, increased the life expectancy of the mice by greater than threefold. In these same studies, it was shown that the often fatal hyperinflammatory response to *P. carinii*, known to follow adoptive transfer of component T cells to SCID mice, could be averted by pretreating the mice with the hyperimmune serum (28). Thus, data are accumulating indicating that antibodies to *P. carinii* play a significant role in the host's ability to resist or recover from *P. carinii* infections. It is possible that they act as opsonins, enhancing the ingestion and destruction of *P. carinii* by alveolar macrophages (56).

Several studies have been done using the immunoblotting technique to determine which specific *P. carinii* antigenic moieties induce the serum IgG antibody response in the host (29,32,45,57–61). Most studies used sera that were obtained from hosts after recovery from the overt disease and from normal hosts after prolonged environmental exposure to *P. carinii*. The rat, mouse and, to a smaller extent, the ferret, are the major experimental animal models used in these studies. Considerable variation has been found among individual animals as well as in results obtained from one laboratory to another; this may be attributed to differences in technique, *P. carinii* isolates used, source of antibody, and possibly other factors. However, three general conclusions can be drawn from immunoblotting studies in which *P. carinii* preparations were solubilized with sodium dodecyl sulfate (SDS) and analyzed under reducing conditions (Table 2). First, rats develop IgG antibodies to *P. carinii* antigens in the relative molecular mass (M_r) ranges of

Table 2 Major *P. carinii* Antigenic Moieties Detected by Immunoblotting Using Convalescent Polyclonal Antisera

Source of *P. carinii*	M_r major reactive antigens (kDa)	Ref.
Rat	42–65	32,45,57–59,61
	110–120	
Ferret	120	61–63
	70	
Mouse	100–120	60,61
	45–50	
Human	35–45,95	29,32,57–59,85
	110–120	
	22,24	

M_r, relative molecular mass.

42–65 and 110–120 kDa (32,45,57–61). In one study in which sequential changes in IgG antibody formation were measured over time of recovery, specific antigens of 45, 50, and 116 kDa were detected, with the 50-kDa entity being recognized slightly earlier than the other two (45). Second, the major mouse *P. carinii* antigenic components recognized by mouse recovery serum or pooled serum from normal mice have M_r of approximately 45–50 kDa (60) and 116–120 kDa (60–62). Third, the major immunoreactive ferret *P. carinii* component appears to be an antigen with an M_r of approximately 120 kDa (63). However, in a recent preliminary study using convalescent antisera, the major antigenic component of ferret *P. carinii* had an M_r of approximately 70 kDa (61). Cross-reactive epitopes have been found on several of the major antigens from different species of *P. carinii* and are discussed in Chapter 5 of this book. The importance of these immunoreactive moieties in the pathogenesis of *P. carinii* is unknown, but purification of these antigens and the production of monoclonal antibodies to them will facilitate structural–functional studies.

B. Studies in Humans

Although the exact role of antibodies in the host response to *P. carinii* infection is unknown, a specific humoral response has been documented in association with this infection. Antibodies to *P. carinii* are present in most of the population (29,34–37). Anti-*P. carinii* antibodies increase in frequency in early childhood, suggesting exposure to the organism at an early age (29,34,35).

Specific anti-*P. carinii* antibody responses have also been demonstrated in the setting of clinical disease. Antibody responses were investigated by IFA in 23 cases of proven or clinically suspected pneumocystosis among patients of a British oncology unit (64). In the group, 10 patients demonstrated titers higher than 1:32, 5 patients showed a fivefold rise in antibody titer, 3 converted from negative to a 1:8 titer, and 1 proven case remained negative. Among 91 controls, 56% demonstrated antibodies, with the highest titer being 1:32. A subsequent study (65), using the same infected human lung sections as antigen, detected antibodies at a titer of 1:8, or higher, in 48% of nonimmunosuppressed children. A trend to more of the older children having higher levels of antibody was noted.

A study performed in Denmark, using IFA, found similar IgG and IgA antibody titers to *P. carinii* among AIDS patients with pneumocystosis and healthy controls (37). However, the *P. carinii* patients with AIDS had a markedly lower frequency of serum IgM antibodies (13 vs 62%). These responses were detected using human-derived *P. carinii* cysts as antigen.

Two further IFA studies have been reported from Scotland using rat-derived *P. carinii* as antigen. In one report, antibodies were detected at a titer of 1:8, or higher, in 58.3% of 24 immunosuppressed patients with histologically proven or strongly suspected cases of *P. carinii* pneumonia, in only 8.8% of normal controls, and in 13.4% of 464 patients symptomatic with pulmonary symptoms or fever (66). No IgM antibodies were detected in the sera from the cases or control groups. Another study evaluated immunosuppressed patients (AIDS, lymphoid and myeloid malignancies) and controls by IFA using frozen sections of *P. carinii*-infected rat lung as antigen (67). Antibodies were detected in 63.2% of AIDS patients, in 70.2% of non-AIDS patients, and in 80% of controls. Some patients had sequential sera examined. Five patients demonstrated a fall in antibody titers before the development of an episode of *P. carinii* pneumonia. Three additional patients demonstrated increasing concentrations of antibody coincident with treatment and clinical recovery from infection.

A report in the United States examined serum antibodies of children and adults in low- and high-risk groups for *P. carinii* pneumonia by IFA and immunoblotting (29). Antibodies to the 40-kDa antigen were the most common antibody response detected in all groups. Antibodies to any *P. carinii* antigen were found in 86% of children by 30 months of age. Antibodies to *P. carinii* were found in 74% of adults, but were detected more frequently in healthy controls than in immunosuppressed patients (71 vs 48%, $p < 0.05$). Patients with AIDS who experienced one or more episodes of *P. carinii* pneumonia were studied sequentially for changes in the antibody response. Active serum IgM or IgG antibody responses, as defined by the appearance of a new band or an increase in staining intensity of an existing band, were detected in 12–93% of patients, depending on the antigen examined.

Another study investigated serological (IgG) responses to purified gp95, the major surface antigen of human *P. carinii* (68). The frequency of serum antibodies to this antigen was significantly higher in HIV patients with pneumocystosis than in HIV patients without the disease or in healthy controls. Sequential analysis of the *P. carinii* patients demonstrated that 43% of these individuals mounted an antibody response to gp95.

Thus, although the significance of the humoral response is unknown in human disease, some patients mount an active response in the presence of infection. The antibody response in the presence of acute disease can include both IgM and IgG antibodies. Characterization of the response to specific purified or recombinant antigens may serve to enhance our understanding of the pathobiology of the disease and may be of diagnostic or prognostic value.

III. Cellular Immunity

In most of the cases of human pneumocystosis, the disease occurs in hosts with underlying conditions that depress the humoral or cellular immune functions (see Table 1). The cell-mediated branch of the immune system is now considered the major component in the host's ability to resist *P. carinii* pneumonia. Studies in animal models of pneumocystosis have provided inferential as well as direct experimental data supporting this conclusion. Some of the more pertinent aspects of these studies are presented in the following sections.

A. Studies in Animal Models

Rats or mice that have been treated with corticosteroids (69,70), cytoxic drugs, such as cyclophosphamide and cyclosporin (71), or malnourished by being administered a low-protein diet (2,72), provide excellent models for studying pneumocystosis. These treatments primarily interfere with the cell-mediated immunity of the animals (73). Unfortunately, these models do not allow detailed analysis of the importance of the cellular components of the host defense against *P. carinii*. The effects of these treatments are complex, and both the cellular and humoral branches of the hosts immune system may be impaired (73,74). Induction of pneumocystosis in the nu/nu mice, nu/nu rats, or SCID mice during which no exogenous immunosuppressants are used provides further inferential evidence that T–cell-mediated processes are important in host defense against this organism (42,75–77).

Until recently, the most compelling evidence that T cells play a critical role in resistance to *P. carinii* infections came from adoptive transfer experiments (43,44). The transfer of spleen T lymphocytes from phenotypically normal heterozygote (nu/+) littermates into *P. carinii*-infected nude (nu/nu) mice reduced the number of *P. carinii* cysts in the lungs and resolved pneumocystosis, whereas the transfer of immune serum into the infected mice had little or no effect (44). Results from these studies led the investigators to study the immune response, specifically the delayed-type hypersensitivity (DTH) to *P. carinii*, in normal rats and mice (42,43). In these latter studies, spleen T cells from infected animals mediated the DTH reaction when transferred intravaneously into normal recipients and reduced the number of *P. carinii* cysts in the lungs when transferred intravenously into *P. carinii*-infected animals. The DTH response was lost when the T cells were treated with antitheta serum and complement before transfer. Another group of investigators demonstrated that the DTH response could be transferred to naive syngeneic BALB/c mice by adoptively transferring spleen cells from mice that had been sensitized with whole *P. carinii* for 7 days before transfer (78). By using monoclonal antibodies to L3T4 and Lyt-2.2 (surface antigens found on mouse T cells that are equivalent to CD4 and CD8 markers on human T cells, respectively) in in vitro cytolysis experiments, these investigators were able to demonstrate that the DTH response appeared to require the cooperation between both L3T4+ and Lyt-2.2+ subsets of T lymphocytes (Fig. 2). A similar finding has been found for *Listeria monocytogenes*, in which a mixture of L3T4+ and Lyt-2+ cells from *L. monocytogenes*-sensitized mice were required to transfer DTH (79). Recent studies, however, indicate that the L3T4+ cells and not the

Humoral and Cellular Immunity 277

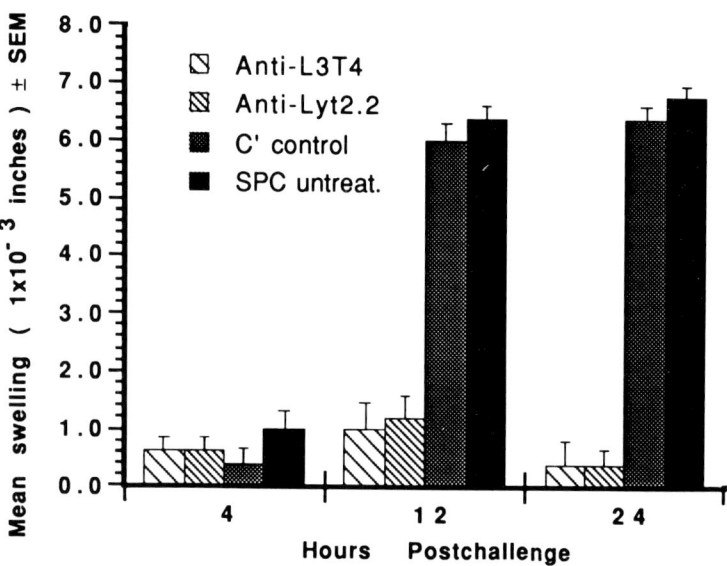

Figure 2 The DTH response in BALB/c mice following adoptive transfer of anti-L3T4 and anti-Lyt 2.2 treated splenocytes from *P. carinii*-sensitized syngeneic donor mice. Before transfer of splenocytes into naive recipient mice, the splenocytes were treated with either anti-L3T4 and complement (◨), anti-Lyt 2.2 and complement (◨), no antibody and complement (◨), or untreated (■). Animals were footpad-challenged with 10 μg of rat *P. carinii* antigen in the right pad after transfer of splenocytes. Footpad swelling was measured at 4-, 12-, and 24-hr postchallenge. The mean swelling and SEM for each group ($n = 5$) was determined. (From Ref. 78.)

Lyt-2+ cells are responsible for the DTH response in mice to *L. monocytogenes*, although the Lyt-2+ cells appear to be necessary for expression of acquired resistance to this organism (80,81). It is feasible that the function of the L3T4+ T cells is regulated by the Lyt-2+ subset of T-suppressor cells in the *P. carinii* model of DTH. This would go along with the hypothesis that in all forms of DTH, the function of the CD4+ cells is regulated by another T-cell subset, the CD8+ T-suppressor cell (82). In any event, results from the adoptive transfer experiments further imply that T cells mediate the DTH response and have an important role in resistance and recovery from *P. carinii* infection. However, further studies are needed to determine the exact mechanisms of interactions between the various subsets of T cells in the DTH response to *P. carinii*.

The most persuasive evidence that T cells, specifically CD4+ cells, play a major role in the host's ability to resist or recover from *P. carinii* infection, has come from recent mouse studies using antibodies to CD4+ cells or adoptive transfer studies in SCID mice (23–25). In one study, monoclonal antibodies to the CD4+ cells were used to chronically deplete helper T lymphocytes in normal conventional BALB/c mice inoculated with *P. carinii*, which resulted in *P. carinii* pneumonitis (24). These studies not only indicated that CD4+ cells are essential for resistance to *P. carinii* infection, but also provided an experimental model of *P. carinii* infection that permits a more detailed analysis of cell-mediated functions in the host's defense against this pathogen. In still another study, SCID mice that acquired *P. carinii* infection from their environment were resolved of the infection after they were given cells from immunocompetent donors (23). In addition, investigators of this study showed that when reconstituted SCID mice were treated with anti-CD4 monoclonal antibody, the ability of the mice to resolve the *P. carinii* pneumonitis was eliminated. Similar studies using treatment with anti-CD8 monoclonal antibody had no effect. In still another adoptive transfer study using SCID mice and fluorescence-activated cell sorter (FACS)-sorted CD4+ and CD8+ T-cell subsets from congenic normal donors, it was shown that CD4+, but not CD8+, cells were effective in resistance to and control of *P. carinii* in these mice (25). Thus, these studies clearly demonstrate that CD4+ cells play a critical role in the host's ability to resist and recover from *P. carinii* infections. However, the functions of these cells, the specific *P. carinii* antigens involved in stimulating a cellular response, and the potential interactions with macrophages or other subsets of T cells have not been clearly defined. Additional studies are needed to better understand the mechanism of interaction between the different subsets of T cells in the host's response to *P. carinii*.

It is possible that the CD4+ cells function as helper cells in the induction of antibody response to *P. carinii*. Recent preliminary studies have shown that *P. carinii*-infected SCID mice, given infusions of thymus cells or spleen cells depleted of cells containing Ig+ or Ia+ cells (e.g., B cells), did not resolve their *P. carinii* infection (26). These results suggest that it was necessary to have B cells present, not just T cells, for the SCID mice to resolve their *P. carinii* pneumonitis. The importance of the humoral response in recovery from *P. carinii* infections has been implicated in other studies (25,27–29,44,62). Thus, more information is needed on the role of B cells in recovery from *P. carinii* infections.

The T-cell proliferative response studies have been performed using splenocytes from rats with and without prolonged environmental exposure to *P. carinii* to further study the cellular immune response (83). In these studies, only the splenocytes from the animals that had prolonged environmental exposure exhibited a significant stimulation index, which indicated that natural exposure to *P. carinii* results in a cellular response. Purified major surface antigen from ferret *P. carinii* has also been used in proliferative response studies (62). In this study, a specific T-cell response was elicited with the purified gp120 surface component from ferrets using T cells isolated from mice that had been immunized with the gp120 antigen (62). In this same study, T cells obtained from reconstituted SCID mice, after recovery from natural infection with *P. carinii*, elicited a blastogenic response to gp120 isolated from mouse *P. carinii*. Furthermore, both groups of mice elicited a significant antibody response to the gp120 antigen. Results from this study suggest that both the cellular as well as the humoral branch of the immune system responds to the major surface antigen of ferret *P. carinii*.

B. Human Studies

In vitro proliferative responses of lymphocytes from normal and immunocompromised human subjects to *P. carinii* have been conducted to gain insight into the host's cellular immune response to this organism (37,83–85). *Pneumocystis carinii* obtained from rats and grown in tissue culture were used to test proliferative responses of peripheral blood mononuclear cells (PBMC) of normal individuals and of patients at different stages of human immunodeficiency (HIV) infection (37,83,84). The PBMC from the normal adults showed a good response to the cultured *P. carinii*; HIV class II (asymptomatic) and class III (lymphadenopathy) patients showed a lower response; and class IV patients (AIDS) demonstrated the lowest response. The fact that PBMC from normal individuals responded suggests that most humans have been sensitized to *P. carinii* antigens. This observation is consistent with serological studies that show that most normal adults have detectable antibody against the organism (34–37). A significant proliferative response was observed in PBMC from 83% of normal individuals when a *P. carinii* antigen preparation was obtained from infected human lung tissue and used in a blastogenic assay (37). No response was seen in PBMC from any of the AIDS patients tested in this study, even though a high percentage of these individuals were diagnosed as having *P. carinii* pneumonia. In studies in which levels of serum antibodies were tested, no correlation between the serum antibody titers and the degree of proliferative responses to *P. carinii* in individual patients was found, suggesting that the humoral and cellular responsive elements may be directed toward different epitopes of the organism (83).

In preliminary studies using a purified gp95 antigen from human *P. carinii* as the test antigen, no blastogenic response was observed in PBMC obtained from normal individuals (85). These results are in contrast with the observations made by previous investigators using relatively crude antigen preparations (37,83). It is possible that the response seen by other investigators (37,83) was due to other *P. carinii* antigens. It is also possible that relevant epitopes on the purified gp95 antigen were destroyed during purification. In this same study, nearly all of the individuals without a history of *P. carinii* pneumonia had no detectable humoral immune response to this major surface antigen.

It is very difficult to compare the results obtained and make conclusions from proliferative response studies that have been done thus far because different host cells and antigen preparations have been used. However, future blastogenic response studies using various T-cell populations from different hosts and purified antigen preparations (possibly recombinant antigens) should provide valuable information about the specific epitopes involved in T-cell immunity to *P. carinii*.

The role of macrophages and other nonspecific effector mechanisms, such as polymorphonuclear leukocytes, natural killer cells, and the complement system, in the host's defense to *P. carinii* infections has not been well defined. Few studies have been done on human macrophages, and no information has been published on using experimental animal models for analyzing the clearance of *P. carinii* that has been exogenously administered. Most of the experiments have been done in vitro using rat alveolar and mouse peritoneal macrophages, and will be discussed in Chapter 15 (56,86,87). However, two recent studies have been reported using human macrophages and *P. carinii* (88,89). In one report, it was shown that when human macrophages and human *P. carinii* were coincubated in the presence of either autologous or heterologous heat-inactivated serum over a period of 72 hr, *P. carinii* were surrounded by the macrophages, giving the appearance of granuloma formation (88). When native (not heat-inactivated) serum was used, no interaction between the macrophage and *P. carinii* was noticed. These results suggested that there was a heat-labile factor in serum that interferes with the interaction of macrophages with *P. carinii*. This factor does not appear to be complement-related, since the addition of anticomplement receptor antibodies (anti-CR1-3) to the incubation mixture in the presence of native or heat-inactivated sera had no effect on the granuloma formation.

In another study, using rat and human alveolar macrophages and rat *P. carinii*, it was shown that the macrophage mannose receptor is important to the cell's ability to bind and uptake *P. carinii* (89). It is possible that in the diseased state, the mannose-rich surface proteins on *P. carinii* are inaccessible; this could be due to blocking components (e.g., antibodies, surfactant), or the proteins could be lost by shedding. Instead of antibodies to *P. carinii* acting as opsonins (and facilitating *P. carinii* ingestion), they could interfere with the binding of the mannose receptor of the macrophages to the organism. Furthermore, potential shedding of the major protein could down-regulate the expression and activity of the macrophage mannose receptor, causing inhibition of the parasite–host interaction (89). Thus, the interaction between macrophages and *P. carinii* is complex, and additional in vitro as well as in vivo studies are needed to better define the factors that play a role in the ultimate outcome of this interaction.

The role(s) of specific cytokines, such as tumor necrosis factor and interferon gamma, have on the *P. carinii*-killing activity of macrophages will be discussed in Chapter 15.

Information about the role of polymorphonuclear leukocytes in the host defenses against *P. carinii* is limited. There have been a few cases reported in which *P. carinii* pneumonia has been seen in patients with granulomatous disease (90). In yet another report, leukocyte transfusion resulted in recovery from the pneumonia (91). On the other hand, an increase in neutrophils in bronchoalveolar lavages of some *P. carinii*-infected patients is often associated with advanced disease and poor prognosis (92–94). It is obvious that further studies are needed to determine what function, if any, polymorphonuclear leukocytes have in the hosts response to *P. carinii* pneumonia.

The role that natural killer cells in defending against *P. carinii* infections is also poorly understood. A case of severe *P. carinii* pneumonia was reported in a patient with depressed natural killer cell cytotoxicity and hypogammaglobulinemia (decreased levels of IgG and IgA) (53). From these findings, the authors suggested that natural killer cells may be important in defense against *P. carinii* infections. The fact that natural killer cells have roles in killing pathogens, including fungi, such as *Cryptococcus*, and also in the regulation of the immune response, indicate that more studies are needed on the contribution of these cells to the innate resistance to pneumocystosis (95).

IV. Conclusion

The limited ability to propagate *P. carinii* in vitro will continue to hamper progress in obtaining a detailed understanding of the immunobiology of this organism. However, with the use of the newly established mouse models that do not need to be treated with corticosteroids for induction of *P. carinii* pneumonia and use of recombinant DNA technology for expression of *P. carinii* antigens, a finer dissection of the humoral and cell-mediated responses to *P. carinii* can be achieved. These new models and techniques should allow researchers to better define the major epitopes of *P. carinii* antigens that induce a humoral immune response and those that are recognized by the cellular arm of the immune system. Results from such studies could lead to the development of a more sensitive, specific, and economical diagnostic assay; a better understanding of epidemiological patterns of *P. carinii* isolates; and to the development of immunological reagents that could be used for therapy or prophylaxis.

References

1. Gajdusek DC. *Pneumocystis carinii*—etiologic agent of interstitial plasma cell pneumonia of premature and young infants. Pediatrics 1957; 19:543–565.
2. Hughes WT, Price RA, Sisko F, Havron WS, Kefatos AG, Schonland M, Smythe PM. Protein calorie malnutrition: a host determinant for *Pneumocystis carinii* infection. Am J Dis Child 1974; 128:44–52.
3. Gleason WA Jr, Roodman ST. Reversible T cell depression in malnourished infants with *Pneumocystis* pneumonia. J Pediatr 1977; 90:1032–1033.
4. Burke BA, Good RA. *Pneumocystis carinii* infection. Medicine 1973; 52:23–51.
5. Walzer PD, Schultz MG, Western KA, Robbins JF. *Pneumocystis carinii* pneumonia and primary immune deficiency disease. Natl Cancer Inst Monogr 1976; 43:65–74.

6. Jose DG, Gatti RA, Good RA. Eosinophilia and *Pneumocystis carinii* pneumonia and immune deficiency syndrome. J Pediatr 1971; 79:748–754.
7. Saulsbury FT, Berstein MT, Winkelstein JA. *Pneumocystis carinii* pneumonia as the presenting infection in congenital hypogammaglobulinemia. J Pediatr 1979; 95:559–561.
8. Rao CP, Gelfand EW. *Pneumocystis carinii* pneumonitis in patients with hypogammaglobulinemia and intact T cell immunity. J Pediatr 1983; 103:410–412.
9. Chandra RK. Cell-mediated immunity in nutritional imbalance. Fed Proc 1980; 39:3088–3092.
10. Walzer PD, Perl DP, Krogstad DJ, Rawson PG, Schultz MG. *Pneumocystis carinii* pneumonia in the United States. Epidemiologic, diagnostic, and clinical features. Ann Intern Med 1974; 80:83–90.
11. Slade JD, Hepburn B. Prednisone-induced alterations of circulating human lymphocyte subsets. J Lab Clin Med 1983; 101:479–487.
12. Hardy AM, Wajszczuk CP, Suffredini AF, Hakala TR, Ho M. *Pneumocystis carinii* pneumonia in renal-transplant recipients treated with cyclosporin and steroids. J Infect Dis 1984; 149:143–147.
13. Ballardie FW, Winearls CG, Williams G. Cyclosporin and steroids in renal transplantation: risk of *Pneumocystis carinii* pneumonia. Lancet 1984; 2:638–639.
14. Hofflin JM, Potasman I, Baldwin JC, Oyer PE, Sinson EB, Remington JM. Infectious complications in heart transplant recipients receiving cyclosporin and corticosteroids. Ann Intern Med 1987; 106:209–216.
15. Bujes D, Hardt C, Rollinghoff M, Wagner H. Cyclosporin A mediates immunosuppression of primary cytotoxic T cell responses by impairing the release of interleukin 1 and interleukin 2. Eur J Immunol 1981; 11:657–661.
16. Browne MT, Hubbard SM, Longo DL, Fisher R, Wesley R, Ihde DH, Pizzo PA. Excess prevalence of *Pneumocystis carinii* pneumonia in patients treated for lymphoma with combination chemotherapy. Ann Intern Med 1986; 104:338–344.
17. Miller JJ, Williams GF, Leissring JD. Multiple late complications of therapy with cyclophosphamide, including ovarian destruction. Am J Med 1971; 50:530–535.
18. Perruquet JL, Harrington TM, Davis DE. *Pneumocystis carinii* pneumonia following methotrexate for rheumatoid arthritis. Arthritis Rheum 1983; 26:1291–1292.
19. Gottlieb MS, Schroff R, Schanker HM, Weisman JD, Fan PT, Wolf RA, Saxon A. *Pneumocystis carinii* pneumonia and mucosal candidiasis in previously healthy homosexual men: evidence of a new acquired cellular immunodeficiency. N Engl J Med 1981; 305:1425–1431.
20. Masur H, Michelis MA, Greene JB, Onorato I, Stouwe RA, Holzman RSW, Wormser W, Brettman L, Lange M, Murray HW, Cunningham-Rundles S. An outbreak of community-acquired *Pneumocystis carinii* pneumonia: initial manifestations of cellular immune dysfunction. N Engl J Med 1981; 305:1431–1438.
21. Walzer PD, Kim CK, Cushion MT. *Pneumocystis carinii*. In: Walzer PD, ed. Parasitic Infections in the Compromised Host. New York: Marcel Dekker, 1989:83–178.
22. Phair J, Munoz A, Detels R, et al. The risk of *Pneumocystis carinii* pneumonia among men infected with human immunodeficiency virus type 1. N Engl J Med 1990; 322:161–165.

23. Harmsen AG, Stankiewicz M. Requirement for CD4+ cells in resistance to *Pneumocystis carinii* pneumonia in mice. J Exp Med 1990; 172:937–945.
24. Shellito J, Suzara VV, Blumenfeld W, Beck JM, Steger HJ, Ermak TH. A new model of *Pneumocystis carinii* infection in mice selectively depleted of helper T lymphocytes. J Clin Invest 1990; 85:1686–1693.
25. Roths B, Sidman CL. Immunity and hyper-responsiveness to *Pneumocystis carinii* resulting from CD4+ but not CD8+ T cells. J Clin Invest 1992; (in press).
26. Harmsen AG, Stankiewicz M. T cells are not sufficient for resistance to *Pneumocystis carinii* pneumonia in mice. J Parasitol 1991; 38:44–45S.
27. Gigliotti F, Hughes WT. Passive immunoprophylaxis with specific monoclonal antibody confers partial protection against *Pneumocystis carinii* pneumonitis in animal models. J Clin Invest 1988; 81:1666–1668.
28. Roths JB, Sidman CL. Single and combined antibody and cell-mediated immune therapy of *Pneumocystis carinii* pneumonia in immunodeficient SCID mice. (submitted).
29. Peglow SL, Smulian AG, Linke MJ, Pogue CL, Nurre S, Crisler J, Phair J, Gold JWM, Armstrong D, Walzer PD. Serologic responses to *Pneumocystis carinii* antigens in health and disease. J Infect Dis 1990; 161:296–306.
30. Walzer P. Experimental models of *Pneumocystis carinii* infections. In: Young LS, ed. *Pneumocystis carinii* Pneumonia: Pathogenesis, Diagnosis, Treatment. New York: Marcel Dekker, 1984:7–76.
31. Hughes WT. *Pneumocystis carinii* pneumonitis. Vol. 2. Boca Raton: CRC Press, 1987:40–48.
32. Graves DC. Immunological studies of *Pneumocystis carinii*. J Protozol 1989; 36:60–69.
33. Pifer LL. *Pneumocystis carinii*. In: Jeljaszewics, ed. Medical Microbiology. London: Academic Press, 1986:121–171.
34. Meuwissen JH, Tauber I, Leeuwenberg AD, Beckers PJ, Sieben M. Parasitologic and serologic observations of infection with *Pneumocystis* in humans. J Infect Dis 1977; 136:43–49.
35. Pifer LL, Hughes WT, Stagno S, Woods D. *Pneumocystis carinii* infection: evidence for high prevalence in normal and immunosuppressed children. Pediatrics 1978; 61:35–41.
36. Maddison SE, Hayes GW, Slemenda SB, Norman LG, Ivey MH. Detection of specific antibody by enzyme-linked immunosorbent assay and antigenemia by counterimmunoelectrophoresis in humans infected with *Pneumocystis carinii*. J Clin Microbiol 1982; 15:1036–1043.
37. Hofmann B, Nielsen PB, Odum N, Gerstoft J, Platz P, Ryder LP, Poulsen A, Mathiesen L, Dickmeiss E, Norrild B, Andersen HK, Westergaard BF, Nielsen CM, Holten-Andersen W, Mojon M, Nielsen JO, Svejgaard A. Humoral and cellular responses to *Pneumocystis carinii*, CMV, and herpes simplex in patients with AIDS and in controls. Scand J Infect Dis 1988; 20:389–394.
38. Walzer PD, Rutledge ME. Humoral immunity in experimental *Pneumocystis carinii* infection: I. Serum and bronchial lavage fluid antibody responses in rats. J Lab Clin Med 1981; 97:820–833.

39. McNabb SJN, Graves DC, Kosanke SD, Moyer MJ, Ivey MH. *Pneumocystis carinii* antigen detection in rat serum and lung lavage. J Clin Microbiol 1988; 26:1763–1771.
40. Walzer PD, Rutledge ME. Serum antibody responses to *Pneumocystis carinii* among different strains of normal and athymic mice. Infect Immun 1982; 35:620–626.
41. Walzer PD, Rutledge ME, Yoneda K. Experimental *Pneumocystis carinii* pneumonia in C3H/HeJ and C3HeB/FeJ mice. J Reticuloendothel Soc 1983; 33:1–9.
42. Furuta T, Ueda K, Fujiwara K. Experimental *Pneumocystis carinii* infection in nude rats. Jpn J Exp Med 1984; 54:65–72.
43. Furuta T, Ueda K, Fujiwara K, Yamanouchi K. Cellular and humoral immune responses of mice subclinically infected with *Pneumocystis carinii*. Infect Immun 1985; 47:544–548.
44. Furuta T, Ueda K, Kyuwa S, Fujiwara K. Effect of T-cell transfer on *Pneumocystis carinii* infection in nude mice. Jpn J Exp Med 1984; 54:57–64.
45. Walzer PD, Stanforth D, Linke MJ, Cushion MT. *Pneumocystis carinii*: immunoblotting and immunofluorescent analysis of serum antibodies during rat infection and recovery. Exp Parasitol 1987; 6:319–328.
46. Furuta T, Fujiwara K, Yamanouchi K. Detection of antibodies to *Pneumocystis carinii* by enzyme-linked immunosorbent assay in experimentally infected mice. J Parasitol 1985; 71:522–523.
47. Brzosko WJ, Madalinski K, Nowoslawski A. Fluorescent antibody and immunoelectrophoretic evaluation of the immune reaction in children with pneumonia induced by *Pneumocystis carinii*. Med Microbiol 1967; 19:397–405.
48. Giron JA, Martinez S, Walzer PD. Should inpatients with *Pneumocystis carinii* be isolated? Lancet 1982; 2:46–48.
49. Dutz W. *Pneumocystis carinii* pneumonia. Pathol Annu 1970; 5:309–313.
50. Hofmann B, Odum N, Platz P, Ryder LP, Svejgaard A, Nielsen PB, Holten-Andersen W, Gerstoft J, Nielsen JO, Mojon M. Humoral responses to *Pneumocystis carinii* in patients with acquired immunodeficiency syndrome and immunocompromised homosexual men. J Infect Dis 1985; 152:838–840.
51. Brzosko WJ, Madalinski K, Crawczynski K, Nowoslawski A. Immunochemistry in studies on the pathogenesis of pneumocystis pneumonia in infants. Ann NY Acad Sci 1971; 177:156–170.
52. Blumenfeld W, Mandrell RE, Jarvis GA, Griffis JM. Localization of host immunoglobulin G to the surface of *Pneumocystis carinii*. Infect Immun 1990; 58:456–463.
53. Staugas REM, Beard LJ, Simmer K, Ferrante A. Hypogammaglobulinemia and depressed natural killer cell cytotoxicity in a patient with *Pneumocystis carinii* infection. Pediatr Infect Dis J 1988; 7:724–728.
54. Dutz W, Post C, Vessal K, Kohut E. Endemic infantile *Pneumocystis carinii* infection: the Shiraz study. Natl Cancer Inst Monogr 1976; 43:31–38.
55. Hughes WT, Ho-Kyun K, Price R, Miller C. Attempts at prophylaxis for murine *Pneumocystis carinii* pneumonitis. Curr Ther Res 1973; 15:581–587.
56. Masur H, Jones TC. The interaction in vitro of *Pneumocystis carinii* with macrophages and L cells. J Exp Med 1978; 147:157–170.
57. Graves DC, McNabb SJN, Worley MA, Downs TD, Ivey MH. Analysis of rat

Pneumocystis carinii antigens recognized by human and rat antibodies by using Western immunoblotting. Infect Immun 1986; 54:96–103.
58. Walzer PD, Linke MJA. A comparison of the antigenic characteristics of rat and human *Pneumocystis carinii* by immunoblotting. J Immunol 1987; 138:2257–2265.
59. Kovacs JA, Halpern JL, Swan JC, Moss J, Parillo JE, Masur H. Identification of antigens and antibodies specific for *Pneumocystis carinii*. J Immunol 1988; 140: 2023–2031.
60. Walzer PD, Kim CK, Linke MJ, Pogue CL, Huerkamp MJ, Chrisp CE, Lerro AV, Wixson SK, Hall E, Shultz LD. Outbreaks of *Pneumocystis carinii* pneumonia in colonies of immunodeficient mice. Infect Immun 1989; 57:62–70.
61. Bauer NL, Paulsrud JR, Bartlett MS, Smith JW, Wilde CE III. Immunological comparisons of *Pneumocystis carinii* strains obtained from rats, ferrets, and mice using convalescent sera from the same sources. J Protozol 1991; 38:166–168S.
62. Fisher DJ, Giglotti F, Zauderer M, Harmsen AG. Specific T-cell response to a *Pneumocystis carinii* surface glycoprotein (gp120) after immunization and natural infection. Infect Immun 1991; 59:3372–3376.
63. Gigliotti F, Ballou LR, Huges WT, Mosley BD. Purification and initial characterization of a ferret *Pneumocystis carinii* surface antigen. J Infect Dis 1988; 158:848–854.
64. Sheperd V, Jameson B, Knowles GK. *Pneumocystis carinii* pneumonitis: a serological study. J Clin Pathol 1979; 32:773–777.
65. Gerrard MP, Eden OB, Jameson B, Craft AW. Serological study of *Pneumocystis carinii* infection in the absence of immunosuppression. Arch Dis Child 1988; 62: 177–179.
66. Chatterton JM, Joss AW, Williams H, Ho-Yen DO. *Pneumocystis carinii* antibody testing. J Clin Pathol 1989; 42:865–868.
67. Burns SM, Read JA, Yap PL, Brettle RP. Reduced concentrations of IgG antibodies to *Pneumocystis carinii* in HIV-infected patients during active *Pneumocystis carinii* infection and the possibility of passive immunization. J Infect 1990; 20:33–39.
68. Lundgren B, Lundgren JD, Mathiesen L, Nielsen JO, Nielsen T, Kovacs JA. Antibody responses to a major *Pneumocystis carinii* antigen in human immunodeficiency virus—infected patients with and without *Pneumocystis carinii* pneumonia. J Infect Dis 1992; 165:1151–1155.
69. Frenkel JK, Good JT, Schultz JA. Latent *Pneumocystis* infection in rats, relapse and chemotherapy. Lab Invest 1966; 15:1559–1577.
70. Walzer PD, Powell RD, Yoneda K. *Pneumocystis carinii* pneumonia in different strains of cortisonized mice. Infect Immun 1979; 24:939–947.
71. Hughes WT, Smith B. Provocation of infection due to *Pneumocystis carinii* by cyclosporin A. J Infect Dis 1982; 145:767.
72. Walzer PD, Powell RD, Yoneda K, Rutledge ME, Milder JE. Growth characteristics and pathogenesis of experimental *Pneumocystis carinii* pneumonia. Infect Immun 1980; 27:929–937.
73. Ruskin J, Hughes WT. *Pneumocystis carinii*. In: Remington JS, Klein JO, eds. Infectious Diseases of the Fetus and Newborn Infant. Philadelphia: WB Saunders, 1983:507–543.
74. Walzer PD, LaBine M, Redington TJ, Cushion M. Lymphocyte changes during

chronic administration of a withdrawal from corticosteroids: relevance to *Pneumocystis carinii* pneumonia. J Immunol 1984; 133:2502–2508.
75. Walzer PD, Schnell V, Armstrong D, Rosen PP. The nude mouse: a new experimental model for *Pneumocystis carinii* infection. Science 1977; 197:177–179.
76. Ueda K, Goto Y, Yamazaki S, Fujiwara K. Chronic fatal pneumocystosis in nude mice. Jpn J Exp Med 1977; 47:475–482.
77. Walzer PD, Kim CK, Linke MJ, Pogue C, Huerkamp WJ, Chrisp CE, Lerro AV, Wixson SK, Hall E, Shultz LD. Outbreaks of *Pneumocystis carinii* pneumonia in colonies of immunodeficient mice. Infect Immun 1989; 57:62–70.
78. Graves DC, Li X, Paiva W. Delayed-type hypersensitivity response in mice to *Pneumocystis carinii*. J Protozol 1991; 38:49–52S.
79. Kaufmann SHE, Hug E, Vath U, Muler I. Effective protection against *Listeria monocytogenes* and delayed-type hypersensitivity to listerial antigens depend on cooperation between specific L3T4+ and Lyt 2+ cells. Infect Immun 1985; 48: 263–266.
80. Czuprynski CJ, Brown JF, Young KM, Cooley AJ. Administration of purified anti-L3T4 monoclonal antibody impairs the resistance of mice to *Listeria monocytogenes* infection. Infect Immun 1989; 57:100–109.
81. Mielke MEA, Ehlers S, Hahn H. T-cell subsets in delayed-type hypersensitivity, protection, and granuloma formation in primary and secondary listeria infection in mice: superior role of Lyt-2+ cells in acquired immunity. Infect Immun 1988; 56: 1920–1925.
82. Meltzer MS, Nacy CA. Delayed-type hypersensitivity and the induction of activated, cytotoxic macrophages. In: Paul WE, ed. Fundamental Immunology. 2nd ed. New York: Raven Press, 1989:765–777.
83. Hagler DN, Deepe GS, Pogue CL, Walzer PD. Blastogenic responses to *Pneumocystis carinii* among patients with human immunodeficiency (HIV) infection. Clin Exp Immunol 1988; 74:7–13.
84. Herrod HG, Valenski WR, Woods DR, Pifer LL. The in vitro response of human lymphocytes to *Pneumocystis carinii* antigen. J Immunol 1981; 126:59–61.
85. Lundgren B, Lipchik GY, Kovacs JA. Purification and characterization of a major human *Pneumocystis carinii* surface antigen. J Clin Invest 1991; 87:163–170.
86. Von Behren LA, Pesanti EL. Uptake and degradation of *Pneumocystis carinii* by macrophages in vitro. Am Rev Respir Dis 1978; 118:1051–1059.
87. Masur H. Interactions between *Pneumocystis carinii* and phagocytic cells. In: Young LS, ed. *Pneumocystis carinii* Pneumonia Pathogenesis, Diagnosis, Treatment. New York: Marcel Dekker, 1984:77–95.
88. Blumenfeld W, McCook O, Griffis JM. In vitro aggregation of macrophages around human-derived *Pneumocystis carinii*. J Protozol 1991; 38:32–33S.
89. Ezekowitz RAB, Williams DJ, Koziel H, Armstrong MYK, Warner A, Richards FF, Rose RM. Uptake of *Pneumocystis carinii* mediated by the macrophage mannose receptor. Nature 1991; 351:155–158.
90. Adinoff AD, Johnston RB, Dolen S, South MA. Chronic granulomatous disease and *Pneumocystis carinii* pneumonia. Pediatrics 1982; 69:133.
91. Pedersen FK, Johansen KS, Rosenkvist J, Tygstrup I, Valerius NH. Refractory

Pneumocystis carinii infection in chronic granulomatous disease: successful treatment with granulocytes. Pediatrics 1979; 64:935–938.
92. Limper AH, Offord KP, Smith TF, Martin WJ II. *Pneumocystis carinii* pneumonia: differences in lung parasite number and inflammation in patients with and without AIDS. Am Rev Respir Dis 1989; 140:1204–1209.
93. Mason GR, Hasimoto CH, Dickman PS, Foutty LF, Cobb CJ. Prognostic implications of bronchoalveolar lavage neutrophilia in patients with *Pneumocystis carinii* pneumonia and AIDS. Am Rev Respir Dis 1989; 139:1336–1342.
94. Smith RL, El-Sadr WM, Lewis ML. Correlation of bronchoalveolar lavage cell populations with clinical severity of *Pneumocystis carinii* pneumonia. Chest 1988; 92:60–64.
95. Murphy JW. Mechanisms of natural resistance to human pathogenic fungi. Annu Rev Microbiol 1991; 45:509–538.

15

Host Defense Effector Mechanisms and *Pneumocystis carinii*

EDWARD L. PESANTI

Veterans Affairs Medical Center
and University of Connecticut
Newington, Connecticut

I. Introduction

Although *Pneumocystis carinii* has been recognized for most of the current century, studies of host defenses against *P. carinii* have been undertaken only in the last 30 years, and in vitro studies began less than 15 years ago. The mechanisms involved in host resistance to *P. carinii* and those that the parasite uses to evade host defenses are only beginning to be characterized.

II. Background

In attempting to formulate an overview of the cellular basis of host defense mechanisms against *P. carinii*, I have attempted to integrate data derived from experiments involving *P. carinii* with data from experiments using other microbes that seem to share a particular feature with *P. carinii*. Although thoroughly reviewed in another chapter in this volume, certain of the in vivo (human and animal) observations deserve special emphasis as having particular relevance to the focus of attempts to define the cellular and biochemical bases of host defense mechanisms in *P. carinii* infection. Even though *P. carinii* infection is common in most mammals (1), disease caused by this organism is rare and is extremely so in adults without severe immunodeficiency (2). Defective humoral immunity [e.g., agammaglobulinemia (3–5)] or defective cellular immunity [e.g., DiGeorge's syndrome (3), athymic rodents (6,7)] predisposes to *P. carinii* infection. Combined immune system defects [SCID mice (8); human (9) or simian (10) immunodeficiency virus infection] further increase the severity or persistence of the infection. The ease with which *P. carinii* pneumonia may be induced in animals [e.g., rabbits (8), rats (9), ferrets (11), but apparently not hamsters (1)] solely by immunosuppression with steroids or other agents suggests that the parasite establishes a latent infection that persists for the life of the host. Stated another way, after the primary infection, *P. carinii* becomes part of the normal flora of the mammal, to cause clinical illness only when the normal control mechanisms are rendered ineffective. Relapsing *P. carinii* pneumonia is common in only two clinical conditions: congenital agammaglobulinemia (3) and acquired immunodeficiency syndrome (AIDS) (12,13). Malnutrition in humans or experimental animals amplifies the effects of defective immunity (14,15). In the earliest cases and the major epidemics of *P. carinii* infection, malnutrition was the primary cause of the disease. Whether this relates to the effects of starvation on cellular immune functions or is more directly related to the availability of certain nutrients is unclear.

Glucocorticoids appear to be uniquely potent in induction of *P. carinii* disease in patients and are the standard drugs used to promote the disease in laboratory animals. Numerous patients with Cushing's disease (not the iatrogenic variant) have been reported to have *P. carinii* pneumonia (16–21). It is probably premature to assume that this glucocorticoid effect is mediated solely by "immunosuppression," which, even if correct, conveys little concerning the actual mechanisms of the process.

Although most attention is focused on conditions that predispose to *P. carinii* pneumonia, certain other pulmonary diseases may act to reduce the possibility of *P. carinii* disease. In a search of the Medline data base from 1966–1992, I could find only three citations concerning *P. carinii* pneumonia in patients receiving high-dose glucocorticoids for asthma (22–24). One patient also received methotrexate (22); another had a T-cell leukemia caused by HTLV-I (23).

Rats that received intratracheal injections of *Pseudomonas aeruginosa* before initiation of glucocorticoid administration were protected from development of *P. carinii* pneumonia (25), a protection that does not appear to result from immunization with *P. carinii*. Among other possibilities, this set of observations suggests the possibility that one of the elements of nonspecific immunity to *P. carinii* may be an accidental effect of specific or nonspecific reactions to other potential pulmonary pathogens.

Patients at highest risk of *P. carinii* pneumonia are also subject to candidiasis, cryptosporidiosis, seborrheic dermatitis, and all the varieties of tinea. All of these infections are caused by pathogens of low virulence, which initiate noninvasive or superficially invasive infections of the epithelial surfaces. These microbes are well adapted to a parasitic life style, are highly species-specific, have no reservoir outside the mammalian host, and only rarely cause progressive disease. *Pneumocystis carinii* appears to be similar to these pathogens; it is a noninvasive obligate parasite of alveolar type I epithelial cells that is restricted to one host species. A coherent explanation of host–parasite interactions in *P. carinii* disease should be able to offer at least tentative explanations for these features of pneumocystosis.

III. Functions of Phagocytic Cells Against *Pneumocystis carinii*

In reviewing studies of mechanisms of host defense, I will focus initially on studies dealing with means by which host defenses could kill *P. carinii*, because, historically, those were the first aspects of the process studied. Before 1980, nearly all cases of pneumocystosis occurred in infants and children who were at risk because of congenital immunodeficiency states (3). The relatively infrequent cases seen on the adult wards were primarily drawn from patient populations with severely compromised cellular immunity. Those adults were also subject to infections with intracellular pathogens, such as *Mycobacterium tuberculosis* and *Toxoplasma gondii*. Effective immunity against those pathogens is known to be mediated by cellular immunity, with the complex interaction among T-lymphocyte populations, macrophages, cytokines, and the pathogen determining the outcome of the infection (26,27). In the most straightforward analysis, lymphocyte activation of macrophages leads to restriction of growth and, perhaps death, of the offending intracellular parasite. Laboratory investigations have confirmed the essential role of cellular immunity in host defenses against *P. carinii*. Athymic rodents (6) and SCID mice (28) can develop overt *P. carinii* infection without additional immunosuppression. Although *P. carinii* causes disease in the same clinical and experimental settings as do the intracellular pathogens, there are notable differences between *P. carinii* and the classic intracellular pathogens.

Pneumocystis carinii does not reside within mammalian cells (10,29–31). There appears to be no intracellular phase of the organism. Unlike the intracellular pathogens with which *P. carinii* is clinically associated, *P. carinii* was not resistant to the antimicrobial activity of normal, unstimulated macrophages, either alveolar or peritoneal (32,33). Phagocytosis of *P. carinii* by normal alveolar macrophages could be improved by addition of specific opsonins (33), but did occur in its absence (32,33). Freshly explanted alveolar macrophages are inefficient in phagocytosis of *P. carinii* in the absence of specific opsonins, but this appears to be an attribute of freshly harvested alveolar macrophages per se, with no specific relevance to host defenses against *P. carinii* (34). This generalized deficiency of nonimmune phagocytosis by freshly explanted alveolar macrophages may reflect the profound surface changes that occur when alveolar macrophages are changed from an environment rich in alveolar lining fluid to one containing serum (35) and is of uncertain relevance to the in vivo state. Once interiorized by normal macrophages, *P. carinii* are rapidly degraded (32,33). Intracellular growth of *P. carinii* does not occur, and steroid treatment of macrophages does not appear to impair their action against *P. carinii* (32,33). Thus, although overt infection with *P. carinii* occurs in the same patient populations that are susceptible to disease caused by intracellular pathogens, *P. carinii* has little in common with those pathogens.

These studies of phagocytic interaction showed that normal macrophages could be effectors in host defenses against *P. carinii* and, more importantly, that *P. carinii* could be studied in vitro. It has not been possible to evaluate the viability of *P. carinii* after phagocytosis by macrophages or other phagocytes, and current knowledge of the fate of interiorized *P. carinii* is based solely on the observation that the organisms are digested within macrophages (32). It remains possible that activation of macrophages enhances intracellular-killing activity against ingested *P. carinii*. However, technical obstacles have prevented studies of the viability of interiorized *P. carinii*.

Procedures that lyse macrophages also render *P. carinii* metabolically inactive. For metabolic pathways that both host cell and parasite possess, the metabolic activity of the macrophages greatly exceeds any known activities of *P. carinii*. It is possible that the recently described system for measuring incorporation of [^{3}H]aminobenzoic acid into folate (36), a metabolic pathway not found in mammalian cells, will allow accurate delineation of the intracellular fate of *P. carinii*, but such experiments have not yet been undertaken. Other conclusions about the susceptibility of *P. carinii* to phagocytic cell processes have been based upon in vitro studies of partially purified preparations of *P. carinii* to which the compounds of interest have been added. In these studies, measures of viability have included supravital stains (37) and measurement of metabolic conversion of [^{14}C]glucose to [^{14}C]CO$_2$ (38). The former suffers from technical difficulty, subjective interpretation, and overwhelming tediousness, although use of flow cytometry with fluorescent vital dyes may offer a more quantitative approach. The metabolic approach suffers from being an assay of a metabolic activity that all aerobic cells undertake, mammalian cells and bacteria, as well as *P. carinii*, and must be rigidly controlled for contaminating host cells and other microbes.

Studies of the effects of various host effector molecules on viability of *P. carinii* have shown that *P. carinii* is only poorly able to scavenge oxidants (39) and is susceptible to peroxidative kill as well as to hydroxyl radical-mediated kill (39). More recently, soluble components of the *P. carinii* cell wall major glycoprotein (gp120,) have been found to stimulate the oxidative burst of normal macrophages (40). *Pneumocystis carinii* also stimulates arginine uptake and nitric oxide production by macrophages (41). The organisms are rendered metabolically inactive after brief exposure to either low (<5.0) or high (>7.8) pH. Compared with the effects at pH 7.5, oxidant stress is more toxic to the organisms at pH 6.5 (39). At pH 5.5, metabolic activity of *P. carinii* ceases and does not return when returned to medium with a higher pH (39). These data appear to be discordant with the observations that in vitro growth of *P. carinii* was enhanced at low pH (42). But, it is not known which morphological forms of *P. carinii* contribute most strongly to each observation; the disagreement may be less serious than it appears. Taken together, these observations suggest that the intracellular environment of phagocytes, both macrophages and polymorphonuclear leukocytes, is inimicable to *P. carinii* and that normal phagocytes possess the biochemical pathways to kill *P. carinii*. It is of interest that cases of *P. carinii* have been reported in patients with chronic granulomatous disease, the hereditary disorder of polymorphonuclear leukocyte (PMN) function in which the oxidative burst and generation of reactive oxygen intermediates does not occur (43). In one of these patients, cure of *P. carinii* pneumonia could not be effected until normal PMN were transfused (44).

Available data, then, suggest, but do not prove, that phagocytic cells resident within the alveolar airspaces or responding to an inflammatory stimulus, can kill *P. carinii*. The efficacy of these nonspecific effector mechanisms in the normal mammal may contribute to the rarity of progressive *P. carinii* infection in immunologically intact individuals. It is also possible that such host defense mechanisms may be relevant to understanding the rarity of *P. carinii* pneumonia in immunosuppressed patients with chronic inflammatory lung diseases.

Although innate resistance is an important factor in defense against *P. carinii*, it is also clear that it must be supplemented by specific immune responses. *Pneumocystis carinii* occasionally causes a benign, self-limited disease in healthy infants, presumably representing primary infection (45,46). In this aspect, *P. carinii* infection may be analogous to other infections (e.g., tuberculosis) in which the usually asymptomatic primary infection is controlled and the parasite is not eliminated, but rendered dormant. The obvious role of immunodeficiency states in predisposition to reactivation of infection emphasizes the importance of specific immune surveillance in maintaining the dormant state. The interactions of innate and specific immunity in resistance to disease caused by *P. carinii* will be addressed more fully in a subsequent section.

IV. Nonphagocytic Mechanisms of Host Defense Against *Pneumocystis carinii*

In the early in vitro studies of *P. carinii*, it was found that fresh complement, with immune rat serum, does not cause either death or lysis of *P. carinii* (37). Complement can contribute to immune opsonization of *P. carinii* for phagocytosis by macrophages (33). Although it remains possible that complement, through either the classic or the alternative pathway, contributes to the rarity of extrapulmonary *P. carinii* disease, there seems no reason to suggest that these serum factors serve more than a supportive role in host defenses against the organism. The more recently recognized serum mannose-binding protein (47,48), a nonspecific opsonin with broad reactivity and structural similarity to surfactant apoprotein A (49), is another serum factor that may be involved in resistance to systemic infection with glycoprotein-rich organisms like *P. carinii*. This, so far untested, possibility seems particularly relevant in light of the recent observation that nonimmune phagocytosis of *P. carinii* is mediated by mannose receptors on macrophages (50).

Although the focus of the initial investigations was on mechanisms by which host effector mechanisms could kill *P. carinii*, other antimicrobial activities could be of much greater import. Host defenses against *P. carinii* can be envisioned to act at several key steps in the intra-alveolar growth of the parasite. Although it cannot be considered to be firmly established, I will view *P. carinii* as a parasite that can (and probably does) undergo all essential portions of its life cycle within the alveolar airspace. It has long been known that *P. carinii* could be found in extrapulmonary locations (3,51), but only since AIDS has become common and use of aerosolized pentamidine prophylaxis widespread has extrapulmonary pneumocystosis become well recognized (51). Nonetheless, the primary focus on understanding defenses against *P. carinii* must remain at the level of the pulmonary alveoli.

As is schematically illustrated in Figure 1, there are several key steps in the growth of *P. carinii* in which effective host defenses could be involved, only some of which would involve phagocytes and result in immediate death of the organism. These defenses, which could interrupt the life cycle of *P. carinii* might be, in the jargon of antibiotic action, either static or cidal mechanisms. The most effective host defenses need not be directed toward death of the offending pathogen. It is probable that the two general mechanisms are complementary, essential, and mediated by multiple, redundant effector systems. It is difficult to be confident that the mechanisms so far identified (e.g., macrophage phagocytosis, lethality of oxygen radicals) are of primary import in control of *P. carinii* infection. I suggest that the available experimental data, from in vivo and in vitro experiments, combined with extrapolations from natural infections, is most compatible with a host defense strategy in which various stages of development of *P. carinii* are controlled by different effector systems. In this hypothesis, cellular immune effectors contribute to control of *P. carinii* both by killing metabolically active parasites, a *cidal* effect, and, also, by reducing the flux of nutrients available to the parasite from host cells, a *static* effect. Humoral immunity could act to prevent attachment to alveolar type I epithelial cells and subsequent multiplication of the parasite within the lungs (52), a static effect. In this view, the cidal effect, in which *P. carinii* is killed by host effector cells, is secondary to, and supportive of, the primary defense, the static or growth-limiting

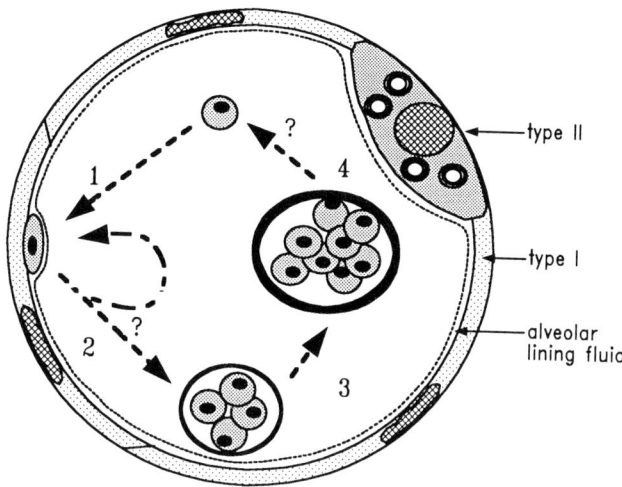

Figure 1 In this simplified outline of an alveolar airspace, the phases of *P. carinii*'s life cycle that seem to be relevant to an understanding of host defense effector mechanisms are highlighted. The normal alveolar airspace is lined by alveolar epithelial cells, composed of type I (gas-exchanging) cells and type II (surfactant-secreting) cells. Covering the surface of these cells is a thin layer of alveolar lining fluid, composed of surfactant and other constituents, secreted largely by the alveolar type II epithelial cells. After inhalation or aspiration of the infectious form (which has not been identified), *P. carinii* establishes a parasitic life-style (1). At this stage, host effector mechanisms that prevent the initial attachment (e.g., antibody to a key attachment protein) or kill the infectious particle (e.g., alveolar macrophages) could intervene. In the nonimmune host exposed to a suitable inoculum, attachment to alveolar type I epithelial cells occurs, and the parasite firmly attaches to the type I alveolar epithelial cell membrane in what appears to be an essential aspect of the intra-alveolar life cycle of *P. carinii* (2). There may be a population of *P. carinii* that grow and divide as "trophozoites" within the alveolar lining fluid, parasitizing alveolar epithelial cells throughout their life. Although *P. carinii* is tightly apposed to alveolar type I epithelial cells, it is covered by a layer of alveolar lining fluid, consisting of surfactant and other substances. *P. carinii* may be relatively inaccessible to phagocytes and immunoglobulins at this stage, but cytokine stimulation of type I epithelial cells may result in inhibition of growth of *P. carinii*. Only at this stage of the life cycle does *P. carinii* bear some resemblance to intracellular pathogens and, it is at this stage, that cellular immunity may be most effective in defenses against it. Subsequently, *P. carinii* multiples and breaks free from the now dead or dying epithelial cell. Further multiplication within the alveolar airspaces then occurs, eventually resulting in the characteristic cysts containing eight daughter cells (3). During this phase of its life cycle, *P. carinii* behaves more like more common facultative pathogens and appears to grow abundantly within the alveolar airspaces. In this phase, host defense mechanisms typically employed against facultative extracellular parasites, such as phagocytes and opsonizing antibody, could contribute to defense of the airspace. The organisms differentiate their cell walls, developing into encysted forms containing eight daughter cells, each of which has a cell wall typical of the nonencysted forms. If encystment is part of the replicative life cycle of *P. carinii*, potent and specific saccharidases or proteinases would presumably be necessary for excystment to occur (4), and antibody to those enzymes could interrupt the life cycle.

effect. The key aspect of host immunity to *P. carinii* is envisioned as operative at the steps that prevent attachment of *P. carinii* to alveolar epithelial cells or that alter the metabolism of the cells so that they are no longer hospitable to *P. carinii*. This view of host defenses against *P. carinii* can, I hope to the reader's satisfaction, provide a structure for better understanding the clinical presentation of *P. carinii* pneumonia and possible future approaches to prevention and treatment of the disease.

Although the life cycle of *P. carinii* is poorly understood, it is generally thought that the trophozoites must parasitize type I alveolar epithelial cells for at least a portion of their life. The reason for such a noninvasive attachment is unknown (nor is it even known if it must occur). Interruption of an apparently mandatory phase of the life cycle is an obvious target for host defense mechanisms. Such defenses could restrict access of *P. carinii* to suitable domains of the alveolar epithelial cell surface, render the cells inhospitable to *P. carinii*, or both. Although recent publications have dealt with possible mechanisms of attachment of *P. carinii* to rat lung cells in vitro (53–56), the existence of defense mechanisms active against *P. carinii* attachment remains unproved.

The importance of antibodies interfering with specific attachment is recognized for many other pathogenic microbes. Interruption of parasitism, the phase of initial contact with the host cell, is important in immunity to viral, bacterial, and protozoan infections. Electron micrographs show that *P. carinii* trophozoite cell membranes are tightly interdigitated with alveolar type I cell membranes (29,57); the possibility that such membrane interactions may facilitate transfer of vital nutrients is obvious—and also unproved. Other phases of the life cycle may also be anchored to the surrounding alveolar cells by filopodia (10). Studies of attachment mechanisms in *P. carinii* are difficult to interpret since the "attachment organelle," if such exists, has not been identified. The cell type primarily parasitized by *P. carinii*, the type I alveolar epithelial cell, has only recently been isolated (58) and has not been successfully cultured in vitro.

Recently, studies have suggested that *P. carinii*'s dominant surface glycoprotein (gp120) mediates specific attachment to host epithelial cells (53,54,56). Avid binding of fibronectin by gp120 appears to be an intermediary step in attachment of *P. carinii* in vitro to cultured cells. It is unclear whether the attachment is identical, or even similar, to that observed within infected lungs. Furthermore, the antigen that has been incriminated in that attachment (gp120) (56,59) is the most widely prevalent structural antigen found in *P. carinii* of any morphological variant (60–68). Available data do not suggest gp120 is a phase-specific antigen, but that it is present on most or all forms of *P. carinii*, including trophozoites, immature cysts, and mature cysts. The means by which such an ubiquitous parasite antigen could mediate specific attachment of a single phase to host cells is inapparent. The dominant surface antigen (gp120) appears to be the ligand responsible for binding of fibronectin (56) and surfactant apoprotein A (69); it is also involved in binding of tumor necrosis factor, albumin and, presumably, other macromolecules (70; unpublished observations). It is possible that gp120, through interaction with fibronectin, is involved in the specific interaction between *P. carinii* trophozoites and alveolar type I epithelial cells (54–56). The observation that monoclonal antibody against gp120 partially protects experimental animals from *P. carinii* pneumonia is consistent with this interpretation (71). Protection, however, was incomplete. This suggests that humoral immunity can provide only partial protection, or that antibody to gp120 is not *the* critical antibody involved in prevention of cell attachment by *P. carinii*. The ubiquity of gp120 indicates that caution must be exercised when any particular stage-specific function is assigned to the antigen. [I am unaware of any data confirming its presence on "trophozoites" attached to alveolar type I cells of infected lungs, but assume it may be present. However, it is possible that it is conspicuously absent in the small minority of *P. carinii* in the alveoli that most obviously parasitize alveolar type I epithelial cells.] In my view, if any function is to be assigned to gp120, the possible contribution of the glycoprotein to the tenacious filopodial network anchoring *P. carinii* to mammalian cells in vitro (10) and in vivo (72) merits much more attention.

A better understanding of the key antigens involved in the parasite's life cycle and of the basis of immunity to those antigens is necessary if we are to rationally explain such observations as the striking similarity of the clinical course of *P. carinii* disease in patients with congenital agammaglobulinemia and in patients with AIDS. Although hypogammaglobulinemia appears to contribute to the risk of *P. carinii* pneumonia in infants, with or without AIDS (73), it does not appear to be an additional risk factor for adults with AIDS. These are the only clinical situations in which recurrent bouts of *P. carinii* are known to occur. In adults with AIDS, as in the infants with either AIDS or agammaglobulinemia, the propensity of *P. carinii* pneumonia to recur may reflect a failure of antibody formation. In this view, the critical antibody could be that which would function primarily to interfere with the first step in the parasitic cycle—attachment to alveolar epithelial cells (see Fig. 1). Absence of the antibody would be expected to allow unrestricted access of this critical phase of the life cycle of *P. carinii* to the alveolar epithelial cells. In patients with agammaglobulinemia, this absent antibody is a direct result of inability to synthesize antibody. In AIDS patients, it may be a manifestation of humoral immune deficiency in which the key *P. carinii* antigen is a T-dependent antigen, or the most effective antibody is of a class that requires T-cell participation in its formation (e.g., IgA) (59). A focus on the antibody type seems unwarranted, since patients with IgA deficiency, the most common immunoglobulin deficiency in humans, who may be afflicted with *Cryptosporidium parvum* or *Giardia lamblia*, do not develop *P. carinii* pneumonia (74). [A search of the Medline data base, 1966–1991, yielded no citations describing infected patients when "pneumocystis" and "IgA" were used as search terms.] Thus, it seems that the focus should be placed on identification of T-dependent antigens of *P. carinii* to define this critical stage in host defenses. Although it is possible that gp120 will be determined to be such a critical antigen, the data are not such as to generate great confidence that the search has been completed.

V. Cellular Immunity, Cytokines, and Epithelial Cells

Cellular immune effectors may contribute to effective host defenses in many ways other than through activation of macrophages, leading to improved phagocytosis and intracellular killing of a parasite. Such effectors may alter the metabolism of alveolar type I epithelial cells such that they no longer support growth of *P. carinii*, or they may stimulate alveolar cells to secrete products that kill or inhibit the growth of *P. carinii* that have not actually contacted the activated cell. The total lack of information concerning the first mechanism relates not to the implausibility of the concept, but to the lack of a suitable model in which to study the phenomenon. It is relevant to these considerations that other pathogens affecting AIDS patients have phases of their life cycle that are best understood if it is assumed that T cells or their products enhance "epithelial immunity" and assure the integrity of the barrier function of normal epithelial surfaces. *Cryptosporidium parvum* is, like *P. carinii*, a parasite that remains restricted to the luminal surface of epithelial cells (75). Similar to *P. carinii*, *C. parvum* is a widely prevalent pathogen in AIDS patients. In addition to *C. parvum* and *P. carinii* infections of the gut and lung epithelial cells, AIDS patients are susceptible to mucocutaneous invasion by *Candida albicans* and to chronic skin infections with other fungi, including *Tinea* sp. and the agent of seborrheic dermatitis. Cellular immunity enhances the resistance of nonphagocytic host cells against parasites through the effects of cytokines and other immune cell products on functions of those cells. Transfer factor, a complex mixture of cytokines released by stimulated T lymphocytes, has resulted in dramatic improvement in a small number of AIDS patients with cryptosporidiosis (76). The invasiveness and intracellular behavior of shigellae within gut epithelial cells can be altered by cytokines (77,78), and AIDS patients may be susceptible to recurrent bouts of shigellosis, despite demonstrably intact humoral immunity (79). Growth of *T. gondii* within relevant cells from tissues affected by the parasite is altered by incubation of the cells with T–cell-derived cytokines (80–83). Lymphocytes or cytokines could act to make the alveolar type I epithelial cells resistant to *P. carinii* parasitism or to enhance alveolar type II cell secretion of substances toxic to *P. carinii*. Although such considerations result in an attractive hypothesis concerning the role of cellular immunity in infection with *P. carinii*, there are no data confirming or refuting the suggestions.

Activation of macrophages has long been known to enhance production and activity of numerous intracellular and extracellular processes. In addition to the first-described effect of lymphocyte activation on the fate of intracellular microbes, first delineated by Mackaness (84), more recent studies have demonstrated that activation leads to greatly increased release of potentially antimicrobial substances (85–88). Such secreted products could contribute to suppression or elimination of parasites, without there being a requirement that physical contact and phagocytosis occur. Principal among such secretory products of macrophages are oxygen radicals (89–91), nitric oxides (41,88), and tumor necrosis factor (TNF) (92–94). When *P. carinii* is incubated in a dual chamber system that permits circulation of medium, but prohibits actual contact of macrophages with *P. carinii*, products secreted by activated macrophages lead to loss of viability of the parasite (95). These data extend previous observations that peroxide as well as superoxide and hydroxyl radical-generating systems are lethal to *P. carinii* (Fig. 2) and that *P. carinii* has limited antioxidant enzymes (39).

Whereas normal macrophages can ingest and kill *P. carinii* (32), they do not kill *P. carinii* in the extracellular environment (95). Activation of macrophages by interferon gamma plus endotoxin, a combination that leads to production and secretion of oxidants (96,97), converts the macrophage to cells capable of killing extracellular *P. carinii* (see Fig. 2). That microbicidal activity is inhibited by coincubation with catalase plus superoxide dismutase (95). In the same experiments, it was found that TNF is directly lethal to *P. carinii* (see Fig. 2), an effect which has not been observed for other pathogenic microbes. Although less sensitive to TNF effects than are standard target cells (L929 cells), *P. carinii* is killed by concentrations of TNF that can occur in tissues in vivo (93,98–100), and the effect is blocked by antiserum to TNF. The lethal effect of secretions of interferon-activated macrophages is inhibited by either anti-TNF antiserum or by antioxidants (95). Similarly, antioxidants inhibit TNF-induced lethality (95). Anti-TNF antiserum does not inhibit oxidant-induced lethality (unpublished observations). *Pneumocystis carinii* has been shown to induce TNF secretion by normal human monocytes (101), an induction that was inhibited by *P. carinii* immune serum, but not by polymixin B. Tumor necrosis factor is present in bronchoalveolar lavage fluid in acute lung disease of a variety of causes (98,100). In one recent study, alveolar macrophages from AIDS patients were found to constitutively secrete TNF (102). When isolated, the cells were maximally secreting TNF, and additional stimuli resulted in no further increase. But, another group found that the levels of TNF in alveolar lavage fluid from AIDS patients with *P. carinii* pneumonia were roughly predictive of the parasite burden; those with high TNF levels had fewer *P. carinii* in the lavage fluid than did those with lower levels (103). Further support of a fundamental role for TNF in host defenses against *P. carinii* was provided by the observation that the cytokine may be pivotal in the initial host responses to *P. carinii* in mice. When SCID mice are reconstituted with normal T cells, they

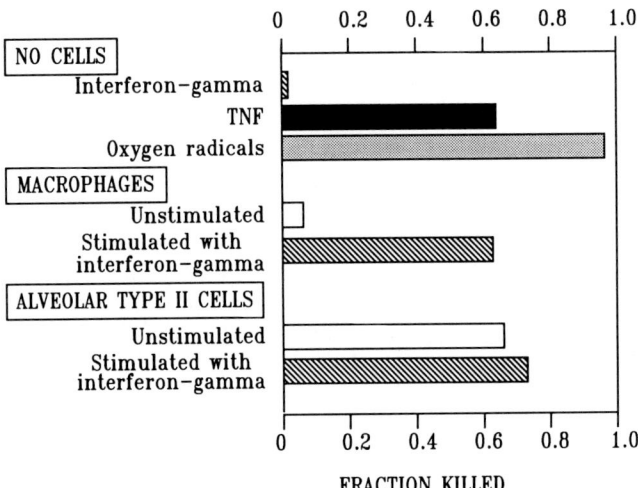

Figure 2 The effects of soluble host defense mediators against *Pneumocystis carinii* are summarized. *P. carinii* from the lungs of steroid treated rats were exposed to the potentially toxic systems and tested for subsequent metabolic activity. *P. carinii* which are no longer capable of converting glucose into CO_2 are considered dead. When no mammalian lung cells are present, TNF-α and oxygen radical-generating systems are lethal to *P. carinii*. Normal alveolar type II cells, but not normal alveolar macrophages, secrete products that kill *P. carinii* that is cultured with the cells in a well insert that allows circulation of medium, but prevents contact of *P. carinii* with the mammalian cells. In this same system, interferon gamma plus endotoxin stimulates alveolar macrophages to secrete products that kill *P. carinii*, but does not further enhance the activity of alveolar type II cells. Inclusion of catalase plus superoxide dismutase in the incubation mixture protects *P. carinii* from toxicity from oxygen radicals, TNF-α, or stimulated macrophage secretions. Inclusion of antibody to TNF-α protects *P. carinii* from the toxic effects of TNF-α or stimulated macrophage secretions. Data showing the approximate fraction of *P. carinii* killed are summarized from references 39 and 95.

eliminate *P. carinii* from their lungs within 3 weeks (104). When antibody to TNF is administered immediately after reconstitution of the animals that harbor *P. carinii*, the clearance is blocked. It appears that initiation of infection is most effectively prevented by macrophages and natural killer (NK) cells (i.e., "innate" immunity). Thus, available data suggest that TNF is of fundamental importance in host defenses against *P. carinii*, supplementing other, more specific, modalities. These authors could find no effect of interferon gamma, the other cytokine with demonstrable, in vitro activity against *P. carinii*. However, other groups found that interferon gamma was therapeutic when administered by aerosolization (105) and that it was a potent adjunct to trimethoprim–sulfamethoxazole (106). All of these studies have been undertaken in rodents. Great caution must be exercised in extrapolating effects of interferon gamma in rodents to other mammals. Data such as these illustrate the complex interactions among elements of innate and specific immunity in resistance to infection and disease.

The available data suggest that macrophage surveillance of the alveolar airspaces is more complex and flexible than that implied in models that restrict the major activities of the cells to phagocytosis and intracellular killing. An activated macrophage may be able to exert antimicrobial effects in its immediate environment, without having to come into direct contact with the target. And, an activated macrophage that is ingesting a microbe or particulate, may release products that damage nearby organisms which, for whatever reason, are not recognized as being foreign.

Since alveolar macrophages can be converted by lymphocyte products into secretory cells that are lethal to *P. carinii*, it is reasonable to examine the primary secretory cells of the alveolar airspaces, the alveolar type II epithelial cells (107). These cells have a tantalizing relation to the pathogenesis of *P. carinii* pneumonia. Alveolar type II epithelial cells, the most numerous epithelial cells in the lung (108), are normally secretory cells that produce alveolar surfactant and apoprotein (107). After lethal injury to the alveolar type I epithelial cells, the alveolar type II cells dedifferentiate and repopulate the epithelial lining of the alveolar airspace (107).

In adults, before the AIDS epidemic, glucocorticoids had been administered prior to onset of *P. carinii* pneumonia in almost all cases (3), and the appearance of pneumocystosis in patients with idiopathic Cushing's syndrome (16–20) has been noted. The alveolar type II cell is a hormone-sensitive cell, responsive to glucocorticoids and thyroid hormone (109–111). The responsiveness of surfactant secretion by alveolar type II epithelial cells to glucocorticoids has resulted in a clinically useful treatment modality: the lung function of premature fetuses can be improved by administration of high-potency steroids to the mother before premature delivery (112). In view of the effects of malnutrition on susceptibility to *P. carinii* disease, it may be relevant that one of the biochemical changes of starvation is alteration of alveolar surfactant secretion by type II cells (113). Also, one of the cells most widely used in in vitro culture of *P. carinii*, the A549 cell, was originally described as having type II cell characteristics (114). We have shown that alveolar type II cells obtained from healthy adult rats can cause destruction of *P. carinii* in vitro (95,115). If the *P. carinii* inoculum is very high, *P. carinii* appear to survive and the type II cells die (115). When cell-to-cell contact is permitted, type II alveolar cells exert a microbicidal against *P. carinii* causing disappearance (?lysis) of *P. carinii* from the medium (115). When contact is prevented, as in the experiments described earlier with cytokine-activated macrophages, the microbicidal effect is slower or less complete, and lysis does not occur (95). Coincubation of alveolar type II cells with cytokines has not yet been shown to significantly increase their activity against *P. carinii* (95); however, the design of the experiments was such that dose–response effects of either cytokine dose or cell number could not be assessed. The lack of a dramatic effect of interferon on type II cell lethality to *P. carinii* is neither surprising nor damaging to the hypothesis that cellular immune effectors may exert controlling influences on alveolar type II cells. Cytokines other than interferon gamma may be the principal effectors. And, the epithelial immunity that is stimulated by cytokines, if it is to contribute to the integrity of epithelial surfaces, should exert a continued enhancement of the antimicrobial resistance of the cells.

The normal state of adult alveolar epithelial cells could be one of "tonic" resistance to *P. carinii*. Epithelial cells obtained from immunodeficient animals, on the other hand, may demonstrate reduced activity against *P. carinii*; coincubation with cytokines should partially restore that activity. Such experiments have not yet been completed, nor has the anti-*P. carinii* activity of alveolar type II cells derived from continuously steroid-treated rats been studied. There is a sizable body of data suggesting a role for alveolar lining fluid, secreted in part by alveolar type II cells, in host defenses against several pathogenic microbes, including the pneumococcus (116) and *C. albicans* (117). Several investigators have demonstrated abnormalities in alveolar phospholipids (118,119) and apoprotein A (49) during *P. carinii* pneumonia in AIDS patients. Whether these abnormalities contributed to the development of disease or are merely a reflection of diffuse epithelial damage is unknown.

Thus, laboratory data and clinical observations suggest several means by which known immunologic effector mechanisms could contribute to host defenses against *P. carinii*. As I hope I have made clear, the evidence that such mechanisms actually do participate in those defenses is generally far from firm. The studies so far reviewed have dealt with phagocytes, lymphocytes, and their products. The possible role of another important immune effector arm, the natural killer cells (NK cells) has not been addressed in *P. carinii* infection until very recently. This primitive immune effector cell appears to contribute to resistance to infection in a variety of conditions in which cellular immunity is thought to be primary and contributes to the ability of severely immunodeficient animals [e.g., SCID mice (120)] to survive. Recent data (4,121,104) suggest that NK cells contribute to host defenses against *P. carinii*.

Any discussion of the cellular mechanisms of steroid action in disease caused by *P. carinii* would be incomplete without mention of the recent data suggesting that glucocorticoids, although contributory to susceptibility to pneumocystosis, also may be useful in therapy of patients critically ill with *P. carinii* pneumonia (122–129; 130 found no benefit). These clinical observations probably have less relevance to considerations of defenses against *P. carinii* than to approaches to patients with diffuse alveolar injury. In patients with tuberculosis who receive good antimicrobial drugs, steroids may improve oxygenation enough to dramatically improve the outcome (131,132). A similar effect has been observed in other models of pulmonary injury in which indomethacin, which can augment the cellular immune response in common variable immunodeficiency syndrome patients (133), has been beneficial (134,135). In all these situations, the clinical effect probably results from inhibition of prostaglandin synthesis, with consequent improvement of ventilation and perfusion matching.

VI. Evasion of Host Defense Effectors by *Pneumocystis carinii*

In the preceding, I have attempted to review available data directly related to the mechanisms operative against *P. carinii* and selected aspects of the much more extensive literature dealing with other, more or less similar, pathogens that might be relevant to understanding host defenses against *P. carinii*. That approach focuses almost exclusively on the host; the parasite is merely a "target." However, as with other obligate parasites, it is critical for *P. carinii* that at least a portion of the organisms survive the efforts of the host to eliminate them. The tactics employed range from the ability to frequently change antigens (136) to avoiding the extracellular milieu entirely by adapting to intracellular residence. Many parasites appear to blunt, if not entirely circumvent, host effectors by accreting to themselves host molecules, essentially cloaking themselves with "self"-determinants from the host (137–139). Understanding the mechanisms employed by the parasite to evade host responses can lead to valuable inferences concerning the host defense mechanisms most harmful to the parasite.

Available date suggest possible mechanisms that may be employed by *P. carinii* to evade host defenses. Photomicrographs that show *P. carinii* to be an extracellular, intra-alveolar parasite are widely available (e.g., 29,57). However, when careful attention is paid to methods of fixation, to preserve the lung in a state as close to that in the living animal as possible, it is evident that *P. carinii* trophozoites are totally blanketed by a layer of alveolar lining fluid and surfactant (30). In vitro, *P. carinii* readily binds surfactant (115), mediated in large part by the binding of surfactant apoprotein A to *P. carinii*'s gp120 (69). Such binding of phospholipid by the parasite may complement the normal tendency of surfactant to cover exposed surfaces within the alveoli. A parasite that is enveloped within the normal alveolar lining fluid should be less recognizable as foreign; no data exist to confirm or refute that speculation. Depending on the assay system, surfactant can be shown to augment or inhibit host defenses against other potential pathogens (117,140–146). Alveolar macrophage response to *C. albicans* is variably influenced by surfactant obtained from experimental animals at different ages after birth (117). The relevance to these considerations of the data indicating substantial changes in lung phospholipid and surfactant properties in experimental and human

P. carinii infection (49,118,119) is unclear. It is likely that the surfactant system contributes to pulmonary host defenses, and it is possible that the obligately parasitic P. carinii can subvert it.

The surface of P. carinii is laden with a variety of glycoproteins and lectin-reactive moieties (62–66), some of which behave as lectins (147). The avidity of the reactive surface for other, host-derived molecules has only recently been investigated. To date, I am familiar with data that show avid binding to the surface of P. carinii of fibronectin (56), albumin (70), and tumor necrosis factor (70). Fibronectin binds to the predominant P. carinii surface glycoprotein (56), and preliminary data indicate that albumin and TNF also bind to glycoproteins, including gp120 (unpublished observations). It is likely that such a list will be expanded considerably as more investigators begin to study the interaction of P. carinii with host macromolecules. These observations suggest that, in common with many parasites, prokaryotic and eukaryotic, P. carinii utilizes at least the simplest of three recognized host molecule mimicry mechanisms, the accretion of host macromolecules to its surface (139). Although such accumulating data provide circumstantial evidence that P. carinii makes use of host molecules in its efforts to evade host defenses, definitive proof is lacking and will be most difficult to provide.

In addition to providing a substrate for acquisition of host macromolecules, the glycoproteinaceous external layer of P. carinii may contribute to evasion of host defenses by more directly immunosuppressive activities. Candida albicans invasiveness may be facilitated by surface glycoproteins and mannan derivatives that inhibit T-lymphocyte function (148). Pneumocystis carinii probably contains substantial quantities of glucan (149), a related starch. The extensive network of the glycoprotein-rich (62) filamentous extensions of the external wall of P. carinii, observable in vivo (30) and in vitro (71) would greatly increase the surface area of the parasite's external wall and might result in increased solubilization of compounds that impair the reactivity of host cells against P. carinii. Both macrophage phagocytosis, which is a saturable phenomenon, and T-cell recognition functions could be subverted by excess particulate or soluble cell wall fragments.

Just as there is frustratingly little information on which to base conclusions concerning how P. carinii survives within an immunocompetent host, there are only faintly suggestive hints about the biochemical basis for its obligately parasitic nature. Investigations into the biochemical attributes of P. carinii suggest that it conducts normal cyanide-sensitive aerobic glycolysis when oxygen is available, but that it survives prolonged periods of microaerophilic ($P_{O_2} < 15$ torr) incubation (39). Although P. carinii primarily resides in the most oxygen-rich environment in its mammalian hosts, the alveolar airspace, the organism is poorly equipped for dealing with oxidative stress, having low concentrations of catalase, superoxide dismutase, and glutathione peroxidase, the major scavengers of toxic oxygen derivatives (39,150). It is possible that *P. carinii* is at least partially dependent on host cells for such reactive oxidant scavenging systems. It is capable of ribonucleic acid, protein, and phospholipid synthesis from simple precursors (38), with folic acid metabolism similar to that observed in other pathogenic microbes (36).

As is true for all known prokaryotic and eukaryotic organisms, *P. carinii* engages in active polyamine metabolism (151). Difluoromethylornithine (DFMO), a specific inhibitor of the rate-limiting enzyme ornithine decarboxylase (ODC), appears to be active against *P. carinii* in some (152), but not all (153,154), studies. However, *P. carinii* has no detectable ODC activity (151,155). The apparent efficacy of DFMO against *P. carinii* is difficult to explain, unless it is postulated that the lack of detectable ODC is an experimental artifact or that the inhibitor's effects is not directly against *P. carinii*. We have speculated that one possible explanation is based on the assumption that DFMO inhibits host cell polyamine synthesis; *P. carinii* is damaged because it requires preformed polyamines for its function (155). If *P. carinii* must import preformed polyamines, the organism will almost certainly have highly active transport mechanisms. It is tempting to speculate that such polyamine transport mechanisms would be susceptible to damage by host defense mediators or by compounds related to the critical polyamines, such as pentamidine (156).

To extend this speculation further, it is possible that one of the effects of intact cellular immunity is limitation of access to polyamines or to other vital host-derived nutrients. Such limitation of nutrient availability is postulated to contribute to the control of other infections for which cellular immunity is critical. *Chlamydia* (157,158) appears to be inhibited by efficient exclusion of tryptophan by activated macrophages and *Legionella* sp. by competition for iron (159). Iron is vital to survival of all organisms, and many bacteria have highly developed chelator systems for its acquisition. No such compounds have yet been identified in *P. carinii*, but growth of *P. carinii* is inhibited by iron chelation (160), and it is possible that iron chelation contributes to host defenses against *P. carinii*, as it does for other pathogenic microbes.

VII. Conclusions

Host defenses against *P. carinii* are complex, with the various arms of the immune system interacting in an almost uniquely intertwined manner. The interaction between host and parasite has resulted in a parasitic relation that, until severely compromised host defenses intervene, is finely tuned to promote an almost model parasitic relation. Neither the host nor the parasite is damaged in the parasite's need for a hospitable environment; *P. carinii* is, practically speaking, part of the normal flora of the immunocompetent mammal. As a result, an ubiquitous, obligate parasite causes disease only in conditions of profound immunosuppression. Available data, derived directly from in vitro experiments with *P. carinii*, have provided only a bare sketch of the mechanisms involved. Cellular immune surveillance contribute by arming macrophages for extracellular killing of *P. carinii*. It may also alter the functions of epithelial cells. Alveolar phagocytes can ingest and degrade *P. carinii* in vitro; whether that activity occurs in the non-aqueous alveolar airspace environment cannot be determined.

Determination of the mechanisms involved in host defenses against an ubiquitous obligate extracellular parasite, which causes disease in states of profound immunosuppression of cellular *or* humoral immunity, but which resists neither phagocytosis nor intracellular killing by nonimmune phagocytes, will require sustained effort, imagination, and keen observation.

Note Added in Proof

Since submission of this manuscript, the observation that prior bacterial infection could affect the intra-alveolar fate of *P. carinii*, noted in reference 25, has been further studied. The authors found that aerosols of killed Gram-negative bacteria accelerate resolution of *P. carinii* pneumonia, primarily, if not solely, through stimulation of release of TNF and other cytokines (161).

References

1. Matsumoto Y, Yoshida Y. Advances in pneumocystis biology. Parasitol Today 1986; 2:137–142.
2. Simon HB, Guerry D, Breslow A, Kirkpatrick CH. Opportunistic pathogens in the immunologically hyperresponsive host. *Pneumocystis carinii* infection in a patient with allergic bronchopulmonary aspergillosis. Am J Med 1973; 55:856–864.
3. Burke BA, Good RA. *Pneumocystis carinii* infections. Medicine 1973; 52:23–51.
4. Bonagura VR, Cunningham-Rundles S, Edwards BL, Ilowite NT, Wedgwood JF, Valacer DJ. Common variable hypogammaglobulinemia, recurrent *Pneumocystis carinii* pneumonia on intravenous gamma-globulin therapy, and natural killer cell deficiency. Clin Immunol Immunopathol 1989; 51:216–231.
5. Rao CP, Gelfand EW. *Pneumocystis carinii* pneumonitis in patients with hypogammaglobulinemia and intact T cell immunity. J Pediatr 1983; 103:410–412.
6. Walzer PD, Schnelle V, Armstrong DA, Rosen PP. Nude mouse: a new experimental model for *Pneumocystis carinii* infection. Science 1977; 197:177–179.
7. Lapinsky SE, Glencross D, Car NG, Kallenbach JM, Zwi S. Quantification and assessment of viability of *Pneumocystis carinii* organisms by flow cytometry. J Clin Microbiol 1991; 29:911–915.
8. Sheldon WH. Experimental pulmonary *Pneumocystis carinii* infection in rabbits. J Exp Med 1959; 110:147–159.

9. Frenkel JK, Good JT, Shultz JA. Latent *Pneumocystis* infection of rats, relapse, and chemotherapy. Lab Invest 1966; 15:1559–1577.
10. Baskerville A, Dowsett AB, Dennis MJ, Cranage MP, Greenaway PJ. *Pneumocystis carinii* pneumonia in simian immunodeficiency virus infection: immunohistological and scanning and transmission electron microscopical studies. J Pathol 1991; 164: 175–184.
11. Stokes DC, Gigliotti F, Rehg, JE, Snellgrove RL, Hughes WT. Experimental *Pneumocystis carinii* pneumonia in the ferret. Br J Exp Pathol 1987; 68:267–276.
12. Shelhamer JH, Ognibene FP, Macher AM, Tuazon C, Steiss R, Longo D, Kovacs JA, Parker MA, Natanson C, Lane HC, Fauci AS, Parrillo JE, Masur H. Persistence of *Pneumocystis carinii* in lung tissue of acquired immunodeficiency syndrome patients treated for pneumocystis pneumonia. Am Rev Respir Dis 1984; 130:1161–1165.
13. Girard P-M, Landman R, Gaudebout C, Lepretre A, Lottin P, Michon C, DeTruchis P, Matheron S, Camus F, Farinottin R, Marche D, Coulaud J, Saimot A. Prevention of *Pneumocystis carinii* pneumonia relapse by pentamidine aerosol in zidovudine-treated AIDS patients. Lancet 1989; 1:1348–1352.
14. Walzer PD, LaBine M, Redington TJ, Cushion MT. Predisposing factors in *Pneumocystis carinii* pneumonia: effects of tetracycline, protein malnutrition, and corticosteroids on hosts. Infect Immun 1984; 46:747–753.
15. Hughes WT, Price RA, Sisko F, Havron S, Kafatos AG, Schonland M, Smythe PM. Protein–calorie malnutrition. A host determinant for *Pneumocystis carinii* infection. Am J Dis Child 1974; 128:44–52.
16. Graham BS, Tucker WS. Opportunistic infections in endogenous Cushing's syndrome. Ann Intern Med 1984; 101:334–338.
17. Sieber SC, Dandurand R, Gelfman N, Iannini P, Braza F. Three opportunistic infections associated with ectopic corticotropin syndrome. Arch Intern Med 1989; 149:2589–2591.
18. Fulkerson WJ, Newman JH. Endogenous Cushing's syndrome complicated by *Pneumocystis carinii* pneumonia. Am Rev Respir Dis 1984; 129:188–189.
19. Anthony LB, Greco FA. *Pneumocystis carinii* pneumonia: a complication of Cushing's syndrome. Ann Intern Med 1981; 94:488–489.
20. Salas M, Angulo O. A case of carcinoma of the adrenal gland and *Pneumocystis carinii* pneumonia. Gac Med Mex 1971; 101:93–100.
21. McQuillen DP, Schroy PC, Hesketh PJ, Sugar AM. *Pneumocystis carinii* pneumonia complicating somatostatin therapy of Cushing's syndrome in a patient with metastatic pancreatic islet cell carcinoma and Zollinger–Ellison syndrome. Am J Gastroenterol 1991; 86:512–514.
22. Ersurum SC, Leff JA, Cochran JE, Ackerson JE, Szefler SJ, Martin RJ, Cott GR. Lack of benefit of methotrexate in severe, steroid-dependent asthma. A double-blind, placebo-controlled study. Ann Intern Med 1991; 114:353–360.
23. Udaka M, Maehara N, Tamaki K, et al. A case of *Pneumocystis carinii* pneumonia with hyperinfection of *Strongyloides stercoralis* complicated with smoldering adult T-cell leukemia. Kansenshogaku Zasshi 1990; 64:630–635.
24. El-Sebai MM, El-Helaly SM, Aly AG, Faris L. Correlation between the level of IgA and *Pneumocystis carinii* infection. J Egypt Soc Parisitol 1991; 21:771–777.

25. Pesanti EL. Effects of bacterial pneumonitis on development of pneumocystosis in rats. Am Rev Respir Dis 1982; 125:723–726.
26. Johnson JE, Philp JR. The defense of the lung: studies of the role of cell-mediated immunity. Johns Hopkins Med J 1977; 141:126–134.
27. Crowle AJ. Immunization against tuberculosis: what kind of vaccine? Infect Immun 1988; 56:2769–2773.
28. Walzer PD, Kim CK, Linke MJ, Pogue CL, Huerkamp MJ, Chrisp CE, Lerro AV. Outbreaks of *Pneumocystis carinii* pneumonia in colonies of immunodeficient mice. Infect Immun 1989; 57:62–70.
29. Lanken PN, Minda M, Pietra GG, Fishman AP. Alveolar response to experimental *Pneumocystis carinii* pneumonia in the rat. Am J Pathol 1980; 99:561–578.
30. Yoshida Y, Matsumoto Y, Yamada M, Okabayashi K, Yoshikawa H, Nakasawa M. *Pneumocystis carinii*: electron microscopic investigation on the interaction of trophozoite and alveolar lining cell. Zentralbl Bakteriol Hyg [A] 1984; 256: 390–399.
31. Beckers PJA. Infections with *Pneumocystis*: Aspects of the Intriguing Relationship with Its Host. Nijmegen, Holland: Studentpers, 1984.
32. VonBehren LA, Pesanti EL. Uptake and degradation of *Pneumocystis carinii* by macrophages in vitro. Am Rev Respir Dis 1978; 118:1051–1059.
33. Masur H, Jones TC. The interaction of *Pneumocystis carinii* with macrophages and L-cells. J Exp Med 1978; 147:157–170.
34. Pesanti EL. Kinetics of phagocytosis of *Staphylococcus aureus* by alveolar and peritoneal macrophages. Infect Immun 1979; 26:479–486.
35. Horio S, Ando M, Ukeshima A, Sugimoto M, Tokuomi H. Surface morphology and function of alveolar macrophages exposed to lung lavage fluids and serum from normal rabbits. J Reticuloendothel Soc 1981; 29:137–152.
36. Kovacs JA, Allegra CJ, Beaver J, Boarman D, Lewis M, Parillo JE, Chabner B, Masur H. Characterization of de novo folate synthesis in *Pneumocystis carinii* and *Toxoplasma gondii*: potential for screening therapeutic agents. J Infect Dis 1989; 160:312–320.
37. Pesanti EL. In vitro effects of antiprotozoan drugs and immune serum on *Pneumocystis carinii*. J Infect Dis 1980; 141:775–780.
38. Pesanti EL, Cox C. Metabolic and synthetic activities of *Pneumocystis carinii* in vitro. Infect Immun 1981; 34:908–914.
39. Pesanti EL. *Pneumocystis carinii*: oxygen uptake, antioxidant enzymes, and susceptibility to oxygen-mediated damage. Infect Immun 1984; 44:7–11.
40. Hidalgo H, Helmke RJ, German VF, Mangos JA. Zymolyase-sensitive sites of *Pneumocystis carinii*: their role in induction of an oxidative burst in macrophages. J Protozool 1991.
41. Sherman MP. *Pneumocystis carinii* induces L-arginine oxidation in lung macrophages. J Protozool 1991.
42. Cushion MT, Ebbets D. Growth and metabolism of *Pneumocystis carinii* in axenic culture. J Clin Microbiol 1990; 28:1385–1394.
43. Gallin JI, Buescher ES, Seligmann BE, Nath J, Gaither T, Katz P. Recent advances in chronic granulomatous disease. Ann Intern Med 1983; 99:657–674.

44. Pedersen FK, Johansen KS, Rosenkvist J, Tygstrup I, Valerius NH. Refractory *Pneumocystis carinii* infection in chronic granulomatous disease: successful treatment with granulocytes. Pediatrics 1979; 64:935–938.
45. Stagno S, Pifer LL, Hughes WT, Brasfield DM, Tiller RE. *Pneumocystis carinii* pneumonia in young immunocompetent infants. Pediatrics 1980; 66:56–62.
46. Soulez B, Dei-Cas E, Charet P, Mougeot G, Caillaux M, Damus D. The young rabbit: a nonimmunosuppressed model for *Pneumocystis carinii* pneumonia. J Infect Dis 1989; 160:355–356.
47. Sumiya M, Super M, Tabona P, Levinsky RJ, Arai T, Turner MW, Summerfield JA. Molecular basis of opsonic defect in immunodeficient children. Lancet 1991; 337: 1569–1570.
48. Schweinle JE, Ezekowitz AB, Tenner AJ, Kuhlman M, Joiner KA. Human mannose-binding protein activates the alternative complement pathway and enhances serum bactericidal activity on a mannose-rich isolate of *Salmonella*. J Clin Invest 1989; 84:1821–1829.
49. Phelps DS, Rose RM. Increased recovery of surfactant protein A in AIDS-related pneumonia. Am Rev Respir Dis 1991; 143:1072–1075.
50. Ezekowitz RAB, Williams DJ, Koziel H, Armstrong MYK, Warner A, Richards FF, Rose RM. Uptake of *Pneumocystis carinii* mediated by the macrophage mannose receptor. Nature 1991; 351:155–158.
51. Raviglione MC. Extrapulmonary pneumocystosis: the first 50 cases. Rev Infect Dis 1990; 12:1127–1138.
52. Walzer PD. Attachment of microbes to host cells: relevance of *Pneumocystis carinii*. Lab Invest 1986; 54:589–592.
53. Limper AH, Martin WJ. *Pneumocystis carinii*: inhibition of lung cell growth mediated by parasite attachment. J Clin Invest 1990; 85:391–396.
54. Pottratz ST, Martin WJ. Role of fibronectin in *Pneumocystis carinii* attachment to cultured lung cells. J Clin Invest 1990; 85:351–356.
55. Pottratz S, Martin WJ. Mechanism of *Pneumocystis carinii* attachment to cultured rat alveolar macrophages. J Clin Invest 1990; 86:1678–1683.
56. Pottratz ST, Paulsrud J, Smith JS, Martin WJ. *Pneumocystis carinii* attachment to cultured lung cells by pneumocystis gp120, a fibronectin binding protein. J Clin Invest 1991; 88:403–407.
57. Long EG, Smith JS, Meier JL. Attachment of *Pneumocystis carinii* to rat pneumocytes. Lab Invest 1986; 54:609–615.
58. Weller NK, Karnovsky MJ. Isolation of pulmonary alveolar type I cells from adult rats. Am J Pathol 1986; 124:448–456.
59. Fisher DJ, Gigliotti F, Sauderer M, Harmsen AG. Specific T-cell response to *Pneumocystis carinii* surface glycoprotein (gp120) after immunization and natural infection. Infect Immun 1991; 59:3372–3376.
60. Graves DC, McNabb SJN, Worley MA, Downs TD, Ivey MH. Analysis of rat *Pneumocystis carinii* antigens recognized by human and rat antibodies by using Western immunoblotting. Infect Immun 1986; 54:96–103.
61. Gigliotti F, Ballou LR, Hughes WT, Mosley BD. Purification and initial characterization of a ferret *Pneumocystis carinii* surface antigen. J Infect Dis 1988; 158:848–854.

62. Pesanti EL, Shanley JD. Glycoproteins of *Pneumocystis carinii*: characterization by electrophoresis and microscopy. J Infect Dis 1988; 158:1353–1359.
63. Cushion MT, DeStefano JA, Walzer PD. *Pneumocystis carinii* surface reactive carbohydrates detected by lectin probes. Exp Protozool 1988; 67:137–147.
64. Yoshikawa H, Tegoshi T, Yoshida Y. Detection of surface carbohydrates on *Pneumocystis carinii* by fluorescein-conjugated lectins. Parasitol Res 1987; 74:43–49.
65. Yoshikawa H, Morioka H, Yoshida Y. Ultrastructural detection of carbohydrates in the pellicle of *Pneumocystis carinii*. Parasitol Res 1988; 74:537–543.
66. Radding JA, Armstrong MYK, Ullu E, Richards FF. Identification and isolation of a major cell surface glycoprotein of *Pneumocystis carinii*. Infect Immun 1989; 57:2149–2157.
67. Cushion MT, DeStefano JA, Walzer PD. *Pneumocystis carinii*: surface reactive carbohydrates detected by lectin probes. Exp Parasitol 1988; 67:137–147.
68. Lundgren B, Lipschik GY, Kovacs JA. Purification and characterization of a major human *Pneumocystis carinii* surface antigen. J Clin Invest 1991; 87:163–170.
69. Zimmerman PE, Voelker DR, McCormack FX, Paulsrud JR, Martin WJ. 120-kD Surface glycoprotein of *Pneumocystis carinii* is a ligand for surfactant protein A. J Clin Invest 1992; 89:143–149.
70. Pesanti EL, Tomicic T, Donta ST. The binding of I125-labelled tumor necrosis factor to *Pneumocystis carinii* and insoluble cell wall fraction. J Protozool 1991.
71. Murphy MJ, Pifer LL, Hughes WT. *Pneumocystis carinii* in vitro. A study by scanning electron microscopy. Am J Pathol 1977; 86:387–402.
72. Gigliotti F, Hughes W. Passive immunoprophylaxis with specific monoclonal antibody confers partial protection against *Pneumocystis carinii* pneumonitis in animal models. J Clin Invest 1988; 81:1666–1668.
73. Rutstein R. Predicting risk of *Pneumocystis carinii* pneumonia in human immunodeficiency virus-infected children. Am J Dis Child 1991; 145:922–924.
74. Spickett GP, Misbah SA, Chapel HM. Primary antibody deficiency in adults. Lancet 1991; 337:281–284.
75. Fayer R, Ungar BLP. *Cryptosporidium* spp. and cryptosporidiosis. Microbiol Rev 1986; 50:458–483.
76. McMeeking A, Borkowsky W, Klesius PH, Bonk S, Holzmann RS, Lawrence HS. A controlled trial of bovine dialyzable leukocyte extract for cryptosporidiosis in patients with AIDS. J Infect Dis 1990; 161:108–112.
77. Niesel DW, Hess CB, Cho YJ, Klimpel KD, Klimpel GR. Natural and recombinant interferons inhibit epithelial cell invasion by *Shigella* spp. Infect Immun 1986; 52:828–833.
78. Bukholm G, Degre M. Effect of human leukocyte interferon on invasiveness of *Salmonella* species in HEp-2 cell cultures. Infect Immun 1983; 42:1198–1202.
79. Blaser MJ, Hale TL, Formal SB. Recurrent shigellosis complicating human immunodeficiency virus infection: failure of pre-existing antibodies to confer protection. Am J Med 1988; 86:105–107.
80. Chinchilla M, Frenkel JK. Mediation of immunity to intracellular infection (*Toxoplasma* and *Besnoitia*) within somatic cells. Infect Immun 1978; 19:999–1012.
81. Jones TC, Bienz KA, Erb P. In vitro cultivation of *Toxoplasma gondii* cysts in astrocytes in the presence of gamma interferon. Infect Immun 1986; 51:147–156.

82. Pfefferkorn ER, Eckel M, Rebhun S. Interferon-gamma suppresses the growth of *Toxoplasma gondii* in human fibroblasts through starvation for tryptophan. Mol Biochem Parasitol 1986; 20:215–224.
83. Pferrerkorn ER, Guyre PM. Inhibition of growth of *Toxoplasma gondii* in cultured fibroblasts by human recombinant gamma interferon. Infect Immun 1984; 44:211–216.
84. Mackaness GB. The immunology of antituberculous immunity. Am Rev Respir Dis 1968; 97:337–344.
85. Wozencraft AO, Dockrell HM, Taverne J, Targett GA, Playfair JH. Killing of human malaria parasites by macrophage secretory products. Infect Immun 1984; 43:664–669.
86. Montealegre F, Levy MG, Ristic M, James MA. Growth inhibition of *Babesia bovis* in culture by secretions from bovine mononuclear phagocytes. Infect Immun 1985; 50:523–526.
87. Davies P, Bonney RJ. Secretory products of mononuclear phagocytes: a brief review. J Reticuloendothel Soc 1979; 26:37–47.
88. Flesch IEA, Kaufmann SHE. Mechanisms involved in mycobacterial growth inhibition by gamma interferon-activated bone marrow macrophages: role of reactive nitrogen intermediates. Infect Immun 1991; 59:3213–3218.
89. Klebanoff SJ. Oxygen metabolism and the toxic properties of phagocytes. Ann Intern Med 1980; 93:480–489.
90. Maridonneau-Parini I, Errasfa M, Russo-Marie F. Inhibition of superoxide generation by dexamethasone is mimicked by lipocortin I in alveolar macrophages. J Clin Invest 1989; 83:1936–1940.
91. Brozna JP, Hoan M, Rademacher JM, Pabst KM, Pabst MJ. Monocyte responses to sulfatide from *Mycobacterium tuberculosis*: inhibition of priming for enhanced release of superoxide, associated with increased secretion of interleukin-1 and tumor necrosis factor alpha, and altered protein phosphorylation. Infect Immun 1991; 59: 2542–2548.
92. Grau GE, Fajardo LF, Piguet P, Allet B, Lambert P, Vassali P. Tumor necrosis factor (cachectin) as an essential mediator in cerebral malaria. Science 1987; 237:1210–1212.
93. Taverne J, Bate CAW, Kwiatkowski D, Jakobsen PH, Playfair JHL. Two soluble antigens of *Plasmodium falciparum* induce tumor necrosis factor release from macrophages. J Infect Dis 1990; 58:2923–2928.
94. Martinet Y, Yamauchi K, Crystal RG. Differential expression of the tumor necrosis factor/cachectin gene by blood and lung mononuclear phagocytes. Am Rev Respir Dis 1988; 138:659–665.
95. Pesanti EL. Interaction of cytokines and alveolar cells with *Pneumocystis carinii* in vitro. J Infect Dis 1991; 163:611–616.
96. Sharp AK, Banerjee DK. Effect of gamma interferon on hydrogen peroxide production by cultured mouse peritoneal macrophages. Infect Immun 1986; 54:597–599.
97. Fast DJ, Shannon BJ, Herriott MJ, Kennedy MJ, Rummage JA, Leu RW. Staphylococcal exotoxins stimulate nitric oxide-dependent murine macrophage tumoricidal activity. Infect Immun 1991; 59:2987–2993.
98. Millar AB, Foley NM, Singer M, Johnson NMcI, Meager A, Rook GAW. Tumor necrosis factor in bronchopulmonary secretions of patients with adult respiratory distress syndrome. Lancet 1989; 2:712–713.

99. Takashima T, Ueta C, Tsuyuguchi I, Kishimoto S. Production of tumor necrosis factor alpha by monocytes from patients with pulmonary tuberculosis. Infect Immun 1990; 58:3286–3292.
100. Smith HG, Magee DM, Williams DM, Graybill HR. Tumor necrosis factor-α plays a role in host defense against *Histoplasma capsulatum*. J Infect Dis 1990; 162:1349–1353.
101. Tamburrini E, DeLuca A, Ventura G, Maiuro G, Siracusano A, Ortona E, Antinori A. *Pneumocystis carinii* stimulates in vitro production of tumor necrosis factor-alpha by human macrophages. Med Microbiol Immunol 1991; 180:15–20.
102. Agostini C, Zambello R, Trentin L, Garbisa S, DiCelle PF, Bulian P, Onisto M, Poletti V, Spiga L, Raise E, Foa R, Semenzato G. Alveolar macrophages from patients with AIDS and AIDS-related complex constitutively synthesize and release tumor necrosis factor alpha. Am Rev Respir Dis 1991; 144:195–201.
103. Krishnan VL, Meager A, Mitchell DM, Pinching AJ. Alveolar macrophages in AIDS patients: increased spontaneous tumor necrosis factor-alpha production in *Pneumocystis carinii* pneumonia. Clin Exp Immunol 1990; 80:156–160.
104. Chen W, Havell EA, Harmsen AG. Importance of endogenous tumor necrosis factor alpha and gamma interferon in host resistance against *Pneumocystis carinii* infection. Infect Immun 1992; 60:1279–1284.
105. Beck JM, Liggitt HD, Brunette EN, Fuchs HJ, Shellito JE, Debs RJ. Reduction in intensity of *Pneumocystis carinii* pneumonia in mice by aerosol administration of gamma interferon. Infect Immun 1991; 59:3859–3862.
106. Shear HL, Valladares G, Narachi MA. Enhanced treatment of *Pneumocystis carinii* pneumonia in rats with interferon-gamma and reduced doses of trimethoprim/sulfamethoxazole. J AIDS 1990; 3:943–948.
107. Gail DB, Lenfant CJM. Cells of the lung: biology and clinical implications. Am Rev Respir Dis 1983; 127:366–387.
108. Bertram JF, Bolender RP. Counting parenchymal cells in the goat lung with serial section reconstruction and stereology. Am Rev Respir Dis 1986; 133:891–896.
109. Kotas RV, Avery ME. The influences of sex on fetal rabbit lung maturation and on the response to glucocorticoid. Am Rev Respir Dis 1980; 121:377–381.
110. Smith LJ, Brody JS. Influence of methylprednisolone on mouse alveolar type 2 cell response to acute lung injury. Am Rev Respir Dis 1981; 123:459–464.
111. Adamson IYR, Bowden DH. Reaction of cultured adult and fetal lung to prednisolone and thyroxine. Arch Pathol 1975; 99:80–85.
112. Jobe A, Ikegami M. Surfactant for the treatment of respiratory distress syndrome. Am Rev Respir Dis 1987; 1361:1256–1275.
113. Sahebjami H, MacGee J. Effects of starvation and refeeding on lung biochemistry in rats. Am Rev Respir Dis 1982; 126:483–487.
114. Smith B, Szakal A, Nelwon-Rees W, Todaro G. A continuous tumor-cell line from a human lung carcinoma with properties of type II alveolar epithelial cells. Int J Cancer 1976; 17:62–70.
115. Pesanti EL. Phospholipid profile of *Pneumocystis carinii* and its interaction with alveolar type II epithelial cells. Infect Immun 1987; 55:736–741.
116. Coonrod JD, Lester RL, Hsu LC. Characterization of the extracellular bactericidal factors of rat alveolar lining material. J Clin Invest 1984; 74:1269–1279.

117. Zeligs BJ, Nerurkar LS, Bellanti JA. Chemotactic and candidacidal responses of rabbit alveolar macrophages during postnatal development and modulating roles of surfactant in these responses. Infect Immun 1984; 44:379–385.
118. Kernbaum S, Masliah J, Alcindor LG, Bouton C, Christol D. Phospholipase activities of bronchoalveolar lavage fluid in rat *Pneumocystis carinii* pneumonia. Br J Exp Pathol 1983; 64:75–80.
119. Sheehan PM, Stokes DC, Yeh Y, Hughes WT. Surfactant phospholipids and lavage phospholipase A_2 in experimental *Pneumocystis carinii* pneumonia. Am Rev Respir Dis 1986; 134:526–531.
120. Wherry JC, Schreiber RD, Unanue ER. Regulation of gamma interferon production by natural killer cells in SCID mice: roles of tumor necrosis factor and bacterial stimuli. Infect Immun 1991; 59:1709–1715.
121. Harmsen AG, Stankiewicz M. T cells are not sufficient for resistance to *Pneumocystis carinii* in mice. J Protozool 1991.
122. MacFadden DK, Hyland RH, Inouye T, Edelson JD, Rodriguez CH, Rebuck AS. Corticosteroids as adjunctive therapy in treatment of *Pneumocystis carinii* pneumonia in patients with acquired immunodeficiency syndrome. Lancet 1987; 1:1477–1479.
123. Rankin JA, Pella JA. Radiographic resolution of *Pneumocystis carinii* pneumonia in response to corticosteroid therapy. Am Rev Respir Dis 1987; 136:182–183.
124. Amundson DE, Murray KM, Brodine S, Oldfield EC. High-dose corticosteroid therapy for *Pneumocystis carinii* pneumonia in patients with acquired immunodeficiency syndrome. South Med J 1989; 82:711–714.
125. Gagnon S, Boota AM, Fischl MA, Baier H, Kirsky OW, LaVoie L. Corticosteroids as adjunctive therapy for severe *Pneumocystis carinii* pneumonia in the acquired immunodeficiency syndrome. N Engl J Med 1990; 323:1444–1450.
126. Bozzette SA, Sattler FR, Chiu J, Wu AW, Gluckstein D, Kemper C, Bartok A, Niosi J, Abramson I, Corrman J, Hughlett C, Loya R, Cassens B, Akil B, Meng T, Boylen CT, Nielsen D, Richman DD, Tilles JG, Leedom J, McCutchan HA, the California cooperative treatment group. A controlled trial of early adjunctive treatment with corticosteroids for *Pneumocystis carinii* pneumonia in the acquired immunodeficiency syndrome. N Engl J Med 1990; 323:1451–1457.
127. Wachter RM, Russi MB, Bloch DA, Hopewell PC, Luce JM. *Pneumocystis carinii* pneumonia and respiratory failure in AIDS. Improved outcomes and increased use of intensive care units. Am Rev Respir Dis 1991; 143:251–256.
128. Montaner JSG, Lawson L, Nevitt N, Belzberg A, Schechter MT, Ruedy J. Corticosteroids prevent early deterioration in patients with moderately severe *Pneumocystis carinii* pneumonia and the acquired immunodeficiency syndrome (AIDS). Ann Intern Med 1990; 113:14–20.
129. Friedman Y, Franklin C, Freels S, Weil MH. Long-term survival of patients with AIDS, *Pneumocystis carinii* pneumonia, and respiratory failure. JAMA 1991; 266:89–92.
130. Schiff MJ, Farber BF, Kaplan MH. Steroids for *Pneumocystis carinii* pneumonia and respiratory failure in the acquired immunodeficiency syndrome. A reassessment. Arch Intern Med 1990; 150:1819–1821.
131. Horne NW. A critical evaluation of corticosteroids in tuberculosis. Adv Tuberc Res 1966; 15:1–54.

132. Johnson JR, Taylor BC, Morrissey JF, Jenne JW, MacDonald FM. Corticosteroids in pulmonary tuberculosis. I. Over-all results in the Madison–Minneapolis Veterans Administration hospitals steroid study. Am Rev Respir Dis 1965; 92:376–391.
133. Goodwin JS, Bankhurst AD, Murphy SA, Selinger DS, Messner RP, Williams RC. Partial reversal of the cellular immune defect in common variable immunodeficiency with indomethacin. J Clin Lab Immunol 1978; 1:197–199.
134. Hanly PJ, Dobson K, Roberts D, Light RB. Effect of indomethacin on arterial oxygenation in critically ill patients with severe bacterial pneumonia. Lancet 1987; 1:351–354.
135. Light RB. Indomethacin and acetylsalicylic acid reduce intrapulmonary shunting in experimental pneumococcal pneumonia. Am Rev Respir Dis 1986; 134:520–525.
136. Donelson JE, Rice-Ficht A. Molecular biology of trypanosome antigenic variation. Microbiol Rev 1985; 49:107–125.
137. Diffley P. Comparative immunological analysis of host plasma proteins bound to bloodstream forms of *Trypanosoma brucei* species. Infect Immun 1978; 21:605–612.
138. Bloom BR. Games parasites play: how parasites evade immune surveillance. Nature 1979; 279:21–26.
139. Greenblatt CL. Molecular mimicry and the carbohydrate language of parasitism. ASM News 1983; 49:488–493.
140. Ansfield MJ, Benson BJ, Kaltreider HB. Immunosuppression by surface-active material: lack of species specificity. Am Rev Respir Dis 1979; 120:949–951.
141. Coonrod JD, Jarrells MC, Yoneda K. Effect of rat surfactant lipids on complement and Fc receptors of macrophages. Infect Immun 1986; 54:371–378.
142. LaForce FM. Effect of alveolar lining material on phagocytic and bactericidal activity of lung macrophages against *Staphylococcus aureus*. J Lab Clin Med 1976; 88:691–699.
143. O'Neill S, Lesperance E, Klass DJ. Rat lung lavage surfactant enhances bacterial phagocytosis and intracellular killing by alveolar macrophages. Am Rev Respir Dis 1984; 130:225–230.
144. Juers JA, Rogers RM, McCurdy JB, Cook WW. Enhancement of bactericidal activity of alveolar macrophages by human alveolar lining material. J Clin Invest 1976; 58:271–275.
145. O'Neill SJ, Lesperance EL, Klass DJ. Human lung lavage surfactant enhances staphylococcal phagocytosis by alveolar macrophages. Am Rev Respir Dis 1984; 130:1177–1179.
146. Coonrod JD, Yoneda K. Detection and partial characterization of antibacterial factor(s) in alveolar lining material of rats. J Clin Invest 1983; 71:129–141.
147. Vierbuchen M, Ortmann M, Uhlenbruck G. Endogenous carbohydrate-binding proteins in *Pneumocystis carinii*. J Infect Dis 1990; 58:3142–3146.
148. Domer J, Elkins K, Ennist D, Baker P. Modulation of immune responses by surface polysaccharides of *Candida albicans*. Rev Infect Dis 1988; 10(S2):S419–S422.
149. Schmatz DM, Romanchek MA, Pitrarelli LA, Schwartz RE, Fromtling RA, Nollstadt KH, Vanmiddlesworth FL, Wilson KE, Turner MJ. Treatment of *Pneumocystis carinii* pneumonia with 1,3-α-glucan synthesis inhibitors. Proc Natl Acad Sci USA 1990; 87:5950–5954.

150. Pesanti EL. Enzymes of *Pneumocystis carinii*: electrophoretic mobility on starch gels. J Protozool 1989; 36:2S–3S.
151. Lipschik GY, Masur H, Kovacs JA. Polyamine metabolism in *Pneumocystis carinii*. J Infect Dis 1991; 163:1121–1127.
152. Golden JA, Sjoerdsma A, Santi DV. *Pneumocystis carinii* pneumonia treated with difluoromethylornithine. West J Med 1984; 141:613–623.
153. Cushion MT, Stanforth D, Linke MJ, Walzer PD. Method of testing the susceptibility of *Pneumocystis carinii* to antimicrobial agents in vitro. Antimicrob Agents Chemother 1985; 28:796–801.
154. Hughes WT, Smith BL. Efficacy of diaminodiphenylsulfone and other drugs in murine *Pneumocystis carinii* pneumonitis. Antimicrob Agents Chemother 1990; 26: 436–440.
155. Pesanti EL, Bartlett MS, Smith JW. Lack of detectable activity of ornithine decarboxylase in *Pneumocystis carinii*. J Infect Dis 1988; 158:1137–1138.
156. Read GW, Hong SM, Kiefer EF. Competitive inhibition of 48/80-induced histamine release by benzalkonium chloride and its analogs and the polyamine receptor in mast cells. J Pharmacol Exp Ther 1982; 222:652–657.
157. Byrne GI, Lehmann LK, Landry GJ. Induction of tryptophan catabolism is the mechanism for gamma-interferon-mediated inhibition of intracellular *Chlamydia psittaci* replication in T24 cells. Infect Immun 1986; 53:347–351.
158. Shermer-Avni Y, Wallach D, Sarov I. Inhibition of *Chlamydia trachomatis* growth by recombinant tumor necrosis factor. Infect Immun 1988; 56:2503–2506.
159. Byrd TF, Horwitz MA. Interferon gamma-activated human monocytes down-regulated transferrin receptors and inhibit the intracellular multiplication of *Legionella pneumophilia* by limiting the availability of iron. J Clin Invest 1989; 83:1457–1465.
160. Weinberg GA, Shaw MM. Suppressive effect of deferoxamine on the growth of *Pneumocystis carinii* in vitro. J Protozool 1991.
161. Harmsen AG, Chen W. Resolution of *Pneumocystis carinii* pneumonia in CD4+ lymphocyte-depleted mice given aerosols of heat-treated *Escherichia coli*. J Exp Med 1992; 176:881–886.

Part Four

CLINICAL FEATURES

16

Clinical Manifestations in Children

WALTER T. HUGHES

St. Jude Children's Research Hospital
Memphis, Tennessee

I. Introduction

The first humans discovered to have *Pneumocystis carinii* pneumonitis were infants. In 1942, van der Meer and Brug found *P. carinii* in the lungs of 3- and 4-month-old infants (1). However, a decade later more convincing data were reported by Vanek et al. (2) linking *P. carinii* with diffuse interstitial plasma cell pneumonitis in humans. They described autopsy findings in 32 infants. Before these reports, *P. carinii* was an obscure parasite found in lower primates.

Although epidemics of interstitial plasma cell pneumonitis occurred in Europe before, during, and after World War II, few detailed reports of these cases are available. In general, the clinical features were those described by Vanek et al. (2). The illness began in a subtle manner, with increasing severity of tachypnea, dyspnea, and cyanosis. The patients were afebrile, and physical findings were limited to weight loss and crackling rales. The course to death or recovery was about 4–6 weeks.

When immunosuppressive therapeutics came into general use in the mid-1950s, *P. carinii* pneumonitis was encountered in the immunocompromised child and adult. Both clinical and histological differences have been observed between the infantile form and that occurring in the child and adult.

The clinical types of *P. carinii* infection can be categorized into four groups:

1. Asymptomatic infection
2. Infantile interstitial plasma cell pneumonitis
3. Child–adult sporadic pneumonitis in the immunosuppressed host
4. Extrapulmonary infection

These types are influenced generally by age and the underlying disease process causing the immunodeficiency.

II. Asymptomatic Infection

Because antibody is detectable in the sera of at least 75% of normal individuals by 4 years of age (3–5) and most of these children have not had discernible pneumonitis, it has been assumed that *P. carinii* may establish an infection, but because of normal immune response, no disease occurs. Furthermore, it is assumed that *P. carinii* may persist in the lung in a latent state. If the host becomes immunodeficient, the organism replicates and provokes disease. This hypothesis has never been proved or disproved. Also, no careful studies of normal children have been done to determine whether or not some mild signs and symptoms of infection might not occur with this primary infection, very much like infections with histoplasmosis, Epstein-Barr virus, or cytomegalovirus.

III. Infantile Interstitial Plasma Cell Pneumonitis

The clinical features of interstitial plasma cell pneumonitis caused by *P. carinii* have been described in reports of the epidemics of this infection in debilitated European infants. The outset is usually subtle, with poor feeding and sometimes diarrhea. An increase in the respiratory rate may be the first sign of respiratory tract involvement. Cough, coryza, and fever may be absent. After 1–2 weeks, respiratory distress becomes obvious, with severe tachypnea, dyspnea, circumoral cyanosis, intercostal and sternal retraction, and diffuse crepitant rales by auscultation. About one-fourth of the infants will die if untreated, but survival without treatment will occur in most infants after a prolonged course of 4–6 weeks. Most infants remain afebrile through the course. A few infants may have an abrupt onset with a rapidly downhill course within a few days (6).

This type of *P. carinii* pneumonitis is encountered infrequently since the epidemics of interstitial plasma cell pneumonitis have subsided (7). Some infants with the acquired immunodeficiency syndrome (AIDS) may have clinical features of this type, but the histological pattern differs.

IV. Child–Adult Sporadic Pneumonitis in the Immunocompromised Host

Currently, *P. carinii* pneumonitis in infants and children is limited almost exclusively to individuals with severe compromise of the immune system, especially impaired cell-mediated responses. Of the congenital immunodeficiency syndromes, the highest rates of *P. carinii* pneumonitis are in infants and children with severe combined immunodeficiency disorder (40%), but cases have occurred, with less frequency, in most of the other congenital disorders (8,9).

Infants and children with cancer acquire *P. carinii* pneumonitis more because of intensive immunosuppressive therapy than because of the malignancy. Organ transplant recipients are at increased risk for this pneumonitis, as well as a variety of other individuals who require immunosuppressive drugs as a part of their therapy.

Almost all of the studies of clinical manifestations of *P. carinii* pneumonitis in infants and children with cancer, organ transplantation, and primary congenital immunodeficiency disorders antedate 1980, when the AIDS era began. The clinical features of the pneumonitis in children with these underlying disorders have been reviewed in detail elsewhere (7) and will not be discussed further here to deal more extensively with *P. carinii* pneumonitis in infants and children with AIDS. Table 1 summarizes the general trend of clinical manifestations in categories of patients with *P. carinii* pneumonitis.

Table 1 General Trend of Clinical Manifestations in Categories of Patients with *P. carinii* Pneumonitis

	Clinical types of *P. carinii* pneumonia			
			Child–adult	
Clinical feature	Subclinical	Infantile	Non-AIDS	AIDS
Fever	−	−	+	+
Tachypnea	−	+	+	+
Rales	−	+	−	−
Cough	−	+	+	+
Intercostal retractions	−	+	−	−
Insidious onset	−	+	−	+
Mortality (untreated)	−	<50%	ca. 100%	ca. 100%

Source: Ref. 7.

A. *Pneumocystis carinii* Pneumonitis in Infants and Children with Acquired Immunodeficiency Syndrome

As in adults, *P. carinii* pneumonitis is the most common serious human immunodeficiency virus (HIV)-associated infection among infants and children. Of the 2786 pediatric AIDS patients reported to the Centers for Disease Control (CDC) through 1990, *P. carinii* was diagnosed in 1080 children (39%) (10). This pneumonitis is frequently the initial clinical sign of HIV.

Risk Factors

The incidence of *P. carinii* pneumonitis in HIV-infected infants and children is related to age, although the pneumonitis can occur at any age. Figure 1 shows the distribution of *P. carinii* pneumonitis by age of the HIV-infected host. Most cases occur between 3 and 6 months of age, and the occurrence in infants younger than 1 month of age is rare. Only one documented case of *P. carinii* pneumonia in an HIV-infected infants younger than 1 month of age has been reported (11). This 2770-g infant had meconium aspiration at birth, followed by respiratory distress and pulmonary infiltrates. A lung biopsy on day 19 of age showed multiple *P. carinii* organisms and interstitial infiltration.

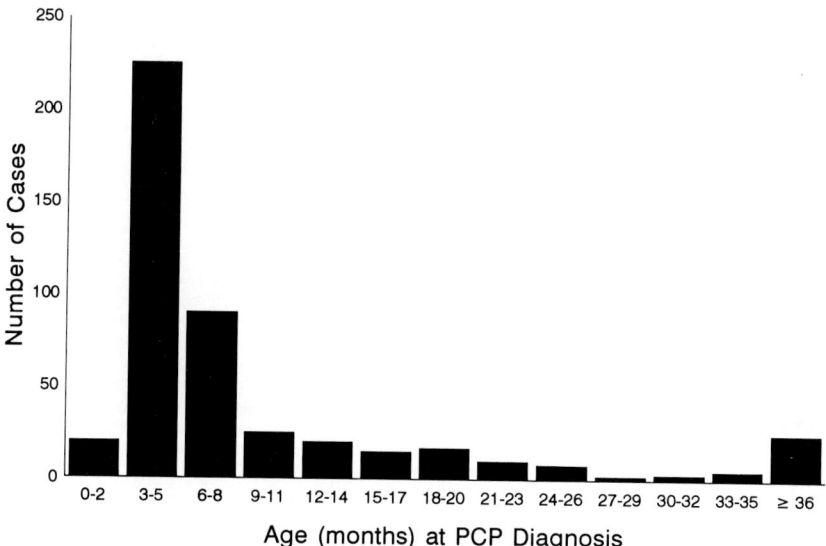

Figure 1 Age at *Pneumocystis carinii* pneumonitis diagnosis for perinatally acquired AIDS cases, for which definitively diagnosed *P. carinii* pneumonitis was the only reported diseases, United States, 1981–1990. $N = 444$ cases. (From Ref. 10.)

CD4 Lymphocyte Count

Studies in adults with HIV infection show a strong predictive value for the CD4 lymphocyte cell count of fewer than 200/mm^3 and the incidence of *P. carinii* pneumonitis, although some cases occur with higher counts (12). However, these data are not applicable to HIV-infected infants. Two studies demonstrate the differences in adult and pediatric cases. In 49 episodes of *P. carinii* pneumonitis in adults, the CD4 lymphocyte cell counts ranged from 1 to 365/mm^3 (13). However, of 22 HIV-infected infants and children with *P. carinii* pneumonitis, 8 (36%) had CD4 lymphocyte-cell counts of more than 450/mm^3 at the time of diagnosis (14). One explanation for this difference is the variation in quantities of lymphocytes between normal infants and adults. Studies have shown that healthy children's CD4 lymphocyte counts are higher than those of adults (15,16). Table 2 provides a guide to the CD4 lymphocyte counts and percentages for healthy individuals. These data are useful in placing the HIV-infected patient in a risk perspective for *P. carinii* pneumonia.

The relation between CD4 lymphocyte counts and the subsequent occurrence of *P. carinii* pneumonitis in HIV-infected infants and children can be appreciated from several studies, although no study has provided the comprehensive and conclusive information desired. Table 3 summarizes these reports and provides a guide to the risk relation of CD4 lymphocyte counts, age, and the occurrence of *P. carinii* pneumonitis (PCP) in HIV-infected infants and children.

Table 2 Age-Adjusted CD4+ Lymphocyte Parameters for Normal, Healthy Children and Adults

	Age				
	1–6 mo	7–12 mo	13–24 mo	25–74 mo	Adults
Number tested	106	28	46	29	327
Absolute CD4+ count					
Median (cells/mm^3)	3211	3128	2601	1668	1027
5–95 percentile (cells/mm^3)	1153–5285	967–5289	739–4463	505–2831	237–1817
Percentage CD4+ cells					
Median (%)	51.6	47.9	45.8	42.1	50.9
5–95 percentile (%)	36.3–67.1	32.8–63.0	31.2–60.4	32.2–52.0	34.7–67.1
CD4/CD8 ratio					
Median	2.2	2.1	2.0	1.4	1.7
5–95 percentile	0.9–3.5	0.8–3.4	0.6–3.4	0.7–2.1	0.4–3.0

Source: Ref. 10.

Table 3 HIV-Infected Children < 1 Year of Age with PCP, by CD4+ Cell Count

Study (Ref.)	No. cases total	CD4+ count (cells/mm^3)		
		< 1000	1000–1499	≥ 1500
Scott et al. (17)	4	3	1	0
Bernstein et al. (18)	10	5	3	2
Leibovitz et al. (14)	15	9	5	1
Sanders-Laufer et al. (19)	9	8	0	1
Connor et al. (20)	13	12	0	1
Kovacs et al. (21)	20	15	3	2
Total (%)	71 (100)	52 (73)	12 (17)	7 (10)

Source: Ref. 10.

For example, approximately three-fourths of children with PCP have CD4 lymphocyte cell counts of fewer than 1000/mm^3.

Prior Episode of Pneumocystis carinii Pneumonitis

Patients who have had one episode of *P. carinii* pneumonitis and recover with treatment are at high risk for a recurrence of the pneumonitis. The incidence of recurrent episodes of the pneumonitis in infants with AIDS has not been precisely established, but at least 40% of adults with AIDS who have recovered from the first episode will have a recurrent episode within 6 months if no prophylactic medication is given.

B. Clinical Features

As with all immunosuppressed patients with *P. carinii* pneumonitis, the predominant clinical features are tachypnea, dyspnea, fever, and cough. The dyspnea may progress to cyanosis. Intercostal retractions occur, and breath sounds are often diminished to auscultation. Rales are usually not audible, but wheezing may occur in some patients.

The onset may be acute or insidious. The acute onset is usually associated with fever and tachypnea. In other cases, the onset is subtle, without fever, and the increase in respiratory rats and shortness of breath progress over the period of a week or so. Connor et al. reported the clinical manifestations of *P. carinii* pneumonitis in 27 children with AIDS (20). Table 4 summarizes their findings at the time of presentation.

Hypoxia is evident as symptoms of dyspnea and tachypnea develop and is almost always evident by blood gas studies by the time diffuse pneumonitis is

Table 4 Findings at Presentation with *Pneumocystis carinii* Pneumonia

Clinical presentation of PCP	Number of cases (%)
Fever	19/24 (79)
Cough	18/21 (86)
Dyspnea	22/25 (88)
Tachypnea	22/25 (88)
Alveolar–arterial gradient > 30 mmHg	21/22 (95)
Elevated lactate dehydrogenase level (mean, 1997 U/L)	10/18 (56)
Hypergammaglobulinemia	17/23 (74)
CD4/CD8 lymphocyte ratio < 1	12/21 (57)
CD4 lymphocyte counts < 400/mm^3	10/17 (59)

Source: Ref. 20.

present in the chest radiograph. The arterial oxygen tension (Pao_2) is usually less than 90 mmHg and the room air alveolar–arterial oxygen pressure gradient is usually elevated with an $A-a(DO_2)$ greater than 30 torr. The arterial carbon dioxide tension ($Paco_2$) is usually within normal limits until terminal phases of the infection.

The chest radiograph shows bilateral diffuse alveolar disease in most cases. The pneumonitis begins in the perihilar area and progresses peripherally. Some atypical forms include lobar and nodular lesions, and occasionally, pleural effusion may be found.

The white blood cell counts are often normal and provide little help with diagnosis.

Several investigators find the serum lactate dehydrogenase (LDH) activity helpful in the management of *P. carinii* pneumonitis, even though the increase encountered is nonspecific and may occur with other types of pneumonia. In the study of Connor et al. (20), only one-half the patients had abnormal LDH values at the time of presentation (see Table 3).

C. Diagnostic Methods

When possible, the same methods used to diagnose *P. carinii* pneumonia in adults and in non-AIDS patients can be applied to infants and children. These include the collection of material from the lower respiratory tract in search of *P. carinii* organisms by bronchoalveolar lavage, induced sputum, tracheal aspirate, transbronchial biopsy, and open-lung biopsy. However, with small children and infants, induced sputum samples are not possible, and bronchoalveolar lavage may not be easily accomplished unless special equipment and a skilled bronchoscopist are available. Birriel et al. (22) found the procedure successful in infants of 3 months of age and older.

The most definitive diagnostic method is by open-lung biopsy by which the type and extent of *P. carinii* infection can be visualized. The major complication is pneumothorax, but bleeding may occur in a few cases. Open-lung biopsy is usually the procedure of choice for infants and small children.

Specimens should be stained with Gomori–Grocott methenamine silver nitrate, toluidine blue O, and Giemsa stains. A fluorescein-labeled monoclonal antibody to *P. carinii* is also useful in the identification of the organism.

V. Extrapulmonary *Pneumocystis carinii* Infection

Extrapulmonary lesions with *P. carinii* have been found primarily in adults and rarely in infants and children. The significance of these lesions and the mechanism by which they occur are unclear. Infected sites reported from all ages include spleen, lymph nodes, bone marrow, pancreas, thymus, retina, appendix, middle ear, mastoid, liver, heart, adrenal glands, kidneys, chorioid, thyroid, and ear (23,24).

VI. Treatment

Trimethoprim–sulfamethoxazole and parenteral pentamidine isethionate are equally effective in the treatment of *P. carinii* pneumonia. Because the adverse effects are less frequent with trimethoprim–sulfamethoxazole than with pentamidine, the former drug is preferred. Patients with AIDS have a higher rate of adverse reactions to either of these drugs than do non-AIDS patients. Usually treatment is initiated with an intravenous dose of 15–20 mg trimethoprim and 75–100 mg sulfamethoxazole per kilogram per day in three or four equally divided doses. Once the disease is under control, and if the patient can easily tolerate oral medication, the trimethoprim–sulfamethoxazole can be changed to the oral route of administration, using the highest aforementioned dose. The therapeutic course is usually about 10 days in non-AIDS patients and 2–3 weeks in children with AIDS. A maculopapular rash and neutropenia are the most frequent of the serious adverse effects.

Intravenous pentamidine is indicated for those patients who do not respond to, or cannot tolerate, trimethoprim–sulfamethoxazole. The dose is 4.0 mg/kg per day, administered as a single dose. If venous access is not available, the same dose can be given by deep intramuscular injection, but injection site reactions may be severe. Other adverse reactions are renal and hepatic toxicity, hypo- or hyperglycemia, rash, and hematological disorders.

The administration of prednisone has been effective in adults with moderate and severe forms of *P. carinii* pneumonitis, but no data are available for children.

The outcome of *P. carinii* is dependent on the extent and type of the underlying disease and the stage of pneumonitis at which treatment is started. In non-AIDS patients with cancer, the mortality rate with treatment is about 25% (7). The mortality rate for infants and children with AIDS and *P. carinii* pneumonitis is about 40% for the episode of the pulmonary infection (18).

VII. Prevention

Chemoprophylaxis is highly effective for the prevention of *P. carinii* pneumonitis and should be used in patients known to be at high risk for this disease. The preferred regimen is trimethoprim–sulfamethoxazole given daily or 3 days per week. The dosage in 5.0 mg trimethoprim and 25 mg sulfamethoxazole per kilogram per day in two equally divided doses.

Certain categories of patients with cancer, organ transplant, congenital immune deficiency disorders, and AIDS should receive prophylaxis for *P. carinii* pneumonitis. Guidelines have been established by an expert task force for the use of chemoprophylaxis in infants and children with AIDS. These recommendations are based on age:

1. Infants 30 days to 12 months of age with mother who is HIV-positive: (a) If CD4 lymphocyte level is unknown, (b) HIV infectivity unknown, or (c) CD4 cells fewer than 1500/mm^2 and HIV seropositive
2. Infants 12–24 months of age and HIV seropositive plus CD4 cells fewer than 750/mm^3
3. Two to 6 years of age and HIV seropositive plus CD4 cells at 500/mm^2 or less
4. Over 6 years of age and HIV seropositive plus CD4 cells fewer than 200/mm^2
5. Any age: prior episode of *P. carinii* pneumonia

For those patients who cannot take trimethoprim–sulfamethoxazole, aerosol pentamidine can be used in children of about 5 years and older. Younger patients may be given dapsone 1.0 mg/kg per dose given orally once daily, not to exceed 200 mg/day. None of the prophylactic regimens have been adequately studied in children.

References

1. Van der Meer G, Brug SL. Infection par Pneumocystis chez l'homme et chez les animaux. Am Soc Belge Med Trop 1942; 22:301–304.
2. Vanek J, Jirovec O, Lukes J. Interstitial plasma cell pneumonia in infants. Ann Paediatr 1953; 180:1–10.

3. Pifer LL, Hughes WT, Stagno S, Woods D. *Pneumocystis carinii* infection: evidence for high prevalence in normal and immunosuppressed children. Pediatrics 1978; 61: 35–40.
4. Meuwissen JHET, Tanker I, Leeuwenberg ADEM, Beckers PJA, Sieben M. Parasitology and serologic observation of infection with *Pneumocystis carinii* in humans. J Infect Dis 1977; 136:43–48.
5. Kovacs JA, Halpern JL, Swan JC, Mass J, Parrillo JE, Masur H. Identification of antigens and antibodies specific for *Pneumocystis carinii*. J Immunol 1988; 140: 2023–2031.
6. Gajdusek DC. *Pneumocystis carinii*—etiologic agent of interstitial plasma cell pneumonia or premature and young infants. Pediatrics 1957; 19:543–565.
7. Hughes WT. *Pneumocystis carinii* Pneumonitis. Vol. 2. Boca Raton: CRC Press, 1987:1–34.
8. Leggiadro RJ, Winkelstein JA, Hughes WT. Prevalence of *Pneumocystis carinii* pneumonitis in severe combined immunodeficiency. J Pediatr 1981; 88:96–98.
9. Walzer PD, Perl DP, Krogstad DJ, Rawson PG, Schultz MG. *Pneumocystis carinii* pneumonia in the United States: epidemiologic, diagnostic and clinical features. Ann Intern Med 1974; 80:83–89.
10. Centers for Disease Control. Guidelines for prophylaxis against *P. carinii* pneumonia for children infected with human immunodeficiency virus. MMWR 1991; 40:1–13.
11. Beach RS, Garcia ER, Sosa R, Good RA. *Pneumocystis carinii* pneumonia in a humans immunodeficiency virus 1-infected neonate with meconium aspiration. Pediatr Infect Dis J 1991; 10:953–955.
12. Phair J, Monoz A, Detels R, Kaslo R, Rinaldo C, Saah A, and multicenter AIDS cohort study group. The risk of *Pneumocystis carinii* pneumonia among men infected with human immunodeficiency virus type 1. N Engl J Med 1990; 322:161–165.
13. Centers for Disease Control. Guidelines for prophylaxis against *Pneumocystis carinii* pneumonia for persons infected with human immunodeficiency virus. MMWR 1989; 38:1–9.
14. Leibovitz E, Rigaud M, Pollack H, Lawrence R, Cahdwani S, Krasinoki K, Borkowsky W. *Pneumocystis carinii* pneumonia in infants infected with the human immunodeficiency virus with more than 450 CD4 T lymphocytes per cubic multimeter. N Engl J Med 1990; 323:531–535.
15. Denny T, Yogev R, Gelman R, Skuza C, Oleske J, Chadwick E, Cheng S-C, Connor E. Lymphocyte subsets in healthy children during the first 5 years of life. JAMA 1992; 267:1384–1488.
16. Giorgi JV. Lymphocyte subset measurements: significance in clinical medicine. In: Rose NR, Friedman H, Fahey JL, eds. The Manual of Clinical Laboratory Immunology. Washington DC: American Society for Microbiology, 1986:236–246.
17. Scott G, Buck BE, Leterman JG, Bloom FL, Parks WP. Acquired immunodeficiency syndrome in infants. N Engl J Med 1984; 310:76–81.
18. Bernstein LJ, Bye MR, Rubinstein A. Prognostic factors and life expectancy in children with acquired immunodeficiency syndrome and *Pneumocystis carinii* pneumonia. Am J Dis Child 1989; 143:775–778.
19. Sanders-Laufer D, Burroughs M, Marshall F, Blankenship C, Hinds G, Noel GJ,

Edelson PJ. *Pneumocystis carinii* pneumonia (PCP) in "low-risk" HIV infected children [abstract 1080]. Pediatr Res 1990; 27:183a.
20. Connor E, Garaazzi M, McSherry G, Holland B, Boland M, Denny T, Oleske J. Clinical and laboratory correlates of *Pneumocystis carinii* pneumonia in children infected with HIV. JAMA 1991; 265:1693–1697.
21. Kovacs A, Frederick T, Church J, Eller A, Oxtoby M, Mascola L. CD4 T-lymphocyte counts and *Pneumocystis carinii* pneumonia in pediatric HIV infection. JAMA 1991; 265:1698–1703.
22. Birriel JA, Adams JA, Saldana MA, Mavunda K, Goldfinger S, Vernon D, Holzman B, McKay RM. Role of flexible bronchoscopy and bronchoalveolar lavages in the diagnosis of pediatric acquired immunodeficiency syndrome-related pulmonary disease. Pediatrics 1991; 87:897–899.
23. Cohen OJ, Stoeckle MY. Extrapulmonary *Pneumocystis carinii* infections in the acquired immunodeficiency syndrome. Arch Intern Med 1991; 151:1205–1214.
24. Raviglione MC. Extrapulmonary pneumocystosis: the first 50 cases. Rev Infect Dis 1990; 12:1127–1138.

17

Clinical Manifestations in Adults

MICHAEL N. DOHN and PETER T. FRAME

University of Cincinnati College of Medicine
Cincinnati, Ohio

I. Introduction

The clinical presentation of active disease caused by *Pneumocystis carinii* is often subtle. A high index of suspicion when treating patients at risk is necessary to pursue the making of a definitive diagnosis. Early diagnosis by demonstration of *P. carinii* organisms in biopsies or clinical specimens, with prompt therapy initiation, can improve the prognosis and reduce the severity of complications associated with *P. carinii* pneumonia.

In this chapter, we will discuss clinical issues involved with *P. carinii* pneumonia in adults. We will consider the populations at risk for development of acute pneumonia and the differences in clinical presentations that have been noted between human immunodeficiency virus (HIV)-infected patients and those who are not HIV-infected. Also discussed are laboratory tests that have been proposed for evaluation and follow-up of *P. carinii* pneumonia, and their possible initial prognostic significance. The clinical course of patients treated for pneumonia, and possible complications, are included later in the chapter.

Although we will touch on many topics that are covered in more detail elsewhere in this book, it is our intent to provide within this chapter information that will be of assistance to the clinician and of interest to the basic scientist concerning *P. carinii* pneumonia.

II. Risk Groups for *Pneumocystis carinii* Pneumonia

A. Overview

Although mistaking it for a variant of *Trypanosome cruzi*, Chagas gave the first pathological description of a lung infection with *P. carinii* in guinea pigs (1). A clinical respiratory syndrome occurring in children in Europe and Asia led to the realization that *P. carinii* could cause disease in humans. The recognition that the disease in these children was the same as observed by Chagas in guinea pigs (2) was followed by identification of *P. carinii* as the causative organism (3). Malnutrition is a risk factor for development of clinical disease caused by *P. carinii* (4–6) and was a likely factor in these early recognized cases. Epidemics of *P. carinii* occurred in Central Europe from the close of World War II through the 1950s, when the general health and nutritional status improved (7). Reports of sporadic disease, representing the endemic rate of clinical disease from *P. carinii*, began to appear in the mid-1950s and demonstrated a worldwide distribution. These reports are well catalogued by Burke and Good (8).

Before the acquired immunodeficiency syndrome (AIDS) epidemic, *P. carinii* pneumonia was a low-incidence disease in the United States, with fewer than 100 cases annually (9). The affected populations were preponderantly patients with advanced malignancy or those receiving immunosuppressive therapy (8–12). An increase in the incidence of *P. carinii* pneumonia was one of the first signs of the beginning of the AIDS epidemic in the United States (13,14). Investigation of these patients led to the identification of the now well-known cellular immunodeficiency caused by human immunodeficiency virus (HIV)-infection (15–17). It has been estimated that the number of cases of *P. carinii* pneumonia in AIDS patients may exceed an average of 50,000 annually (18,19). Although the common factor among these groups is immunosuppression related to T-lymphocyte dysfunction, occasional reports of the occurrence of *P. carinii* pneumonia in adults without any known preexisting immunosuppression have also appeared. In the following paragraphs, risk groups who are not HIV-infected are discussed first, followed by the rare reports of disease in adults without predisposing conditions. Consideration is then turned to the HIV-infected population.

B. Non–Human Immunodeficiency Virus-Infected, Immunosuppressed Patients

Among individuals not infected with HIV, 98% of those who develop *P. carinii* pneumonia have an immunodeficiency disorder, received immunosuppressive therapy, or received cytotoxic therapy (9). The highest incidence rates are in children; among adults, those in the 50- to 59-year-old age range have the highest incidence (9). Before the AIDS epidemic, Hodgkin's disease and renal transplantation were the conditions most associated with *P. carinii* pneumonia in younger adults; in older adults, chronic lymphatic leukemia was the most associated underlying condition (9).

Adult patients receiving intensive cytotoxic chemotherapy for malignancy or immunosuppressive therapy for a variety of conditions continue to be at increased risk. Therapy for different types of solid tumors can predispose patients to development of *P. carinii* pneumonia (8,9,20–22). Symptoms often develop in patients receiving corticosteroid therapy while it is being tapered or just after it is discontinued, which is a well-recognized pattern (8,9,20,22). Endogenous production of corticosteroids also can predispose to *P. carinii* pneumonia, and cases are reported in patients with Cushing's syndrome, especially when morning cortisol levels exceed 120 μg/dL (3300 nmol/liter) (23). Patients receiving cytotoxic therapy and corticosteroids for connective tissue disease are also at risk (9,24–26).

Patients immunosuppressed after organ or bone marrow transplantation constitute another risk group. The greatest experience has followed renal transplantation. Immunosuppression using cyclosporine in place of azathioprine resulted in almost a tripling of the rate of *P. carinii* pneumonia after renal transplantation at one center (27). However, immunosuppressive regimens after renal transplantation commonly employ corticosteroids, and it is difficult to separate the effects of the individual drugs. Other series do not demonstrate an increased risk of *P. carinii* pneumonia with cyclosporine use after renal transplantation (28–30), and some show lower overall mortality related to infections in patients receiving lower doses of steroids (30). Another apparent clustering of *P. carinii* pneumonia cases in renal transplant patients (31) has lead to speculation that the previously reported cluster of *P. carinii* pneumonias was fortuitously observed in conjunction with the change to a regimen containing cyclosporine (32). In heart transplantation, there was a lower incidence of acute *P. carinii* pneumonia associated with cyclosporine compared with conventional immunosuppression using azathioprine (33). Among a group of patients after heart–lung transplantation, *P. carinii* organisms were found in bronchoalveolar lavage fluid, with a reported prevalence rate of 88% (34). In 41% of these cases, the patients were asymptomatic when the *P. carinii* was found. Cyclosporine does not apparently predispose to *P. carinii* infection after liver transplantation (35). Infection can occur after bone marrow transplantation if there is an interruption in prophylactic therapy against *P. carinii* (36).

Protein and calorie malnutrition is a recognized cause of immunosuppression (4–6). Malnutrition has a number of effects. Both quantitative changes with fewer circulating T lymphocytes and qualitative changes in response to lymphocyte stimulation tests occur (6). Some of these qualitative defects reverse with

immunosuppressing factor sufficient to increase the risk of *P. carinii* pneumonia in children. Malnutrition may also be contributing to the development of *P. carinii* pneumonia in adult patients. Nutrition is frequently suboptimal in these adult patients who are being treated with immunosuppressive therapy, and attention should be directed toward their nutritional support.

In some predisposing conditions, the timing of *P. carinii* pneumonia can be predicted. As noted earlier, the tapering or discontinuation of steroid therapy is often associated with the onset of symptoms. Following bone marrow transplantation, the median time until clinical infection is 9 weeks (37).

C. "Normal Hosts"

The occurrence of fatal *P. carinii* pneumonia demonstrated at autopsy in a set of parents after a prolonged, undiagnosed respiratory illness in their 7-year-old daughter raised the question of the development of clinical disease in a normal adult host after person-to-person spread from a possible symptomatic primary infection in a child (38). Although the father had acute lymphocytic leukemia in remission, the mother had no known predisposing conditions. Other adults with *P. carinii* pneumonia and without any known predisposing immunodeficiency have been described (39–43). One of the larger series is a cluster of five elderly patients diagnosed with *P. carinii* pneumonia within a 3-month period at one institution (44). Quantitative study of peripheral blood mononuclear cells from three of these patients were normal; however, qualitative studies showed a functional decrease in T-cell activity. The small number of *P. carinii* organisms demonstrated in these patients and their atypical clinical courses have caused some to question the accuracy of the diagnoses (45–47). Three patients with quantitative and qualitative T-cell defects of unknown origin had documented *P. carinii* pneumonia successfully treated (48). Two of these patients were elderly (but one was 30 years old), and none of them had other serious concurrent disease. Although it appears to be possible for previously healthy adults to contract symptomatic *P. carinii* pneumonia, it would still seem to be a rare event and to be associated with qualitative defects in T- cell function.

D. Human Immunodeficiency Virus-Infected Patients

Individuals infected with HIV represent the most susceptible group of patients in whom *P. carinii* pneumonia occurs. Early in the AIDS epidemic, more than 60% of patients presented with *P. carinii* pneumonia (49), and more than 80% of patients were estimated to have at least one episode of *P. carinii* during their clinical courses (50,51). The risk of the contraction of symptomatic *P. carinii* pneumonia is directly related to the degree of immunosuppression produced by the HIV infection (52–54). With the CD4 lymphocyte count per cubic millimeter or the percentage of circulating lymphocytes that are CD4-positive as a marker of immunosuppression, AIDS patients who develop an initial episode of *P. carinii* pneumonia have a median CD4 count fewer than 50 and a median CD4 percentage less than 5% (Fig. 1). In the absence of prophylactic therapy, the cumulative incidence of *P. carinii* pneumonia for individuals with baseline CD4 counts of fewer than or equal to 200 is 8.4% at 6 months, 18.4% at 12 months, and 33.3% at 36 months (54). Most patients with CD4 counts higher than 200 who develop *P. carinii* pneumonia within 6 months are symptomatic from the HIV infection, particularly with fever or oral candidiasis; fever and oral candidiasis function as independent risk factors for *P. carinii* pneumonia in individuals with fewer than 200 CD4 cells (54). Also for those patients with CD4 counts of fewer than 200, symptoms of persistent fatigue and unintentional weight loss contribute to the risk of developing pneumonia (54). In general, individuals with HIV infection are at risk of developing *P. carinii* pneumonia when the CD4 count is fewer than 200 or when there are symptoms of HIV disease (particularly thrush and fever) at whatever level of CD4 cell depletion.

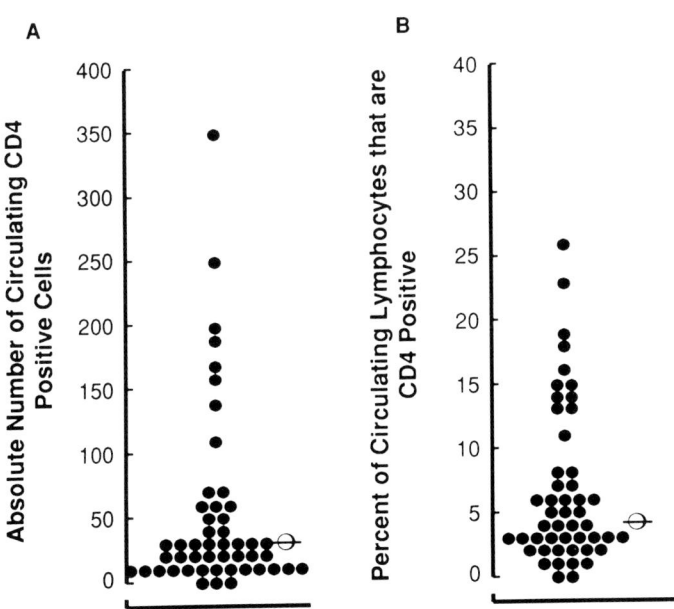

Figure 1 *Pneumocystis carinii* pneumonia and the degree of immunosuppression in AIDS. Both (A) and (B) show values obtained within 60 days of the diagnosis of *P. carinii* pneumonia. Each solid circle represents one *P. carinii* pneumonia diagnosis. Median values are shown by the open circle. (A) Distribution of absolute CD4 counts. (B) Distribution of CD4-positive cells as a percentage of circulating lymphocytes. (Adapted with permission from Masur H, et al. CD4 counts as predictors of opportunistic pneumonias in human immunodeficiency virus (HIV) infection. Ann Intern Med 1989; 111:223–231.)

Pneumocystis carinii has apparently been a less prevalent pathogen among HIV-infected populations outside of North America and Europe. The high prevalence of *Mycobacterium tuberculosis* in Africa alters the observed patterns of opportunistic diseases. For instance, *M. tuberculosis* is a cause of death four times more frequently than *P. carinii* in West Africa (55).

Just as for other immunosuppressed patients, malnutrition may be contributing to poor T-lymphocyte function (4–6). The correlation of low albumin values with a poorer prognosis for AIDS patients with *P. carinii* pneumonia suggests that malnutrition is a factor (56–58). For these patients, whether malnutrition is adding to the immunosuppression or simply related to the severity of the underlying disease is uncertain.

E. Transmission Among Risk Groups

The epidemiology of *P. carinii* infection is discussed in detail in Chapters 7 and 8, however a few comments are pertinent here. Because it is still unclear in humans whether clinical disease from *P. carinii* is reactivation or reinfection, there is concern about the spread of disease to an immunosuppressed patient from someone who has active pneumonia. Evidence suggesting person-to-person transmission has come from outbreaks among malnourished infants at orphanages and in immunosuppressed patients at some institutions (59–61). With the higher prevalence of *P. carinii* pneumonia since the AIDS epidemic, some reports have noted an increasing incidence of disease in other risk groups (62,63). Increases in *P. carinii*-specific IgG antibody occurs in immunocompetent persons after exposure to an individual with acute *P. carinii* pneumonia, suggesting that person-to-person spread may occur (64). Although the data are limited, we isolate patients with acute *P. carinii* pneumonia from other immunocompromised patients and recommend this action as a prudent measure for infection control (64,65).

III. Clinical Presentation and Markers for Disease Severity and Prognosis

A. Clinical History, Signs, Symptoms, and Differences with Human Immunodeficiency Virus Status

The clinical presentation of *P. carinii* pneumonia is characterized by increasing dyspnea. Dyspnea may occur only with exertion initially, but may progress to the point it occurs with talking or at rest. The mechanism of dyspnea is probably related to hypoxemia produced when alveoli are filled with *P. carinii* organisms and their related exudate. Fevers and cough are also common in both patients with and without HIV infection (66). The cough is usually nonproductive, but some patients have sputum (9,66). Presenting symptoms also can include chest tightness or pain (sometimes related to a pneumothorax) and hemoptysis (9,16,66–68).

Physical findings may include fine crackles with advanced disease, but the pulmonary examination is most frequently normal (9,18).

However, there are differences in the clinical presentation of *P. carinii* pneumonia, depending on the patient's HIV status (66,69,70). In non–HIV-infected populations, the onset of symptoms may be followed within days by severe dyspnea and hypoxemia. For adults with immunosuppression unrelated to HIV, the median duration from onset of symptoms until diagnosis is in the range of 5–10 days, compared with a median of 25 or more days in AIDS patients (Fig. 2) (66,69). Whereas AIDS patients have a more prolonged and insidious development of clinical disease, they have better oxygenation and smaller alveolar-to-arterial oxygen differences at the time of diagnosis than patients with other causes of immunosuppression (66,70). Findings in bronchoalveolar lavage fluid from AIDS patients include a larger number of *P. carinii* organisms, but less lung inflammation, with fewer neutrophils than in non–HIV-infected patients with *P. carinii* pneumonia (71).

Among historical and clinical factors that can be determined at the time of admission to the hospital with *P. carinii* pneumonia, some are related to prognosis.

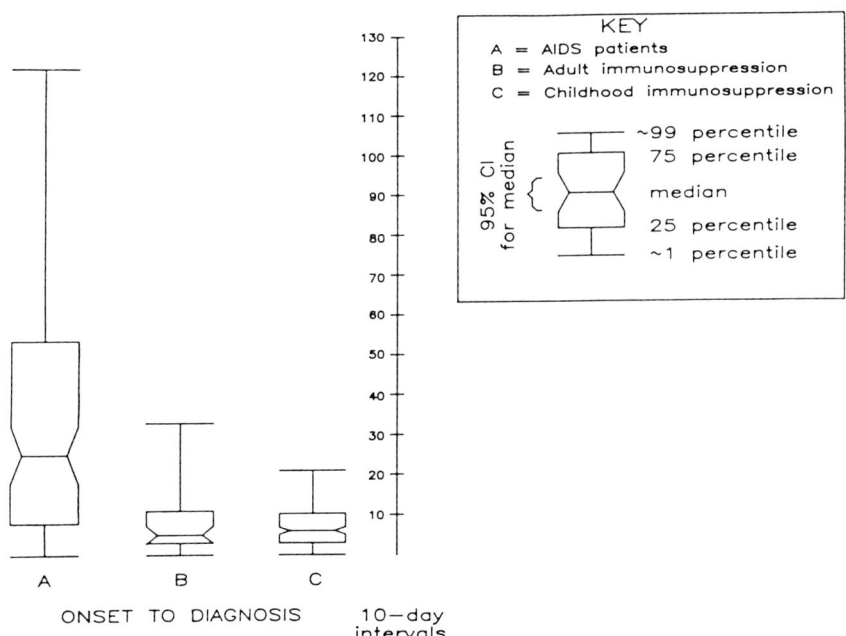

Figure 2 Lengths of time from onset of symptoms to diagnosis of *P. carinii* pneumonia for three different patient groups. (Adapted from Ref. 69.)

A normal respiratory rate and normal lung examination are good prognostic signs (56). Patients with AIDS who have prior hospitalizations, who enter the hospital through the emergency department, or who are admitted after transfer from another facility have higher mortality (72,73).

Although bacterial pneumonia will worsen the prognosis (56), concurrent cytomegalovirus pneumonia probably does not adversely effect the outcome of *P. carinii* pneumonia in AIDS patients (74–77). In fact, a generally less severe clinical course during treatment for *P. carinii* pneumonia is observed in patients with concurrent cytomegalovirus infection (78). A decreased inflammatory response has been hypothesized to occur when both pathogens are present.

In general, the presence or severity of specific symptoms do not consistently relate to whether or not patients survive the acute episode (66). However, APACHE II scores do correlate with survival and response to therapy for an acute episode of *P. carinii* pneumonia (58), although underestimating the mortality of patients requiring mechanical ventilation for respiratory failure (79).

Previous episodes of *P. carinii* pneumonia have also been a poor prognostic sign. For example, early in the AIDS epidemic in a contemporaneous group of patients with *P. carinii* pneumonia, whose overall survival was 77%, the subgroup of patients with a second episode had only 59% survival (69). Second and subsequent episodes of *P. carinii* came to be regarded as having a poorer prognosis than initial episodes (51,80). However, our experience at the University of Cincinnati before the use of adjunctive corticosteroids from 1986 through 1990 did not show a significant difference among the survival rates of first, second, and third episodes, which were 85, 84, and 88%, respectively (Fig. 3) (81).

B. Clinical Tests

A variety of tests have been proposed as helpful in the diagnosis and the determination of the prognosis in *P. carinii* pneumonia. Diagnosis, which is discussed in detail in Chapter 19, ultimately depends on the demonstration of *P. carinii* organisms in biological samples. However, the prognosis depends on the severity of the pneumonia, and the underlying or concurrent illnesses. The most consistently reproducible clinical tests demonstrating prognostic value at the time of diagnosis of *P. carinii* pneumonia are measures of hypoxemia.

Hypoxemia, often expressed as the alveolar-to-arterial oxygen difference (P_A–aO_2), has generally been the best prognostic test (82,83). Room air arterial blood gas evaluations (ABG) are often performed as part of the routine assessment of patients with respiratory complaints and, thus, are readily available for use. Lower arterial oxygen pressures on an ABG at the time of diagnosis have a poorer prognosis (56). Higher initial P_A–aO_2 values (especially greater than 30 mmHg) are correlated with higher mortality during the acute treatment period (66,82–85). The room air P_A–aO_2 has evolved as a convenient standard to classify acute

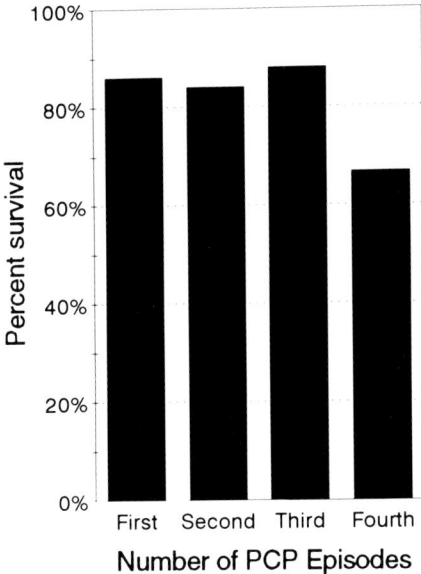

Figure 3 Survival rates of acute *P. carinii* pneumonia by episode number. Survival rates for first, second, and third episodes are not significantly different (Chi square 0.287, $p = 0.87$). The number of patients for each episode are: 143 first, 55 second, 17 third, and 6 fourth. Abbreviations: PCP indicates *P. carinii* pneumonia. (Adapted from Arch Intern Med, December 1992; 152:2465–2470. Copyright 1992, American Medical Association.)

episodes of *P. carinii* pneumonia into mild ($P_A-a_{O_2}$, <35), moderate ($P_A-a_{O_2}$, 36–45), and severe ($P_A-a_{O_2}$, >45) categories, which can be used clinically, such as in the decision to give adjunctive steroid therapy (86). Other methods to quantitate the degree of hypoxemia (such as the hypoxemia ratio) are used in some studies (87), but the room air $P_A-a_{O_2}$ is preferable as a more generally recognizable and representative measurement.

With recurrent *P. carinii* pneumonia, there is a trend for the patients to present with milder disease as categorized by the $P_A-a_{O_2}$. At the University of Cincinnati Medical Center, from 1986 through 1990, a larger proportion of patients with acute *P. carinii* pneumonia presented with mild disease by the $P_A-a_{O_2}$ in second and third episodes than initial episodes (Table 1). Hypothetical reasons for this pattern are multiple. Closer medical follow-up of patients now known to be HIV-positive after an initial episode of *P. carinii* pneumonia could contribute to earlier diagnosis of another acute problem, such as a subsequent *P. carinii* pneumonia episode (82). Also, patients may recognize the development of the same symptoms as accompanied their first episode of pneumonia and present for evaluation with milder disease. Prophylaxis for *P. carinii* pneumonia may also be playing a role by modifying the development of incubating disease and allowing earlier diagnosis when the pneumonia is less fulminant.

Related to the pathophysiology of hypoxemia, evaluations of the change in oxygenation with exercise (88,89) and of the diffusing capacity (90–93) have

Table 1 Initial Arterial Blood Gas Evaluations in *P. carinii* Pneumonia

Episode	Initial RA ABG available	$P_{A-a}O_2$ (torr)			
Order (*n*)	*n* (%)	Mean (SD)	≤ 35[a]	> 35–> 45	≥ 45
First (143)	110 (77%)	43.0 (16.7)	36 (33%)	24 (22%)	50 (45%)
Second (55)	43 (78%)	31.6 (15.0)	23 (53%)[b]	13 (30%)	7 (16%)
Third (17)	14 (82%)	32.2 (20.2)	9 (64%)[b]	2 (14%)	3 (21%)
Fourth (6)	5 (83%)	28.0 (10.5)	4 (80%)	1 (20%)	0
Fifth (1)	0				

[a]Shown as *n* (%), where *n* is the number of patients in that $P_{A-a}O_2$ group and the percent is of the total patients in that episode with room air arterial blood gas evaluations.
[b]Significantly larger proportions of patients had mild disease in second and third episodes compared with first episode (Chi square 15.1, $p = 0.0046$).
Abbreviations: RA ABG, room air arterial blood gas evaluation; $P_{A-a}O_2$, alveolar-to-arterial oxygen tension difference.
Source: Arch Intern Med, Dec 1992; 152:2465–2470. Copyright 1992, American Medical Association.

shown diagnostic, but not prognostic, usefulness. A decrease of 5 mmHg or more in the $P_{A-a}O_2$ with a simple exercise test excluded *P. carinii* pneumonia from the differential diagnosis in one study (89). Nearly all AIDS patients with *P. carinii* pneumonia have an abnormal diffusing capacity; all 14 patients in one series had a diffusing capacity less than 70% of predicted, and 54 of 55 patients in another series had an abnormal diffusing capacity (92,93). While being sensitive, the diffusing capacity is not specific and may be abnormal for a number of reasons, unrelated to *P. carinii* pneumonia. However, in patients with a normal ABG, an abnormal diffusing capacity may direct the clinician to pursue further studies.

The lactate dehydrogenase (LDH) level has been studied extensively in *P. carinii* pneumonia (56,58,84,85,94–98). From blood and bronchoalveolar lavage fluid from AIDS patients with *P. carinii* pneumonia, comparison of LDH isoenzyme levels suggests that LDH produced in the lung is selectively filtered by the alveolar–capillary membrane before appearing in the serum (95). The LDH levels are higher in *P. carinii* pneumonia than in other respiratory conditions. Survivors of acute *P. carinii* pneumonia have lower LDH levels than those who die of the acute episode. For patients successfully treated, serial LDH levels decrease during therapy; therapeutic failure produces steady or increasing LDH levels as treatment progresses. The overlap of LDH levels (between individuals with and without *P. carinii* pneumonia, and between survivors and nonsurvivors of *P. carinii* pneumonia) is sufficiently large that considerable caution must be used in the interpretation of an LDH level for a particular patient (94,96). However, LDH elevations are highly sensitive, high levels are moderately specific in the correct clinical setting, and low values have a high negative predictive value when used in the diagnosis of acute *P. carinii* pneumonia; in addition, they provide prognostic information and, through serial sampling, a method to check for treatment efficacy and disease resolution.

The radiographic presentation of *P. carinii* pneumonia can be quite variable (99), and is discussed in detail in Chapter 21. The pattern of a diffuse interstitial infiltrate is most common, but atypical patterns occur frequently, including pleural effusions, cavities, pneumatoceles, and nodules. Patients with *P. carinii* pneumonia may also have a normal chest radiograph, which is a good prognostic sign (100). Any HIV-infected individual who presents with a pneumothorax should have *P. carinii* pneumonia excluded as the cause (67). The severity of abnormalities on the initial chest radiograph are prognostic. When findings are graded on a scale from normal to extensive interstitial and alveolar infiltrates, there is a correlation between the worsening chest radiograph findings and higher mortality (82). Not surprisingly, there is also a correlation between the severity of abnormalities on the chest radiograph and the P_A-aO_2.

Other tests have been associated, either singly or in combinations, with a poorer outcome in AIDS patients with *P. carinii* pneumonia. These tests include leukocytosis (56), decreased total lymphocyte count (57), decreased hemoglobin values (57), decreased serum albumin level (56–58), and bronchoalveolar lavage fluid neutrophilia (71,85,101,102). A larger number of *P. carinii* organisms recovered by bronchoalveolar lavage correlates with higher P_A-aO_2 and higher LDH levels (103), and is associated with a higher mortality (104).

Among the more novel tests used for diagnosis and prognostication have been angiotensin-converting enzyme (ACE) levels, anticardiolipin antibodies, total thyroxine (T_4) levels, total triiodothyronine (T_3) levels, and serum carcinoembryonic antigen (CEA).

The ACE levels are higher in patients with acute *P. carinii* pneumonia than in normal controls (105–106) and are highest in smokers with acute *P. carinii* pneumonia (105). Although apparently sensitive, elevations of ACE levels are nonspecific, having also been reported in *Mycobacterium avium-intracellulare* infection and Kaposi's sarcoma.

An initial report showed anticardiolipin antibodies to be very specific for *P. carinii* infection and stated that no positive assays were found in 14 AIDS patients with other opportunistic infections (107). The anticardiolipin antibody positivity is postulated to arise from shared determinants between *P. carinii* and cardiolipin (108). However, other researchers have not been able to reproduce the original results and conclude that anticardiolipin antibodies have no diagnostic value (109).

Thyroid hormone indices are known to have predictive value in seriously ill patients. Decreased total T_3 and T_4 levels were correlated with higher mortality from acute *P. carinii* pneumonia in AIDS patients in one study (57). Of a number of laboratory factors examined in this study, the T_3 was the best single predictor of acute mortality.

The CEA levels are higher in AIDS patients with *P. carinii* pneumonia than in those with another cause of pneumonia or a nonpulmonary infection (110). Among patients with *P. carinii* pneumonia, CEA levels are higher in those with a $P_{A}-a_{O_2}$ greater than 50 mmHg. Among these sicker patients, the CEA levels were significantly different between survivors and nonsurvivors, even though the initial mean arterial oxygen pressures and LDH levels were not different.

Some estimation of oxygenation is often done as part of the usual clinical evaluation of patients with respiratory disease. Considering how rapidly ABG results can be available for clinical decision-making (and the ease with which an $P_{A}-a_{O_2}$ can be calculated), it is unlikely that other blood tests will replace measures of oxygenation as the primary initial test with prognostic significance. An ABG is necessary for accurate classification of a patient as mild, moderate, or severe disease for purposes of determining the need for adjunctive corticosteroid therapy for treatment of *P. carinii* pneumonia (86). With the demonstration that adjunctive corticosteroid therapy decreases mortality (87,111), it is now uncertain how well any of the foregoing described tests can still predict mortality. However, it seems likely that the ABG with a calculated $P_{A}-a_{O_2}$ will remain the most commonly obtained initial test with clinical and prognostic usefulness. Among the available clinical tests, we routinely use only the initial room air ABG to guide clinical decision-making, and repeat ABGs (along with the chest x-ray film) to follow the patient's clinical course.

C. Influence of Clinical Experience with Acquired Immunodeficiency Syndrome Patients

In addition to test results, the prognosis for the outcome of an acute episode of *P. carinii* pneumonia in an AIDS patient is affected by the familiarity of the treating facility with HIV-related disease. Bennett and co-workers classified 15 hospitals as either high or low AIDS familiarity (7 and 8, respectively) based on whether there were more or less than 30 AIDS-related discharge diagnoses per 10,000 hospital discharges (72,73). There was a significant relation between AIDS experience and mortality from *P. carinii* pneumonia. After adjusting for severity, the chances of dying in a low AIDS familiarity hospital were about 3.6 times higher than in a high-familiarity hospital (95% CI 1.9–6.3). Although average charges and resource use in the care of patients with *P. carinii* pneumonia did not differ between the two categories of institutions, the pattern of resource use was different. High-familiarity hospitals tended to apply resources earlier and more aggressively.

D. Recurrence and Long-term Prognosis

Some measurements taken as part of the evaluation of an episode of *P. carinii* pneumonia have prognostic significance beyond the acute episode itself. There are factors that are correlated with early recurrence of *P. carinii* pneumonia and with long-term prognosis.

Following an initial episode of *P. carinii* pneumonia, AIDS patients are at risk of recurrent pneumonia. Early in the epidemic, an initial episode was followed within 18 months by subsequent episodes of *P. carinii* pneumonia in more than 60% of AIDS patients (112,113). Prophylaxis therapy for *P. carinii* pneumonia has cut this recurrence rate substantially (81,112,114,115). Our experience has been that another episode of *P. carinii* pneumonia can be prevented equally well after either a first or a second episode (Fig. 4).

However, even among AIDS patients who are apparently successfully treated for an acute episode, there may be early recurrences within 6 months. Following successful therapy for pneumonia, *P. carinii* organisms can still be found by bronchoscopy up to 35 days or more (116). Although the finding of any

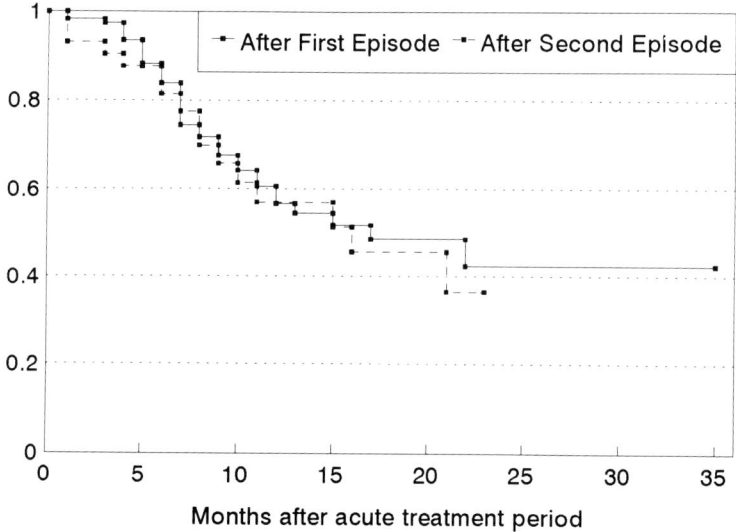

Figure 4 The probability of remaining free of a recurrence after successful therapy of acute *P. carinii* pneumonia. The probability of being free of recurrence is shown for 121 patients after a first episode (solid line) and 44 patients after a second episode (dashed line). The two groups are not significantly different for the probability of recurrence of PCP ($p = 0.62$). The number of evaluable patients drops below 10 in month 20 for the first episode group and in month 15 for the second episode group. (From Arch Intern Med, December 1992; 152:2465–2470. Copyright 1992, American Medical Association.)

residual *P. carinii* organisms at follow-up bronchoscopy is not predictive of early recurrence (82), applying a semiquantitative technique to estimate the organism burden in bronchoalveolar lavage fluid can define a high-risk group for early recurrence. By using the estimate of *P. carinii* burden at the time of diagnosis as the baseline, patients who have less than a 50% clearance of organisms at the end of therapy are at increased risk of early recurrence of disease (117). This method of staining and semiquantitation cannot distinguish between viable *P. carinii* organisms and those that are dead; nevertheless, it is a quick and reproducible technique providing clinically useful information.

Decreased long-term survival after an episode of *P. carinii* pneumonia is correlated with the severity of the illness at presentation, as reflected in the degree of interstitial edema on transbronchial lung biopsy and elevation of the $P_A-a_{O_2}$ (82). Persistence of *P. carinii* cysts in the lung on follow-up evaluation after 3 weeks of therapy is also a poor long-term prognostic sign (82). However, overall the long-term prognosis after an initial episode of *P. carinii* pneumonia in HIV-infected individuals has improved. For patients having a first episode of *P. carinii* pneumonia, 1-year survival increased from 33% in 1981 to 48% by 1985, during a period before the use of antiretroviral therapy or *P. carinii* pneumonia prophylaxis in this patient population (118). For our 1986–1990 cohort of AIDS patients,

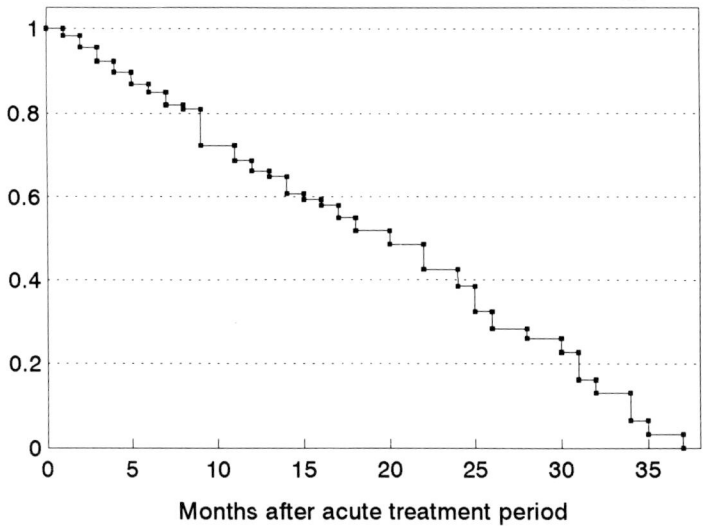

Figure 5 The probability of survival after a first episode of *P. carinii* pneumonia. Of 121 original patients, the number of evaluable patients drops below 20 during month 25 and below 10 in month 28. (From Arch Intern Med, December 1992; 152:2465–2470. Copyright 1992, American Medical Association.)

(Fig. 5). Similar improved estimates of 1-year survival come from another contemporaneous series in which *P. carinii* pneumonia was not a predictor of either the short-term or long-term mortality in multivariate analysis of HIV-infected patients with atypical pneumonia (78).

IV. Clinical Course of *Pneumocystis carinii* Pneumonia

A. Natural Course, Treated Course, and "Treatment Failure"

Serological studies demonstrate that *P. carinii* infection occurs in immunocompetent people (119–121); if there is a self-limited clinical syndrome that accompanies such infections, it is unrecognized. A small prospective serology study of immunocompetent people exposed to an active case of *P. carinii* pneumonia shows that their *P. carinii*-specific IgG antibody increases significantly compared with controls (implying that an infection occurred sufficient for an antibody response) without any clinical disease noted (64). Unlike immunocompetent hosts, the natural course of clinical *P. carinii* pneumonia in immunosuppressed patients is progressive dyspnea and hypoxemia, resulting in death by suffocation.

The AIDS epidemic has dramatically increased experience with the treated course of *P. carinii* pneumonia. Therapy is covered in detail in other portions of this book, but a few comments are offered here. The efficacy of therapy for *P. carinii* pneumonia is equal for patients with and without HIV infection. However, in contrast with non–HIV-infected patients, those with AIDS have more therapy-related adverse effects, and survivors may take a longer time until defervescence and to show radiographic improvement (66,69). Also noted have been the longer durations of therapy for AIDS patients.

Patients who are not responding to antipneumocystis therapy warrant investigation for other pulmonary diseases. Approximately half of these patients have continuing *P. carinii* pneumonia found at repeat bronchoscopy as the cause of the continuing symptoms, and we generally alter antipneumocystis treatment at that point. However, the remaining half frequently have another pulmonary infection (117) and are responding well to therapy for pneumocystosis with decreasing semiquantitative estimates of *P. carinii* organism burden (Fig. 6). Among a group of AIDS patients at the University of Cincinnati Medical Center, symptomatic secondary infections discovered at repeat bronchoscopy have included bacterial pneumonia, fungal pneumonia, cytomegalovirus pneumonia, and nocardiosis (117).

In AIDS patients with respiratory failure secondary to *P. carinii* pneumonia who are not improving on therapy, a similar pattern with persistent *P. carinii* and new pulmonary infections is seen (122). However, these patients are more likely to have no specific etiology found for the continuing respiratory failure and to have a high prevalence of severe pulmonary fibrosis on biopsy or at autopsy. The fibrosis

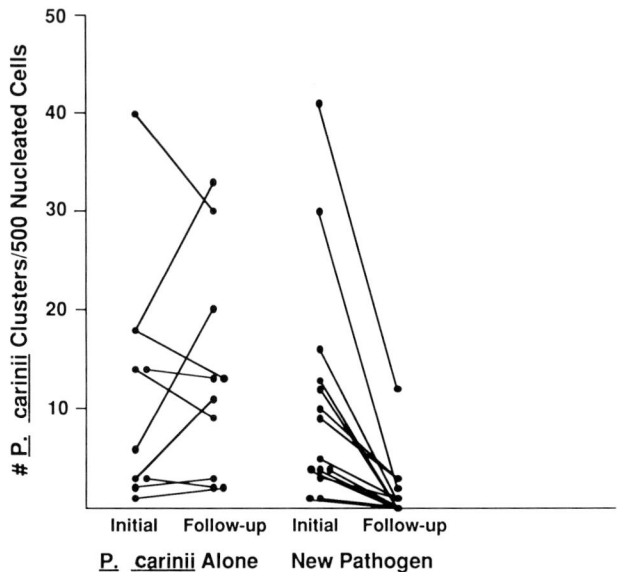

Figure 6 Results of follow-up bronchoscopy on patients not improving while receiving therapy for *P. carinii* pneumonia. Of 24 patients undergoing follow-up bronchoscopy with bronchoalveolar lavage for failure to respond to antipneumocystis therapy, 13 had other infections identified as the cause of the continuing respiratory symptoms (the new pathogen group). Ten patients had only *P. carinii* found (the *P. carinii* alone group). One patient (included in the new pathogen group) had congestive heart failure without any demonstrable lung infection. The vertical axis shows a semiquantitative estimate of the lung's *P. carinii* burden and the change in this value is illustrated. (From Ref. 117.)

may result from the high oxygen concentrations that these patients require or as a consequence of the *P. carinii* infection itself.

B. Complications: Hypoxemia, Pneumothorax, and Respiratory Failure

Several complications may occur during the course of therapy for *P. carinii* pneumonia. The most common adverse experience in AIDS patients is worsening hypoxemia in the first 3–5 days after therapy initiation (123). The etiology of this deterioration in oxygenation is unknown, but it has been hypothesized that an accelerated inflammatory reaction occurs in the lung in response to dead *P. carinii* organisms after antipneumocystis therapy begins (86). For patients with moderate or severe disease, the worsening hypoxemia often produces respiratory failure, requiring intensive care unit (ICU) admission and possible mechanical ventilation.

Corticosteroid use prevents the early deterioration in oxygenation (123), and this effect is most likely responsible for the improvement in morbidity and mortality demonstrated when they are used in moderate and severe *P. carinii* pneumonia in AIDS patients (87,111).

Whether a similar worsening of oxygenation occurs in non–HIV-infected patients is uncertain. Deterioration in oxygenation with treatment initiation has not been reported specifically, and case reports with sufficient information for evaluation do not demonstrate this pattern. As patients without HIV infection already have more lung inflammation initially (71), the hypothesis that an accelerated inflammatory response occurs secondary to treatment initiation may not apply to these patients.

Another problem related to *P. carinii* pneumonia that may have serious repercussions is the occurrence of a pneumothorax. Reported pneumothorax incidence rates related to *P. carinii* pneumonia range from 3 to 9% (124,125). Pneumothoraces related to acute *P. carinii* pneumonia are associated with significant morbidity, a tendency to recur, bilateral incidence, and mortality (67,126–131). The overall incidence of spontaneous pneumothorax in AIDS patients is 2–3%, which is approximately 450 times the rate in the general population (67,125). A spontaneous pneumothorax in an HIV-infected individual should prompt an attempt to exclude *P. carinii* pneumonia as the cause (67,125). A previous episode of *P. carinii* pneumonia and the use of aerosol pentamidine prophylactic therapy increases the risk of pneumothorax (67). In addition to pneumothorax, pneumomediastinum and subcutaneous emphysema may also occur (132). These complications are likely related to the reported destruction of lung tissue that accompanies *P. carinii* pneumonia in patients with and without HIV infection (8,127,129).

Probably because of the associated lung tissue destruction, a pneumothorax occurring in relation to an episode of *P. carinii* pneumonia can be particularly difficult to manage. Air leaks frequently persist even with thoracostomy tube evacuation of the pleural space. Conservative management may be the best alternative, as most patients' pneumothoraces will resolve spontaneously without thoracostomy tube placement (124). For recalcitrant air leaks, measures including endobronchial instillation of fibrin glue, pleurodesis, and thoracotomy have been tried with variable success (128,133–136).

Respiratory failure requiring mechanical ventilation secondary to *P. carinii* pneumonia relates to a poorer prognosis (72). Early reports of mortality rates for AIDS patients with respiratory failure secondary to *P. carinii* who required mechanical ventilation ranged from 86 to 94% (137–140). Subsequent to the publication of these high-mortality rates, a decreasing use of intensive care and mechanical ventilation for AIDS patients was noted (139). Reasons for the lower use of intensive care were apparently related to the poor prognosis and a sense of futility.

Pneumocystis carinii pneumonia produces respiratory failure through a physiological mechanism similar to adult respiratory distress syndrome (ARDS) (141,142). The response to positive end-expiratory pressure is the same, and *P. carinii* patients display the same pathological relation with oxygen consumption being dependent on oxygen delivery. In a rat model of *P. carinii* pneumonia, surfactant replacement improved oxygenation and produced aerated alveoli on histological examination, in contrast with alveoli filled with foamy exudate in untreated animals (143). Trials of surfactant as adjunctive therapy for *P. carinii* pneumonia in humans are presently ongoing.

Although clinical and laboratory information at ICU admission is not generally predictive of survival, higher admission serum albumin level is a good prognostic sign (144), and development of a metabolic acidemia with pH less than 7.35 or base deficit more than 4 mEq/liter at any point during the ICU stay is a poor prognostic sign (145).

Series showing a better prognosis for AIDS patients with *P. carinii*-related respiratory failure requiring mechanical ventilation began to appear in 1988. These reports demonstrated substantially improved survival rates (Table 2) (83,123,144–150). Besides better acute prognoses, respiratory failure secondary

Table 2 Outcome of Respiratory Failure Secondary to *P. carinii* Pneumonia in AIDS Patients

Ref.	Year	n	Survival (%)[a]
137	1986	16	6
138	1986	25	16
139	1986	45	13
140	1987	49	9
83	1988	19	42
146	1989	75	47
123	1989	24	50
147	1989	33	55
79	1989	37	14
148	1989	24	38 (Alive at ICU discharge)
			21 (Alive at 3 months)
149	1990	7	71
150	1990	13	46
144	1991	35	14 (1981–85 cohort)
		42	40 (1986–88 cohort)
145	1991	27	30

[a]Survival is defined differently in different reports. As best as can be determined, *survival* in this table is the percentage surviving to hospital discharge. Exceptions are noted on the table.

to *P. carinii* pneumonia is not necessarily a poor prognostic event heralding a terminal phase of HIV infection. Overall 1-year survival is 37%, and nearly 75% of hospital survivors are still alive at 1 year (151). In light of these reports, more recent recommendations encourage consideration of ICU care for patients with respiratory failure secondary to *P. carinii* pneumonia (152–155). With initiation of adjunctive steroid therapy for moderate and severe *P. carinii* pneumonia, many of the previous transfers to the ICU for increasing hypoxemia during the third to fifth day of therapy are now avoided entirely.

V. Conclusion

Effective prophylaxis is available against the development of *P. carinii* pneumonia and is discussed in Chapter 22. Prophylaxis is effective for patients on immunosuppressive therapy and with non-HIV immunodeficient states (156). For patients with HIV infection, prophylaxis is effective for both primary (157,158) and secondary (112,114,115) prevention of clinical disease. Many cases of clinical *P. carinii* pneumonia are now prevented from developing. Although the number of cases in AIDS patients may not reach the levels previously predicted, *P. carinii* pneumonia continues to occur in an ever-increasing population of susceptible individuals. At the University of Cincinnati Medical Center, for the years 1986 through 1990, about a third of the acute *P. carinii* pneumonias each year occurred in individuals who found that they were HIV-positive less than 1 month before the *P. carinii* pneumonia diagnosis, despite that HIV testing has been available throughout this time period (159). These patients had not availed themselves of any prophylactic therapy.

With more aggressive chemotherapeutic regimens and development of new pharmaceuticals for immunomodulation, *P. carinii* pneumonia is likely to remain as a threat for patients receiving these drugs. Predisposition to symptomatic *P. carinii* infection may be unpredictable as recombinant technology makes possible the production of cytokines and other new therapeutic agents. Future waves of *P. carinii* infection may have clinical characteristics distinctive from either of the present patterns in non–HIV- and HIV-infected individuals.

With increasing numbers of patients receiving treatment or prophylaxis for *P. carinii* pneumonia, the possibility of drug resistance arises. This may also alter the future clinical presentation and course of *P. carinii* infection. Our ability to continue to better understand and to more effectively manage clinically apparent infections with *P. carinii* will depend on advances in our knowledge of the biochemistry of the *P. carinii* organism and of its basic epidemiology.

References

1. Chagas C. Nova trypanomiazaea humana. Mem Inst Cruz 1909; 1:159.

2. Van der Meer G, Brug SL. Infection par pneumocystis chez l'homme et chez les animaux. Ann Soc Belge Med Trop 1942; 22:301.
3. Vanek J, Jirovec O. Parasitaere pneumonie. Interstitielle plasmazellen pneumonie der fruegheborenen verursacht durch *Pneumocystis carinii*. Abl Bakteriol 1952; 158:120–127.
4. Hughes WT, Price RA, Sisko F, Havron WS, Kafatos AG, Schonland M, Smythe PM. Protein–calorie malnutrition: a host determinant for *Pneumocystis carinii* infection. Am J Dis Child 1974; 128:44–52.
5. Gleason WA, Roodman ST. Reversible T cell depression in malnourished infants with pneumocystis pneumonia [letter]. J Pediatr 1977; 90:1032–1033.
6. Chandra RK. Cell-mediated immunity in nutritional imbalance. Fed Proc 1980; 39:3088–3092.
7. Dutz W. *Pneumocystis carinii* pneumonia. Pathol Annu 1979; 5:309–331.
8. Burke BA, Good RA. *Pneumocystis carinii* infection. Medicine 1973; 52:23–51.
9. Walzer PD, Perl DP, Krogstead DJ, Rawson PG, Schultz MG. *Pneumocystis carinii* pneumonia in the United States; epidemiologic, diagnostic, and clinical features. Ann Intern Med 1974; 80:83–93.
10. LeClair RA. Descriptive epidemiology of interstitial pneumocystic pneumonia. Am Rev Respir Dis 1969; 99:542–547.
11. Bradshaw M, Myerowitz RL, Schneerson R, Whisnant JK, Robbins JB. *Pneumocystis carinii* pneumonitis. Ann Intern Med 1970; 73:775–777.
12. Rosen P, Armstrong D, Ramos C. *Pneumocystis carinii* pneumonia: a clinicopathologic study of twenty patients with neoplastic diseases. Am J Med 1972; 53:428–436.
13. Centers for Disease Control. *Pneumocystis* pneumonia—Los Angeles. MMWR 1981; 30:250–252.
14. Centers for Disease Control. Kaposi's sarcoma and *Pneumocystis* pneumonia among homosexual men—New York City and California. MMWR 1981; 30:305–308.
15. Gottlieb MS, Schroff, R, Schanker HM, Weisman JD, Fan PT, Wolf RA, Saxon A. *Pneumocystis carinii* pneumonia and mucosal candidiasis in previously healthy homosexual men: evidence of a new acquired cellular immunodeficiency. N Engl J Med 1981; 305:1425–1431.
16. Masur H, Michelis MA, Greene JB, Onorato I, Stouwe RAV, Holzman RS, Wormser G, Brettman L, Lange M, Murray HW, Cunningham-Rundles S. An outbreak of community-acquired *Pneumocystis carinii* pneumonia: initial manifestation of cellular immune dysfunction. N Engl J Med 1981; 305:1431–1438.
17. Masur H, Michelis MA, Wormser GP, Lewin S, Gold J, Tapper ML, Giron J, Lerner CW, Armstrong D, Setia U, Sender JA, Siebken RS, Nicholas P, Arlen Z, Maayan S, Ernst JA, Siegel FP, Cunningham-Rundles S. Opportunistic infection in previously healthy women; initial manifestations of a community-acquired cellular immunodeficiency. Ann Intern Med 1982; 97:533–539.
18. Hopewell PC. *Pneumocystis carinii* pneumonia: diagnosis. J Infect Dis 1988; 157:1115–1119.
19. Masur H, Lane HC, Kovacs JA, Allegra CJ, Edman JC. Pneumocystis pneumonia: from bench to clinic. Ann Intern Med 1989; 111:813–826.

20. Poplin EA, Gordon CJ, Piskorowski TJ, Chandrasekar PH. *Pneumocystis carinii* pneumonia in patients with solid tumors without acquired immune deficiency syndrome. Cancer 1991; 68:193–194.
21. Brunvand MW, Collins C, Livingston RB, Raghu G. *Pneumocystis carinii* pneumonia associated with profound lymphopenia and abnormal T-lymphocyte subset ratios during treatment for early-stage breast carcinoma. Cancer 1991; 67:2407–2409.
22. Henson JW, Jalaj JK, Walker RW, Stover DE, Fels AOS. *Pneumocystis carinii* pneumonia in patients with primary brain tumors. Arch Neurol 1991; 48:406–409.
23. Graham BS, Tucker WS. Opportunistic infections in endogenous Cushing's syndrome. Ann Intern Med 1984; 101:334–338.
24. Western KA, Perera DR, Schultz ME. Pentamidine isethionate in the treatment of *Pneumocystis carinii* pneumonia. Ann Intern Med 1970; 73:695–702.
25. Peters SG, Prakash UBS. *Pneumocystis carinii* pneumonia: review of 53 cases. Am J Med 1987; 82:73–78.
26. Crayton HE, Sundstrom WR. *Pneumocystis carinii* pneumonia following corticosteroid therapy for giant cell arteritis. Wis Med J 1991; 90:170–171.
27. Hardy AM, Wajszczuk CP, Suffredini AF, Hakala TR, Ho M. *Pneumocystis carinii* pneumonia in renal transplant recipients treated with cyclosporine and steroids. J Infect Dis 1984; 149:143–147.
28. European multicentre trial group. Cyclosporin in cadaveric renal transplantation: one-year follow-up of a multicentre trial. Lancet 1983; 2:986–989.
29. Canadian multicentre transplant study group. A randomized clinical trial of cyclosporine in cadaveric renal transplantation. N Engl J Med 1983; 309:809–815.
30. Canadian multicentre transplant study group. A randomized clinical trial of cyclosporine in cadaveric renal transplantation. N Engl J Med 1986; 314:1219–1225.
31. Ballardie FW, Winearls CG, Cohen J, Carr DH, Rees AJ, Williams G. *Pneumocystis carinii* pneumonia in renal transplant recipients—clinical and radiographic features, diagnosis and complications of treatment. Q J Med 1985; 57:729–747.
32. Ballardie FW, Winearls CG, Williams G. Cyclosporin and steroids in renal transplantation: risk of *Pneumocystis carinii* pneumonia [letter]? Lancet 1984; 2:638–639.
33. Hofflin JM, Potasman I, Baldwin JC, Oyer PE, Stinson EB, Remington JS. Infectious complications in heart transplant recipients receiving cyclosporine and corticosteroids. Ann Intern Med 1987; 106:209–216.
34. Gryzan S, Paradis IL, Seevi A, Duquesnoy RJ, Dummer JS, Griffith BP, Hardesty RL, Trento A, Nalesnik MA, Dauber JH. Unexpectedly high incidence of *Pneumocystis carinii* infection after lung–heart transplantation. Am Rev Respir Dis 1988; 137:1268–1274.
35. Busuttil RW, Goldstein LI, Danovitch GM, Ament ME, Memsic LDF. Liver transplantation today. Ann Intern Med 1986; 104:377–389.
36. Kay HEM, Watson JG, Jameson B, Morgenstern GR, Powles RL. Infections after bone marrow transplantation using cyclosporine. Transplantation 1983; 36:491–495.
37. Meyers JL, Thomas ED. Infection complicating bone marrow transplantation. In:

Rubin RH, Young LS, eds. Clinical Approach to Infection in the Compromised Host. 2nd ed. New York: Plenum Publishing, 1988:525–556.
38. Watanabe JM, Chinchinian H, Weitz C, McIlvanie SK. *Pneumocystis carinii* pneumonia in a family. JAMA 1965; 193:685–686.
39. Anderson CD, Barrie HJ. Fatal pneumocystis pneumonia in an adult. Am J Clin Pathol 1960; 34:365–370.
40. Hennigar GR. *Pneumocystis carinii* pneumonia in an adult. Am J Clin Pathol 1961; 35:353.
41. Lyons HA, Vinijchaikul K, Henningar GR. *Pneumocystis carinii* pneumonia unassociated with other disease. Arch Intern Med 1961; 108:929–936.
42. Robinson JJ. Two cases of pneumocystosis. Arch Pathol 1961; 71:156–159.
43. Kaftori JK, Bassan H, Gellei B, Griffel B. *Pneumocystis carinii* pneumonia in an adult. Arch Intern Med 1962; 109:438–446.
44. Jacobs JL, Libby DM, Winters RA, Gelmont DM, Fried ED, Hartman BJ, Laurence J. A cluster of *Pneumocystis carinii* pneumonia in adults without predisposing illnesses. N Engl J Med 1991; 324:246–250.
45. Goetz A, Yu VL. *Pneumocystis carinii* pneumonia in adults without predisposing illnesses [letter]. N Engl J Med 1991; 325:1313–1314.
46. Katzenstein A-LA. *Pneumocystis carinii* pneumonia in adults without predisposing illnesses [letter]. N Engl J Med 1991; 325:1314.
47. O'Connor S. *Pneumocystis carinii* pneumonia in adults without predisposing illnesses [letter]. N Engl J Med 1991; 325:1314.
48. Gautier V, Chanez P, Vendrell JP, Pujol JL, Lacoste JY, de Faucal H, Godard P, Michel FB. Unexplained CD4-positive T-cell deficiency in non-HIV patients presenting as a *Pneumocystis carinii* pneumonia. Clin Exp Allergy 1991; 21:63–66.
49. Centers for Disease Control. Update: acquired immunodeficiency syndrome—United States. MMWR 1986; 35:757–766.
50. Centers for Disease Control. Update: acquired immunodeficiency syndrome (AIDS)—United States. MMWR 1986; 35:17–21.
51. Allegra CJ, Chabner BA, Tuazon CU, Ogata-Arakaki D, Baird B, Drake JC, Simmons T, Lack EE, Shelhamer JH, Balis F, Walker R, Kovacs JA, Lane HC, Masur H. Trimetrexate for the treatment of *Pneumocystis carinii* pneumonia in patients with acquired immunodeficiency syndrome. N Engl J Med 1987; 317: 978–985.
52. Kaslow RA, Phair JP, Friedman HB, Lyter D, Solomon RE, Dudley J, Polk BF, Blackwelder W. Infection with human immunodeficiency virus: clinical manifestations and their relationship to immune deficiency. Ann Intern Med 1987; 107:474–480.
53. Masur H, Ognibene FP, Yarchoan R, Shelhamer JH, Baird BF, Travis W, Suffredini AF, Deyton L, Kovacs JA, Falloon J, Davey R, Polis M, Metcalf J, Baseler M, Wesley R, Gill VJ, Fauci AS, Lane HC. CD4 counts as predictors of opportunistic pneumonias in human immunodeficiency virus (HIV) infection. Ann Intern Med 1989; 111:223–231.
54. Phair J, Munoz A, Detels R, Kaslow R, Rinaldo C, Saah A. The risk of *Pneumocystis carinii* pneumonia among men infected with human immunodeficiency virus type 1. N Engl J Med 1990; 322:161–165.

55. Abouya YL, Beaumel A, Lucas S, Dago-Akribi A, Coulibaly G, N'Dhatz M, Konan JB, Yapi A, de Cock KM. *Pneumocystis carinii* pneumonia. An uncommon cause of death in African patients with acquired immunodeficiency syndrome. Am Rev Respir Dis 1992; 145:617–620.
56. Kales CP, Murren JR, Torres RA, Crocco JA. Early predictors of in-hospital mortality for *Pneumocystis carinii* pneumonia in the acquired immunodeficiency syndrome. Arch Intern Med 1987; 147:1413–1417.
57. Fried JC, LoPresti JS, Micon M, Bauer M, Tuchschmidt JA, Nicoloff JT. Serum triiodothyronine values: prognostic indicators of acute mortality due to *Pneumocystis carinii* pneumonia associated with the acquired immunodeficiency syndrome. Arch Intern Med 1990; 150:406–409.
58. Benson CA, Spear J, Hines D, Pottage JC Jr, Kessler HA, Trenholme GM. Combined APACHE II score and serum lactate dehydrogenase as predictors of in-hospital mortality caused by first episode *Pneumocystis carinii* pneumonia in patients with acquired immunodeficiency syndrome. Am Rev Respir Dis 1991; 144:319–323.
59. Singer C, Armstrong D, Rosen PP, Schottenfeld D. *Pneumocystis carinii* pneumonia: a cluster of eleven cases. Ann Intern Med 1975; 82:772–777.
60. Bensousan T, Garo B, Islam S, Bourbigot B, Cledes J, Garre M. Possible transfer of *Pneumocystis carinii* between kidney transplant recipients [letter]. Lancet 1990; 336:1066–1067.
61. Goesch TR, Gotz G, Stellbrinck KH, Albrecht H, Weh HJ, Hossfeld DK. Possible transfer of *Pneumocystis carinii* between immunodeficient patients [letter]. Lancet 1990; 336:627.
62. Haron E, Bodey GP, Luna MA, Dekmezian R, Elting L. Has the incidence of *Pneumocystis carinii* pneumonia in cancer patients increased with the AIDS epidemic [letter]? Lancet 1988; 2:904–905.
63. Chave J-P, David S, Wauters J-P, Van Melle G, Francioli P. Transmission of *Pneumocystis carinii* from AIDS patients to other immunosuppressed patients: a cluster of *Pneumocystis carinii* pneumonia in renal transplant recipients. AIDS 1991; 5:927–932.
64. Giron JA, Martinez S, Walzer PD. Should patients with *Pneumocystis carinii* be isolated [letter]? Lancet 1982; 2:46.
65. Walzer PD. *Pneumocystis carinii*—new clinical spectrum? N Engl J Med 1991; 323:263–265.
66. Kovacs JA, Himenez JW, Macher AM. *Pneumocystis carinii* pneumonia: a comparison between patients with acquired immunodeficiency syndrome and patients with other immunodeficiencies. Ann Intern Med 1984; 100:633–671.
67. Sepkowitz KA, Telzak EE, Gold JWM, Bernard EM, Blum S, Carrow M, Dickmeyer M, Armstrong D. Pneumothorax in AIDS. Ann Intern Med 1991; 114:455–459.
68. Mascarenhas DAN, Vasudevan VP, Vaidya KP. *Pneumocystis carinii* pneumonia. Rare cause of hemoptysis. Chest 1991; 99:251–253.
69. Haverkos HW. Assessment of therapy for *Pneumocystis carinii* pneumonia. Am J Med 1984; 76:501–508.

70. Ziefer A, Abramowitz JA. *Pneumocystis carinii* pneumonia in HIV-positive and HIV-negative patients. S Afr Med J 1989; 76:308–313.
71. Limper AH, Offord KP, Smith TF, Martin WJ II. *Pneumocystis carinii* pneumonia. Differences in lung parasite number and inflammation in patients with and without AIDS. Am Rev Respir Dis 1989; 140:1204–1209.
72. Bennett CL, Garfinkle JB, Greenfield S, Draper D, Rogers W, Mathews WC, Kanouse DE. The relation between hospital experience and in-hospital mortality for patients with AIDS-related PCP. JAMA 1989; 261:2975–2979.
73. Bennett CL, Gertler P, Guze PA, Garfinkle JB, Kanouse DE, Greenfield S. The relation between resource use and in-hospital mortality for patients with acquired immunodeficiency syndrome-related *Pneumocystis carinii* pneumonia. Arch Intern Med 1990; 150:1447–1452.
74. Bower M, Barton SE, Nelson MR, Bobby J, Smith D, Youle M, Gazzard BG. The significance of the detection of cytomegalovirus in bronchoalveolar lavage fluid in AIDS patients with pneumonia. AIDS 1990; 4:317–320.
75. Miles PR, Baughman RP, Linnemann CC. Cytomegalovirus in the bronchoalveolar lavage fluid of patients with AIDS. Chest 1990; 97:1072–1076.
76. Millar AB, Patou G, Miller RF, Grundy JE, Katz DR, Weller IV, Semple SJ. Cytomegalovirus in the lungs of patients with AIDS. Respiratory pathogen or passenger? Am Rev Respir Dis 1990; 141:1474–1477.
77. Jacobson MA, Mills J, Rush J, Peiperl L, Seru V, Mohanty PK, Hopewell PC, Hadley WK, Broaddus VC, Leoung G, Feigal DW. Morbidity and mortality of patients with AIDS and first-episode *Pneumocystis carinii* pneumonia unaffected by concomitant pulmonary cytomegalovirus infection. Am Rev Respir Dis 1991; 144:6–9.
78. Bozzette SA, Arcia J, Bartok AE, McGlynn LM, McCutchan JA, Richman DD, Spector SA. Impact of *Pneumocystis carinii* and cytomegalovirus on the course and outcome of atypical pneumonia in advanced human immunodeficiency virus disease. J Infect Dis 1992; 165:93–98.
79. Smith RL, Levine SM, Lewis ML. Prognosis of patients with AIDS requiring intensive care. Chest 1989; 96:857–861.
80. Sattler FR, Cowan R, Nielsen DM, Ruskin J. Trimethoprim–sulfamethoxazole compared with pentamidine for treatment of *Pneumocystis carinii* pneumonia in the acquired immunodeficiency syndrome. Ann Intern Med 1988; 109:280–287.
81. Dohn MN, Baughman RP, Vigdorth EM, Frame DL. Equal survival rates for first, second, and third episodes of *Pneumocystis carinii* pneumonia in AIDS patients. Arch Intern Med 1992; 152:2465–2470.
82. Brenner M, Ognibene FP, Lack EE, Simmons JT, Suffredini AF, Lane HC, Fauci AS, Parrillo JE, Shelhamer JH, Masur H. Prognostic factors and life expectancy of patients with acquired immunodeficiency syndrome and *Pneumocystis carinii* pneumonia. Am Rev Respir Dis 1987; 136:1199–1206.
83. Ed-Sadr W, Simberkoff MS. Survival and prognostic factors in severe *Pneumocystis carinii* pneumonia requiring mechanical ventilation. Am Rev Respir Dis 1988; 137:1264–1267.
84. Garay SM, Greene J. Prognostic indicators in the initial presentation of *Pneumocystis carinii* pneumonia. Chest 1989; 95:769–772.

85. Speich R, Weber R, Kronauer CHM, Opravil M, Luthy R, Russi EW. Prognostic score for *Pneumocystis carinii* pneumonia. Respiration 1990; 57:259–263.
86. National Institutes of Health—University of California expert panel for corticosteroids as adjunctive therapy for pneumocystis pneumonia. Consensus statement on the use of corticosteroids as adjunctive therapy for pneumocystis pneumonia in the acquired immunodeficiency syndrome. N Engl J Med 1990; 323:1500–1504.
87. Bozzette SA, Sattler FR, Chiu J, Wu AW, Gluckstein D, Kemper C, Bartok A, Niosi J, Abramson I, Coffman J, Hughlett C, Loya R, Cassens B, Akil B, Meng T-C, Boylen CT, Nielsen D, Richman DD, Tilles JG, Leedom J, McCutchan JA. A controlled trial of early adjunctive treatment with corticosteroids for *Pneumocystis carinii* pneumonia in the acquired immunodeficiency syndrome. N Engl J Med 1990; 323:1451–1457.
88. Zaman MK, Beyer D, Bernard E, Morgan R, Bhat S, White DA. Pulse oximetry exercise testing: role in detection of *Pneumocystis carinii* pneumonia (PCP) in AIDS patients [abstract]. Am Rev Respir Dis 1989; 139:A148.
89. Stover DE, Greeno RA, Gagliardi AJ. The use of a simple exercise test for the diagnosis of *Pneumocystis carinii* pneumonia in patients with AIDS. Am Rev Respir Dis 1989; 139:1343–1346.
90. Murray JF. Pulmonary complications of the acquired immune deficiency syndrome: a report of a National Heart, Lung and Blood Institute workshop. N Engl J Med 1984; 310:1682–1688.
91. Coleman DL, Dodek PM, Golden JA, Luce JM, Golden E, Gold WM, Murray JF. Correlation between serial pulmonary function tests and fiberoptic bronchoscopy in patients with *Pneumocystis carinii* pneumonia and the acquired immunodeficiency syndrome. Am Rev Respir Dis 1984; 129:491–493.
92. Stover DE, White DA, Romano PA, Gellene RA, Robeson WA. Spectrum of pulmonary diseases associated with the acquired immunodeficiency syndrome. Am J Med 1985; 78:429–437.
93. Hopewell PC, Luce JM. Pulmonary involvement in the acquired immune deficiency syndrome. Chest 1985; 87:104–112.
94. Kagawa FT, Kirsch CM, Yenokida GG, Levine ML. Serum lactate dehydrogenase activity in patients with AIDS and *Pneumocystis carinii* pneumonia: an adjunct to diagnosis. Chest 1988; 94:1031–1033.
95. Smith RL, Ripps CS, Lewis ML. Elevated lactate dehydrogenase values in patients with *Pneumocystis carinii* pneumonia. Chest 1988; 93:987–992.
96. Zaman MK, White DA. Serum lactate dehydrogenase levels and *Pneumocystis carinii* pneumonia: diagnostic and prognostic significance. Am Rev Respir Dis 1988; 137:796–800.
97. Boudes P, Fuhrman C, Verra F, Sobel A. Interet de la determination du taux des LDH au cours de la pneumopathie a *Pneumocystis carinii* chez les patients infectes par le virus de l'immunodeficience humaine. Ann Med Interne 1990; 141:175–178.
98. Katz MH, Baron RB, Grady D. Risk stratification of ambulatory patients suspected of pneumocystis pneumonia. Arch Intern Med 1991; 151:105–110.
99. DeLorenzo LJ, Huang CT, Maguire GP, Stone DJ. Roentgenographic patterns of *Pneumocystis carinii* pneumonia in 104 patients with AIDS. Chest 1987; 91:323–327.

100. Tow TWY, Rosen MJ, Tierstein AS. Normal chest roentgenogram as a prognostic factor in *Pneumocystis carinii* pneumonia in patients with acquired immunodeficiency syndrome [abstract]. Am Rev Respir Dis 1984; 129:A54.
101. Smith RL, El-Sadr WM, Lewis ML. Correlation of bronchoalveolar lavage cell populations with clinical severity of *Pneumocystis carinii* pneumonia. Chest 1988; 92:60–64.
102. Mason GR, Hashimoto CH, Dickman PS, Foutty LF, Cobb CJ. Prognostic implications of bronchoalveolar lavage neutrophilia in patients with *Pneumocystis carinii* pneumonia and AIDS. Am Rev Respir Dis 1989; 139:1336–1342.
103. Greco MJ, Heimann A, Steigbigel RT, Smaldone GC. Severity of *Pneumocystis carinii* pneumonia (PCP) correlates with number of organisms recovered from lavage [abstract]. Am Rev Respir Dis 1989; 139:A149.
104. Colangelo G, Baughman R, Dohn M, Connolly M, Frame PT. Pneumocystis burden as a risk factor for mortality in AIDS patients with *Pneumocystis carinii* pneumonia [abstract]. Am Rev Respir Dis 1990; 141:A270.
105. Singer F, Talavera W, Zumoff B. Elevated levels of angiotensin-converting enzyme in *Pneumocystis carinii* pneumonia. Chest 1989; 95:803–806.
106. O'Brien RF, Cohn DL. Serum angiotensin converting enzyme levels in AIDS [letter]. Chest 1990; 97:1021–1022.
107. DiPrima MA, Sorice M, Vullo V, Mastroianni CM, Amendolea MA, Masala C. Anticardiolipin antibody in the acquired immunodeficiency syndrome: a marker of *Pneumocystis carinii* infection [letter]? J Infect 1989; 18:100–101.
108. Masala C, Sorice M, DiPrima MA, Lenti L, Misasi R, Contini C, Vullo V. Anticardiolipin antibodies and *Pneumocystis carinii* pneumonia [letter]. Ann Intern Med 1989; 110:749.
109. Coll J, Yazbeck H, Garces JM, Berges A, Trats F, Rubies-Prat J. Anticardiolipin antibodies and *Pneumocystis carinii* pneumonia in patients with AIDS [letter]. J Infect 1990; 21:120.
110. Bedos JP, Lucet JC, Hignette C, Wolff M, Casalino E, Matheron S, Leport C, Vachon F. Serum carcinoembryonic antigen (CEA): a new prognostic marker in HIV-related *Pneumocystis carinii* pneumonia (PCP) [abstract]. Am Rev Respir Dis 1991; 143:A712.
111. Gagnon S, Boota AM, Fischl MA, Baier H, Kirksey OW, La Voie L. Corticosteroids as adjunctive therapy for severe *Pneumocystis carinii* pneumonia in the acquired immunodeficiency syndrome. N Engl J Med 1990; 323:1444–1450.
112. Centers for Disease Control. Guidelines for prophylaxis against *Pneumocystis carinii* pneumonia for persons infected with human immunodeficiency virus. MMWR 1989; 38(suppl 5):1S–9S.
113. Rainer CA, Feigel DW, Leoung G, Clement M, Wofsy C. Prognosis and natural history of *Pneumocystis carinii* pneumonia: indicators for early and late survival [abstract THP.154]. In: Third International Conference on AIDS Abstracts. Frederick, Md: University Publishing Group, 1988:189.
114. Wormser GP, Horowitz HW, Duncanson FP, Forseter G, Javaly K, Alampur SK, Gilroy SA, Lenox T, Rappaport A, Nadelman RB. Low-dose intermittent trimethoprim–sulfamethoxazole for prevention of *Pneumocystis carinii* pneumonia in pa-

tients with human immunodeficiency virus infection. Arch Intern Med 1991; 151: 688–692.
115. Martin MA, Cox PH, Beck K, Styer CM, Beall GN. A comparison of the effectiveness of three regimens in the prevention of *Pneumocystis carinii* pneumonia in human immunodeficiency virus-infected patients. Arch Intern Med 1992; 152: 523–528.
116. Shelhamer JH, Ognibene FP, Macher AM, Tuazon C, Steiss R, Longo D, Kovacs JA, Parker MM, Natanson C, Lane HC, Fauci AS, Parrillo JE, Masur H. Persistence of *Pneumocystis carinii* in lung tissue of acquired immunodeficiency syndrome patients treated for pneumocystis pneumonia. Am Rev Respir Dis 1984; 130;1161–1165.
117. Colangelo G, Baughman RP, Dohn MN, Frame PT. Follow-up bronchoalveolar lavage in AIDS patients with *Pneumocystis carinii* pneumonia: *Pneumocystis carinii* burden predicts early relapse. Am Rev Respir Dis 1991; 143:1067–1071.
118. Rothenberg R, Woelfel M, Stoneburner R, Milberg J, Parker R, Truman B. Survival with the acquired immunodeficiency syndrome. Experience with 5833 cases in New York City. N Engl J Med 1987; 317:1297–1302.
119. Meuwissen JHET, Tauber I, Leeuwenberg ADEM, Beckers PJA, Sieben M. Parasitologic and serologic observations of infection with *Pneumocystis* in humans. J Infect Dis 1977; 136:43–49.
120. Pifer LL, Hughes WT, Stagno S, Woods D. *Pneumocystis carinii* infection: evidence for high prevalence in normal and immunosuppressed children. Pediatrics 1978; 61: 35–41.
121. Maddison SF, Hayes GV, Slemenda SB, Norman LG, Ivey MH. Detection of specific antibody by enzyme-linked immunosorbent assay and antigenemia by counterimmunoelectrophoresis in humans infected with *Pneumocystis carinii*. J Clin Microbiol 1982; 15:1036–1043.
122. Garay S. Respiratory failure in AIDS [abstract]. Am Rev Respir Dis 1986; 133:A344.
123. Montaner JSG, Russell JA, Lawson L, Ruedy J. Acute respiratory failure secondary to *Pneumocystis carinii* pneumonia in the acquired immunodeficiency syndrome; a potential role for systemic corticosteroids. Chest 1989; 95:881–884.
124. McClellan MD, Miller SB, Parsons PE, Cohn DL. Pneumothorax with *Pneumocystis carinii* pneumonia in AIDS: incidence and clinical characteristics. Chest 1991; 100:1224–1228.
125. Truitt T, Bagheri K, Safirstein BH. Spontaneous pneumothorax in *Pneumocystis carinii* pneumonia: common or uncommon [letter]? AJR 1992; 158:916–917.
126. Goodman PC, Daley C, Minagi H. Spontaneous pneumothorax in AIDS patients with *Pneumocystis carinii* pneumonia. AJR 1986; 147:29–31.
127. Eng RHK, Bishburg E, Smith SM. Evidence for destruction of lung tissues during *Pneumocystis carinii* infection. Arch Intern Med 1987; 147:746–749.
128. Byrnes TA, Brevig JK, Yeoh CB. Pneumothorax in patients with acquired immunodeficiency syndrome. J Thorac Cardiovasc Surg 1989; 98:546–550.
129. Beers MF, Sohn M, Swartz M. Recurrent pneumothorax in AIDS patients with pneumocystis pneumonia. Chest 1990; 98:266–270.

130. Shanley DJ, Luyckx BA, Haggerty MF, Murphy TF. Spontaneous pneumothorax in AIDS patients with recurrent *Pneumocystis carinii* pneumonia despite aerosolized pentamidine prophylaxis. Chest 1991; 99:502–504.
131. Sherman M, Levin D, Breidbart D. *Pneumocystis carinii* pneumonia with spontaneous pneumothorax. Chest 1986; 90:609–610.
132. del Arco Galan C, Lopez Rodriquez C, Santos I, Sanchez Molini P. Neumothorax, neumomediastino y enfisema subcutaneo en la neumonia por *P. carinii*. Rev Clin Esp 1991; 188:68–69.
133. Fleisher AG, McElvaney G, Lawson L, Gerein AN, Grant D, Tyers FO. Surgical management of spontaneous pneumothorax in patients with acquired immunodeficiency syndrome. Ann Thorac Surg 1988; 45:21–23.
134. Hnatiuk OW, Dillard TA, Oster CN. Bleomycin sclerotherapy for bilateral pneumothoraces in a patient with AIDS. Ann Intern Med 1990; 113:988–990.
135. Scannel KA. Pneumothoraces and *Pneumocystis carinii* pneumonia in two AIDS patients receiving aerosolized pentamidine. Chest 1990; 97:479–480.
136. Tunon-de-Lara J-M, Constans J, Vincent M-P, Receveur M-C, Conri C, Taytard A. Spontaneous pneumothorax associated with *Pneumocystis carinii* pneumonia. Successful treatment with talc pleurodesis. Chest 1992; 101:1177–1178.
137. Schein RM, Fischl MA, Pitchenik AE, Aprung CL. ICU survival of patients with the acquired immunodeficiency syndrome. Crit Care Med 1986; 14:1026–1027.
138. Rosen MJ, Cucco RA, Tierstein AS. Outcome of intensive care in patients with the acquired immunodeficiency syndrome. J Intensive Care Med 1986; 1:55–60.
139. Wachter RM, Luce JM, Turner J, Volberding P, Hopewell PC. Intensive care of patients with the acquired immunodeficiency syndrome: outcome and changing patterns of utilization. Am Rev Respir Dis 1986; 134:891–896.
140. Baggott LA, Baggott BB. *Pneumocystis carinii* pneumonia in AIDS patients in intensive care [abstract]. Chest 1987; 92:133S.
141. Maxfield RA, Sorkin B, Fazzini EP, Rapoport DM, Stenson WM, Goldring RM. Respiratory failure in patients with acquired immunodeficiency syndrome and *Pneumocystis carinii* pneumonia. Crit Care Med 1986; 14:443–449.
142. Ronco JJ, Montaner JSG, Fenwick JC, Ruedy J, Russell JA. Pathologic dependence of oxygen consumption on oxygen delivery in acute respiratory failure secondary to AIDS-related *Pneumocystis carinii* pneumonia. Chest 1990; 98:1463–1466.
143. Eijking EP, van Daal G-J, Tenbrinck R, Luijendijk A, Sluiters JF, Hannappel E, Lachmann B. Effect of surfactant replacement on *Pneumocystis carinii* pneumonia in rats. Intensive Care Med 1991; 17:475–478.
144. Wachter RM, Russi MB, Bloch DA, Hopewell PC, Luce JM. *Pneumocystis carinii* pneumonia and respiratory failure in AIDS: improved outcomes and increased use of intensive care units. Am Rev Respir Dis 1991; 143:251–256.
145. Peruzzi WT, Skoutelis A, Shapiro BA, Murphy RM, Currie DL, Cane RD, Noskin GA, Phair JP. Intensive care unit patients with acquired immunodeficiency syndrome and *Pneumocystis carinii* pneumonia: suggested predictors of hospital outcome. Crit Care Med 1991; 19:892–900.
146. Friedman Y, Franklin C, Rackow EC, Weil MH. Improved survival in patients with AIDS, *Pneumocystis carinii* pneumonia, and severe respiratory failure. Chest 1989; 96:862–866.

147. Efferen LS, Nadarajah D, Palat DS. Survival following mechanical ventilation for *Pneumocystis carinii* pneumonia in patients with the acquired immunodeficiency syndrome: a different perspective. Am J Med 1989; 87:401–404.
148. Rogers PL, Lane HC, Henderson DK, Parrillo J, Masur H. Admission of AIDS patients to a medical intensive care unit: causes and outcomes. Crit Care Med 1989; 17:113–117.
149. Lee P, Dow FT, Bryant CG, Roy TM. AIDS: intensive care utilization and outcome. J Ky Med Assoc 1990; 88:17–19.
150. Larpin R, Chave J-P, Schaller MD, Perret C. Survival of HIV positive patients admitted to intensive care with respiratory failure secondary to *Pneumocystis carinii* pneumonia. Schweiz Med Wochenschr 1990; 120:1928–1933.
151. Friedman Y, Franklin C, Freels S, Weil MH. Long-term survival of patients with AIDS, *Pneumocystis carinii* pneumonia, and respiratory failure. JAMA 1991; 266: 89–92.
152. Luce JM, Wachter RM, Hopewell PC. Intensive care of patients with the acquired immunodeficiency syndrome: time for a reassessment [editorial]? Am Rev Respir Dis 1988; 137:1261–1263.
153. Wachter RM, Luce JM, Lo B, Raffin TA. Life-sustaining treatment for patients with AIDS. Chest 1989; 95:647–652.
154. Singer P, Askanazi J, Akiva L, Bursztein S, Kvetan V. Reassessing intensive care for patients with the acquired immunodeficiency syndrome. Heart Lung 1990; 19: 387–394.
155. Wachter RM, Luce JM, Hopewell PC. Critical care of patients with AIDS. JAMA 1992; 267:541–547.
156. Hughes WT, Kuhn S, Chaudhary S, Feldman S, Verzosa M, Aur RJA, Pratt C, George SL. Successful chemoprophylaxis for *Pneumocystis carinii* pneumonia. N Engl J Med 1977; 297:1419–1423.
157. Hirschel B, Lazzarin A, Chopard P, Opravil M, Furrer H-J, Ruttimann S, Vernazza P, Chave J-P, Ancarani F, Gabriel V, Heald A, King R, Malinverni R, Martin J-L, Mermillod B, Nicod L, Simoni L, Vivirito MC, Zerboni R, Swiss group for clinical studies on AIDS. A controlled study of inhaled pentamidine for primary prevention of *Pneumocystis carinii* pneumonia. N Engl J Med 1991; 324:1079–1083.
158. Blum RN, Miller LA, Gaggini LC, Cohn DL. Comparative trial of dapsone versus trimethoprim/sulfamethoxazole for primary prophylaxis of *Pneumocystis carinii* pneumonia. J AIDS 1992; 5:341–347.
159. Vigdorth EM. Epidemiology of *Pneumocystis carinii* pneumonia at the University of Cincinnati AIDS Treatment Center, 1986–1989. Doctoral dissertation. Department of Environmental Health, College of Medicine, University of Cincinnati, Cincinnati, Ohio, 1992.

18

Extrapulmonary Infection and Other Unusual Manifestations of *Pneumocystis carinii*

EDWARD E. TELZAK

Bronx–Lebanon Hospital Center
and Albert Einstein College of Medicine
Bronx, New York

DONALD ARMSTRONG

Memorial Sloan–Kettering Cancer Center
and Cornell University Medical College
New York, New York

I. Introduction

Pneumocystis carinii is the most common microorganism causing opportunistic infection in patients with the acquired immunodeficiency syndrome (AIDS). Almost 200,000 cases of AIDS have been reported to the Centers for Disease Control as of September 1991 (1). Before the use of prophylaxis for *P. carinii* pneumonia (PCP), it was estimated that 60% of human immunodeficiency virus (HIV)-infected patients presented with PCP as their AIDS-defining illness, and an additional 20% developed PCP later in the course of their illness (2). With the advent of effective prophylaxis for *P. carinii* pneumonia, fewer patients are developing this infection. Nevertheless, a conservative estimate would be that over 120,000 cases of *P. carinii* pneumonia have occurred in patients with AIDS in the United States.

Typically, *P. carinii* infection is a bilateral and diffuse pneumonitis. Before the AIDS epidemic, unusual pulmonary presentations for *P. carinii* pneumonia were described (3), as was extrapulmonary spread (4–12). The annual number of reported cases of pneumocystosis, however, was fewer than 100 per year (13). As this number has risen, so has the number of cases that do not present in the typical fashion. In addition, widespread use of prophylaxis, especially aerosol pentamidine, in patients at highest risk for *P. carinii* pneumonia, is making atypical presentations more common. The following chapter will review the unusual presentations of *P. carinii* infections, concentration on extrapulmonary spread and unusual pulmonary presentations including pneumothorax and focal pulmonary disease.

II. Extrapulmonary Infection

There have been four recent clinical reviews on extrapulmonary *P. carinii* infection (14–17). Each review stresses that, although PCP is the most common opportunistic infection in AIDS, extrapulmonary spread of this organism is either infrequent or rare. Although, in all probability, this crude prevalence estimate is correct, more cases are being reported. In addition, many cases are not reported. For example, at a weekly New York City infectious disease meeting in which case presentations are made, several unpublished cases of extrapulmonary infection have been presented. Similarly, in a recent review from San Francisco, the authors state that numerous unreported cases have occurred in that city as well (16). Despite this "underreporting," sufficient numbers of cases have been reported such that distinct clinical patterns may be emerging.

III. Frequency of Extrapulmonary *Pneumocystis carinii*

The prevalence of extrapulmonary *P. carinii* infection is difficult to determine; *P. carinii* is rarely looked for as a cause of lymphadenopathy, hepatosplenomegaly, bone marrow depression, or the numerous other clinical manifestations that have been associated with extrapulmonary disease. Nevertheless, several studies may help us estimate the prevalence of this entity.

Gajdusek, in a review of approximately 200 autopsies from an apparently epidemic form of *P. carinii* infection in postwar Central Europe, did not report a single case of extrapulmonary involvement (18). In a 1973 review by Burke and Good, 46 cases of PCP were reviewed, and at least 28 autopsies were performed; 1 case of extrapulmonary infection involving the hilar lymph nodes and thymus was noted (19). At Memorial Sloan–Kettering Cancer Center (MSKCC) 140 patients without HIV infection have had morphologically proved PCP in the 12-year period between 1978 and 1989 (20). Thirty-two (23%) of these patients died with active PCP and had autopsies performed; no evidence of extrapulmonary infection was found in any case (unpublished data).

Extrapulmonary infection with *P. carinii* in patients infected with HIV might be more common than in other severely immunocompromised patients. At a community hospital in New York City, five cases of extrapulmonary infection have been documented during the course of the AIDS epidemic (15). Concurrently, there were 940 cases of PCP. The author projected a "rate" of 0.5%, although clearly acknowledged the limitations of this estimate, including the lack of autopsy data and the possibility that patients may have had extrapulmonary disease without lung infection.

At MSKCC we estimate the risk of extrapulmonary *P. carinii* infection in patients with AIDS to be 2–3% (14). Of the more than 1000 patients with AIDS who have received care at our institution since January 1980, 641 have died. Autopsies have been obtained on 253, or 39%. Seven (2.8%) of these autopsied cases have had extrapulmonary *P. carinii* infection. One of these cases was initially diagnosed antemortem. In all likelihood, this represents the minimum estimate for extrapulmonary infection. As previously stated, *P. carinii* is rarely considered as a potential etiological agent for a clinical sign or symptom outside the lung when a patient is alive. Therefore, silver stains would not routinely be obtained on autopsy material, unless the characteristic foamy eosinophilic material associated with *P. carinii* is apparent on hematoxylin–eosin (H&E) staining. In addition, patients with PCP may have concurrent extrapulmonary disease; systemic treatment for the pneumonia would likely cure extrapulmonary disease as well.

IV. Clinical Presentation

There have been at least 12 published cases of extrapulmonary *P. carinii* since 1960 in patients without known HIV infection (4–12). Eight of the 12 patients were male, and their ages ranged from 5 months to 75 years; there were 4 infants between 5 months and 16 months, and a 5-year-old boy. The mean age of the 7 adults was 51 years. Risk factors for the development of extrapulmonary *P. carinii* infection included congenital hypogammaglobulinemia, thymic alymphoplasia, chronic myelogenous leukemia, Hodgkin's disease, lymphoma, immunosuppression in association with renal transplantation, and steroid use. For 1 case a risk factor was not reported.

Of these 12 patients, 9 (75%) had their diagnosis of extrapulmonary infection made at autopsy. Only 3 patients were diagnosed before death and, in all 3, the extrapulmonary site was the bone marrow.

The organ distribution of extrapulmonary sites of infection is detailed in Table 1. The most common extrapulmonary site was the lymph nodes, followed by the bone marrow, the spleen, and the liver. In all 12 cases, concurrent pulmonary infection with *P. carinii* was present.

There have been over 80 reported cases of patients with HIV infection who have had extrapulmonary *P. carinii* infection. More than half are detailed clinical case reports, with the remainder being in the radiology literature or in abstract form (21–51). The spectrum of disease has ranged from asymptomatic lymph-

Table 1 Extrapulmonary Sites of *P. carinii* Infection

Extrapulmonary site	AIDS $n = 40$ (%)	Non-AIDS $n = 12$ (%)	Total $n = 52$ (%)
Lymph nodes	14 (35)	9 (75)	23 (44)
Spleen	13 (33)	4 (33)	17 (33)
Liver	13 (33)	3 (25)	16 (31)
Bone marrow	12 (30)	5 (42)	17 (33)
Adrenal glands	9 (23)	1 (8)	10 (19)
Gastrointestinal tract	8 (20)	2 (17)	10 (19)
Genitourinary tract	7 (18)	2 (17)	9 (17)
Thyroid	8 (20)	1 (8)	9 (17)
Heart	6 (15)	2 (17)	8 (15)
Pancreas	6 (15)	1 (8)	7 (13)
Eyes	6 (15)	0	6 (12)
Ears	6 (15)	0	6 (12)
Skin	2 (5)	0	2 (4)
Cerebral cortex	1 (3)	0	1 (2)
Pituitary gland	1 (3)	0	1 (2)
Parathyroid glands	1 (3)	0	1 (2)
Paraspinal mass	1 (3)	0	1 (3)

adenopathy to fulminant and overwhelming infection. The later presentation is well represented in the following case.

V. Case Reports

The patient was a 33-year-old man, with a history of progressive Kaposi's sarcoma requiring systemic chemotherapy and three previous episodes of PCP treated with 21-day courses of pentamidine. After his third episode of PCP he was started on aerosol pentamidine prophylaxis. Five months after his third episode of PCP and 8 days before his death, the patient was admitted to Memorial Hospital for evaluation of fever, lethargy, and substernal chest pain. On admission he was hypotensive, in acute respiratory distress, and hypothermic. The remainder of his physical examination was notable for widespread Kaposi's sarcoma, oral thrush, and a mildly tender abdomen without hepatosplenomegaly. Pulmonary and cardiac examinations were unremarkable. Laboratory data was notable for a white blood cell count of 2300, with a left shift; a hematocrit of 35%, and a platelet count of 80,000. Prothrobin time (PT) and partial thromboplastin time (PTT) were markedly elevated, and renal function was severely compromised with a blood urea nitrogen (BUN) of 50 mg/dL and a creatinine of 2.9 mg/dL. His total protein was

3.3 g/dL; albumin 0.7 g/dL; and liver function tests were grossly abnormal with an alkaline phosphatase of 433 U/liter, and an aspartate aminotransferase of 269 U/liter. An arterial blood gas had a pH of 7.19 with a P_{O_2} of 38 mmHg and a P_{CO_2} of 45 mmHg. A chest roentgenogram was notable for perihilar infiltrates, with perihilar adenopathy. Despite vigorous support with intravenous fluids, pressors, high-dose adrenocorticosteroids, broad-spectrum antibacterial agents, and empiric pentamidine, the patient became progressively less responsive and died within 1 week of his hospitalization.

Postmortem examination revealed widespread Kaposi's sarcoma. Microscopic examination of the lungs revealed diffuse involvement with fluffy eosinophilic intra-alveolar infiltrates. Gomori–methenamine silver (GMS) stain demonstrated cyst forms of *P. carinii*. Examination of the liver revealed sinuses expanded by foamy eosinophilic material associated with Kupffer cells and focal hepatocellular necrosis (Fig. 1a); GMS stains were positive for *P. carinii* (see Fig. 1b). The spleen had multiple areas of cell loss, with replacement by foamy eosinophilic material that stained for *P. carinii* on GMS stain. The bone marrow was striking in that it was almost entirely replaced by fluffy eosinophilic material and *P. carinii* (Fig. 2). *Pneumocystis carinii* was seen on GMS staining of both kidneys and was associated with areas of necrosis of the glomerular tufts. Other areas of pneumocystis involvement included the pituitary, skin, trachea, lymph nodes, and heart (Fig. 3).

In contrast with the case just presented is one that was reported by Schinella (36). A 36-year-old man, who was a former intravenous drug user and known to be HIV-antibody positive, presented with a subacute course of progressive hearing loss. On physical examination, the patient's left tympanic membrane showed scarring with a 3-mm × 5-mm polyp at the junction of the external auditory canal and the pars flaccida. The remainder of the physical examination was normal, with normal blood values, a normal chest roentgenogram, and a negative gallium scan. The patient was not anergic, with a 15-mm area of induration to intradermal candida testing. The aural polyp was biopsied and light microscopy showed foamy eosinophilic material; silver stains revealed *P. carinii*. Symptoms resolved on an oral trimethoprim–sulfamethoxasole regimen.

These two cases represent the extremes in the clinical presentation of extrapulmonary pneumocystosis: the first, a widely disseminated and invasive infection causing multiple organ dysfunction and death in a profoundly immunocompromised patient; the second, a single site of infection causing localized symptoms and responding to oral therapy.

Of the 40 well-described HIV-infected patients, 38 were men and 2 were women and the age range was 24–74 years, with a mean age of approximately 35 years; no children have been reported with extrapulmonary disease. The distribution of extrapulmonary *P. carinii* by risk factor for HIV is approximately representative of the distribution of risk factors for AIDS cases for the epidemic.

Table 1 shows the organ distribution of 40 cases of extrapulmonary pneumo-

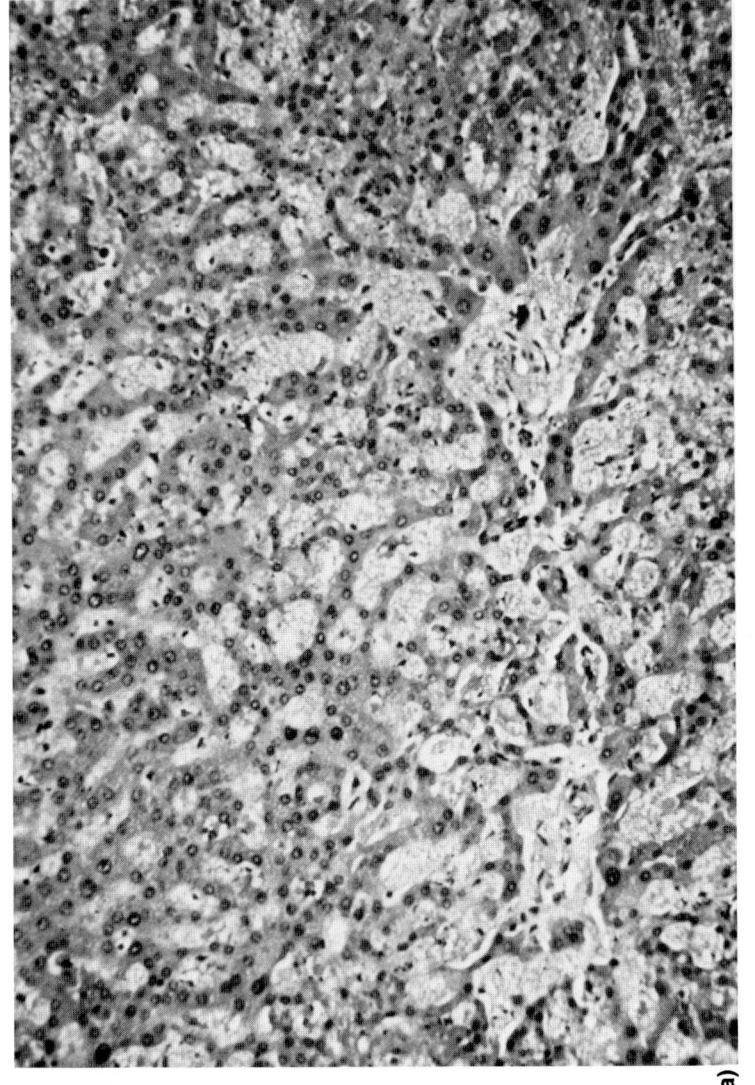

Figure 1 (a) H&E stain of liver; sinuses expanded by foamy eosinophilic material and hepatic necrosis. (b) GMS stain of liver: cyst form of *P. carinii*.

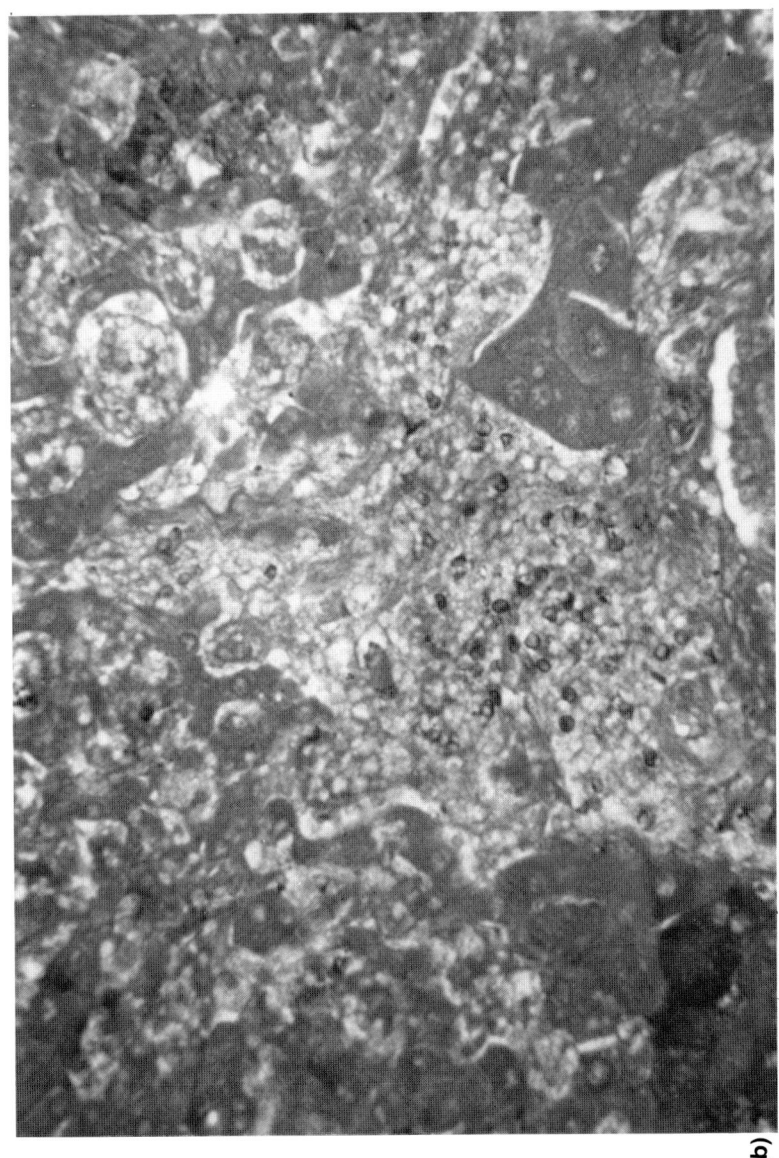

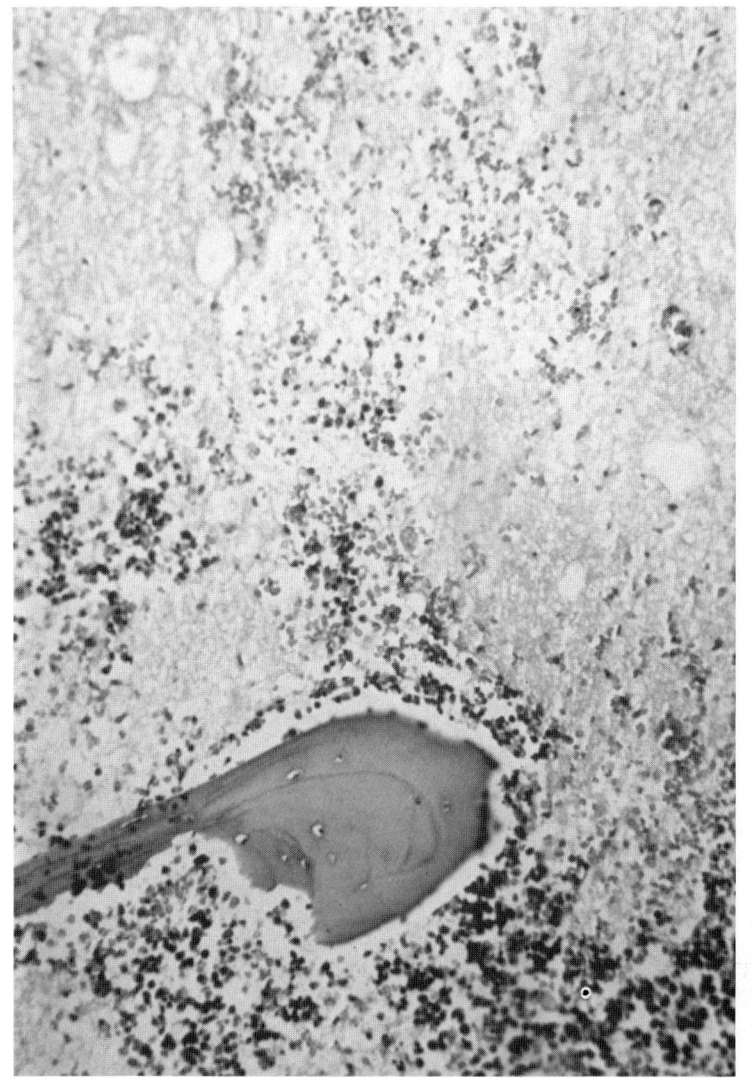

Figure 2 (a) H&E stain of bone marrow; almost complete replacement of normal elements by eosinophilic material. (b) GMS stain of bone marrow: cyst form of *P. carinii*.

Extrapulmonary Infection

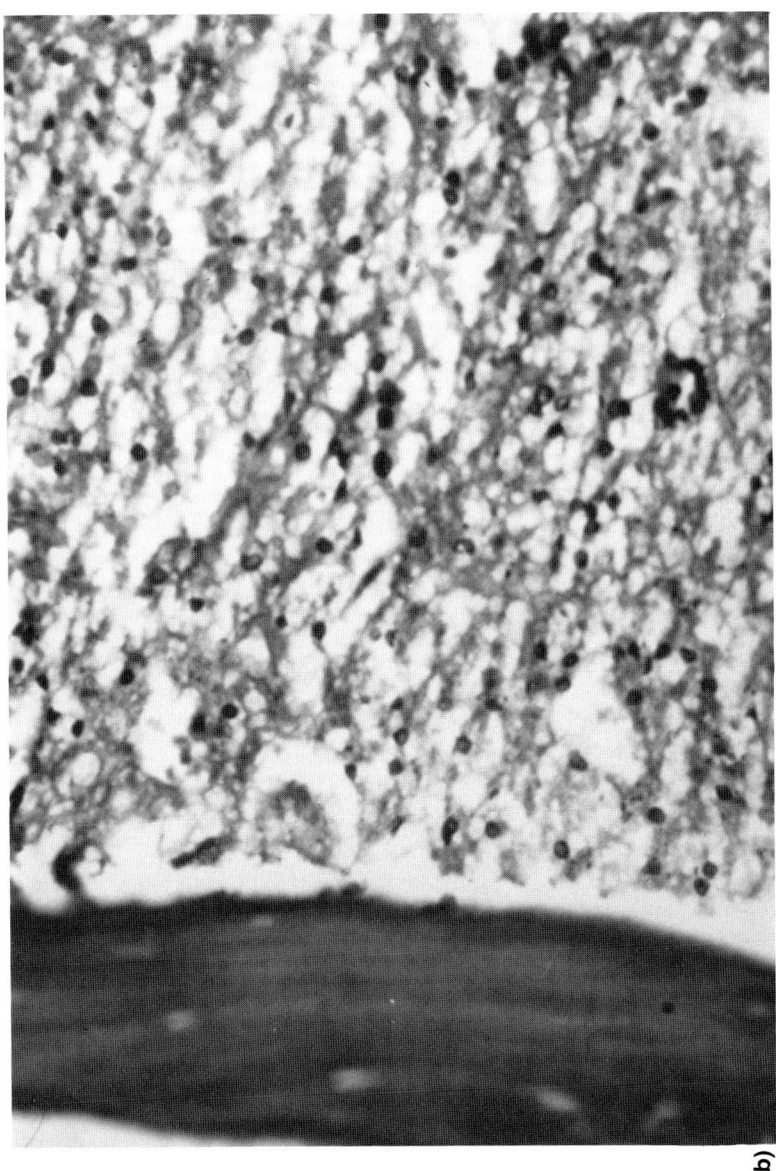

(b)

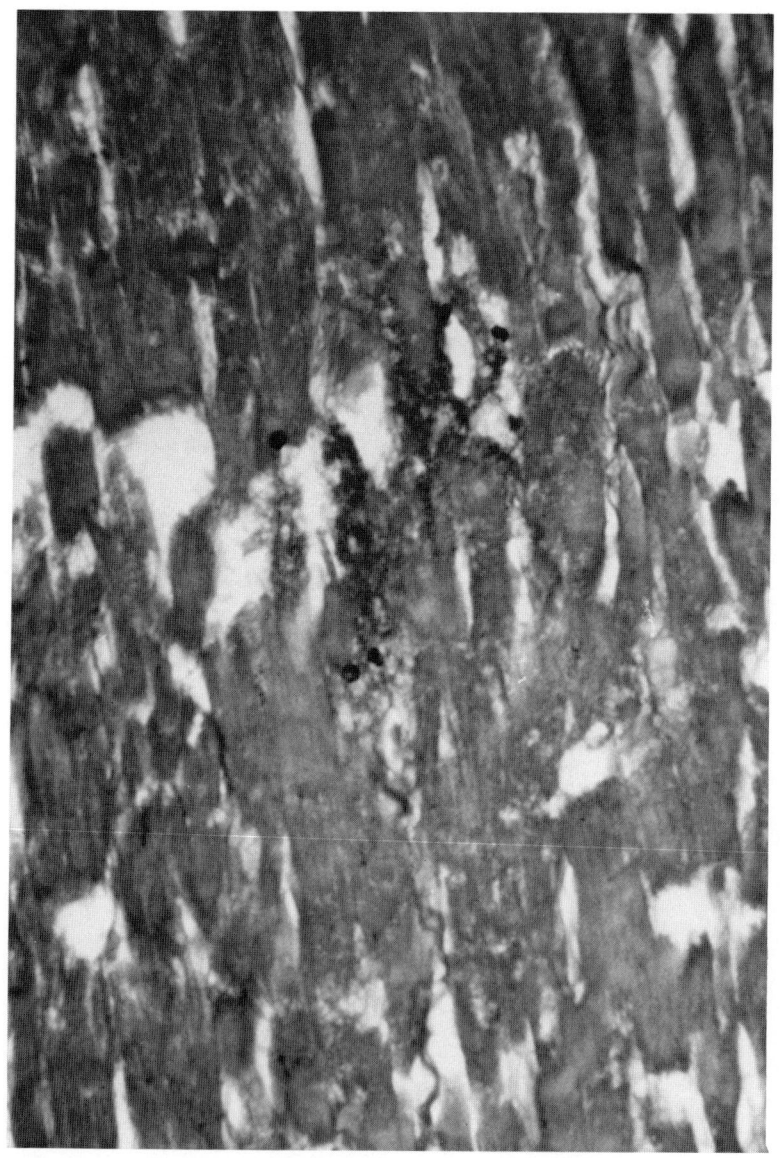

Figure 3 GMS stain of cardiac tissue revealing *P. carinii*.

cystosis in AIDS patients compared with patients who were not infected with HIV. As is apparent in cases without HIV infection, the organ systems most commonly involved are the lymph nodes, the spleen and liver, and the bone marrow. Whereas no patient without HIV had eye involvement, six (15%) patients with AIDS had involvement of this organ. Similarly, external otitis or middle ear *P. carinii* infections were not described before the AIDS epidemic; subsequently, six cases have been published. Unusual areas of involvement include the pituitary gland, the parathyroid glands, the skin, and the cerebral cortex. One patient presented with three paraspinal masses in the thoracic region that responded to medical management.

The clinical presentation in reported cases has varied widely as already noted. In nearly all cases, nonspecific signs and symptoms of infection, such as fever and malaise, were present. Eighteen (45%) patients presented with concurrent *P. carinii* pneumonia, and many had symptoms suggestive of pulmonary involvement. Even with extensive extrapulmonary involvement, however, some patients remained relatively asymptomatic. This was particularly evident for infection of the spleen, lymph nodes, and adrenal glands. In contrast, *P. carinii* infections of the liver, the bone marrow, the choroid or retina, and the ears were generally associated with signs and symptoms referable to that organ. In addition, two patients seen at MSKCC have had pneumocystosis of the small bowel, resulting in perforation (unpublished). Despite prolonged courses of intravenous pentamidine, both patients died.

VI. Diagnosis and Pathology

Obtaining of an adequate tissue sample through biopsy of the involved organ is the most effective means of making a diagnosis of extrapulmonary *P. carinii* infection. However, these organisms have been seen on pleural and ascitic fluid specimens and from aspirated material of masses (16,50). On gross pathological inspection the involved tissues are frequently described as containing firm and tan nodules, some of which may contain necrotic material or calcification. The diagnosis has usually been suspected because the histopathology seen on hematoxylin–eosin stain resembles that seen in the lung: foamy eosinophilic exudate replacing normal tissue. Gomori–methenamine silver stain reveals the cyst form of *P. carinii* within the foamy eosinophilic material. Some authors have suggested that immunohistochemical techniques be used in addition to the GMS stain to identify *P. carinii* organisms (46).

The radiologic literature contains descriptions of the sonographic and computed tomographic (CT) findings in extrapulmonary infection (50,51). On CT scans, focal low-attenuation lesions are seen in involved organs; these lesions become progressively calcified in either a rim-like or punctate fashion. Similarly, involvement of pleural and peritoneal spaces resulted in subsequent calcification of the pleural and peritoneal surfaces. With sonography, calcifications, comparable with the CT findings have been noted in abdominal organs.

VII. Outcome

Of the 40 patients with AIDS detailed in this review, 23 (58%) died as a result of their pneumocystosis and 17 survived. Of the 18 patients who were thought to have only a single extrapulmonary site of infection without concurrent PCP, 13 (72%) survived compared with 4 of 22 patients who had more than one site of *P. carinii* infection (OR = 11.7, $p < 0.002$).

VIII. Risk Factors

In many of the recent articles on extrapulmonary *P. carinii* infection, aerosol pentamidine is cited as a risk factor or a probable risk factor for the development of extrapulmonary disease. Implicating aerosol pentamidine appears biologically reasonable, given the primarily pulmonary distribution of this method of delivery. However, only 20 (50%) of the patients were receiving aerosol pentamidine. Most of these patients had two or more organs involved.

Twenty patients were not receiving aerosol pentamidine at the time their extrapulmonary disease was diagnosed and many of these patients presented with relatively localized infection. In addition, none of the non–HIV-infected patients who developed extrapulmonary disease were using aerosol pentamidine. Obviously, aerosol pentamidine is not necessary for the development of extrapulmonary disease. Even if this agent is associated with an elevated risk of extrapulmonary infection, it is unclear whether aerosol pentamidine use itself is a risk; whether patients using the drug are more immunosuppressed compared with those not receiving it and, therefore, at higher risk; or, finally, whether aerosol pentamidine allows patients to survive longer, and increased survival puts them at higher risk for the development of multiple adverse outcomes, including extrapulmonary *P. carinii* infection.

Until recently, no case of extrapulmonary infection had been reported in patients receiving systemic prophylaxis for PCP. A case was presented at the VIIth International AIDS Conference of hepatosplenic pneumocystosis in a patient with a previous history of *P. carinii* pneumonia who had been receiving trimethoprim–sulfamethoxasole for 7 weeks (49).

Other potential risk factors for extraalveolar *P. carinii* infection have not been characterized. Whether there are local pulmonary factors, systemic factors, or perhaps even variations in the invasiveness of organisms is completely unknown. Recently, *P. carinii* has been detected in serum of AIDS patients with PCP by the polymerase chain reaction (PCR) (52). By using a nucleotide sequence of the *P. carinii* dihydrofolate reductase gene, 5 of 11 adults with PCP had evidence of *P. carinii* DNA in their serum detectable by PCR. Although additional studies are needed, the preliminary implication of the foregoing study is that *P. carinii* circulates in the serum of almost 50% of patients with PCP.

IX. Unusual Pulmonary Manifestations of *Pneumocystis carinii* Pneumonia

Before the AIDS epidemic, unusual pulmonary presentations, both clinical and radiologic, were well described (3,53). In one review of 30 morphologically confirmed cases of *P. carinii* pneumonia, only 13 patients had a classic radiologic presentation. Seventeen (56%) presented with at least one atypical radiologic finding during the course of their illness, which included unilateral distribution, lobar involvement, abscess formation, fulminant progression, and atelectatic changes. Others had described pleural effusions and sparing of previously irradiated areas of lung (53) and localized nodular densities (54).

Roentgenographic abnormalities in patients with AIDS attributed to *P. carinii* infection before the introduction of aerosol pentamidine have been reviewed (55). DeLorenzo et al. observed that localized infiltrates were present in 47 of 104 cases of PCP. Lower lung field infiltrates were present in 35 patients, upper lung field infiltrates were present in 6 patients, and an additional 6 patients had midlung field infiltrates. Cysts, pneumothoraces, and hilar adenopathy were noted in a few patients.

The effect of aerosol pentamidine on the presentation and diagnosis of PCP has been well demonstrated in patients with AIDS (56). Of 21 patients receiving prophylactic aerosol pentamidine only 11 (52%) had the classic roentgenogram of diffuse infiltrates, compared with 29 (90%) of 31 patients not receiving aerosol pentamidine ($p < 0.05$). In comparison, 38% of patients receiving aerosol pentamidine had predominantly upper lobe infiltrates compared with only 2 of the 31 patients not receiving aerosol pentamidine. Cystic lesions were noted in both groups and pneumothoraces occurred in 3 patients, all of whom were receiving aerosol pentamidine. Others have also noted that patients receiving aerosol pentamidine were more likely to have infection isolated or preponderantly in the upper lobes (57).

Multiple recent radiologic reviews have emphasized atypical manifestations of PCP in patients with AIDS. Cavitary lesions involving both nodular and more diffuse infiltrates are increasingly recognized (58–60). In addition, pneumatoceles, or pulmonary air-filled cysts have been identified in up to 10% of chest roentgenograms of patients with documented PCP (61). The cysts are described as typically thin walled and without intracystic material or a propensity for any particular lobe of the lung. Small unilateral and bilateral pleural effusions also occur.

X. Pneumothorax

Given the rarity of spontaneous pneumothorax in the general population, there has been a growing appreciation, as evidenced by case reports, of a higher than expected rate of pneumothorax in patients with AIDS. At Memorial Sloan–Kettering Cancer Center 20 (2%) of 1030 patients with AIDS developed pneumothorax unrelated to trauma, including bronchoscopy or mechanical ventilation from the period January 1, 1980 through September 30, 1989 (62). Use of aerosol pentamidine (relative risk, 17.6) and a previous episode of PCP (relative risk, 14.5) were significant risk factors for the development of pneumothorax by bivariate analysis. Patients with a greater number of previous episodes of PCP, however, were more likely to be receiving aerosol pentamidine prophylaxis. By Mantel–Haenszel multivariate analysis only a history of aerosol pentamidine use proved to be a statistically significant independent risk factor for the development of pneumothorax. The synergistic contribution of aerosol pentamidine use and a history of *P. carinii* pneumonia toward the development of pneumothorax is shown in Table 2. There were no cases of pneumothorax among 365 patients who had neither risk factor, whereas 6.3% of patients with both risk factors developed pneumothorax. In addition, of the 20 patients who developed pneumothorax, 19 (95%) had compelling evidence of concurrent active pneumocystis infection.

It appeared biologically plausible that patients receiving aerosol pentamidine were at higher risk for developing pneumothorax. Aerosol pentamidine may be deposited at low concentrations in the lung periphery (63). We have hypothesized, therefore, that those patients who develop PCP while receiving aerosol pentamidine are more likely to develop a peripheral low-grade pneumonitis; with extension to the pleural surface and necrosis by actively proliferating *P. carinii*, a pneumothorax results.

Table 2 The Combined Effects of Aerosol Pentamidine and Prior History of PCP upon the Development of Pneumothorax (PTX)

Prior history of PCP	Aerosol pentamidine use	PTX	(rate)
No	No	0/365	(0%)
Yes	No	2/317	(0.6%)
No	Yes	1/80	(1.3%)
Yes	Yes	17/268	(6.3%)

Source: Ref. 62.

Given the very strong association of concurrent PCP with pneumothorax (19 of 20 patients) we have recommended that any patient with AIDS who develops a pneumothorax should be treated as if the patient were actively infected with PCP.

XI. Summary

There has long been an appreciation of the diversity of clinical presentation of both pulmonary and extrapulmonary infection with *P. carinii*. The true prevalence of bloodstream invasion and dissemination by *P. carinii* is unknown. Sensitive techniques to detect the presence of *P. carinii* DNA should overcome the inability to isolate the organism. Given the frequency of PCP that is currently seen and the routine use of aerosol pentamidine prophylaxis in patients at highest risk for *P. carinii* infection, it is likely that the numbers of cases who present in an atypical fashion will increase, and the diversity of clinical presentation will continue. This chapter has reviewed the unusual manifestations of *P. carinii* infection in both patients infected and uninfected with HIV.

Acknowledgments

Dr. Kent Sepkowitz for his critical review of the manuscript and Dr. Richard Cote for photographs.

References

1. Centers for Disease Control. HIV/AIDS surveillance report, September 1991:1–18.
2. Selik RM, Starcher ET, Curran JW. Opportunistic diseases reported in AIDS patients: frequencies, associations, and trends. AIDS 1987; 1:175–182.
3. Doppman JL, Geelhoed GW, DeVita VT. Atypical radiographic features in *Pneumocystis carinii* pneumonia. Radiology 1975; 114:39–44.
4. Anderson CD, Barrie HJ. Fatal pneumocystis pneumonia in an adult. Am J Clin Pathol 1960; 34:365–370.
5. Livingstone CS. Pneumocystis pneumonia occurring in a family with agammaglobulinemia. Can Med Assoc J 1964; 90:1223–1225.
6. Jarnum S, Rasmussen EF, Ohlsen AS, Sorenson AWS. Generalized *Pneumocystis carinii* infection with severe idiopathic hypoproteinemia. Ann Intern Med 1968; 68:138–145.
7. Barnett RN, Hull JG, Vortel V, Kralove H, Schwartz J. *Pneumocystis carinii* in lymph nodes and spleen. Arch Pathol 1969; 88:175–180.
8. Awen CF, Baltzan MA. Systemic dissemination of *Pneumocystis carinii* pneumonia. Can Med Assoc J 1971; 104:809–812.
9. Henderson DW, Humeniuk V, Meadows R, Forbes IJ. *Pneumocystis carinii* pneu-

monia with vascular and lymph node involvement. Pathology 1974; 6:235–241.
10. LeGolvan DP, Heidelberger KP. Disseminated granulomatous *Pneumocystis carinii* pneumonia. Arch Pathol 1973; 95:344–348.
11. Rahimi SA. Disseminated *Pneumocystis carinii* in thymic alymphoplasia. Arch Pathol 1974; 97:162–165.
12. Rossi JF, Dubois A, Bengler C, Arich C, Gervais C, Delage A, Janbon C. *Pneumocystis carinii* in bone marrow [letter]. Ann Intern Med 1985; 102:868.
13. Walzer PD, Perl DP, Krogstad DJ, Rawson PG, Schulz MG. *Pneumocystis carinii* pneumonia in the United States. Ann Intern Med 1974; 80:83–93.
14. Telzak EE, Cote RJ, Gold JWM, Campbell SW, Armstrong D. Extrapulmonary *Pneumocystis carinii* infections. Rev Infect Dis 1990; 12:380–386.
15. Raviglione MC. Extrapulmonary pneumocystosis: the first 50 cases. Rev Infect Dis 1990; 12:1127–1138.
16. Northfelt DW, Clement MJ, Safrin S. Extrapulmonary pneumocystosis: clinical features in human immunodeficiency virus infection. Medicine 1990; 69:392–398.
17. Cohen OJ, Stoeckle MY. Extrapulmonary *Pneumocystis carinii* infections in the acquired immunodeficiency syndrome. Arch Interm Med 1991; 151:1205–1214.
18. Gajdusek DC. *Pneumocystis carinii*: etiologic agent of interstitial plasma-cell pneumonia of premature and young infants. Pediatrics 1957; 19:543–565.
19. Burke BA, Good RA. *Pneumocystis carinii* infection. Medicine 1973; 52:23–51.
20. Sepkowitz KA, Brown AE, Telzak EE, Gottlieb S, Armstrong D. *Pneumocystis carinii* pneumonia among patients without AIDS at a cancer hospital. JAMA (in press).
21. Kwok S, O'Donnell JJ, Wood IS. Retinal cotton-wool spots in a patient with *Pneumocystis carinii* infection [letter]. N Engl J Med 1982; 307:184–185.
22. Grimes MM, LaPook JD, Bar MH, Wasserman HS, Dwork A. Disseminated *Pneumocystis carinii* infection in a patient with acquired immunodeficiency syndrome. Hum Pathol 1987; 18:307–308.
23. Macher AM, Bardenstein DS, Zimmerman LE, Steigmsn CK, Pastore L, Poretz DM, Eron LJ. *Pneumocystis carinii* choroiditis in a male homosexual with AIDS and disseminated pulmonary and extrapulmonary *P. carinii* infection [letter]. N Engl J Med 1987; 316:1092.
24. Heyman MR, Rasmussen P. *Pneumocystis carinii* involvement of bone marrow in acquired immunodeficiency syndrome. Am J Clin Pathol 1987; 87:780–783.
25. Pilon VA, Echols RM, Celo JS, Elmendorf SL. Disseminated *Pneumocystis carinii* infection in AIDS [letter]. N Engl J Med 1987; 316:1410–1411.
26. Schinella RA, Breda SD, Hammerschlag PE. Otic infection due to *Pneumocystis carinii* in an apparently healthy man with antibody to the human immunodeficiency virus. Ann Intern Med 1987; 106:399–400.
27. Coulman CU, Greene I, Archibald RWR. Cutaneous pneumocystosis. Ann Intern Med 1987; 106:396–398.
28. Gallant JE, Enriquez RE, Cohen KL, Hammers LW. *Pneumocystis carinii* thyroiditis. Am J Med 1988; 84:303–306.
29. Unger PD, Rosenblum M, Krown SE. Disseminated *Pneumocystis carinii* infection in a patient with acquired immunodeficiency syndrome. Hum Pathol 1988; 19:113–116.

30. Gherman CR, Ward RR, Bassis ML. *Pneumocystis carinii* otitis media and mastoiditis as the initial manifestation of the acquired immunodeficiency syndrome. Am J Med 1988; 85:250–252.
31. Afessa B, Green WR, Williams WA, Hagler NG, Gumbs RV, Hackney RL, Frederick WR. *Pneumocystis carinii* pneumonia complicated by lymphadenopathy and pneumothorax. Arch Intern Med 1988; 148:2651–2654.
32. Breda SD, Gigliotti F, Hammerschlag PE, Schinella R. *Pneumocystis carinii* in the temporal bone as a primary manifestation of the acquired immunodeficiency syndrome. Ann Otol Rhinol Laryngol 1988; 97:427–431.
33. Smith MA, Hirschfield LS, Zahtz G, Siegel FP. *Pneumocystis carinii* otitis media. Am J Med 1988; 85:745–746.
34. Carter TR, Cooper PH, Petri WA, Kim K, Walzer PD, Guerrant RL. *Pneumocystis carinii* infection of the small intestine in a patient with acquired immune deficiency syndrome. Am J Clin Pathol 1988; 89:679–683.
35. Raviglione MC, Garner GR, Mullen MP. *Pneumocystis carinii* in bone marrow [letter]. Ann Intern Med 1988; 109:253.
36. Raviglione MC, Mariuz P, Sugar J, Mullen MP. Extrapulmonary pneumocystis infection [letter]. Ann Intern Med 1989; 111:339.
37. Poblete RB, Rodriguez K, Foust RT, Reddy KR, Saldana MJ. *Pneumocystis carinii* hepatitis in the acquired immunodeficiency syndrome (AIDS). Ann Intern Med 1989; 110:737–738.
38. Richie TL, Yamaguchi E, Virani NA, Quinn BD, Chaisson RE. Extrapulmonary pneumocystis infection [letter]. Ann Intern Med 1989; 11:339–340.
39. Hardy WD, Northfelt DW, Drake TA. Fatal disseminated pneumocystosis in a patient with acquired immunodeficiency syndrome receiving prophylactic aerosolized pentamidine. Am J Med 1989; 87:329–331.
40. Davey TR, Margolis D, Kleiner D, Deyton L, Travis W. Digital necrosis and disseminated *Pneumocystis carinii* infection after aerosolized pentamidine prophylaxis. Ann Intern Med 1989; 111:681–682.
41. Hagopian WA, Huseby JS. Pneumocystis hepatitis and choroiditis despite successful aerosolized pentamidine pulmonary prophylaxis. Chest 1989; 96:949–951.
42. Sparling TG, Dong SR, Hegedis C, Burdge DR. Aerosolized pentamidine and disseminated infection with *Pneumocystis carinii* [letter]. Ann Intern Med 1989; 111:442.
43. Matsuda S, Urata Y, Shiota T, Yamada M, Yoshikawa H, Tegoshi T, Okada M, Nakamura H, Kitaoka T, Ashihara T, Yoshida Y. Disseminated infection of *Pneumocystis carinii* in a patient with acquired immunodeficiency syndrome. Virchows Arch [A] 1989; 414:523–527.
44. Rao NA, Zimmerman PL, Boyer D, Biswas J, Causey D, Beniz J, Nichols PW. A clinical, histopathologic, and electron microscopic study of *Pneumocystis carinii* choroiditis. Am J Ophthalmol 1989; 107:218–228.
45. Sneed SR, Blodi CF, Berger BB, Speights JW, Folk JC, Weingeist TA. *Pneumocystis carinii* choroiditis in patients receiving inhaled pentamidine [letter]. N Engl J Med 1990; 322:936–937.
46. Cote RJ, Rosenblum M, Telzak EE, May M, Unger PD, Cartun RW. Disseminated

Pneumocystis carinii infection causing extrapulmonary organ failure: clinical, pathologic, and immunohistochemical analysis. Mod Pathol 1990; 3:25–30.
47. Ragni MV, Dekker A, DeRubertis FR, Watson CG, Skolnick ML, Goold SD, Finikiotis MW, Doshi S, Myers D. Pneumocystis carinii infection presenting as necrotizing thyroiditis and hypothyroidism. Am J Clin Pathol 1991; 95:489–493.
48. Rossi JF, Eledjam JJ, Delage A, Bengler C, Schved JF, Bonnafoux J. Pneumocystis carinii infection of bone marrow in patients with malignant lymphoma and acquired immunodeficiency syndrome. Arch Intern Med 1991; 150:450–452.
49. Rockstroh J, Ewig S, Luster W, Niese D. Disseminated Pneumocystis carinii infection in an AIDS-patient on trimethoprim/sulfamethoxazole prophylaxis after breakthrough PCI. Seventh International Conference on AIDS, Florence, Italy, 1991.
50. Lubat E, Megibow AJ, Balthazar EJ, Goldenberg AS, Birnbaum BA, Bosniak MA. Extrapulmonary Pneumocystis carinii infection in AIDS: CT findings. Radiology 1990; 174:157–160.
51. Radin DR, Baker EL, Klatt EC, et al. Visceral and nodal calcification in patients with AIDS-related Pneumocystis carinii infection. AJR 1990; 154:27–31.
52. Schluger N, Sepkowitz K, Armstrong D, Rifkin M, Bernard E, Cerami A, Bucala A. Detection of Pneumocystis carinii in serum of AIDS patients with Pneumocystis pneumonia by the polymerase chain reaction. Forty-fourth Annual Meeting of the Society of Protozoologists, Bozeman, Montana, 1991.
53. Forrest JV. Radiographic findings in Pneumocystis carinii pneumonia. Radiology 1972; 103:539–544.
54. Cross AS, Steigbigel RT. Pneumocystis carinii pneumonia presenting as localized nodular densities. N Engl J Med 1974; 291:831–832.
55. DeLorenzo LJ, Huang CT, Maguire GP, Stone DJ. Roentgenographic patterns of Pneumocystis carinii pneumonia in 104 patients with AIDS. Chest 1987; 91:323–327.
56. Jules-Elysee KM, Stover, DE, Zaman MB, Bernard EM, White DA. Aerosolized pentamidine: effect on diagnosis and presentation of Pneumocystis carinii pneumonia. Ann Intern Med 1990; 112:750–757.
57. Chaffey MH, Klein JS, Gamsu G, Blanc P, Golden JA. Radiographic distribution of Pneumocystis carinii pneumonia in patients with AIDS treated with prophylactic inhaled pentamidine. Radiology 1990; 175:715–719.
58. Saldana MJ, Mones JM. Cavitation and other atypical manifestations of Pneumocystis carinii pneumonia. Semin Diag Pathol 1989; 6:273–286.
59. Feuerstein IM, Archer A, Pluda JM, Francis PS, Falloon J, Masur H, Pass HI, Travis WD. Thin-walled cavities, cysts, and pneumothorax in Pneumocystis carinii pneumonia: further observations with histopathologic correlation. Radiology 1990; 174: 697–702.
60. Kuhlman JE, Kavuru M, Fishman EK, Siegelman SS. Pneumocystis carinii pneumonia: spectrum of parenchymal CT findings. Radiology 1990; 175:711714.
61. Sandhu JS, Goodman PC. Pulmonary cysts associated with Pneumocystis carinii pneumonia in patients with AIDS. Radiology 1989; 173:33–35.
62. Sepkowitz KA, Telzak EE, Gold JWM, Bernard EM, Blum S, Carrow M, Dickmeyer M, Armstrong D. Pneumothorax in AIDS. Ann Intern Med 1991; 114:455–459.

Part Five

DIAGNOSIS

19

Current Methods of Diagnosis

ROBERT P. BAUGHMAN

University of Cincinnati Medical Center
Cincinnati, Ohio

I. Introduction

As is discussed elsewhere in this book, *Pneumocystis carinii* is a potential pathogen usually found in the lung (1,2), although extrapulmonary infection has been described (3,4). The infection is usually detected by examination of lung specimens for evidence of *P. carinii* organisms. The methods for detection have been developed in two ways. First, there has been an attempt to use less invasively obtained samples to make a premortem diagnosis of *P. carinii* pneumonia. Therefore, the specimens examined range from open-lung specimens (5,6), through transbronchial biopsies (7,8) and bronchoalveolar lavage (BAL) specimens (9,10) obtained by bronchoscopy, to examination of sputum (11–13). Another area of development has been with new stains. The traditional method to recognize *P. carinii* has been through the use of stains of the cyst wall, such as a silver (14) or toluidine blue O stain (15,16). In patients with a large number of *P. carinii*, the commonly used Papanicolaou or Wright–Giemsa stain can be used to recognize the trophozoites (17,18). These stains are widely used and can be performed in as short as 5 min (19). The characterization of antigens on the *P. carinii* surface has allowed development of antibodies against *P. carinii* and the use of direct fluorescent and indirect immunofluorescent stains (11,20–22). These methods are more sensitive than either the cyst or trophozoite stains; however, the techniques are more expensive and require a certain amount of expertise.

With the identification of antigens specific for *P. carinii*, there has also been the additional possibility of diagnosing *P. carinii* on the basis of antigen or antibody testing in the blood (23,24). Serological testing is of limited value because most people have antibodies to *P. carinii* from childhood onward. However, changes in titer may represent infection, even in asymptomatic persons (25). This technique has been used for epidemiological studies, and may be useful in determining the source and infectivity of *P. carinii*. Pneumocystis carinii antigen has also been detected in the blood of infected patients (26). However, the presence of this antigen may not be specific for *P. carinii* infection or pneumonia (27,28).

The rest of this chapter will be divided into three sections. The first will discuss methods of obtaining specimens to examine for *P. carinii*. The second section will deal with staining techniques and their relative merits. The final sections will deal with other methods to diagnose or suggest *P. carinii*.

II. Obtaining Specimens

The least invasive method for obtaining lower respiratory specimens is sputum examination. Initially, it was felt that *P. carinii* could be diagnosed only by invasive sampling of the lower respiratory tract. In patients infected with human immunodeficiency virus (HIV), there is often a much larger amount of *P. carinii* encountered in airway specimens. Because of this, several groups have reported on the merit of examining sputum for *P. carinii* (11–13). In these studies, it has become clear that most patients with *P. carinii* pneumonia do not spontaneously produce enough sputum for a diagnosis. However, with the use of hypertonic saline, adequate sputum can be induced from patients (12,29). It has also been found that the use of mucolytic agents may help increase yield (30).

The use of sputum induction for diagnosing *P. carinii* has resulted in some variability in the sensitivity for the organism, ranging from less than 30% to as high as 90% (11,12,29,31). The results of several groups who compared sputum examination versus other techniques to diagnose *P. carinii* are summarized in Table 1. The major factor for higher yield appears to be familiarity. As centers do more sputum examinations, the yield appears to rise in greater than 50%. With the use immunofluorescent stains, the yield may be higher than 90% (12). This high yield for sputum examination has mostly been found in patients not receiving aerosol pentamidine prophylaxis. In one study of patients receiving aerosol pentamidine prophylaxis, the yield of induced sputum was reduced, but was still greater than 50% (32).

Another commonly used method to diagnose *P. carinii* is flexible fiberoptic

Table 1 Sensitivity of Sputum for Diagnosis of *P. carinii*

Stain used	Sputum-positive/ number with pneumonia	Percentage positive	Other conditions	Ref.
Wright–Giemsa	11/20	55		12
Wright–Giemsa	14/25	56		13
Wright–Giemsa	10/25	40	Routine sputum	30
Wright–Giemsa	21/25	84	Concentrated sputum	30
Methenamine silver	2/13	15		31
Toluidine blue O	21/25	84		11
Indirect immunofluorescent	23/25	92		11
Wright–Giemsa	66/73	90		22
Direct fluorescent	71/73	97		22

bronchoscopy. Bronchoscopy is a simple procedure done with local anesthesia, often performed in an outpatient setting. The procedure is usually done with the aid of intravenous narcotics and benzodiazepams. Although sedation makes the procedure more tolerable for the patient, it increases the risk. The most frequently encountered problems with bronchoscopy are due to preoperative medication, including oversedation and hypoventilation. Complete assessment of the patient before bronchoscopy will minimize these complications (33–36).

The bronchoscopic examination of the airways provides little direct information. The advantage of bronchoscopy for diagnosing *P. carinii* pneumonia is in the specimens obtained. Bronchial brush specimens can be obtained of the airways or specimens beyond the airways. Bronchial wash is simply the captured secretions suctioned throughout the bronchoscopy. These usually represent large-airway samples. The transbronchial biopsy is a method of obtaining parenchymal lung tissue and can be done either blindly or under fluoroscopic guidance. In either method, the bronchoscopist advances the biopsy forceps along the airways to a small enough airway that the biopsy taken will contain alveolar units. The procedure is associated with a 5–10% incidence of pneumothorax. In a study by Broaddas et al. (7), AIDS patients underwent 253 bronchoscopies with transbronchial biopsies. Twenty-three (9%) had pneumothoraces and 15 (6%) required chest tube placement.

Although the use of BAL to diagnose *P. carinii* was reported as early as 1974 (37), it did not become a widely used technique until the mid-1980s, mostly as a result of the report by Stover et al. (9). Bronchoalveolar lavage is a technique by which the bronchoscope is advanced as far as possible along a natural pathway to a nonindependent lobe (e.g., right middle lobe) (38). Normal saline (100–240 mL) is instilled and immediately withdrawn by either a hand-held syringe or low-pressure suction. The collected fluid is then studied for *P. carinii*.

The various techniques have differing yields for *P. carinii*. Figure 1 demonstrates the yield from several large studies, as well as our own experience (7,9,10,39). One conclusion from this figure is that the bronchial wash and brush specimens are associated with a relatively low yield (40–80%), whereas both BAL and transbronchial biopsy have been associated with a usually greater than 90% yield. The introduction of lavage has significantly increased the yield of bronchoscopy for diagnosing *P. carinii* (40).

Diagnosis of *P. carinii* infection by lavage alone bypasses the toxicity of transbronchial biopsy in patients with possible *P. carinii*. As noted the foregoing, transbronchial biopsy is associated with a significant risk of pneumothorax, which is rare when BAL alone is performed. Pneumothoraces are more common in acquired immunodeficiency syndrome (AIDS) patients with *P. carinii* (41,42), and patients with pneumothoraces may develop bronchopleural fistulas that can be troublesome to treat (41,43). Therefore, many centers prefer to perform bronchoscopy with lavage for initial evaluation (44). Patients who fail to have a diagnostic bronchoscopy undergo repeat bronchoscopy with lavage and transbronchial biopsy.

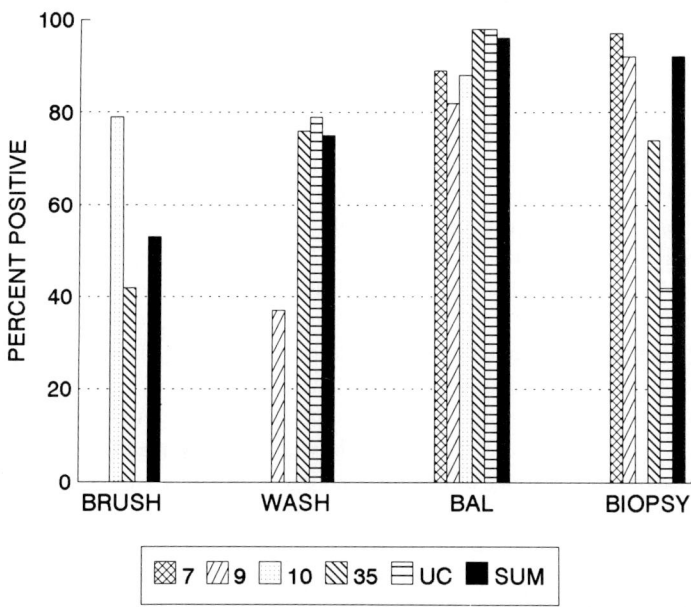

Figure 1 Comparative yield for four bronchoscopic specimens in patients with *P. carinii* pneumonia. Four centers, plus the experience at the University of Cincinnati (UC) are shown, plus the sum of all five studies.

Recently, Jules-Elysee et al. reported that lavage failed to make a diagnosis in 33% of their patients with *P. carinii* who had been receiving pentamidine aerosol prophylaxis (8). In that study, they found that transbronchial biopsy was significantly better. Chest roentgenograms of their patients demonstrated an atypical appearance, usually of upper lobe disease. At another institution, a similarly designed study of patients receiving aerosol pentamidine found a high yield for lavage and no significant benefit for an additional transbronchial biopsy (45). Subsequent reports have suggested that the yield for *P. carinii* could be increased by sampling multiple areas within the lung (46,47). For example, we performed lavage on 50 consecutive patient with *P. carinii* pneumonia. We found an approximate 2:1 preponderance of *P. carinii* in the upper lobe compared with the lower lobe. In 6 cases, there was no *P. carinii* identified in the middle lobe (46). Figures 2 and 3 show the chest roentgenogram and lavage specimens of an AIDS patient, with cough, fever, and shortness of breath, who underwent bronchoscopy and lavage. The patient had been receiving once-a-month aerosol pentamidine prophylaxis. Figure 2 demonstrates a localized infiltrate in the right upper lobe. Figure 3a shows the cells retrieved by lavage of the medial segment of the right middle lobe; no clusters of *P. carinii* were seen. Figure 3b shows the cells and *P. carinii* identified from in the apical segment of the right upper lobe; the clusters of *P. carinii* are easily identified.

An adaptation for AIDS patients has been the use of nonbronchoscopic techniques of sampling the lower airways. These include the insertion of catheters blindly into the lower airway, advancing them as far as possible, and performing a large-volume wash with saline (48,49). The diagnostic yield appears similar to that of lavage, and the procedure may have use in centers trying to reduce the number of bronchoscopies performed. However, there is a requirement for sedation and local anesthesia to a level similar for bronchoscopy and, therefore, the risk to the patient appears to be the same as routine bronchoscopy. In mechanically ventilated patients, Karpel et al. reported that "endobronchial lavage," wherein a large-volume wash was done through the endotracheal tube, resulted in a diagnosis of *P. carinii* in 19 of 20 patients studied (50).

Bronchoscopy does not always make the diagnosis of *P. carinii*. Open-lung biopsy remains the most sensitive test and continues to be used whenever other tests have failed (6,51). The effect of open-lung biopsy on ultimate survival is unclear. In a retrospective study of 66 AIDS patients undergoing open-lung biopsy, *P. carinii* was found in 49 patients; however, successful changes in therapy on the basis of open-lung biopsy was possible in only 1 case (51). A prospective study of immunocompromised cancer patients found no benefit of open-lung biopsy over empiric therapy, even though *P. carinii* was found in half of the patients undergoing open-lung biopsy (5). We have used open-lung biopsy sparingly at our institution (eight cases), usually in the mild to moderately ill patient who has had one or more nondiagnostic bronchoscopies for persistent pulmonary infiltrates. Over half have had a treatable diagnosis: *Mycobacterium*

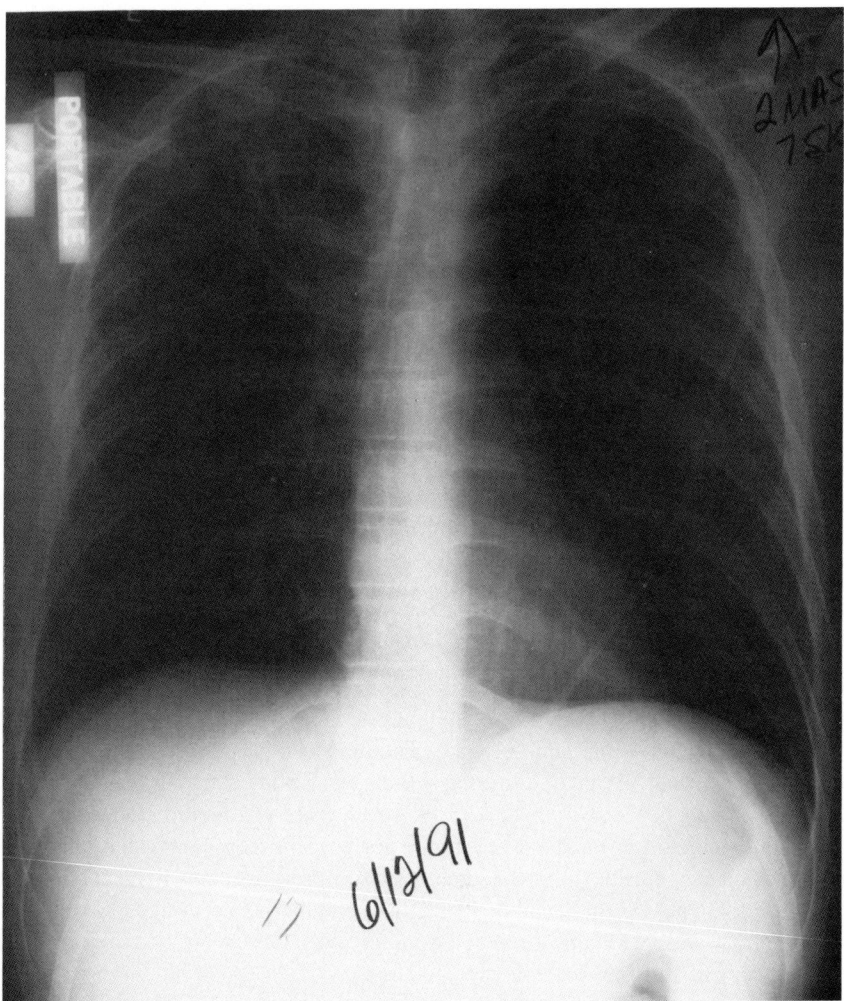

Figure 2 The chest roentgenogram from a patient with HIV infection, receiving aerosol pentamidine prophylaxis for 12 months, who developed cough, fever, and shortness of breath. The right upper infiltrate was not seen on a chest roentgenogram done 6 months before this admission.

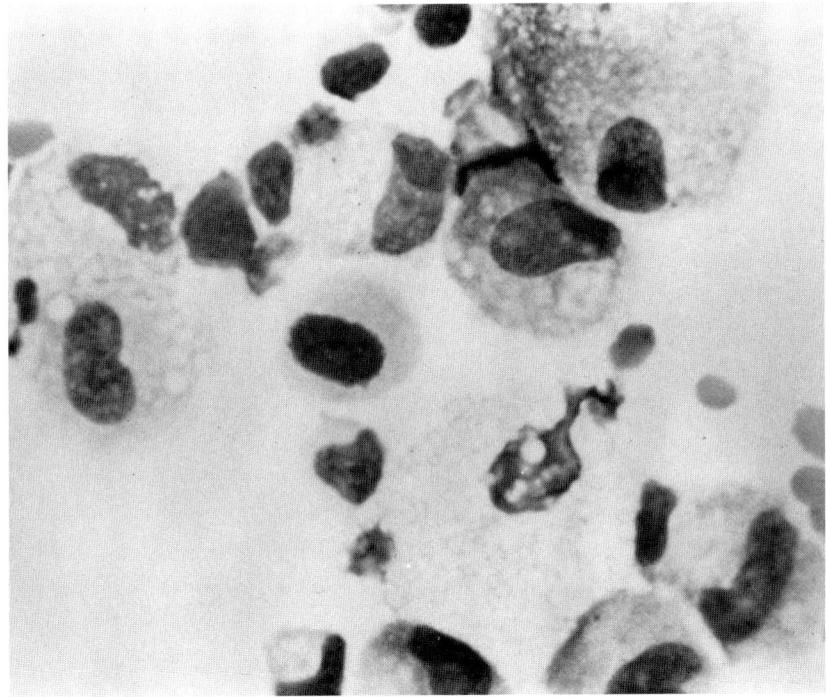

(a)

Figure 3 BAL specimen from the patient described in Figure 2. (a) The high-power (40×) view of the right middle lobe. For the middle lobe, no *P. carinii* clusters were seen. (b) A high-power (40×) view of the clusters of *P. carinii* organisms recovered from the upper lobe. Modified Wright–Giemsa stain (Diff-Quik) was used to stain the cytocentrifuge-prepared slides.

tuberculosis, *Cryptococcus neoformans*, *Rhodococcus* sp., and three patients with *P. carinii*. All five patients responded to changes in their treatment.

Bronchoscopy with lavage has been performed less frequently in children than in adults; however, the diagnostic yield is similar (52,53). It has been well established that human immunodeficiency virus (HIV)-infected adults and older children are at higher risk for *P. carinii* infection once their CD4 lymphocyte cell count goes below $250/mm^3$. Yet, for infants younger than 1 year old with HIV infection, the CD4 lymphocyte counts may not be predictive of risk, and a heightened index of suspicion is necessary (54).

In summary, the approach to diagnose *P. carinii* depends on the patient, their underlying disease, and the level of suspicion. In the HIV-infected patient, induced

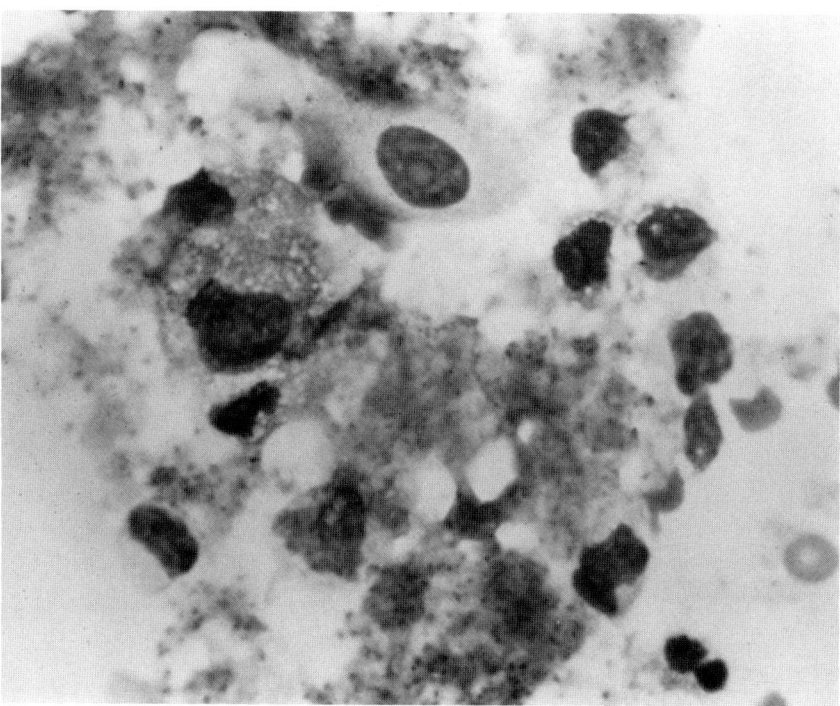

(b)

Figure 3 (Continued)

sputum examination is often recommended as a first step, especially if one's laboratory has reasonable familiarity with the technique. A positive specimen is unequivocal. However, a negative specimen does not rule out *P. carinii*. In patients in whom there is a high index of suspicion, especially for patients receiving aerosol pentamidine prophylaxis, more invasive specimens taken by bronchoscopy, including BAL and transbronchial biopsy, may be necessary.

III. Stains

There are several major issues when discussing the "best" stain of human specimens. One has to consider ease of performance, rapidity of the stain, sensitivity, specificity, and cost. Table 2 summarizes many of the stains currently in use.

For many years, the gold standard of diagnosis has been the methenamine

Table 2 Summary of Stains for *P. carinii*

Stain	Sensitivity (%)	Specificity (%)	Length of time to perform (hr)	Relative cost	Current use
Methenamine silver	>95	>95	6–24	Moderate	Widespread
Papanicolaou	80	90	1–6	Moderate	Widespread
Wright–Giemsa	80	90	<1	Small	Potentially widespread
Toluidine blue	80	>95	1–6	Moderate	Limited
Crysl echt violet	75	>95	1–6	Moderate	Limited
Calcofluor white	>90	>95	1–6	Moderate	Limited
Immunofluorescent	>95	>95	1–6	High	Limited
Polymerase chain reaction	>95	?	24–48	High	Very limited

silver stain. This reagent, originally developed to stain fungi, selectively stains the *P. carinii* cyst wall (40,55,56). Characteristics of *P. carinii* include being about the size of a red blood cell, a central dimpling, and the appearance resembling that of a crushed table tennis ball (56). Usually the *P. carinii* cysts are found in clusters, often with associated foamy material. Although considered the standard test for many years, it is not 100% sensitive. As shown in Table 3, there have been several studies showing false-negative results with the silver stain. In one comparative study, 7 of 63 (11%) BAL specimens from patients with *P. carinii* pneumonia had negative silver stains, but positive foamy material seen on Papanicolaou stain (61). Although the traditional silver stain usually is done overnight, modifications of the stain have led to stains being completed in 1–2 hr (14,61). The use of the silver stain permits the absolute counting of individual cysts, and has been used to provide quantitation of *P. carinii* in the BAL fluid (62).

The Wright–Giemsa stain and its modification (Diff-Quik) have been used for several years to identify *P. carinii*. This stain does not stain the cyst wall, but, in fact, stains the nuclei of trophozoites, cysts, and intermediate stages (19). The stain has been used to quantitate the number of organisms present in BAL specimens by counting the number of clusters present (63). This has been used to follow a patient's response to therapy, since successful therapy for *P. carinii* is associated with a greater than 50% drop in cluster count (64). The stain can be performed on an air-dried sample. Usually it is performed on a cytocentrifuge-prepared specimen (such as BAL) or an air-dried smear (sputum).

The Wright–Giemsa stain or its modification has also been used to characterize the inflammatory response in BAL of many diseases including sarcoidosis and idiopathic pulmonary fibrosis (38). The interpretation of the BAL specimen

Table 3 Yield of Various Stains for P. carinii

Specimen type	Methenamine silver	Wright–Giemsa	Papanicolaou	Calcofluor white	Toluidine blue	Crysl echt violet	Immuno-fluorescent	Ref.
Sputum		12/23 (52)[a]					21/23 (91)	57
Sputum		37/49 (76)			39/49 (80)		45/49 (92)	11
Sputum	34/37 (92)	34/37 (92)					36/37 (97)	58
Sputum				5/10 (50)			9/10 (90)	59
Sputum Total	34/37 (92)	83/109 (76)		5/10 (50)	39/49 (80)		111/119 (93)	
Wash	32/46 (70)	21/35 (60)	29/50 (58)				43/46 (93)	20
Wash	43/50 (86)	38/50 (76)	29/50 (58)			38/50 (76)		60
Wash Total	76/96 (80)	59/85 (69)				38/50 (76)	43/46 (93)	
BAL	58/65 (89)		63/65 (97)					61
BAL		10/13 (77)					13/13 (100)	57
BAL	57/59 (97)	49/58 (84)					57/59 (97)	20
BAL	18/21 (86)	17/21 (81)					18/21 (86)	58
BAL				13/13 (100)			13/13 (100)	59
BAL Total	128/145 (88)	76/92 (83)	63/65 (97)	13/13 (100)			101/106 (95)	

[a]Number positive/number studied (%).

requires some expertise in differentiating the various inflammatory cells, especially differentiation of the lymphocyte from the immature, monocyte-like macrophage often encountered in acute inflammation. With standard criteria, one is able to produce a reliable differential cell count of the cells retrieved by BAL. This differential cell count has been used to characterize the inflammatory response around *P. carinii*. Several authors have found that neutrophils in the BAL are associated with more severe hypoxemia and a worse overall prognosis from the *P. carinii* pneumonia (4,64,65).

The Papanicolaou stain can also be performed on the BAL specimen (18). It has been used mostly for routine cellular evaluation and remains the standard stain used by cytopathologists for evaluating any specimen. Similar to the Wright–Giemsa, it stains the nonspecific foam surrounding large clusters of *P. carinii*. The individual organisms do not stain well and, therefore, it is probably not as specific as the Wright–Giemsa stain; however, it can suggest the diagnosis. Because of its widespread use and ease of staining, it has been useful for screening a large sample of BAL or other pulmonary specimens (61). In addition, the Papanicolaou stain is useful for identifying cellular changes caused by viruses, especially cytomegalovirus (CMV). Cytomegalovirus occurs quite frequently with *P. carinii* infection (67).

Two less commonly used, but specific, stains for *P. carinii* are the toluidine blue O and calcofluor stains. The toluidine blue O stain, which identifies the cyst wall (11,15,16), is more rapid than the routine silver stain and has been used as a screening stain (11). Calcofluor white is a chemifluorescent optical-brightening agent that nonspecifically binds to β-linked polysaccharide polymers found on fungi and other organisms such as *P. carinii* (68). The cresyl echt violet is similar to toluidine blue O stain, with little clinical experience, but has been used in animal studies (69).

Immunofluorescent stains have become widely available for the specific diagnosis of *P. carinii* (70). For the less-than-optimal specimens of sputum and bronchial wash, the fluorescent stains have increased sensitivity over the Wright–Giemsa and silver stain (11,20–22,58). There are several different stains, involving both direct and indirect immunofluorescent techniques. The antibodies used are against major cell wall and surface antigens of *P. carinii*. Many of the kits use the monoclonal antibodies developed by Kovacs et al. at the National Institutes of Health (NIH) (70). Two reports have directly compared the direct versus indirect immunofluorescent techniques. In each study, the direct immunofluorescence antibody assay was more sensitive, but the difference was not significant (58,59).

The current techniques to obtain adequate specimens have led to a high yield for *P. carinii*. However, as new stains are examined, less invasive procedures may be used for diagnosis. For example, the use of oligonuclide probes (71) and polymerase chain reactions (PCR) (72) may allow increased sensitivity of diagnosis. This technology is discussed in greater detail in Chapter 20. In the future,

PCR may increase sensitivity adequately to allow higher yield for sputum examination alone. On the other hand, prophylaxis, such as aerosolized pentamidine, may reduce diagnostic yield for BAL (8); therefore, more sensitive stains may also become more important for bronchoscopy specimens.

These stains can be used in a complementary fashion. At our institution, we routinely stain fresh lavage specimens using a modified Wright–Giemsa as well as a silver stain. In some cases, we have also performed immunofluorescent staining. The modified Wright–Giemsa is available within 30 min of the procedure. This information is used to direct therapy, since a positive stain is fairly specific. However, 10–15% of AIDS cases will be missed when using the modified Wright–Giemsa alone (19,20). The final silver stain result is usually not available for 6–24 hr. This stain is considered our final stain for BAL specimens. We have found the immunofluorescent stain useful in the less-than-optimal specimens, for example, bronchial wash (20). However, we have not used it routinely because of cost.

When obtaining a specimen from the immunocompromised patient, one should look for other pathogens besides *P. carinii*. A significant percentage of immunocompromised patients will have pulmonary infiltrates for reasons other than *P. carinii*, either in combination with *P. carinii* or as the sole cause of the pulmonary symptoms (7,9,64). The use of bronchoscopy with BAL allows the diagnosis of other pathogens such as tuberculosis, fungal infections, bacterial, and viral causes of pneumonia (67,73,74).

The diagnosis of *P. carinii* relies on morphological and not culture criteria. Unfortunately, as a patient is treated for *P. carinii*, there is some lag in clearance of the organism. In at least two-thirds of patients completing successful anti-*P. carinii* therapy, persistent organisms can be found in a repeat lavage (75). Unfortunately, only 80% of patients respond to single therapy for their *P. carinii* pneumonia (76). To determine whether we could identify patients who were failing therapy versus those being successfully treated, we examined a cohort of HIV-infected patients treated with anti-*P. carinii* therapy. We found that in repeat BAL, at 3 weeks, the amount of *P. carinii* was reduced by at least two-thirds (64). We measured this reduction using a previously described semiquantitative technique. In those patients who had a less than 50% reduction in the amount of *P. carinii*, they either had persistent *P. carinii* pneumonia or were likely to have a recurrence of their *P. carinii* pneumonia within the next few months (64).

IV. Indirect Diagnostic Measures

Although the definitive diagnosis of *P. carinii* requires identification of the organism, indirect signs have been described. These have been useful in many ways. They help identify those patients in whom further workup may be useful, identify prognosis of patient with *P. carinii* pneumonia, and can sometimes be used to follow therapy. Table 4 summarizes the relative sensitivity and specificity of the various characteristics from the history, physical examination, and laboratory that suggest the diagnosis of *P. carinii* pneumonia.

The history and physical examination are noninvasive and universally used as part of the evaluation of patients with pulmonary symptoms. It has been noted for several years that the presentation of *P. carinii* pneumonia relies on the patient's underlying disease. Haverkos et al. found that the duration of symptoms were longer and the diagnosis was more subtle in AIDS patients (76). In patients with AIDS and *P. carinii*, dyspnea or fever were seen in over 70% of patients (77,78).

In patients with HIV infection, several studies have shown the value of assessing the immunocompetent state of the patient being evaluated. Over 85% of patients with *P. carinii* pneumonia have a CD4 lymphocyte count of fewer than $250/mm^3$ (79,80). Thus, the patient's CD4 count is often used in assessing the individual patient's risk of having *P. carinii*. For example, an HIV-infected patient with dyspnea and pulmonary infiltrates, but a CD4 count of more than $500/mm^3$ is unlikely to have *P. carinii*. This information may also apply to the non-HIV, but immunocompromised, cancer patient who is receiving chemotherapy (81).

The chest roentgenogram has also been widely used in screening patients for *P. carinii* (78) and is discussed in detail in Chapter 21. Most patients with *P. carinii* pneumonia have an abnormal chest roentgenogram (82,83), although patients may have a normal chest roentgenograms at the time of diagnosis (83,84). The usual chest roentgenogram shows a diffuse, interstitial infiltrate involving both lungs, although alveolar pattern and unilateral localized infiltrates have been described (82,85,86). Pleural effusions are rarely seen (86,87) and, if present, should

Table 4 Evaluation of Patient for *P. carinii*

Diagnostic procedure	Relative sensitivity[a]	Relative specificity[a]
History of dyspnea, cough, or fever	3	2
Known immunocompromised patient		
HIV infection	1	1
CD4 lymphocytes < $250/mm^3$	2	2
Previous Pc	2	2
Abnormal chest roentgenogram	3	3
Hypoxemia	2	2
Hypoxemia with exercise	4	2
Positive gallium scan	4	2
Increased serum LDH	3	3
Sputum examination	3	4
Bronchoscopy with BAL	4	4

[a]On scale of 1–4 (lowest to highest).

suggest a different or additional disease process, such as empyema or Kaposi's sarcoma.

Recently, there have been increasing reports of *P. carinii* presenting with upper lobe infiltrates mimicking tuberculosis (88). Also, spontaneous pneumothoraces have been recognized in increasing frequency in AIDS patients (41,42). Both the upper lobe infiltrates and pneumothoraces appear to occur more frequently in patients who have received prior aerosol pentamidine prophylaxis (8,41,83). Therefore, the chest roentgenogram is a fairly nonspecific test in patients with possible *P. carinii* infection, although any abnormality on chest roentgenogram makes the AIDS patient more likely to have infection with *P. carinii* (77,78).

Another test used to assess patients is the arterial blood gas. Hypoxemia, or at least an increased arterial–alveolar gradient, is seen in over 80% of patients (77,78). *Pneumocystis* pneumonia is an interstitial process, and all interstitial lung diseases cause difficulties in gas exchange. A sensitive test for early interstitial lung disease is the exercise blood gas assessment. Stover et al. reported that exercise desaturation occurred in patients with *P. carinii* (89). Other pulmonary function abnormalities have been reported with *P. carinii* pneumonia (90). Reduced D_{LCO} is the most common abnormality found. However, this test is technically difficult, and reduced D_{LCO} can be seen in many situations, including sarcoidosis, pulmonary fibrosis, and anemia.

The serum lactate dehydrogenase (LDH) will usually rise with the onset of *P. carinii* infection and may also be useful in following a patient's response to therapy (91,92). Unfortunately, elevation of LDH can be seen in many diseases, including lymphoma. In addition, normal LDH levels have been seen in 7–17% of patients with *P. carinii* pneumonia (78,92).

The radionuclide gallium and diethylenetriamine pentaacetic acid (DTPA) scans have been reported to be abnormal in patients with *P. carinii* infection (93–95) and are discussed in greater depth in Chapter 21. Gallium is taken up in areas of acute inflammation by activated macrophages, probably through the transferrin receptor. DTPA is a radioaerosol that is deposited in the alveoli by nebulization, and the rate of uptake into the blood is measured as an estimated of alveolar-capillary permeability. Unfortunately, both gallium and DTPA are abnormal in other inflammatory disease processes, such as sarcoid (96–98). In addition, the gallium scan is relatively expensive and takes at least 72 hr to complete and, therefore, is of limited use. The DTPA scan is less expensive; however, abnormalities are routinely seen in cigarette smokers (99).

V. Conclusion

In conclusion, although several abnormalities can suggest the diagnosis of *P. carinii* by the routine history, physical examination, and laboratory test, none of these are definitive. Diagnosis of *P. carinii* still relies on tissue confirmation. A wide variety of stains are available, with various sensitivity as well as cost and complexity. The choice of stain depends on the specimen to be studied as well as the expertise and preference of the diagnostic laboratory.

References

1. Walzer PD, Perl DP, Krogsta DJ, Rawson PG, Shultz MG. *Pneumocystis carinii* pneumonia in the United States: epidemiologic, diagnostic, and clinical features. Ann Intern Med 1974; 80:83–93.
2. Masur H, Lane C, Kovacs JA, Allegra CJ, Edman JC. Pneumocystis pneumonia: from bench to clinic. Ann Intern Med 1989; 111:813–826.
3. Davey RT, Margolis D, Kleiner D, Deyton L, Travis W. Digital necrosis and disseminated *Pneumocystis carinii* infection after aerosolized pentamidine prophylaxis. Ann Intern Med 1989; 111:681–682.
4. Momose H, Lee S. *Pneumocystis carinii* as foamy exudate in bone marrow. JAMA 1991; 265:1672.
5. Browne MJ, Potter D, Gress J, Cotton D, et al. A randomized trial of open lung biopsy versus empiric antimicrobial therapy in cancer patients with diffuse pulmonary infiltrates. J Clin Oncol 1990; 8:222–229.
6. Fitzgerald W, Bevelaqua FA, Garay SM, Aranda CP. The role of open lung biopsy in patients with the acquired immunodeficiency syndrome. Chest 1987; 91: 659–661.
7. Broaddus C, Dake MD, Stulbarg MS, Blumenfeld LV, Hadley K, Golden JA, Hopewell PC. Bronchoalveolar lavage and transbronchial biopsy for the diagnosis of pulmonary infections in the acquired immunodeficiency syndrome. Ann Intern Med 1985; 102:747–752.
8. Jules-Elysee KM, Stover DM, Zaman MB, Bernard EM, White DA. Aerosolized pentamidine: effect on diagnosis and presentation of *Pneumocystis carinii* pneumonia. Ann Intern Med 1990; 112:750–757.
9. Stover DE, Zaman MB, Hajdu SI, Lange M, Gold J, Armstrong D. Bronchoalveolar lavage in the diagnosis of diffuse pulmonary infiltrates in the immunosuppressed host. Ann Intern Med 1984; 101:1–7.
10. Gal AA, Klatt EC, Koss MN, Strigle SM, Bovlen CT. The effectiveness of bronchoscopy in the diagnosis of *Pneumocystis carinii* and cytomegalovirus pulmonary infections in acquired immunodeficiency syndrome. Arch Pathol Lab Med 1987; 111: 238–241.
11. Kovacs JA, Ng VL, Masur H, et al. Diagnosis of *Pneumocystis carinii* pneumonia: improved detection in sputum with use of monoclonal antibodies. N Engl J Med 1988; 318;589–593.
12. Pitchenik AE, Ganjei P, Torres A, Evans DA, Rubin E, Baier H. Sputum examination for the diagnosis of *Pneumocystis carinii* pneumonia in the acquired immunodeficiency syndrome. Am Rev Respir Dis 1986; 133:226–229.
13. Bigby TD, Margolskee D, Curtis JL, Michael PF, Sheppard D, Hadley WK, Hopewell PC. The usefulness of induced sputum in the diagnosis of immunodeficiency syndrome. Am Rev Respir Dis 1986; 133:515–518.

14. Mahan CT, Sale GE. Rapid methenamine silver stain for pneumocystis and fungi. Arch Pathol Lab Med 1978; 102:351–352.
15. Gosey LL, Howard RM, Witzbsky FG, Ognibene FP, Wu TC, Gill VJ, MacLowry JD. Advantages of a modified toluidine blue O stain and bronchoalveolar lavage for the diagnosis of *Pneumocystis carinii* pneumonia. J Clin Microbiol 1985; 22:803–807.
16. Paradis IL, Ross C, Dekker A, Dauber J. Comparison of methenamine silver and modified toluidine blue stains for the detection of *Pneumocystis carinii* in bronchoalveolar fluid. Acta Cytol (in press).
17. Domingo J, Waksal HW. Wright's stain in rapid diagnosis of *Pneumocystis carinii*. Am J Clin Pathol 1984; 81:511–514.
18. Greaves TS, Strigle SM. The recognition of *Pneumocystis carinii* in routine Papanicolaou-stained smears. Acta Cytol 1985; 29:714–720.
19. Tollerud DJ, Kim CK, Weseler TA, Baughman RP. Use of a rapid differential stain for identifying *Pneumocystis carinii* in bronchoalveolar lavage fluid. Chest 1989; 95: 493–497.
20. Baughman RP, Strohofer SS, Clinton BA, Nickol AD, Frame PT. The use of an indirect fluorescent antibody test for detecting *Pneumocystis carinii*. Arch Pathol Lab Med 1989; 113:1062–1065.
21. Ng VL, Yajko DM, McPhaul LW, et al. Evaluation of an indirect fluorescent-antibody stain for detection of *Pneumocystis carinii* in respiratory secretions. J Clin Microbiol 1990; 28:975–979.
22. Ng VL, Virani NA, Chaisson RE, et al. Rapid detection of *Pneumocystis carinii* using a direct fluorescent monoclonal antibody stain. J Clin Microbiol 1990; 28:2228–2233.
23. Young LS. Antigen detection in *Pneumocystis carinii* pneumonia. Serodiagnosis and immunotherapy. 1987; 1:163–165.
24. Hughes WT. *Pneumocystis carinii* pneumonitis. Chest 1984; 85:810–813.
25. Peglow SL, Smulian G, Linke MJ, et al. Serologic responses to *Pneumocystis carinii* antigens in health and disease. J Infect Dis 1990; 161:296–306.
26. Pifer LL, Hughes WT, Stagno S, Woods D. *Pneumocystis carinii* infection: evidence for high prevalence in normal and immunosuppressed children. Pediatrics 1978; 61: 35–41.
27. Meyers JD, Pifer LL, Sale GE, Thomas ED. The value of *Pneumocystis carinii* antibody and antigen detection for the diagnosis of *Pneumocystis carinii* pneumonia after marrow transplantation. Am Rev Respir Dis 1979; 120:1283–1287.
28. Maddison SE, Hayes GV, Slemenda SB, Norman LG, Ivey ME. Detection of specific antibody to enzyme-linked immunosorbent assay and antigenemia by counter immunoelectrophoresis in humans infected with *Pneumocystis carinii*. J Clin Microbiol 1982; 15:1036–1043.
29. Miller RF, Semple SJG, Kocjan G. Difficulties with sputum induction for diagnosis of *Pneumocystis carinii* pneumonia. Lancet 1990; 1:112.
30. Zaman MK, Wooten OJ, Suprahmanya B, Ankobiah W, Finch PJP, Kamholz SL. Rapid noninvasive diagnosis of *Pneumocystis carinii* from induced liquefied sputum. Ann Intern Med 1988; 109:7–10.
31. Del Rio C, Guarner J, Honig EG, Slade BA. Sputum examination in the diagnosis of

Pneumocystis carinii pneumonia in the acquired immunodeficiency syndrome. Arch Pathol Lab Med 1988; 112:1229–1232.

32. Metersky ML, Cantanzaro A. Diagnostic approach to *Pneumocystis carinii* pneumonia in the setting of prophylactic aerosolized pentamidine. Chest 1991; 100:1345–1349.
33. Pereira W, Kovnat DM, Snider GL. A prospective cooperative study of complications following flexible fiberoptic bronchoscopy. Chest 1978; 73:813–816.
34. Credle XVF, Smiddy JF, Elliott RC. Complication of fiberoptic bronchoscopy. Am Rev Respir Dis 1974; 109:67–69.
35. Strumpf JJ, Feld MK, Cornelius MJ, Keogh BA, Crystal RG. Safety of fiberoptic bronchoalveolar lavage in evaluation of interstitial lung disease. Chest 1981; 80:268–271.
36. Cole P, Turton C, Lanyon H, Collins J. Bronchoalveolar lavage for the preparation of free lung cells: technique and complications. Br J Dis Chest 1980; 74:273–278.
37. Drew WL, Finley TN, Mintz L, Klein HZ. Diagnosis of *Pneumocystis carinii* pneumonia by bronchopulmonary lavage. JAMA 1974; 230:713–715.
38. Reynolds HY. Bronchoalveolar lavage. Am Rev Respir Dis 1987; 135:250–263.
39. Orenstein M, Webber CA, Heurich AE. Cytologic diagnosis of *Pneumocystis carinii* infection by bronchoalveolar lavage in acquired immune deficiency syndrome. Acta Cytol 1985; 29:727–731.
40. Define LA, Saleba KP, Gibson BB, Wesseler TA, Baughman RP. Cytologic evaluation of bronchoalveolar lavage specimens in immunosuppressed patients with suspected opportunistic infections. Acta Cytol 1987; 31:235–242.
41. Sherman M, Levin D, Briedbart. *Pneumocystis carinii* pneumonia with spontaneous pneumothorax: a report of three cases. Chest 1986; 90:609–610.
42. Sepkowitz KA, Telzak EE, Gold JWM, et al. Pneumothorax in AIDS. Ann Intern Med 1991; 114:455–459.
43. Fisher AG, McElvaney G, Lawson L, et al. Surgical management of spontaneous pneumothorax in patients with AIDS. Ann Thorac Surg 1988; 45:21–23.
44. Golden JA, Hollander H, Stulbarg MS, Gamsu G. Bronchoalveolar lavage as the exclusive diagnostic modality for *Pneumocystis carinii* pneumonia: a prospective study among patients with acquired immunodeficiency syndrome. Chest 1986; 90:18–22.
45. Johnson DL, Boylen CT, Barbers R, et al. A reevaluation of bronchoscopy in patients with possible *Pneumocystis carinii* pneumonia [abstract]. Presented at the Third International Conference of Bronchoalveolar Lavage in Vienna, June 1991.
46. Baughman RP, Dohn MN, Shipley R, Buchsbaum JA, Frame PT. Increased *Pneumocystis carinii* recovery from the upper lobes in pneumocystis pneumonia. The effect of aerosol pentamidine prophylaxis. Chest 1993; 103:426–432.
47. Meduri GU, Stover DE, Greeno RA, Nash T, Zaman MB. Bilateral bronchoalveolar lavage in the diagnosis of opportunistic pulmonary infections. Chest 1991; 100;1272–1276.
48. Martin WR, Albertson TE, Siegel B. Tracheal catheters in patients with acquired immunodeficiency syndrome for the diagnosis of *Pneumocystis carinii* pneumonia. Chest 1990; 98:29–32.
49. Caughey G, Wong H, Gamsu G, Golden J. Nonbronchoscopic bronchoalveolar lavage

for the diagnosis for *Pneumocystis carinii* pneumonia in the acquired immunodeficiency syndrome. Chest 1985; 88:659–662.
50. Karpel JP, Prezant D, Appel D, Bezahler G. Endotracheal lavage for the diagnosis of *Pneumocystis carinii* pneumonia in intubated patients with acquired immune deficiency syndrome. Crit Care Med 1986; 14:741.
51. Bonfils-Roberts EA, Nickodem A, Nealon TF. Retrospective analysis of the efficacy of open lung biopsy in acquired immunodeficiency syndrome. Ann Thorac Surg 1990; 49:115–117.
52. Birriel JA, Adams JA, Saldana MA, et al. Role of flexible bronchoscopy and bronchoalveolar lavage in the diagnosis of pediatric acquired immunodeficiency syndrome-related pulmonary diseases. Pediatrics 1991; 87:897–899.
53. Stokes DC, Shenep JL, Parham D, et al. Role of flexible bronchoscopy in the diagnosis of pulmonary infiltrates in pediatric patients with cancer. J Pediatr 1989; 115:561–567.
54. Rutstein RM. Predicting risk of *Pneumocystis carinii* pneumonia in human immunodeficiency virus-infected children. Am J Dis Child 1991; 145:922–924.
55. Grocott RG. A stain for fungi in tissue sections and smears using Gomori methenamine-silver nitrate technique. Am J Clin Pathol 1955; 25:975–979.
56. Pintozzi RL, Blecka LJ, Nanos S. Morphologic identification of *Pneumocystis carinii*. Acta Cytol 1979; 23:35–39.
57. Wolfson JS, Waldron MA, Sierra LS. Blinded comparison of a direct immunofluorescent monoclonal antibody staining method and a Giemsa staining method for identification of *Pneumocystis carinii* in induced sputum and bronchoalveolar lavage specimens of patients infected with human immunodeficiency virus. J Clin Microbiol 1990; 28:2136–2138.
58. Cregan P, Yamamoto A, Lum A, VanDerHeide T, MacDonald M, Pulliam L. Comparison of four methods for rapid detection of *Pneumocystis carinii* in respiratory specimens. J Clin Microbiol 1990; 28:2432–2436.
59. Stratton N, Hryniewicki J, Aarnaes SL, Tan G, de le Maza L, Peterson EM. Comparison of monoclonal antibody and celcofluor white stains for detection of *Pneumocystis carinii* from respiratory specimens. J Clin Microbiol 1991; 29:645–647.
60. Chandra P, Delaney M, Tuazon CU. Role of special stains in the diagnosis of *Pneumocystis carinii* infection from bronchial washing specimens in patients with the acquired immune deficiency syndrome. Acta Cytol 1988; 32:105–108.
61. Schumann GB, Swensen JJ. Comparison of Papanicolaou's stain with Gomori methamine silver (GMS) stain for the cytodiagnosis of *Pneumocystis carinii* in bronchoalveolar lavage (BAL) fluid. Am J Clin Pathol 1991; 95:583–586.
62. Limper AH, Offord KP, Smith TS, Martin WJ II. *Pneumocystis carinii* pneumonia: differences in lung parasite number and inflammation in patients with and without AIDS. Am Rev Respir Dis 1989; 140;1204–1209.
63. Baughman RP, Strohofer S, Colangelo G, Frame PT. Semiquantitative technique for estimating *Pneumocystis carinii* burden in the lung. J Clin Microbiol 1990; 28:1425–1427.
64. Colangelo G, Baughman RP, Dohn MN, Frame PT. Follow-up bronchoalveolar lavage in AIDS patients with *Pneumocystis carinii* pneumonia. *Pneumocystis carinii* burden predicts early relapse. Am Rev Respir Dis 1991; 143:1067–1071.

65. Smith RL, El-Sadr WM, Lewis ML. Correlation of bronchoalveolar lavage cell populations with clinical severity of *Pneumocystis carinii* pneumonia. Chest 1988; 92:60–64.
66. Mason GR, Hashimoto CH, Dickman PS, Foutty LF, Cobb CJ. Prognostic implications of bronchoalveolar lavage neutrophilia in patients with *Pneumocystis carinii* pneumonia and AIDS. Am Rev Respir Dis 1989; 139:1336–1342.
67. Miles PR, Baughman RP, Linnemann CC. Cytomegalovirus in the bronchoalveolar lavage fluid of patients with AIDS. Chest 1990; 97:1072–1076.
68. Baselski VS, Robinson MK, Pifer LW, Woods DR. Rapid detection of *Pneumocystis carinii* in bronchoalveolar lavage samples by using celcofluor staining. J Clin Microbiol 1990; 28:393–394.
69. Walzer PD, Kim CK, Cushion MT. *Pneumocystis carinii*. In: Walzer PD, Genta RM, eds. Parasitic Infections in the Compromised Host. New York: Marcel Dekker, 1989: 83–178.
70. Kovacs JA, Gill V, Swan JC, Ognibene F, Shelhamer J, Parrillo JE, Masur H. Prospective evaluation of a monoclonal antibody in diagnosis of *Pneumocystis carinii* pneumonia. Lancet 1986; 2:1–3.
71. Hayashi Y, Watanabe J, Nakata K, Kukayama M, Ikeda H. A novel diagnostic method of *Pneumocystis carinii*. In situ hybridization of ribosomal ribonucleic acid with biotinylated oligonucleotide probes. Lab Invest 1990; 63:576–580.
72. Wakefield AE, Guiver L, Miller RF, Hopkin JM. DNA amplification on induced sputum samples for diagnosis of *Pneumocystis carinii* pneumonia. Lancet 1991; 1: 337–338.
73. Baughman RP, Dohn MN, Loudon RG, Frame PT. Bronchoscopy with bronchoalveolar lavage in tuberculosis and fungal infections. Chest 1991; 99:92–97.
74. Thorpe JE, Baughman RP, Frame PT, Wesseler TW, Staneck J. Bronchoalveolar lavage for diagnosing acute bacterial pneumonia. J Infect Dis 1987; 155:855–861.
75. Shelhammer JH, Ognibene FP, Macher AM, et al. Persistence of *Pneumocystis carinii* in lung tissue of acquired immunodeficiency syndrome patients treated for pneumocystis pneumonia. Am Rev Respir Dis 1984; 130:1161–1165.
76. Haverkos HW. Assessment of therapy for *Pneumocystis carinii* pneumonia: PCP therapy project group. Am J Med 1984; 76:501–508.
77. Baughman RP, Frame PT. Predicting a positive result for immunocompromised patients undergoing BAL for fever and pulmonary symptoms. Chest 1989; 95:192S–193S.
78. Katz MH, Baron RB, Grady D. Risk stratification of ambulatory patients suspected of *Pneumocystis* pneumonia. Arch Intern Med 1991; 151:105–110.
79. Masur H, Ognibene FP, Yarchoan R, et al. CD4 counts as predictors of opportunistic pneumonias in human immunodeficiency virus infected individuals. Ann Intern Med 1989; 111:223–231.
80. Phair J, Munoz A, Detecs R, Rinaldo C, Saah A. The rise of *Pneumocystis carinii* pneumonia among men infected with human immunodeficiency virus type 1. Multicenter AIDS cohort study group. N Engl J Med 1990; 332:161–165.
81. Siminski J, Kidd P, Phillips GD, Collins C, Ragh G. Reversed helper/suppressor T-lymphocyte ratio in bronchoalveolar lavage fluid from patients with breast cancer and *Pneumocystis carinii* pneumonia. Am Rev Respir Dis 1991; 143:437–440.

82. DeLorenzo LJ, Huang CT, Maguire GP, Stone DJ. Roentgenographic patterns of *Pneumocystis carinii* pneumonia in 104 patients with AIDS. Chest 1987; 91: 323–327.
83. Chaffey MH, Klein JS, Gamsu G, Blanc P, Golden JA. Radiographic distribution of *Pneumocystis carinii* pneumonia in patients with AIDS treated with prophylactic inhaled pentamidine. Radiology 1990; 175:715–719.
84. Israel HI, Gottlieb JE, Schulman ES. Hypoxemia with normal chest roentgenogram due to *Pneumocystis carinii* pneumonia. Diagnostic errors due to low suspicion of AIDS. Chest 1987; 92:857–859.
85. Scott WW, Kuhlman JE. Focal pulmonary lesions in patients with AIDS: percutaneous transthoracic needle biopsy. Radiology 1991; 180:419–421.
86. Barrio JL, Suarez M, Rodriguez JL, Saldana MJ, Pitchenik AE. *Pneumocystis carinii* pneumonia presenting as cavitating and noncavitating solitary pulmonary nodules in patients with acquired immunodeficiency syndrome. Am Rev Respir Dis 1986; 134: 1094–1096.
87. Mariuz P, Raviglione MC, Gould IA, Mullin MP. Pleural disease in *Pneumocystis carinii* infection. Chest 1991; 99:774–776.
88. Milligan SA, Stulberg MS, Gamsu G, Golden JA. *Pneumocystis carinii* pneumonia radiographically simulating tuberculosis. Am Rev Respir Dis 1985; 132:1124–1126.
89. Stover DA, Greeno RA, Gagliardi AJ. The use of a simple exercise test for the diagnosis of *Pneumocystis carinii* pneumonia in patients with AIDS. Am Rev Respir Dis 1989; 139:1343–1346.
90. Coleman DL, Dodek PM, Golden JA, et al. Correlation between serial pulmonary function tests and fiberoptic bronchoscopy in patients with *Pneumocystis carinii* pneumonia and the acquired immune deficiency syndrome. Am Rev Respir Dis 1984; 129:491–493.
91. Zaman MK, White DA. Serum lactate dehydrogenase levels and *Pneumocystis carinii* pneumonia. Diagnostic and prognostic significance. Am Rev Respir Dis 1988; 137: 796–800.
92. Kagawa FT, Kirsch CM, Yenokida GG, Levine ML. Serum lactate dehydrogenous activity in patients with AIDS and *Pneumocystis carinii* pneumonia. An adjunct to diagnosis. Chest 1988; 94:1031–1033.
93. Tuazon CU, Delaney MD, Simon GL, Witorsch P, Varma VM. Utility of gallium-67 scintigraphy and bronchial washings in the diagnosis and treatment of *Pneumocystis carinii* pneumonia in patients with acquired immune deficiency syndrome. Am Rev Respir Dis 1985; 132:1087–1092.
94. Reiss TF, Golden J. Abnormal lung gallium-67 uptake preceding pulmonary physiologic impairment in an asymptomatic patient with *Pneumocystis carinii* pneumonia. Chest 1990; 97:1261–1263.
95. Mason GR, Duane GB, Mena I, Effros RM. Accelerated solute clearance in *Pneumocystis carinii* pneumonia. Am Rev Respir Dis 1987; 135:864–868.
96. Linz BR, Hunninghake GW, Keogh BA, et al. Gallium-67 scanning to stage the alveolitis of sarcoidosis: correlation with clinical studies, pulmonary function studies, and bronchoalveolar lavage. Am Rev Respir Dis 1981; 123:440–446.
97. Baughman, RP, Fernandez M, Bosken CH, Mantil J, Hurtubise P. Comparison of

gallium-67 scanning, bronchoalveolar lavage, and serum angiotensin-converting enzyme levels in pulmonary sarcoidosis. Predicting response to therapy. Am Rev Respir Dis 1984; 129:676–681.
98. Jacobs MP, Baughman RP, Hughes J, Fernandez-Ulloa M. Radioaerosol lung clearance in patients with active pulmonary sarcoidosis. Am Rev Respir Dis 1985; 131: 687–698.
99. Jones JG, Lawler P, Crawley JCW, et al. Increased alveolar epithelial permeability in cigarette smokers. Lancet 1980; 1:66–68.

20

A Molecular Approach to the Diagnosis of *Pneumocystis carinii* Pneumonia

ANN E. WAKEFIELD

Institute of Molecular Medicine
University of Oxford
Oxford, England

JULIAN HOPKIN

Churchill Hospital
Oxford, England

I. Introduction

The application of molecular genetic techniques for microbial diagnosis has great potential. Currently, it seems particularly appropriate to develop such a specific and sensitive method when standard techniques are unsatisfactory or difficult; *Pneumocystis carinii* cannot be effectively cultured in vitro, which eliminates this usually valuable diagnostic amplification step.

The properties of microbes are most precisely expressed at the genetic level, defined by the sequence of nucleic acid bases in their DNA (or sometimes RNA for certain viruses). The sequence is unique to each organism, and this property can be capitalized on to devise highly specific diagnostic methods (1). DNA is a double helix of two complementary polynucleotide chains in which perfect matching is dictated by hydrogen bonding between purine in one chain and pyrimidine in the other. This perfect matching, or hybridization, of specific sequences is the basis for various highly specific molecular genetic techniques for the identification of different gene sequences. DNA provides a universal molecule for microbiological diagnostic study that may be processed by vigorous physical treatments in preparation for hybridization analysis. Double-stranded DNA may be denatured into its two single, complementary strands by treatment with heat or alkali; reannealing or hybridization of single-stranded sequences, therefore, is directed by hydrogen bonding between the DNA bases—guanine with cytosine and adenine with thymine. Conditions of high temperature and low ionic strength demand more perfect matching of DNA bases in the complementary strands before such reannealing or hybridization occurs; therefore, these conditions of high stringency allow tests of great specificity to be performed. For example, appropriate conditions of stringency can distinguish between single-base differences. Variation in the conditions of hybridization and choice of gene sequence for study, whether highly conserved, semiconserved, or highly variable regions of DNA, allow methods to differentiate between organisms of different type, species, or genus.

Great sensitivity of assay can also now be achieved, as well as great specificity, by biochemical amplification of specific gene sequences, analogous to the amplification obtained by the culture of organisms. Such amplification is currently most efficiently achieved by the polymerase chain reaction (PCR) (2), in which a DNA polymerase enzyme and oligonucleotide primers, specific to the DNA target molecule, are used to synthesize complementary strands to this molecule by the three steps of DNA denaturation, oligonucleotide primer annealing, and primer extension. Twenty to 40 cycles of this three-step reaction result in exponential amplification of the sequence of interest. The amplification product can be simply detected by ethidium bromide staining of electrophoretically size-separated DNA, and its identity can be confirmed by hybridization to an oligonucleotide derived from the internal sequence after Southern transfer of DNA. The use of the heat-stable DNA polymerase from *Thermus aquaticus* (Taq polymerase) means that the polymerase chain reaction can be automated using a thermocycler (2).

Application of DNA hybridization techniques in microbial diagnosis is indeed proceeding rapidly and is being extended to epidemiological studies and the identification of antibiotic-resistance genes (3). Before these hopes can be realized, there are demanding requirements to be met: (1) painstaking analysis of the pathogen's DNA sequences of choice. This is especially important for *P. carinii* for which pure, genomic DNA is unobtainable, the parasite always being in the presence of host lung tissue and potentially contaminated with other microbial DNA; (2) careful comparison with sequences from related organisms that may confuse diagnostic and epidemiological studies; and (3) relating the results of any sensitive assay to the expression of clinical disease for the purposes of diagnostic work (1).

II. *Pneumocystis carinii*–Specific DNA Sequences

Deriving DNA sequences that are specific to *P. carinii* has proved difficult because the organism cannot be efficiently cultured. The parasite, therefore, has to be concentrated from lung material, resulting in the concomitant extraction of host DNA sequences or other contaminating microbial sequences; since pure genomic *P. carinii* is unobtainable, an alternative strategy is the use of cloned sequences of *P. carinii* DNA (4).

We derived a parasite-enriched fraction by filtration of lavage fluid from *P. carinii*-infected lung of the steroid immunosuppressed rat. Extracted DNA sequences were cloned, but then screened by colony hybridization using genomic rat DNA to identify and exclude cloned host DNA. Nonreactive colonies, putative *P. carinii* recombinants, were tested by in situ hybridization assay to determine whether they produced patterns of annealing with *P. carinii*-infected lung tissue that were characteristic of the distribution of infection and the morphology of the parasite. Several sequences were isolated showing characteristic in situ hybridization signals; one of these, determined by DNA sequence analysis to be a portion of the mitochondrial gene encoding the large-subunit ribosomal RNA, was chosen as a candidate sequence for the development of specific diagnostic probes (5).

From the sequence analysis and with the purpose of developing DNA amplification as a diagnostic method for *P. carinii*, we constructed priming oligonucleotides for DNA amplification and internal oligonucleotides for subsequent confirmatory hybridization. The sequences of the oligonucleotide primers and internal oligonucleotide probe that we have finally developed for diagnostic purposes are shown in Table 1. DNA was extracted from test samples by proteinase K digestion [1 mg/mL final concentration of proteinase K, in the presence of 10 mM ethylenediaminetetraacetic acid (EDTA), pH 8.0 and 1% (weight/volume) sodium dodecyl sulfate (SDS), at 50°C for 16 hr], followed by extraction with phenol, phenol/chloroform, and chloroform, and precipitation with ethanol. DNA amplification was performed with the oligonucleotide primers, pAZ102-E and pAZ102-H, with denaturation at 94°C for 1.5 min, annealing at 55°C for 1.5 min, and extension at 72°C for 2 min (40 cycles). The amplification products were subjected to electrophoresis in 1.5% agarose gel, and a specific *P. carinii* sequence (346 base pairs) was identified by visualization with ultraviolet light (UV) after ethidium bromide staining or by oligohybridization, after Southern transfer and autoradiography with the internal primer pAZ102-L1.

Table 1 *P. carinii* Oligonucleotide Sequences Used in DNA Amplification and Oligohybridization from Human Clinical Samples

Primer oligonucleotides
   pAZ102-E:-5'-GATGGCTGTTTCCAAGCCCA-3'
   pAZ102-H:-5'-GTGTACGTTGCAAAGTACTC-3'
Internal oligonucleotide
   pAZ102-L2:-5'-ATAAGGTAGATAGTCGAAAG-3'

Priming oligonucleotides, pAZ102-E and pAZ102-H, from rat-derived *P. carinii* DNA sequences also amplified *P. carinii*-specific DNA from the infected lungs of humans, ferrets, and rabbits (5). The sequence differences identified between the rat- and human-derived *P. carinii* gave the opportunity for development of an alternative, host-specific, internal oligonucleotide hybridization probe for studies on human material—pAZ102-L2. Amplified *P. carinii* DNA of specific length can be detected by (1) ethidium bromide staining after gel electrophoresis or (2) autoradiography after probing Southern-transferred DNA with the internal oligonucleotide (Fig. 1). This second step offers an increased sensitivity of detection by approximately 100-fold.

In experiments on uninfected, postmortem human lung tissue seeded with rat-derived *P. carinii*, we have been able to show that detection of amplified DNA on ethidium bromide-stained gel (a strong signal) implied the presence of 100 or more organisms in a test PCR sample, whereas a positive signal detected only by oligonucleotide hybridization (a weak signal) implied the presence of fewer organisms, and indeed, as few as one to two parasites (6), detected despite the high concentration of coextracted human DNA in the samples.

The sensitivity of the assay is conferred by the intrinsic characteristics of the DNA amplification, providing a doubling of the copy number of the relevant DNA sequence after each cycle of amplification; this produces an exponential increase in copy number of the amplified product. Contamination of the test sample with phenol, used in the DNA extraction, or with other less well-defined substance, can inhibit the Taq polymerase and, thereby, the PCR. False-negative results owing to inhibition of amplification may be tested for by conducting parallel PCR on each clinical sample using primers derived from a human sequence (we used antithrombin gene, exon 2) (5), since human genomic DNA will be coextracted from any clinical sample; this test allows monitoring of efficient amplification. The problem of false-positive results arising from contamination during PCR can be addressed by the systematic use of the following: (1) negative control samples with no added template DNA included after each clinical sample; (2) UV irradiation of the PCR reagents before the addition of the template DNA; (3) disposable

---

Figure 1 Amplified DNA sequences demonstrated by ethidium bromide staining in pulmonary samplings from both rat and human hosts. Comparative oligoblotting with rat and human *P. carinii*-specific internal oligonucleotide. Products of DNA amplification using DNA templates prepared from: lanes 2, 3, 4, rat-derived *P. carinii*; lanes 5, 6, 7, human-derived *P. carinii*; lane 8, no template control; lanes 1 and 9, 1-kb molecular mass markers. (a) ethidium bromide-stained gel; (b) autoradiograph of Southern blot probed with pAZ102-L1; (c) autoradiograph of Southern blot probed with pAZ102-L2. Arrows mark bands of amplified DNA specific to *P. carinii*.

Molecular Approach to Diagnosis

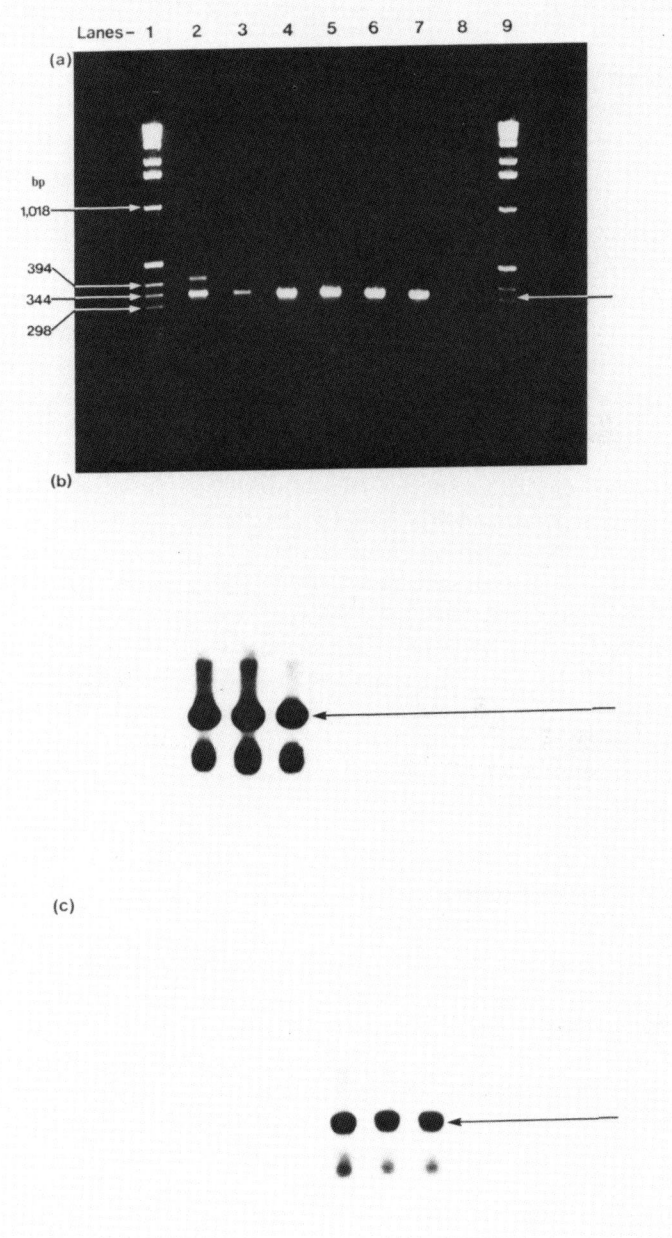

tips, tubes, reagent aliquots, and microcapillaries for the addition of each template DNA.

The specificity of the DNA amplification is determined by the choice of primer oligonucleotides and choice of an appropriate annealing temperature in the PCR cycle; increasing temperature makes the reaction more specific and, in our experiments, we used 55°C which is 3° below the melting temperatures ($T_m - 3°C$) of the primers pAZ102-H and E.

Establishing the specificity of the oligonucleotide primers to *P. carinii* in comparison with a range of other potential pulmonary pathogens and organisms closely related to *P. carinii* is essential. In patients with T-lymphocyte immunodeficiency, many other opportunistic infections occur; therefore, absence of specific amplification product from mycobacteria, viruses, including cytomegalovirus, and fungi, including aspergillus, is vital; none were found to be positive using the *P. carinii*-specific oligonucleotide primers at high stringency (5). Since *P. carinii* has been assigned to the fungal, rather than protozoal, kingdom based on DNA sequence comparison (7–9), it was also essential to demonstrate that primers pAZ102-H and pAZ102-E did not produce amplification from a range of fungal organisms, many of which, by virtue of their biology, might be contaminants of clinical samples or laboratory reagents. We have been able to study DNA amplification using these *P. carinii*-specific primers from 122 fungi taken from the different phyla of the fungal kingdom. We have shown at reduced stringency (PCR-annealing temperature = $T_m - 8°C$) that an amplification product may be obtained from only one group of fungi closely related to *P. carinii* (the ustomycetous red yeast fungi); at conditions of high stringency annealing ($T_m - 3°C$) an amplification product of approximately 350 base pairs is specific for *P. carinii* (10).

III. Clinical Studies

We have now been able to study the results of DNA amplification, applied to different diagnostic samples, in over 100 episodes of acute respiratory illness, with special emphasis on immunosuppressed subjects with AIDS (11,12).

In our study on bronchoscopic alveolar lavage from immunosuppressed subjects with acute respiratory disease and from nonimmunosuppressed subjects, the results of DNA amplification were compared with the results of silver staining for *P. carinii* and with the physician's diagnosis, based on clinical and radiographic feature and responses to treatment (11) (Table 2). No *P. carinii* DNA was found in lavage from 10 immunocompetent subjects and only low levels (weak signals detectable only by oligonucleotide hybridization) were found in 10 of 46 samples from immunosuppressed individuals without *P. carinii* pneumonia. The highest levels, detected by ethidium bromide staining of electrophoresed amplified DNA,

Table 2 One Hundred Subjects Studied by DNA Amplification and Silver Staining for *P. carinii* in Bronchoalveolar Lavage Samples

Patients	(n)	Clinical PCP	Silver staining	DNA amplification	
				Gel	Blot
Immunosuppressed	(90)				
Clinical PCP and silver positive	(30)	30	30	30	30
Clinical PCP, but silver negative	(14)	14	0	10	10
Not PCP, silver negative	(46)	0	0	1a	11
Immunocompetent	(10)	0	0	0	0

aDeveloped PCP within 10 weeks of study.

were found in all of the 30 samples from immunosuppressed patients with *P. carinii* pneumonia confirmed by clinical means and by standard silver staining. In 10 of 14 other patients with clinical *P. carinii* pneumonia, but negative silver stains, strong signals of amplified DNA were detected. The sensitivity of DNA amplification suggests that the pulmonary illness in the 4 remaining patients must be attributable to some other cause, entities such as nonspecific and lymphocytic pneumonitis, which are clinically indistinguishable from *P. carinii* pneumonia and which can remit spontaneously are well recognized (13).

We compared the use of paired induced sputum and bronchoscopic lavage samples, and 37 episodes of respiratory illness in subjects with HIV infection were included (12) (Table 3). In 20 episodes in which the clinical diagnosis was *P. carinii* pneumonia, silver stain was positive in 14 (70%) of lavage samples and in 7 (35%) of sputum samples. In contrast, DNA amplification produced strong signals in 19 of these lavage samples (95%) and in 18 (90%) of the induced sputum samples.

Thus, the presence of a strong signal detected by ethidium bromide staining (implying the presence of 100 organisms or more in the PCR test sample—3×10^4 or more per milliliter of lavage or sputum) is obtained in over 90% of bronchoscopic lavage samples and induced sputum samples from patients with clinical *P. carinii* pneumonia. In only 1 of 50 samples has such a strong signal been obtained in a patient without *P. carinii* pneumonia, and this patient died of disease within 10 weeks. Therefore, DNA amplification for *P. carinii* offers great sensitivity and specificity in clinical diagnostic work; simple calibration of results allow excellent correlation with clinical disease. Although we know the approximate number of organisms that PCR is detecting in a test sample, such as lavage or sputum, and can relate this to clinical disease, it does not provide a formal estimate of the numbers of organisms within the lung, since the vagaries of such

Table 3 Thirty-five Immunosuppressed Subjects Studied by DNA Amplification and Silver Staining for *P. carinii* in Paired Bronchoalveolar Lavage and Induced Sputum Samples

Patients	(n)	Clinical PCP	Lavage			Sputum		
			Silver staining	DNA amplification		Silver staining	DNA amplification	
				Gel	Blot		Gel	Blot
Clinical PCP and silver positive	(15)	15	14[a]	15	15	7[a]	15	15
Clinical PCP, but silver negative	(5)	5	0	4	4	0	3	4
Not PCP, silver negative	(17)	0	0	1[b]	4	0	1[b]	1

[a]One patient was silver positive on sputum, but not lavage.
[b]One patient developed PCP within 10 weeks of study.

sampling are significant. We have, to date, conducted follow-up DNA amplification studies on lavage on only two subjects with successfully treated *P. carinii* pneumonia; both were negative by DNA amplification after 3 weeks of treatment.

It is notable that weaker signals (on oligonucleotide hybridization alone, implying the presence of fewer organisms and perhaps as few as one or two in a PCR test sample—300 organisms per milliliter of lavage or sputum) are detectable in roughly one-fifth of patients with established AIDS with acute respiratory illness attributable to causes other than *P. carinii* pneumonia. The great majority of such subjects had not suffered a previous episode of *P. carinii* pneumonia; therefore, the results represent subclinical colonization. We are currently testing, in clinical follow-up studies on these subjects, whether such a finding is an important prognostic indicator of impending disease.

Primers pAZ102-H and pAZ102-E have been employed by Galan et al. (14) on bronchoalveolar lavage samples from their population of HIV-positive immunosuppressed subjects. Results of PCR analysis were compared with results of conventional stainings and immunofluorescence; PCR was positive in 30 of 35 samples that were positive either by conventional stains or immunofluorescence and was positive in only one of 34 cases for which other methods were negative. Becker-Hapak et al. (15) have reported the use of PCR based on a repetitive DNA sequence from *P. carinii*, and their preliminary clinical studies demonstrate increased sensitivity of the method in comparison with indirect fluorescence assay. Our own studies show that, whereas DNA amplification readily identifies 100 organisms or more after ethidium bromide staining of electrophoresed DNA, reliable diagnosis by immunofluorescence in a health service laboratory may require significantly more organisms per sample (16). Other groups have demonstrated a similar sensitivity of PCR, ranging down to the ability to detect one organism per sample—Kitada et al. (17) used PCR based on 5S rRNA and Schluger et al. (18) used primers based on the *P. carinii* dihydrofolate reductase gene for the detection of rat-derived *P. carinii*. In the latter study, it was shown that DNA amplification for *P. carinii* was positive in the circulating blood of 5 of 14 experimental rats with *P. carinii* and that detectable organism material was present in the cellular fraction of peripheral blood.

The development of molecular methods, based on DNA hybridization and the polymerase chain reaction, in diagnosis of *P. carinii* pneumonia is developing rapidly and effectively. It promises to replace the nonspecific conventional techniques of lower sensitivity and to be more generally applicable to the diagnosis of other pulmonary pathogens when it can be applied to simple samples, such as induced sputum.

IV. Epidemiology

A significant finding in our studies has been the absence of amplified *P. carinii* DNA sequences in the lavage from normal individuals (11,12). In a follow-up study, using DNA amplification directly on postmortem lung samples (19), we have obtained no *P. carinii*-specific DNA amplification in repeated testing of different lobar samples from 15 immunocompetent individuals. Although this is a small sample size, the DNA amplification is specific to *P. carinii*, and this contrasts with the larger studies that have used microscopy after silver staining, which binds to mannan residues from a range of fungal organisms and spores and, therefore, is nonspecific. Postmortem studies using specific monoclonal antibodies have also failed to identify *P. carinii* in the lungs of immunocompetent individuals (20). Therefore, the results, contrary to current opinion, imply that carriage of *P. carinii* does *not* occur in the normal lung and, accordingly, that opportunistic pneumonia in the immunosuppressed is the result of fresh infection.

Comparative studies indicate that there are consistent differences in DNA sequence in amplified DNA between *P. carinii* derived from human, rat, ferret, and rabbit hosts (10,21), implying that infected mammals are not the source of infection for man; this is consistent with the observations that exposure to animals in the home is not a risk factor for the development of *P. carinii* in childhood leukemics (22).

The use of DNA amplification promises to unravel the ill-understood epidemiology of *P. carinii* pneumonia and specifically address the issues of whether fresh infection may occur by contagion from fellow humans with *P. carinii* pneumonia, or from some free-living environmental source.

V. Conclusions

DNA amplification has been developed as a powerful diagnostic tool in the identification of clinical *P. carinii* pneumonia. Specificity for the method has been achieved by careful analysis of the DNA sequence used and, in particular, the testing of a very broad range of related organisms by PCR to ensure confidence in the specificity of products amplified to *P. carinii*. The method has been applied to samples from over 100 subjects, immunosuppressed and immunocompetent, comparing the tests with established silver stain methods from clinical samples and clinical observations, including response to specific treatment, to gauge the relation between positive PCR results and clinical disease. It has been shown that the results of DNA amplification can be simply calibrated into *strong signals* (amplified DNA detectable by simple ethidium bromide staining of electrophoresed DNA, equivalent to 100 or more organisms per PCR sample or 3×10^4 or more per milliliter of lavage or sputum) and *weaker signals* (the identification of amplification product only after Southern hybridization, which has sensitivity down to the recognition of one to two organisms per PCR sample or 300/ml of sputum or lavage). It is of interest that 20% of immunodeficient HIV-positive patients with alternative diagnoses to account for their respiratory symptoms have *weak signals*, suggesting colonization by *P. carinii*, but that no such colonization is observed in clinical samplings on direct tests on lung tissue from immunocompetent subjects. The presence of a *strong signal* from DNA amplification correlates excellently with *P. carinii* pneumonia; more than 95% of *P. carinii* pneumonia cases may be identified by such a signal in induced sputum; our studies indicate that the presence of such a signal indicates clinical *P. carinii* pneumonia in 98% of instances.

Acknowledgments

This work has been supported in Britain by the Wellcome Trust, Medical Research Council and Royal Society.

References

1. Hopkin JM, Wakefield AE. DNA hybridisation for the diagnosis of microbial disease. Q J Med 1990; 75:415–421.

2. Saiki RK, Gelfand DH, Stoffel S, et al. Primer-directed enzymatic amplification of DNA with a thermostable DNA polymerase. Science 1988; 239:487–491.
3. Gootz TD, Tenover FC, Young SA, Gordon KP, Plorde JJ. Comparison of three DNA hybridization methods for detection of the aminoglycoside 2"-O-adenyltransferase gene in clinical bacterial isolates. Antimicrob Agents Chemother 1985; 28:69–73.
4. Wakefield AE, Hopkin JM, Burns J, Hipkiss JA, Stewart TJ, Moxon ER. Cloning of DNA from *Pneumocystis carinii*. J Infect Dis 1988; 158:859–862.
5. Wakefield AE, Pixley FJ, Banerji S, Sinclair K, Miller RF, Moxon ER, Hopkin JM. Amplification of mitochondrial ribosomal RNA sequences from *Pneumocystis carinii* DNA of rat and human origin. Mol Biochem Parasitol 1990; 43:69–76.
6. Peters SE, Wakefield AE, Banerji S, Hopkin JM. Quantifying the detection of *Pneumocystis carinii* by DNA amplification. Mol Cell Probes 1992; 6:115–117.
7. Edman JC, Kovacs JA, Masur H, Santi DV, Elwood HJ, Sogin ML. Ribosomal RNA sequence shows *Pneumocystis carinii* to be a member of the fungi. Nature 1988; 334:519–522.
8. Pixley FJ, Wakefield AE, Banerji S, Hopkin JM. Mitochondrial gene sequences show fungal homology for *Pneumocystis carinii*. Mol Microbiol 1991; 5:1347–1351.
9. Stringer SL, Stringer JR, Blase MH, Walzer PU, Cushion MI. *Pneumocystis carinii*: sequence from ribosomal RNA implies a close relationship with fungi. Exp Parasitol 1989; 68:450–461.
10. Wakefield AE, Peters SE, Banerji S, et al. *Pneumocystis carinii* shows DNA homology with the ustomycetous red yeast fungi. Mol Microbiol 1992; 6:1903–1911.
11. Wakefield AE, Pixley FJ, Banerji S, Sinclair K, Miller RF, Moxon ER, Hopkin JM. Detection of *Pneumocystis carinii* with DNA amplification. Lancet 1990; 336:451–453.
12. Wakefield AE, Guiver L, Miller RF, Hopkin JM. DNA amplification on induced sputum samples for diagnosis of *Pneumocystis carinii* pneumonia. Lancet 1991; 337:1378–1379.
13. Suffredini AF, Ognibene FP, Lack EE, et al. Nonspecific interstitial pneumonitis: a common cause of pulmonary disease in the acquired immunodeficiency syndrome. Ann Intern Med 1987; 107:7–13.
14. Galan F, Olivier JL, Roux P, Poirot JL, Bereziat G. Detection of *Pneumocystis carinii* DNA by polymerase chain reaction in bronchoscopic lavage compared to direct microscopy and immunofluorescence. J Protozool 1991; 38:1995–2005.
15. Becker-Hapak M, Liberator P, Graves D. Detection of *P. carinii* by polymerase chain reaction. J Protozool 1991; 38:1915–1945.
16. Leigh TR, Wakefield AE, Peters SE, Hopkin JM, Collins JV. Comparison of DNA amplification and immunofluorescence for detecting *Pneumocystis carinii* in patients receiving immunosuppressive therapy. Transplantation 1992; 54:468–470.
17. Kitada K, Oka S, Kimura S, Shimada K, Tadao S, Yamada J, Tsunoo H, Egawa K, Nakamura Y. Detection of *Pneumocystis carinii* sequences by polymerase chain reaction: animal models and clinical application to noninvasive specimens. J Clin Microbiol 1991; 29:1985–1990.
18. Schluger N, Sepkowitz K, Armstrong D, Bernard E, Rifkin M, Cerami A, Bucala R. Detection of *Pneumocystis carinii* in serum of AIDS patients with pneumocystis pneumonia by the polymerase chain reaction. J Protozool 1991; 38:2405–2425.

19. Peters SE, Wakefield AE, Sinclair K, Millard PJ, Hopkin JM. A search for latent *Pneumocystis carinii* infection in post-mortem lungs by DNA amplification. J Pathol 1992; 166:195–198.
20. Millard PR, Heryet AR. Observations favouring *P. carinii* pneumonia as a primary infection: a monoclonal antibody study on paraffin sections. J Pathol 1988; 154:365–370.
21. Sinclair K, Wakefield AE, Banerji S, Hopkin JM. *Pneumocystis carinii* organisms derived from rat and human hosts are genetically distinct. Mol Biochem Parasitol 1991; 45:183–184.
22. Hughes WT, Price RA, Ho-Kyun K, et al. *Pneumocystis carinii* pneumonitis in children with malignancies. J Paediatr 1973; 82:404–415.

21

Radiological Approaches to the Diagnosis of *Pneumocystis carinii* Pneumonia

JAY A. FISHMAN

Massachusetts General Hospital
and Harvard Medical School
Boston, Massachusetts

I. Introduction

The diagnosis of *Pneumocystis carinii* pneumonia relies on the histological demonstration of *P. carinii* in pulmonary specimens. The importance of radiological diagnosis as an adjunct to the microscopic detection of organisms has increased despite recent improvements in the noninvasive diagnosis of *P. carinii* pneumonia, including better collection (i.e., sputum induction) and processing (i.e., fluorescent antibodies) of patient samples. The radiological approach to *P. carinii* pneumonia is important because

1. Despite improved antibiotic prophylaxis, *P. carinii* remains a common pathogen in many immunocompromised hosts and is a defining illness of the acquired immunodeficiency syndrome (AIDS).
2. Chest radiographs may help in the initial assessment of the severity of the disease.
3. Radiology is useful in the management of patients during antibiotic therapy or prophylaxis, both in assessing the response of the disease to therapy and investigating concurrent infections in the susceptible host.

4. Despite a lack of specificity, radiographs may indicate the need for invasive diagnostic modalities to establish firm diagnoses.
5. Newer imaging techniques may allow the quantitation of disease caused by *P. carinii*.
6. Extrapulmonary disease may present as obstructive or mass lesions in the absence of known pulmonary disease. These lesions are amenable to aspiration or biopsy under tomographic or ultrasound-directed guidance.

By contrast, the value of radiological techniques is limited by a general lack of specificity of the images obtained, by the time lag that exists between clinical developments and radiological changes, by alterations in images produced by intercurrent infections, (e.g., cytomegalovirus, bacteria) and in the transplanted lung allograft, and by the diminished inflammation seen in the immunocompromised host.

II. The Chest Radiograph in *Pneumocystis carinii* Pneumonia: Acute Infection

The chest radiograph is a useful screening test in the immunocompromised individual with respiratory symptoms and is central to the diagnosis of *P. carinii* pneumonia. No radiographic pattern is pathognomonic for pneumocystis infection, any more than for the other "atypical" pneumonias—interstitial processes on chest radiograph that present with cough, hypoxemia, fever, and without significant sputum production (1–3). The radiographic pattern varies with underlying or accompanying diseases, the state of immunosuppression, and the duration of infection. Sometimes the chest radiograph is normal, despite overt pulmonary disease (1,3–8). More often, the early stage of *P. carinii* pneumonia is manifested by fine, bilateral, perihilar, diffuse "ground-glass" infiltrates that progress to an interstitial alveolar butterfly pattern. From the hilar region, the infiltrates spread to the apices or bases (Fig. 1). Despite therapy, this pattern is often succeeded in 3–5 days by progressive consolidation, the appearance of air bronchograms, and complete opacification of the lung fields. The radiographic image of *P. carinii* pneumonia may emerge as immunosuppressive therapies are reduced during treatment for pneumocystosis or for other conditions. In the acquired immunodeficiency syndrome (AIDS), up to 20% of asymptomatic individuals have pleuropulmonary changes of unknown etiology on chest radiograph (9,10). Infiltrates and hypoxemia tend to evolve more slowly (4–8 weeks) in this population (11).

A. Atypical Patterns

As in many of the atypical pneumonias, unusual courses and patterns are seen (Table 1) (2–4,7,12–19). Atypical roentgenographic appearances of *P. carinii*

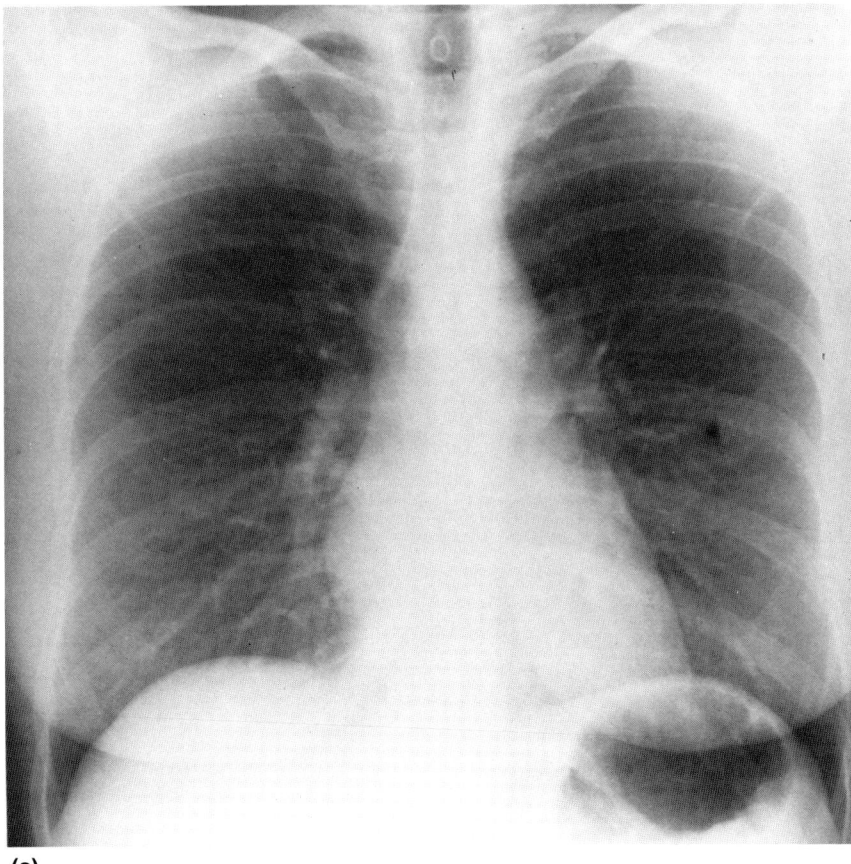

(a)

Figure 1 (a) Chest radiograph of a liver transplantation recipient with *P. carinii* pneumonia. The diffuse interstitial infiltrate has a perihilar predominance. (b) Chest radiograph of child with AIDS and *P. carinii* pneumonia.

pneumonia include localized infiltrates, cystic or honeycomb lesions, hilar enlargement with lymphadenopathy, spontaneous pneumothoraces, isolated disease in the upper lobes or in single lobes, and, occasionally, solitary pulmonary nodules. Small pleural effusions may also occur infrequently. The bilateral ground-glass pattern may be interrupted by linear opacities in some patients (17,20). It is unclear whether or not these represent a unique feature of *P. carinii* pneumonia, or a predisposition to atelectasis in these patients who are subject to shallow and rapid breathing patterns. Generally, one to three of these linear opacities are seen and may measure up to 5 cm in length and 1–2 mm in width.

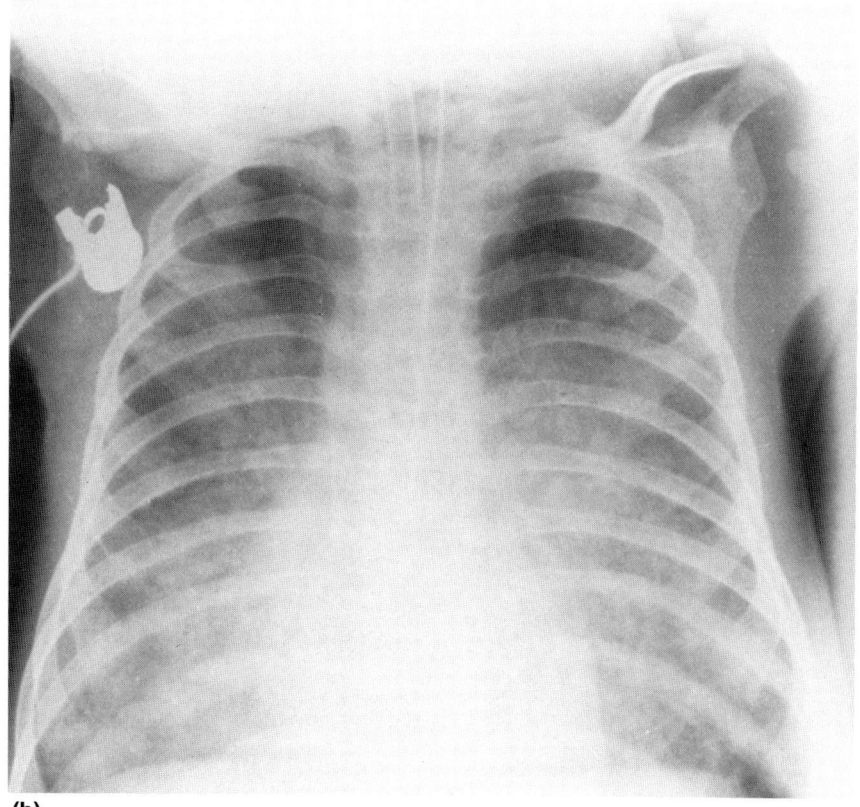

(b)

Figure 1 (Continued)

These opacities disappear during therapy and are seen only in the acutely ill patient. Occasionally, *P. carinii* will present as a solitary pulmonary nodule that may or may not cavitate (2,7,16,21,22) (Fig. 2). Microabscesses that develop may contain either *P. carinii* alone or bacterial or fungal superinfection (2). *Pneumocystis carinii* can also superinfect preexisting cavities caused by prior mycobacterial or fungal disease. Smaller cavities resolve in the patient who responds to therapy for primary *P. carinii* pneumonia.

Hilar or medistinal adenopathy occurs infrequently (up to 5%) in patients with *P. carinii* pneumonia in the absence of other infections such as *Mycobacterium tuberculosis* or *Cryptococcus neoformans* (7,23,24). Of note, peripheral lymphadenopathy is not necessarily associated with hilar mediastinal adenopathy (7). The association of cytomegalovirus (CMV) with *P. carinii* infection of the

Table 1 Radiographic Features: *Pneumocystis carinii*[a]

Common	Uncommon[b]
Interstitial infiltrates	Lymphadenopathy
Perihilar distribution	Abscess or cavity
Cyst/nodules, scattered	Nodules, diffuse
Atelectasis, mild	Atelectasis, severe
Progressive consolidation	Effusions, significant
Normal radiograph (early)	Extrapulmonary masses
Residual fibrosis	Pneumothorax
Diffuse distribution	Lobar or segmental disease
Hyperinflation, infantile	Spontaneous resolution
Progressive consolidation	

[a]Manifestations of *P. carinii* as sole pathogen.
[b]Increased by other infections, therapies, diseases.

lungs does not tend to alter the radiographic pattern at the time of presentation; however, the intensity of infiltrates may be greater in the presence of CMV. Alterations in the radiographic picture are commonly produced by prior radiation, pulmonary fibrosis or inflammation resulting from drug therapies, other concurrent infections, or cancer (25).

The patient with recurrent disease may develop chronic interstitial markings, small cysts, or honeycombing on chest radiograph (4,12,24,26). Interstitial fibrosis may develop after acute pneumonia, resulting in persistent infiltrates. Radiographic changes are common in the intravenous drug abuser in the absence of infection (27,28) and may be difficult to differentiate from *P. carinii* pneumonia. Peripheral or apical bullae may be seen in uninfected intravenous drug abusers, whereas, in pneumocystosis, the distribution of small cysts and bullae, when present, is more often diffuse (15,24,26–29). Nodules (as with lymphadenopathy) may be associated with lymphoma or Kaposi's sarcoma in AIDS patients.

B. Altered Hosts

1. Pentamidine and Pneumothorax

The use of aerosolized pentamidine for the therapy and prophylaxis of *P. carinii* pneumonia in AIDS has created some new problems in the diagnosis and treatment of pneumocystosis (14,30–33) (Fig. 3). The disease may present largely or solely in the upper lobes on chest radiograph, which may reflect the regional distribution of pentamidine in the lungs. Cystic changes are also more common in these patients. The development of spontaneous pneumothorax may indicate the recur-

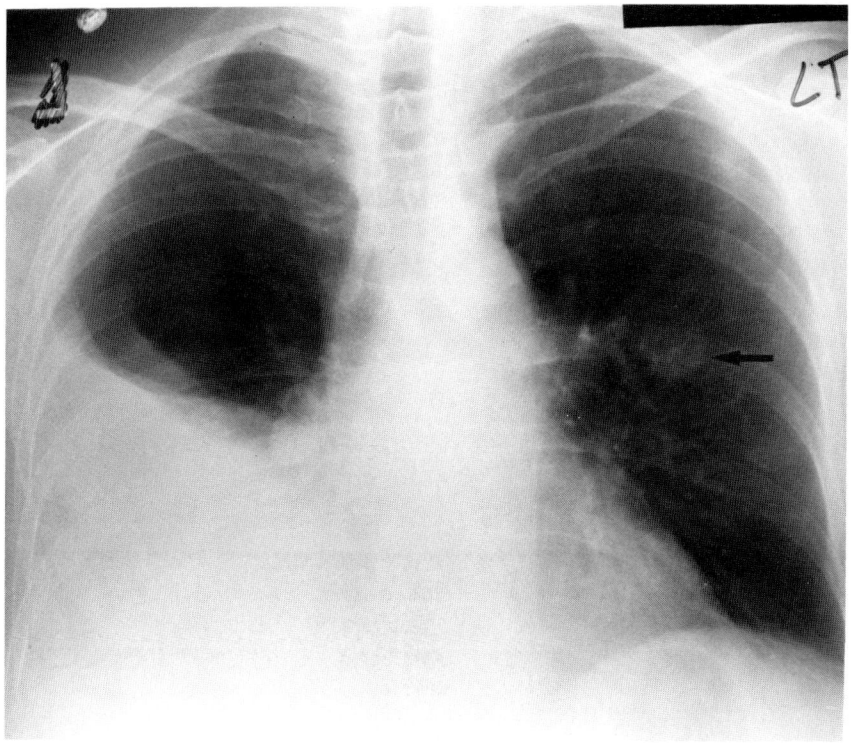

(a)

Figure 2 (a) Reduction in immunosuppression in a liver transplant recipient revealed a pulmonary nodule (arrow) in a patient (see Fig. 1) previously treated for *P. carinii* pneumonia. (b) Cavitation of the nodule (arrow) occurred over the course of a week. Bronchoscopic biopsies revealed both *P. carinii* and *Aspergillus* species.

rence of *P. carinii* infection in the upper lobes, despite on-going prophylactic therapy (31,34). Pneumothorax may also complicate the management of intubated patients with pneumocystosis; in these cases it is due to active pneumonia or fibrosis in the upper lobes (18,31,35,36). If undiagnosed, there is a 50% mortality associated with this complication. Upper zone disease should also suggest mycobacterial disease, especially in the presence of pleural effusions. Extrapulmonary *P. carinii* infection in these patients is discussed below.

2. Transplantation

In transplanted lungs, rejection and infection are both associated with abnormal chest radiographs (37,38). In the first month, rejection of the transplanted lung will

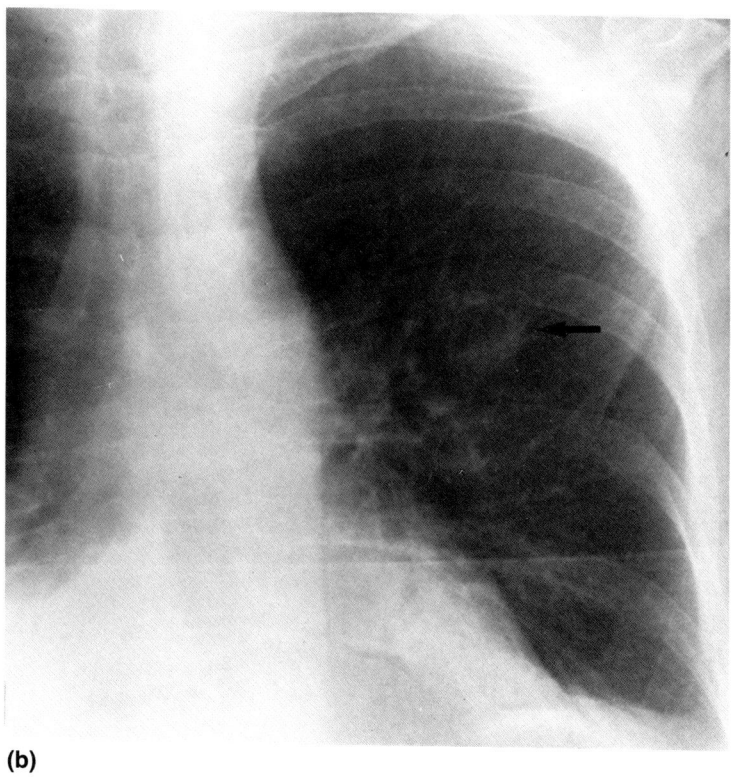

(b)

cause radiographic changes in up to 75% of patients. These changes include nodular and interstitial infiltrates in the perihilar area and in the lower lobes, which may progress to consolidation. These changes may also occur with infection, of which CMV is most common, and may be radiographically indistinguishable from organ rejection (37). After the first month, rejection is less often associated with radiographic changes (about 25%) and the radiographic findings of infection with *P. carinii* are similar to those of other immunocompromised hosts (37,38). Perhaps most striking is the relative paucity of chest radiographic findings in lung allograft recipients with demonstrated *P. carinii* infection (39). Asymptomatic *P. carinii* infections were diagnosed by bronchoalveolar lavage in 10 of 16 lung transplant recipients in whom *P. carinii* was identified in a series from the University of Pittsburgh. Three (of the 6) remaining symptomatic patients also had simultaneous bacterial infections. Whether asymptomatic carriage of *P. carinii* occurs in transplanted lungs, or whether these are merely early infections in an organ with altered vascular, lymphatic, and nervous systems remains unclear. Other non-

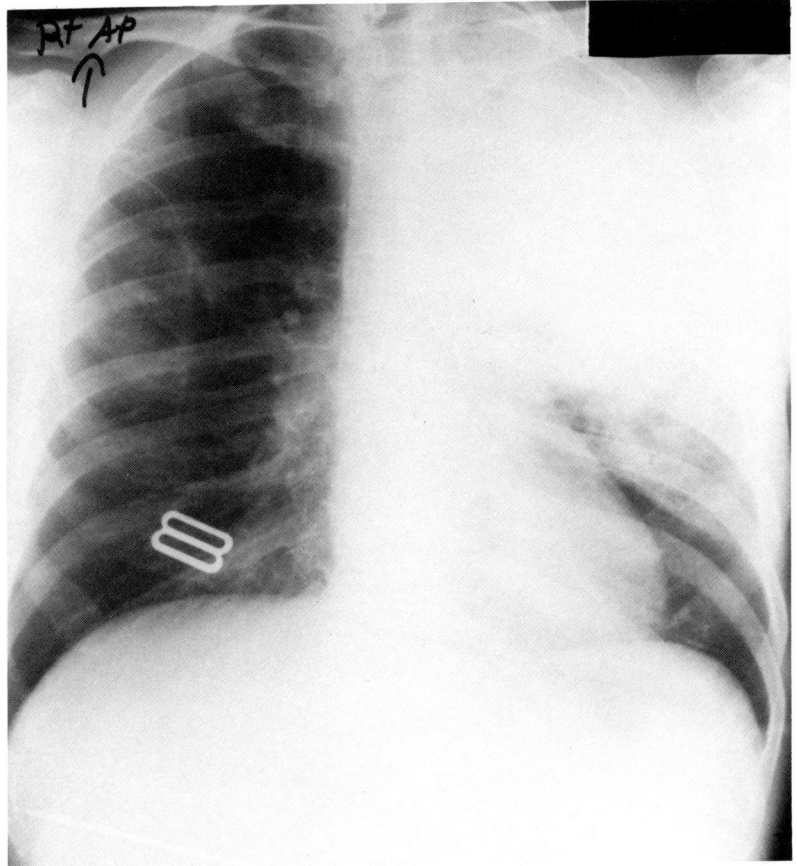

Figure 3 An AIDS patient receiving aerosolized pentamidine prophylaxis developed simultaneous *P. carinii* and *Legionella* pneumonia in the left upper lobe.

pulmonary organ transplantation recipients have radiologic findings similar to those of other immunosuppressed patients (see Fig. 1) (40).

C. Infantile and Pediatric *Pneumocystis carinii* Pneumonia

Children with interstitial plasma cell pneumonitis or the epidemic form of *P. carinii* pneumonia have radiologic manifestations of disease somewhat different from those in adults (41–45). In studies of children in Hungary, the evolution of the chest radiograph occurred over 3–8 weeks (as described by Paldy and Ivady; 46). The progression includes progressively increased vascular and airway markings;

small areas of atelectasis (3–4 weeks); peripheral hyperinflation with flattened diaphragms, interstitial infiltrates, and early consolidation (4–5 weeks); air bronchograms in hyperinflated lungs with increased interstitial infiltrates, scattered nodules, areas of lucency, and intercostal widening (5–6 weeks); and, finally, complete consolidation (8 weeks). This progression is variable. Resolution takes 2–3 weeks when therapy is initiated early; in advanced infections or without specific therapy, radiological improvement occurs over 2–6 months. Respiratory improvement (intercostal widening, diaphragmatic flattening, hyperinflation) precedes resolution of pulmonary infiltrates.

Atypical features are common in epidemic infantile pneumocystosis (2,41–43,45,47). In addition to the typical perihilar or diffuse interstitial infiltrates and hyperinflation, some patients will have normal radiographs or asymmetric infiltrates with cysts, nodules, effusions, atelectasis, or lymphadenopathy. The radiological appearance of *P. carinii* pneumonitis in immunosuppressed children or in those with AIDS is similar to that of the immunocompromised adult (44). Lymphocytic interstitial pneumonitis (LIP) in AIDS will produce an interstitial pattern on x-ray films similar to that of *P. carinii* (44). However, in LIP, systemic (including mediastinal) lymphadenopathy is common. Bacterial pneumonia is more common than *P. carinii* pneumonia in children with AIDS.

III. Computed Tomography and Magnetic Resonance Imaging

The many potential pathogens and tumors that affect immunocompromised individuals have led to the extensive use of more advanced technologies for the evaluation of these patients. These include computed tomography (CT) scan, magnetic resonance imaging (MRI or NMR) scans, as well as several techniques that rely on inflammatory responses (discussed below). Promising techniques, including positron emission tomography (PET scan), have not yet come into common use. The relatively poor signal obtained at the air–tissue interface in the lung has reduced the value of the MRI scan in many pulmonary infections.

Three general patterns of thoracic disease are commonly observed on CT scans: lymphadenopathy, mass lesions, and parenchymal abnormalities. Lymphadenopathy is not common in *P. carinii* pneumonia in the absence of other causes of lymph node hyperplasia (7,23,48). Studies of AIDS patients with lymphadenopathy by CT scanning have demonstrated that lymphadenopathy is due to reactive follicular hyperplasia in up to half of the patients, to non-Hodgkin's lymphoma (20%), Kaposi's sarcoma (10%), and mycobacteria (17%), as well as a variety of other infections, tumors, and conditions (7,23–25,47,49,50). In non-AIDS patients, lymphadenopathy is more often associated with an underlying tumor, or with fungal or viral infections (47). A few conditions merit specific comment. Adverse drug reactions may cause lymph node enlargement in the absence of specific infectious etiologies. In children with AIDS, the syndrome of lymphoid interstitial pneumonitis (LIP) also presents with lymphadenopathy, either localized to the mediastinum or generalized. The chest radiograph in LIP is indistinguishable from that of acute *P. carinii* pneumonia. Generalized lymphadenopathy is common in AIDS and in AIDS-related complex (ARC), in the absence of other diseases.

Parenchymal involvement of the lungs by *P. carinii* pneumonia takes many forms on CT scans. The CT scans may reveal parenchymal disease that is not observed on routine radiographic examination (Fig. 4). The correlation of CT findings with pulmonary histopathology is quite good. Asymmetry is common. The infiltrates can be dense and homogeneous or patchy in both lung fields (24). Frequently, areas of dense involvement will be adjacent to alveoli, segments, or lobes that have been entirely spared. The picture may be further complicated by the existence of previous infection or of coexistent disease. Previous *P. carinii*

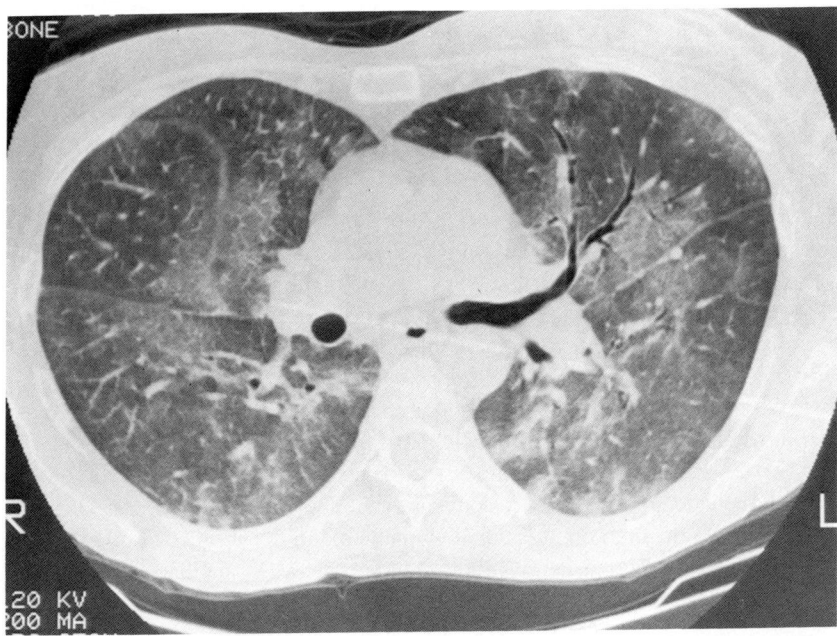

Figure 4 A contrast-enhanced CT examination of the chest of a woman with AIDS (receiving aerosolized pentamidine) reveals diffuse parenchymal disease with patches or "nodular" infiltrates, despite a normal chest radiograph. *Pneumocystis carinii* was demonstrated by induced sputum examination.

infection will frequently leave (up to 50%) dense interstitial markings by CT, which correlate with fibrosis (24,51). Pleural disease or pleural effusions are uncommon in isolated pneumocystis infection and other infections or tumors should be considered in the differential for such findings. Bullae occur frequently in AIDS patients, from mild apical involvement to extensive emphysematous changes (24).

Mass lesions in *P. carinii* infection are uncommon (see Fig. 4). Diffuse small nodules are frequently seen throughout the lung parenchyma by CT scan, and occasionally these small nodules may cavitate or become secondarily infected (12). These changes are often undetected by routine radiography. Small pulmonary cysts have been observed more often in *P. carinii* infection in AIDS patients than in other hosts (4,7,12,26). The cysts tend to be thin-walled and generally free of fluid or debris (4). The roles of preexisting interstitial fibrosis and of mechanical ventilation in the development of small cystic lesions are unclear. It appears that cystic lesions are more common in intravenous drug abusers, especially those with AIDS, then in patients with *P. carinii* pneumonia from other causes. These cysts tend to be diffusely dispersed throughout the lung parenchyma (27,28). Virtually all of the patients with *P. carinii* pneumonia and significant pneumatoceles have had AIDS. It is unclear whether human immunodeficiency virus (HIV) is a cofactor in the development of this particular manifestation of disease. Patients with *P. carinii* who have had only upper lobe disease occasionally develop pneumothoraxes as a complication of a rupture of a cystic lesion into the pleural space.

Infrequently, the radiographic picture moves beyond small cyst and cavities to produce a patient with frank pulmonary cavitation (7,15,52) (see Fig. 3). In some of these cases, it is clear that *P. carinii* has secondarily infected the cavity remaining after treatment for previous tuberculosis or for fungal infection. However, in some of these patients, it appears that the cavity is due to *P. carinii* alone.

A. Extrapulmonary Disease

Extrapulmonary disease caused by *P. carinii* has been reported with increasing frequency over the past few years (53). Careful review of the literature also suggests that some of these were patients without underlying AIDS (53–55). There is usually clear pulmonary involvement by *P. carinii* before the diagnosis of extrapulmonary disease (53). The mechanisms for the extrapulmonary spread of *P. carinii* remain unclear. It is uncertain whether organisms are transported within phagocytic cells or spread independently. At least a part of the spread of disease appears to be through the reticuloendothelial system, with manifestations in the lymph nodes, spleen, bone marrow, and liver (53,56). Multiple organ involvement suggests that a hematogenous route of spread also occurs, with *P. carinii* found in kidneys, pancreas, liver, heart, thymus, and throughout the gastrointestinal tract. Organisms have also been found in the eye, omentum, external auditory canal, thyroid, and adrenal glands, as well as single reports in a variety of other locations. Although the numbers are small, it does appear that the frequency of hematogenous dissemination (as opposed to contiguous or lymphatic spread) is greater in AIDS patients than in other compromised hosts.

Mass lesions caused by *P. carinii* are similar to other mass lesions in that the primary symptoms are those of obstruction. Splenic disease is common (Fig. 5) (56). This needs to be separated from other splenic diseases, including splenic abscesses caused by *M. tuberculosis*, by fungi, or by other bacteria (56,57). The CT scans demonstrate multiple splenic lesions with reduced attenuation varying from several millimeters up to 10 cm in diameter (see Fig. 5). Some of these lesions are calcified at initial presentation, whereas others develop a rim of calcification or punctate calcifications during the course of therapy (53). Some patients also develop calcification of lymph nodes, pleura, or peritoneum.

We have not observed disseminated *P. carinii* infection in individuals receiving systemic therapy with either trimethoprim–sulfamethoxazole or with pentamidine. However, infections outside the lungs have been seen in individuals

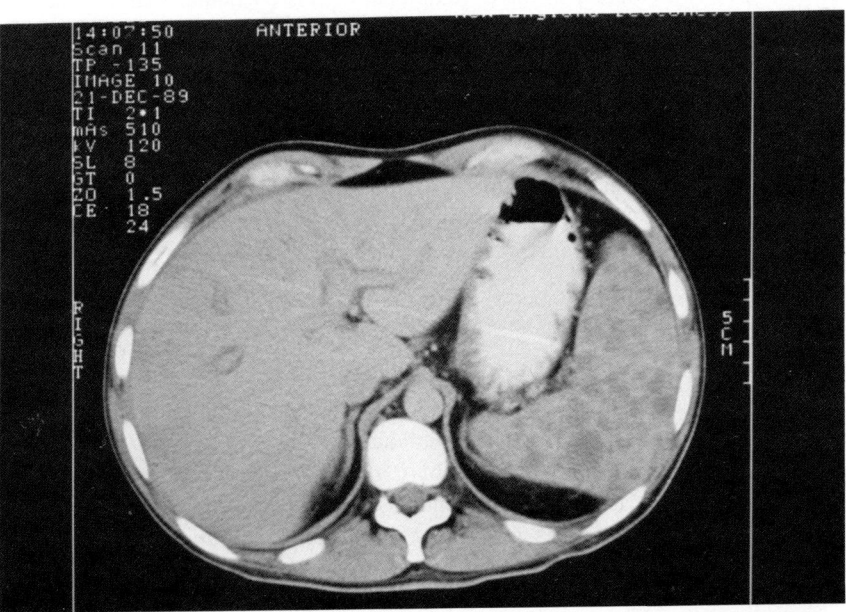

Figure 5 A CT scan of the abdomen of an AIDS patient with acute abdominal pain revealed inhomogeneity of the liver and spleen. Early splenic rupture with hepatic, splenic, and omental masses was observed. The masses contained *P. carinii*. No other pathogens were detected microscopically or in culture.

Radiological Approaches to Diagnosis   427

receiving aerosolized pentamidine and dapsone prophylaxis. Histopathological documentation should be obtained to support the diagnosis of *P. carinii* infection as the cause for extrapulmonary mass lesions.

IV. Ultrasound

Ultrasound may offer an advantage in the anatomical evaluation of extrapulmonary *P. carinii* (33,58,59). Some of the patients with extrapulmonary disease do not have evident pulmonary manifestations; however, several AIDS patients examined by ultrasound have had numerous very small highly echogenic (of greater tissue density than the surrounding parenchyma) foci of *P. carinii* infection in the liver, spleen, kidneys, pancreas, lymph nodes, thyroid, and adrenal organs. These foci are generally clumped and found in association with regions of punctate or rim calcifications on CT scans. The earliest form of these lesions may be hypoechoic (cavities or necrotic tissues), with an echogenic rim developing during therapy. Ultrasound may be used to guide a needle biopsy or aspiration of these masses. Many such masses are not easily visualized by routine CT scans (33). This may suggest that ultrasound is a more sensitive technique than CT in detecting early extrapulmonary *P. carinii* disease.

Ultrasound and fluoroscopy are also used to guide the aspiration of peripheral pulmonary nodules and cysts (60–62). The yield is lower than for bronchoscopic biopsies (or lavage in AIDS patients). This technique cannot be used without correction of any bleeding or coagulation abnormalities. The main complications are pneumothorax (in up to a third of patients) and bleeding. The yields of various diagnostic procedures differ greatly among medical centers. For all procedures, the increased organism burden in AIDS patients improves the detection of *P. carinii*. Ultrasound or fluoroscopic guidance of bronchoscopic procedures (needle or covered brush) does not improve diagnostic yields.

V. "Inflammation Imaging"

Nuclear medicine has produced a series of imaging techniques that take advantage of gamma-emitting radionuclides attached to a variety of substrates useful in the detection of areas of inflammation. These scans include gallium-67 citrate scans, indium–125-labeled white blood cells, technetium-99m and indium–111-labeled human immunoglobulin (IgG) scans. Each of these scans is limited to some extent by the need for tissue inflammation to produce a positive image (23,63). That is, in patients with marked neutropenia or uremia or in infections that generate little inflammation (cryptococcal infection), these scans may be less useful. In each case, imaging depends on capillary permeability in the area of infection and on the local binding of the imaging agent to delay its elimination from the tissue. A major advantage of these methods is that up to 15% of total body scans will detect unanticipated abnormalities.

A. Gallium Scanning

Gallium scanning has been widely used as an adjunct to the diagnosis of *P. carinii* pneumonia (23,63–70). Gallium citrate scanning (^{67}Ga scintigraphy) can be entirely normal in patients with opportunistic pneumonia, with or without AIDS (8,23,63,69,71). Conversely, AIDS patients may have an abnormal gallium scan in the absence of infection other than with HIV. Gallium scans have up to a 91% sensitivity for *P. carinii* pneumonia, but a relatively low specificity (51%) (23,64, 68,72). Lymph node uptake alone may indicate ARC caused by HIV infection (23). Diffuse pulmonary uptake may indicate occult infection, in the asymptomatic immunocompromised patient, that would allow early intervention for therapy or prophylaxis (26,72). In AIDS, T-cell cytotoxicity directed against HIV-infected cells may generate a pattern of interstitial inflammation, resulting in a positive gallium scan (73). Drug reactions, pneumoconiosis, radiation therapy, adult respiratory distress syndrome, and infections caused by cytomegalovirus, cryptococcus, mycobacteria, or chlamydia, all can give a diffusely positive gallium scan in the immunosuppressed host (23,26,69). Focal infection may suggest the presence of the other pathogens, notably *M. avium–intracellulare* complex.

The positive gallium scan will precede the radiographic manifestations of *P. carinii* in many immunocompromised patients by as many as 4–6 weeks (23,62,67,69). Lung uptake of gallium can be demonstrated in up to 100% of AIDS patients with *P. carinii* pneumonia, including those with subclinical infections (23,69,70). In the presence of a negative gallium scan, there is only a small (less than 9%) chance that pneumocystis infection is present (23,64,68,72). However, up to a quarter of patients with a positive scan will not have *P. carinii* pneumonia. The best sensitivity of ^{67}Ga-scanning is seen on images taken at 48–72 hr after injection (Fig. 6). This appears to be true for all of the inflammation-imaging techniques. A normal scan in an extremely ill AIDS patient with known infection seems to correlate with a poor clinical outcome (23,63). The ^{67}Ga scan may also be useful as a measure of therapeutic efficacy. The failure of a gallium scan to return to normal after treatment for *P. carinii* pneumonia should suggest the presence of a therapeutic failure or the presence of other opportunistic infection or malignancy (23,26). Normal uptake should return 3–4 weeks after the start of anti-*P. carinii* therapy. Scanning does not correlate with the presence or absence of organisms. The pattern of gallium uptake in children with lymphoid interstitial pneumonitis (LIP) in AIDS is frequently not distinguishable from that of *P. carinii* pneumonia.

The cost of the routine use of gallium scanning in AIDS probably outweighs its usefulness when compared with the judicious use of antiviral or of anti-*P. carinii* antibiotics based on CD4 cell counts and on other clinical data. The ^{67}Ga

Radiological Approaches to Diagnosis 429

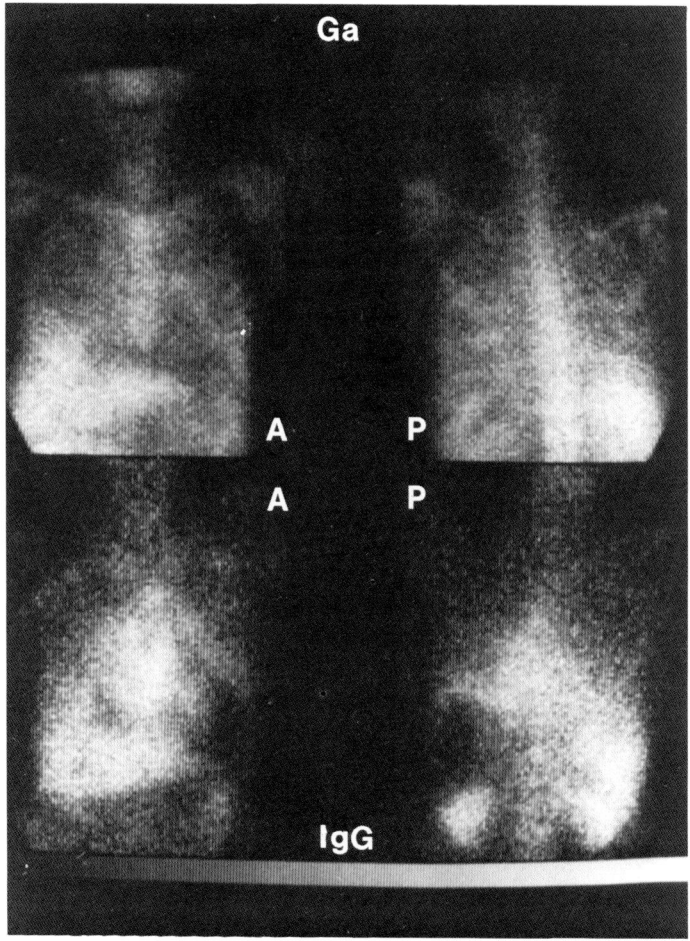

Figure 6 Gallium-67 citrate scan (GA, upper) and indium-111-immunoglobulin scan (IgG lower) of an AIDS patient with *P. carinii* pneumonia. Diffuse pulmonary uptake is seen with both agents. Image intensity is greater in the IgG scans, despite a much smaller dose of administered radioactivity. Hepatic and splenic images are normal. (A, anterior image; P, posterior image). (Courtesy Dr. Alan Fischman, Massachusetts General Hospital.)

scans are particularly useful, however, in the presence of a normal or atypical chest radiograph or when hypoxemia is not present. Some centers make a presumptive diagnosis of *P. carinii* pneumonia in the patient with AIDS when a decrease in diffusing capacity (D_{LCO}) is coupled with an abnormal chest radiograph and gallium scan.

B. Diethylenetriamine Pentaacetic Acid Scans

The clearance of radiolabeled inhaled ^{99m}Tc-DTPA (diethylenetriamine pentaacetate) is also increased in *P. carinii* pneumonia (as in other pneumonitides and in smokers). Some centers have reported a biphasic DTPA clearance during *P. carinii* pneumonia. Clearance reverts to monophasic decay after the successful treatment of the infection. It has not yet been determined how useful this test will be in larger patient populations. Although these tests are usually abnormal in *P. carinii* pneumonia, they lack specificity.

C. Immunoglobulin G Scans

The immunoglobulin scan uses indium- (or technetium)-labeled human serum immunoglobulin and depends on the localization of the Fc fragment of the immunoglobulin in areas of inflammation. The mechanism of this localization is unclear (23,50,74), as it appears to be for other imaging agents. The specificity of the immunoglobulin preparation does not affect the image. The IgG scan has the advantage of low cost and low total radiation dose, with a high-quality image, and the general availability of the necessary materials. This technique also has the advantage of the rapidity with which images can be taken. However, high levels of uptake in the normal liver, spleen, and bladder interfere with the detection of focal processes in these organs.

Imaging with radiolabeled (indium-111) human IgG has proved a useful adjunct to the diagnosis and therapy of *P. carinii* pneumonia for two reasons (74,75) (see Fig. 6): first, in both animal and in human studies the IgG scan appears to be more sensitive to inflammatory changes than is the gallium scan (74). This allows the detection of superimposed focal pulmonary processes caused by other pathogens in addition to the diffuse pattern seen in *P. carinii*. This sensitivity also allows the IgG scan to be used to follow the gradual resolution of inflammation in response to therapy, which has not been possible with gallium. Second, the IgG scan has been useful in detecting extrapulmonary foci of infection; this may be important in the management of AIDS patients with disseminated *P. carinii* or other processes (75). The IgG scan is not useful in the neutropenic patient or the uremic patient with dysfunctional neutrophils. The CT and MRI scans are better-suited to the definition of mass lesions.

Novel techniques are under development that depend on the unique metabolic pathways of the organism and on specific antibodies against *P. carinii*. These will enhance the sensitivity and specificity of radiological diagnosis.

VI. Resolution of Infection

The follow-up of patients treated for *P. carinii* pneumonia is perhaps the greatest deficiency of the radiographic techniques. Although nuclear medicine scanning may indicate the resolution of inflammation in the lungs with some degree of accuracy, the frequencies of coinfection and of false-positive scans make many of these images difficult to interpret (76–78). The routine chest radiograph is unchanged in most patients for the first 2 weeks of disease and may show progression of infiltrates for up to 3 weeks, despite appropriate therapy. In one series, only 17% of patients showed regression in radiographic abnormalities in the first week, with over 30% showing improvement by the end of the second week (4). Although most patients will have radiographic abnormalities resolve over 1–2 months, some patients take up to 5 months to resolve pulmonary infiltrates. Many patients develop various degrees of interstitial fibrosis (51,76,78). These patients may never develop completely normal chest radiographs (78). Some patients are left with residual cysts, although many of the cystic or honeycomb abnormalities will be seen to resolve over the period of the first 8–12 weeks after discharge from the hospital. Hilar enlargement caused by *P. carinii* pneumonia will resolve during the course of therapy. In the absence of resolution, alternative diagnoses need to be entertained (15). Late spontaneous pneumothoraxes and pneumomediastinum are observed occasionally in patients in the absence of diagnostic procedures or the use of mechanical ventilation. These abnormalities appear to be more common in patients maintained on a prophylactic aerosolized pentamidine regimen and in patients with peripherally located cystic lesions.

VII. Conclusions

Radiology remains an important component of the diagnostic approach to infection in the immunocompromised host. Because the manifestations of clinical disease are muted in these hosts, multiple diagnostic modalities are often required to determine the pattern of infectious disease. Traditional-imaging techniques (chest radiographs, CT scans) assist in the detection of disease associated with clinical symptoms. Newer radiologic modalities (antibody-based techniques, radionuclidic imaging, nucleic acid hybridization or amplification) will be applied to the noninvasive quantitation of *P. carinii* pneumonia (infectious burden) and of the response to therapy. Further evolution of these techniques will give the clinician tools with the sensitivity to detect and to allow prevention of infection before the development of significant disease.

References

1. Dee P, Winn W, McKee K. *Pneumocystis carinii* infection of the lung: radiologic and pathologic correlation. AJR 1979; 132:741–746.
2. Doppman JL, Gellhoed GW, DeVita VT. Atypical radiographic features in *Pneumocystis carinii* pneumonia. Diagn Radiol 1975; 114:39.

3. Forrest JV. Radiographic findings in *Pneumocystis carinii* pneumonia. Radiology 1972; 103:539–544.
4. DeLorenzo LJ, Huang CT, Maguire GP, Stone DJ. Roentgenographic patterns of *Pneumocystis carinii* pneumonia in 104 patients with AIDS. Chest 1987; 91:323–327.
5. Falenback KH, Bachmann KD, O'Loughlin BJ. *Pneumocystis carinii* pneumonia. AJR 1961; 85:706–713.
6. Goodman PC, Daley C, Minagi H. Spontaneous pneumothorax in AIDS patients with *Pneumocystis carinii* pneumonia. AJR 1986; 147:29–31.
7. Suster, B, Akerman M, Orenstein M, Wax MR. Pulmonary manifestations of AIDS: review of 106 episodes. Radiology 1986; 161:87–93.
8. Turbiner EH, Yeh SDJ, Rosen PP, Bains MS, Benua RS. Abnormal gallium scintigraphy in *Pneumocystis carinii* pneumonia with a normal chest radiograph. Radiology 1978; 127:437.
9. Cohen BA, Pomeranz S, Rabinowitz JG, Rosen MJ, Train JS, Norton KI, Mendalson DS. Pulmonary complications of AIDS: radiologic features. AJR 1984; 143:115–122.
10. Naidich DP, Garay SM, Leitman BS, McCauley DI. Radiographic manifestations of pulmonary disease in the acquired immunodeficiency syndrome (AIDS). Semin Roentgenol 1987; 22:14–30.
11. Kovacs JA, Hiemenz JW, Macher AM, Stover D, Murray HW, Shelhamer J, Lane NC. *Pneumocystis carinii* pneumonia: a comparison between patients with AIDS and patients with other immunodeficiency. Ann Intern Med 1983; 100:663–671.
12. Barrio JL, Suarez M, Rodriguez JL, Saldana MJ, Pitchenik AE. *Pneumocystis carinii* pneumonia presenting as cavitating and noncavitating solitary pulmonary nodules in patients with acquired immunodeficiency syndrome. Am Rev Respir Dis 1986; 134:1094–1096.
13. Bier S, Halton K, Krivisky B, Leonidas J. *Pneumocystis carinii* pneumonia presenting as a single pulmonary nodule. Paediatr Radiol 1986; 16:59–60.
14. Bradburne RM, Ettensohn DB, Opal SM, McCool FD. Relapse of *Pneumocystis carinii* pneumonia in the upper lobes during aerosol pentamidine prophylaxis. Thorax 1989; 44:591–593.
15. Chechani V, Zaman MK, Finch PJ. Chronic cavitary *Pneumocystis carinii* pneumonia in a patient with AIDS. Chest 1989; 95:1347–1348.
16. Cross AS, Steigbigel RT. *Pneumocystis carinii* pneumonia presenting as localized nodular densities. N Engl J Med 1974; 291:831–832.
17. Gedroyc WM, Reidy JF. Early changes in *Pneumocystis carinii* pneumonia. Clin Radiol 1985; 36:331–334.
18. Luddy RE, Champion LAA, Swartz AD. *Pneumocystis carinii* pneumonia with pneumatocele formation. Am J Dis Child 1977; 131:470.
19. Milligan SA, Stulbarg MS, Gamsu G, Golden JA, Pneumocystis pneumonia radiographically simulating tuberculosis. Am Rev Respir Dis 1985; 132:1124–1126.
20. Page JE, Wilson AG. Linear opacities as a feature of pneumocystis pneumonia. Br J Radiol 1990; 63:597–601.
21. Feldman AH, Donnelly WH. *Pneumocystis carinii* pneumonia in children. South Med J 1979; 72:1404.

22. Hartz JW, Ggeisinger KR, Scharyj M, Muss HB. Granulomatous pneumocystosis presenting as a solitary pulmonary nodule. Arch Pathol Lab Med 1985; 190: 466–469.
23. Bekerman C, Bitran J. Gallium-67 scanning in the clinical evaluation of human immunodeficiency virus infection: indications and limitations. Semin Nucl Med 1988; 18:273–286.
24. Kuhlman JE, Fishman EK, Hruban RH, Knowles M, Zerhouni EA, Siegelman SS. Diseases of the chest in AIDS: CT diagnosis. RadioGraphics 1989; 9:827–857.
25. Lowery WS, Whitlock WL, Dietrich RA, Fine JM. Sarcoidosis complicated by HIV infection: three case reports and a review of the literature. Am Rev Respir Dis 1990; 142:887–889.
26. Gurney W, Bates FT. Pulmonary cystic disease; comparison of *Pneumocystis carinii* pneumatoceles and bullous emphysema due to intravenous drug abuse. Radiology 1989; 173:27–31.
27. Stern W, Subbarao K. Pulmonary complications of drug abuse. Semin Roentgenol 1983; 18:183–197.
28. Tomashefski JF Jr, Hirsch CS. The pulmonary vascular lesions of intravenous drug abuse. Hum Pathol 1980; 11:133–145.
29. Goldstein DS, Karpel JP, Appel D, Williams MH Jr. Bullous pulmonary damage in users of intravenous drugs. Chest 1986; 89:266–269.
30. Baskin MI, Abd AG, Ilowite JS. Regional deposition of aerosolized pentamidine: effects of body position and breathing pattern. Ann Intern Med 1990; 113:677–683.
31. Goodman JL, Tashbin DP. *Pneumocystis* with normal chest x-ray film and arterial oxygen tension. Arch Intern Med 1981; 143:1981.
32. Newsome GS, Ward DJ, Pierce PF. Spontaneous pneumothorax in patients with acquired immunodeficiency syndrome treated with prophylactic aerosolized pentamidine. Arch Intern Med 1990; 150:2167–2168.
33. Spouge AR, Wilson SR, Gopinath N, Sherman M, Blendis LM. Extrapulmonary *Pneumocystis carinii* in a patient with AIDS: sonographic findings. AJR 1990; 155: 76–78.
34. Sherman M, Levin D, Breidbart D. *Pneumocystis carinii* pneumonia with spontaneous pneumothorax. Chest 1986; 90:609–610.
35. Joe L, Gordin F, Parker RH. Spontaneous pneumothorax with *Pneumocystic carinii* infection. Arch Intern Med 1986; 146:1816–1817.
36. Martinez C, Romanelli A, Mullen MP, Lee M. Spontaneous pnumothoraces in AIDS patients receiving aerosolized pentamidine. Chest 1988; 94:1317–1318.
37. Dauber JH, Paradis IL, Dummer JS. Infectious complications in pulmonary allograft recipients. Clin Chest Med 1990; 11:291–308.
38. Millet B, Higenbottam TW, Flower CDR, Stewart S, Wallwork J. The radiographic appearances of infection and acute rejection of the lung after heart–lung transplantation. Am Rev Respir Dis 1989; 140:62–67.
39. Gryzan S, Paradis IL, Zeevi A, Duquesnoy RJ, Dummer JS, Griffith BP, Hardesty RL, Trento A, Nalesnik MA, Dauber JH. Unexpectedly high incidence of *Pneumocystis carinii* infection after lung–heart transplantation. Am Rev Respir Dis 1988; 137:1268–1274.

40. Cooper DKC, Lanza RP, Oliver S, Forder AA, Rose AG, Uys CJ, Novitzky D, Barnard CN. Infectious complications after heart transplantation. Thorax 1983; 38: 822–828.
41. Johnson HD, Johnson WW. *Pneumocystis carinii* pneumonia in children with cancer. JAMA 1970; 214:1069.
42. Kim HK, Hughes WT. Comparison of methods for identification of *Pneumocystis carinii* in pulmonary aspirates. Am J Clin Pathol 1973; 60:462.
43. Kornstein MJ, Pietra GG, Hoxie JA, Conley ME. The pathology and treatment of interstitial pneumonitis in two infants with AIDS. Am Rev Respir Dis 1986; 133: 1196–1198.
44. Schiff RG, Kabat L, Kamani N. Gallium scanning in lymphoid interstitial pneumonitis of children with AIDS. J Nucl Med 1987; 28:1915–1919.
45. Vessal K, Post C, Dutz W, Bandarizadch B. Roentgenographic changes in infantile *Pneumocystis carinii* pneumonia. Am J Roentgenol Radium Ther Nucl Med 1974; 120:254.
46. Paldy L, Ivady G. Roentgenologic diagnosis of interstitial plasma cell pneumonia in infancy. Natl Cancer Inst Monogr 1976; 43:99.
47. Hughes WT, Price RA, Kim HK, Coburn T, Grigsby D, Feldman S. *Pneumocystis carinii* pneumonitis in children with malignancies. J Pediatr 1973; 82:404.
48. Stern RG, Gamsu G, Golden JA, Mirji M, Webb WR, Abrams DI. Intrathoracic adenopathy: differential feature of AIDS and diffuse lymphadenopathy syndrome. AJR 1984; 142:689–692.
49. Nyberg DA, Federic MP, Jeffrey RB. Abdominal CT findings in disseminated *Mycobacterium avium-intracellulare*. AJR 1985; 145:297–299.
50. Pitchenik AE, Robinson HA. The radiographic appearance of tuberculosis in patients with the acquired immune deficiency syndrome (AIDS) and preAIDS. Am Rev Respir Dis 1985; 131:393–396.
51. Whitcomb ME, Schwarz MI, Charles MA, Larson PH. Interstitial fibrosis after *Pneumocystis carinii* pneumonia. Ann Intern Med 1970; 73:761–765.
52. Eng RHK, Bishburg E, Smith SM. Evidence for destruction of lung tissue during *Pneumocystis carinii* infection. Arch Intern Med 1987; 147:746–749.
53. Lubat E, Megibow AJ, Balthazar EJ, Goldenberg AS, Birnbaum BA, Bosniak MA. Extrapulmonary *Pneumocystis carinii* infection in AIDS: CT findings. Radiology 1990; 174:157–160.
54. Byrd RB, Horn BR. Infection due to *Pneumocystis carinii* simulating lobar bacterial pneumonia. Chest 1976; 70:91.
55. LeGolvan DP, Heidelberger KP. Disseminated granulomatous *Pneumocystis carinii* pneumonia. Arch Pathol 1973; 95:344–348.
56. Fishman EK, Magid D, Kuhlman JE. *Pneumocystis carinii* involvement of the liver and spleen: CT demonstration. J Comput Assist Tomogr 1990; 14:146–148.
57. Wolff MJ, Bitran J, Northland RG, Levy IL. Splenic abscesses due to *Mycobacterium tuberculosis* in patients with AIDS. Rev Infect Dis 1991; 13:373–375.
58. Hamper UM, Goldblum LE, Hutchins GM, Sheth S, Dahnert WF, Bartlett JG, Sanders RC. Renal involvement in AIDS; sonographic–pathologic correlations. AJR 1988; 150:1321–1325.

59. Jeffrey RB. Gastrointestinal imaging in AIDS: abdominal computed tomography and ultrasound. Gastroenterol Clin North Am 1988; 17:507–521.
60. Bhatt ON, Miller R, LeRiche J, King EG. Aspiration biopsy in pulmonary opportunistic infections. Acta Cytol 1977; 21:206.
61. Burt ME, Flye MW, Webber BL, Wesley RA. Prospective evaluation of needle aspiration, cutting needle transbronchial, and open lung biopsy in patients with pulmonary infiltrates. Ann Thorac Surg 1981; 32:146.
62. Chaudhary S, Hughes WT, Feldman S, Sanyal SK, Coburn T, Ossi M, Cox F. Percutaneous transthoracic needle aspiration of the lung. Diagnosing *Pneumocystis carinii* pneumonitis. Am J Dis Child 1977; 131:902.
63. Bitran J, Bekerman C, Weinstein R, Bennett C, Ryo U, Pinsky S. Patterns of gallium-67 scintigraphy in patients with acquired immunodeficiency syndrome and AIDS related complex. J Nucl Med 1987; 28:1103–1106.
64. Barron TF, Birnbaum NSA, Shane LB, Goldsmith SJ, Rosen MJ. *Pneumocystis carinii* pneumonia studied by gallium-67 scanning. Radiology 1985; 154:791–793.
65. Coleman DL, Hattner RS, Luce SM, Dodek PM, Golden JA, Murray JF. Correlation between gallium scans and fiberoptic bronchoscopy in patients with suspected *Pneumocystis carinii* pneumonia and the acquired immune deficiency syndrome. Am Rev Respir Dis 1984; 130:1166–1169.
66. Kramer EL, Sanger JJ, Garay SM, Greene JB, Tiu S, Banner H, McCauley DI. Gallium-67 scans of the chest in patients with acquired immunodeficiency syndrome. J Nucl Med 1987; 28:1107–1114.
67. McCauley DI, Naidich DP, Leitman BS, Reede DL, Laubenstein L. Radiographic patterns of opportunistic lung infections and Kaposi sarcoma in homosexual men. AJR 1982; 139:653–658.
68. Siemsen JK, Grebe SF, Sargent EN, Wentz D. Gallium-67 scintigraphy of pulmonary diseases as a complement to radiography. Radiology 1976; 118:371–375.
69. Tuazon CV, Delaney MD, Simon GL, Witorsch P, Varma VM. Utility of gallium-67 scintigraphy and bronchial washings in the diagnosis and treatment of *Pneumocystis carinii* pneumonia in patients with the acquired immune deficiency syndrome. Am Rev Respir Dis 1985; 132:1087–1092.
70. Woolfenden JM, Carrasquillo JA, Larson SM, Simons JT, Masor H, Smith PD, Shelhamer JH, Ognibene FP. Acquired immunodeficiency syndrome: Ga-67 citrate imaging. Radiology 1987; 162:383–387.
71. Stokes DC, Hughes WT, Alderson PO, King RE, Garfinkel DJ. Lung mechanics, radiography and gallium 67 scintigraphy in experimental *Pneumocystis carinii* pneumonia. Am J Exp Pathol 1986; 67:383–393.
72. Coleman DL, Hattner RS, Luce JM, Dodek PM, Golden JA, Murray FJ. Correlation between gallium lung scans and fiberoptic bronchoscopy in patients with suspected *Pneumocystis carinii* pneumonia and acquired immune deficiency syndrome. Am Rev Respir Dis 1984; 130:1166–1169.
73. Meignan M, Guillon JM, Denis M, Joly P, Rosso J, Carette MF, Baud L, Parquin F, Plata F, Debre P, Akoun G, Autran B, Mayaud C. Increased lung epithelial permeability in HIV-infected patients with isolated cytotoxic T-lymphocytic alveolitis. Am Rev Respir Dis 1990; 141:1241–1248.

74. Fishman JA, Strauss HW, Fischman AJ, Nedelman M, Callahan R, Khaw BA, Rubin RH. Imaging of *Pneumocystis carinii* pneumonia with ^{111}In-labelled non-specific polyclonal IgG: an experimental study in rats. Nucl Med Commun 1991; 12: 175–187.
75. Rubin RH, Fischman AJ, Callahan RJ, Khaw BA, Keech F, Ahmad M, Wilkinson R, Strauss HW. ^{111}In-labeled nonspecific immunoglobulin scanning in the detection of focal infection. N Engl J Med 1989; 321:935–940.
76. DeLorenzo LJ, Maguire GP, Wormser GP, Davidian MM, Stone DJ. Persistence of *Pneumocystis carinii* pneumonia in the acquired immunodeficiency syndrome: evaluation of therapy by follow-up transbronchial lung biopsy. Chest 1985; 88:79–83.
77. Seigel R, Wolson AH. Radiographic manifestations of chronic *Pneumocystis carinii* pneumonia. AJR 1977; 128:150–152.
78. Vanley GT, Huberman R, Lufkin RB. Atypical *Pneumocystis carinii* pneumonia in homosexual men with unusual immunodeficiency. Am J Roentgen 1982; 138:1037–1041.

Part Six

TREATMENT AND PREVENTION

22

Current Regimens of Therapy and Prophylaxis

ROBERT E. WALKER

National Institute of Allergy and Infectious Diseases
National Institutes of Health
Bethesda, Maryland

HENRY MASUR

Warren G. Magnuson Clinical Center
National Institutes of Health
Bethesda, Maryland

I. Introduction

Before the 1980s, when *Pneumocystis carinii* pneumonia was an infrequent clinical entity except in select subpopulations of patients, the clinician had few therapeutic options from which to choose. Parenteral pentamidine, first reported to be effective treatment for *P. carinii* pneumonia in the 1950s, pyrimethamine–sulfadiazine, first used successfully in the 1960s, and trimethoprim–sulfamethoxazole (TMP–SMX), first used to treat *P. carinii* pneumonia in the 1970s, were the only available agents with proved safety and efficacy. The current United States and worldwide epidemic of human immunodeficiency virus (HIV) infection has accelerated the field of developmental therapeutics of *P. carinii* pneumonia, and several new and promising drugs and drug combinations are in various stages of clinical development. Yet, it is a testimony to the success of the early clinical investigators that pentamidine and TMP–SMX remain the standard therapeutic agents for this infection, even in the face of intense efforts to discover and develop better drug therapies.

The first decade of the acquired immunodeficiency syndrome (AIDS) epidemic has produced a number of significant advances and refinements in the management of pneumocystosis. For example, newer and less invasive diagnostic techniques, such as bronchoalveolar lavage and induced sputum sampling, are often responsible for more rapid and safer diagnosis, earlier treatment, and reduced morbidity and mortality, compared with the era of open-lung biopsies or transbronchial biopsies. Earlier diagnosis has also permitted a shift away from inpatient parenteral therapy toward more convenient and economical oral or even parenteral home therapy. For those patients with more advanced *P. carinii* pneumonia progressing to respiratory failure, the role of adjuvant corticosteroid therapy has become better defined, with established guidelines for its use based on prospective, controlled clinical data. Perhaps the advances that will have the greatest influence on the epidemiology of *P. carinii* infections are those resulting from investigations in prophylactic therapies. Although *P. carinii* pneumonia prophylaxis has been the standard of care in pediatric oncology since the late 1970s, the relative risks and benefits of preventative regimens for children and adults with HIV infection are still being defined.

II. Treatment

Standard treatment regimens for pneumocystis pneumonia include either TMP–SMX, administered orally or intravenously, or parenteral pentamidine isethionate. Both agents appear to have similar efficacy in both HIV-infected and HIV-uninfected patients, although the spectrum of adverse effects is quite different. In addition, successful therapy for *P. carinii* pneumonia in AIDS generally requires up to 21 days of either agent, rather than the standard 14-day regimen used in other immunosuppressed patients.

A. Pentamidine

Pentamidine belongs to the diamidine class of compounds and has broad-spectrum antiprotozoan activity. It was first used to treat *P. carinii* pneumonia in the late 1950s when, in one study of 212 premature infants with pneumocystis pneumonia, pentamidine reduced the case fatality rate from 50 to 3.5% (1). Subsequent reports have confirmed the efficacy of pentamidine in newborns and in immunosuppressed children and adults with documented *P. carinii* pneumonia (2–8).

In two retrospective reviews that evaluated the efficacy of pentamidine before the HIV epidemic, pentamidine therapy was successful in 63–77% of immunosuppressed patients who could tolerate therapy at least 9 days (2,3). Subsequent prospective studies in pediatric patients with pneumocystis pneumonia have resulted in success rates of 71–87% in those completing a full course of pentamidine therapy (4,5). In patients with AIDS, rates for successful treatment of *P. carinii* pneumonia with pentamidine range from 61 to 95% in prospective series (6–8). Some of this variability can be explained on the basis of differences in patient selection, dosing, duration of therapy, severity of pneumonia, concomitant illnesses and therapies, and aggressiveness of care. For example, in the study reporting a 61% success rate for pentamidine in AIDS-related *P. carinii* pneumonia, pentamidine dosage was reduced by up to 50% according to changes in serum creatinine concentrations during therapy (8). Although this modification allowed successful completion of 17–21 days of therapy in all patients, the reduced dose may conceivably have had a deleterious effect on killing of organisms and, thereby, on the success of treatment.

Pentamidine administered either intravenously or intramuscularly is associated with minor adverse effects in virtually 100% of patients and with major toxicity requiring discontinuation of therapy in up to 47% of patients (2–9). In one retrospective chart review comparing *P. carinii* pneumonia in patients with AIDS with *P. carinii* pneumonia in patients with other immunodeficiencies, 11% of AIDS patients who received pentamidine as initial therapy required institution of an alternative agent because of adverse effects, compared with none of the patients with other causes of immunodeficiency (9). The most severe, dose-limiting toxicities associated with pentamidine include azotemia, pancreatitis, dysglycemia, hypocalcemia, and leukopenia, as well as those less frequently observed, such as thrombocytopenia, orthostatic hypotension, ventricular tachyarrhythmias, nausea, and vomiting. Some of these side effects, such as azotemia, may remit promptly after dose reduction or discontinuation (8). Others, however, such as pancreatic dysfunction, may be profound, irreversible, and life-threatening (10,11). When administered intramuscularly, pentamidine may cause local adverse reactions, such as pain, inflammation, and sterile abscesses, in up to 20% of patients (4). In some instances, these abscesses may progress to ulceration and require skin grafting. Since the safety of slow intravenous administration is now well established, pentamidine should be given intramuscularly only in unusual circumstances.

The mechanism of action of pentamidine is unknown. The standard dosing regimen for both adults and children is 4 mg/kg, in 5% glucose solution, given intravenously over 60–90 min once daily (see Tables 1 and 3). More rapid administration has been associated with hypotension and at least one reported case of cardiac arrest (8). In AIDS patients, reduced dosages (e.g., 3 mg/kg daily) have had a high degree of efficacy and less toxicity than the conventional 4 mg/kg dose (7,8).

B. Trimethoprim–Sulfamethoxazole

The other established treatment for *P. carinii* pneumonia, TMP–SMX, is generally considered the agent of choice in patients without a history of life-threatening intolerance, because of its comparable efficacy but lower incidence of severe adverse effects (4). The efficacy of this agent for treating human *P. carinii* pneumonia was first reported in 1974; in a subsequent prospective, randomized, pediatric study comparing TMP–SMX to pentamidine, TMP–SMX had equivalent efficacy (81% for TMP–SMX vs 71% for pentamidine) and the advantages of oral administration, improved tolerance, and fewer adverse effects (4,12).

Trimethoprim–sulfamethoxazole is a combination of two antimicrobial agents that act at different sites to inhibit folate metabolism. The sulfa component inhibits the enzyme dihydropteroate synthetase, which catalyzes the conversion of *para*-aminobenzoic acid (PABA) to dihydropteroate. Trimethoprim inhibits dihydrofolate reductase, which converts dihydrofolate to tetrahydrofolate. The most important effect of this sequential inhibition is the interruption of thymidine synthesis in susceptible organisms (13). Employing a combination of agents with differing sites of action has the theoretical potential to produce synergistic efficacy while reducing the likelihood of the emergence of resistant organisms. Thus, TMP–SMX possesses several pharmacological features that make it an attractive choice for therapy.

A series of retrospective and prospective studies of patients with *P. carinii* pneumonia, both AIDS- and non–AIDS-related, demonstrates a response rate for TMP–SMX ranging from 60 to 90% (4–6,8,9,12,14–19). As was true for those studies evaluating pentamidine, some of the variability in these response rates may be due to differences in patient selection, extent of illness, and drug administration.

One of the most striking and poorly understood features of TMP–SMX therapy is the high rate of associated allergic-type reactions occurring in patients with AIDS, compared with those in other immunosuppressive conditions. These adverse effects, which may occur in up to 83% of patients and may be dose-limiting in over 50%, include rash, fever, leukopenia, hepatitis, and thrombocytopenia (20). In a retrospective review, these reactions were not reported in 17 patients who developed *P. carinii* pneumonia in association with immunosuppressive diseases other than AIDS and who were treated with TMP–SMX (9). On the basis of these and other studies, there appears to be a unique feature related to HIV immunopathogenesis that predisposes to a higher frequency and enhanced severity of drug intolerance. Typically, TMP–SMX reactions occur 8–12 days after beginning treatment, are almost always reversible when the drug is stopped, and will often resolve even as treatment is continued (20). A prior history of other drug allergies or other atopic illnesses is not predictive for reacting adversely to TMP–SMX (20).

Patients who have a history of adverse reactions to TMP–SMX, and in whom rechallenge is being considered, warrant special consideration. In some series, HIV-infected patients with prior non–life-threatening reactions to therapeutic or prophylactic doses of TMP–SMX (such as rash and fever) were successfully rechallenged; in other patients, rechallenge produced severe, occasionally life-threatening adverse reactions, frequently within hours of administration (20–22). Such severe reactions include a systemic syndrome resembling anaphylaxis or septic shock. In a recent prophylaxis study, the frequencies of severe adverse reactions to TMP–SMX did not differ significantly between patients with (32%) or without (26%) a history of mild intolerance to TMP–SMX (23). These findings support the conviction that a prior mild reaction is not a contraindication to rechallenge with this agent, and that vigilance for possible severe reactions must be maintained in all patients receiving this drug. Some investigators have reported on the successful use of desensitization regimens when rechallenging patients with previous intolerance (24). The risk of recurrent life-threatening reactions upon rechallenge is not well defined. Given the severe nature of the toxicity and the availability of alternative agents, however, patients with a history of severe TMP–SMX toxic reactions should not undergo rechallenge.

Some investigators recommend monitoring serum drug levels in patients receiving oral or intravenous TMP–SMX in an effort to ensure adequate levels and reduce toxicity. Sulfa levels between 100 and 150 μg/mL are desirable, and levels above 200 μg/mL are associated with an increased risk of adverse reactions. In one study, serum TMP levels were measured to help guide therapy (8). By adjusting the dose of TMP–SMX to achieve and maintain TMP levels between 5 and 8 μg/mL, all patients in this study were able to complete a full course of therapy. Success rates for recovery from *P. carinii* pneumonia were equivalent to other published reports, despite the use of lower than conventional dosages of TMP–SMX. The serum levels for TMP and SMX that maximize efficacy and minimize toxicity are unknown, but maintaining sulfa levels between 100 and 150 μg/mL or TMP levels between 5 and 8 μg/mL seems reasonable, based on available information.

The standard adult dose of TMP–SMX for *P. carinii* pneumonia is 15–20 mg/kg per day of the TMP component (or 75–100 mg/kg per day of SMX), administered orally or intravenously in three or four divided doses for 14–21 days. For the average adult, this equates to an oral dose of two double-strength tablets three or four times daily. A total dose of six double-strength tablets daily almost always suffices to attain the desired serum concentrations of drug in the absence of major gastrointestinal dysfunction, such as vomiting or severe diarrhea. Most mild to moderate cases of *P. carinii* pneumonia can be treated orally. Patients with severe pneumonitis (i.e., $PaO_2 < 70$ torr) and any patient in whom gastrointestinal absorption is in question, should receive parenteral therapy until substantial improvement has occurred. The recommended pediatric regimen is 20 mg/kg per day of TMP with 100 mg/kg per day of SMX intravenously in four divided doses for 14–21 days.

Regardless of which agent is chosen as initial therapy, improvement in symptoms and signs usually does not occur until the fourth to eighth day of treatment. In fact, many patients get worse over the first 2–4 days before they begin to improve. In one study of AIDS patients with *P. carinii* pneumonia, for example, dyspnea scores worsened during the first 3 days and required 6 days before returning to pretreatment levels, whereas radiographic infiltrates worsened during the first 6 days as well and required 21 days to show improvement (6). In another report of patients with *P. carinii* pneumonia in the setting of immunodeficiencies other than AIDS, the time before a clinical response was evident ranged from 2 to 9 days (16). Therefore, switching agents during the first 5–10 days of treatment because of failure to improve or clinical deterioration may be unwarranted and has not been proved to result in increased survival (9).

C. Dapsone

Even though TMP–SMX and pentamidine are the only drugs licensed for the treatment of *P. carinii* infections, other agents appear to be safe and are reasonable second-line agents in patients failing or intolerant of standard therapy (Table 1). Dapsone alone and in combination with trimethoprim has been used to treat *P. carinii* pneumonia in patients with HIV infection. In one uncontrolled study of oral dapsone (100 mg/day) used to treat 18 patients with AIDS and microscopically documented *P. carinii* pneumonia, 11 (61%) patients responded within 3–10 days of instituting therapy and successfully completed the 21-day course (25). The nonresponders had more severe pneumonitis (mean Pao_2 of 63.4 torr vs 84 torr for responders) and were switched to alternative therapy after a mean of 5.8 days. A more recent study of dapsone monotherapy in patients with mild to moderate *P. carinii* pneumonia found that none of the seven patients enrolled successfully completed a full course of therapy (26). After receiving 5 or more days of dapsone, 200 mg/day orally, three patients had worsening respiratory failure, requiring mechanical ventilation in two, and four patients developed a severe toxic reaction and required alternative therapy.

D. Trimethoprim–Dapsone

With the addition of TMP to dapsone therapy, more favorable outcomes have been achieved. In an uncontrolled study of 15 AIDS patients with mild to moderate pneumocystis pneumonia, the combination of TMP 20 mg/kg per day in four divided doses and dapsone 100 mg/day, each administered orally, was effective in all (27). A randomized, double-blind study comparing TMP–dapsone with TMP–SMX in 60 patients with AIDS and mild to moderate *P. carinii* pneumonia demonstrated equivalent efficacy and improved tolerance with TMP–dapsone (19). Therapy was successful in 28 (93%) of 30 patients who received TMP–dapsone and in 27 (90%) of 30 patients treated with TMP–SMX, whereas major adverse reactions occurred in 30 and 57% of each group, respectively. Toxic reactions seen with TMP–dapsone in this trial included rash, fever, nausea and vomiting, hyperkalemia, neutropenia, thrombocytopenia, and anemia. Methemoglobinemia occurred in 63% of patients receiving TMP–dapsone, but was greater than 20% in only one patient in whom the drug was stopped. Rash and fever, which

Table 1 Current Regimens for Therapy of *Pneumocystis carinii* Pneumonia in Adults

Drug	Initial dose	Route	Interval	Duration
Conventional agents				
Trimethoprim–sulfamethoxazole	5 mg/kg trimethoprim + 25 mg/kg sulfamethoxazole	iv or po	q 6–8 hr	14–21 days
Pentamidine isethionate	4 mg/kg	iv	Daily over 60–90 min	14–21 days
Investigational agents				
Trimethoprim–dapsone	5 mg/kg trimethoprim + 100 mg dapsone	po po	q 6 hr daily	14–21 days
Trimetrexate + leucovorin with or without sulfadiazine	45 mg/m^2 + 20 mg/m^2 1 g	iv po po	q 6 hr q 6 hr q 6 hr	21 days
566C80 (atovaquone)	750 mg	po	q 8 hr	21 days
Clindamycin–primaquine	450–900 mg clindamycin + 15–30 mg primaquine base	iv or po po	q 6–8hr daily	14–21 days
Difluoromethylornithine (DFMO; eflornithine)	400 mg/kg	iv	Daily by continuous infusion or in four divided doses	14–21 days, followed by 4–6 wk oral therapy
Pentamidine isethionate	600 mg or 8 mg/kg	By Respirgard II nebulizer	Daily	21 days

occurred in 40–47% of patients treated with either agent, appeared 5–11 days into therapy, peaked 1–2 days later, and resolved after another 3–4 days, even when therapy was continued.

Despite its associated adverse effects, TMP–dapsone is better-tolerated than TMP–SMX. Many physicians now consider TMP–dapsone the agent of choice for the initial therapy of mild to moderate *P. carinii* pneumonia. Even in some patients intolerant of TMP–SMX, dapsone has been administered without adverse effects, indicating that cross-reactivity is not universal (28). The known risk of hemolysis in patients with glucose-6-phosphate dehydrogenase (G6PD) deficiency mandates screening for this deficiency before dapsone is instituted, however.

E. Aerosolized Pentamidine

In an attempt to reduce the toxicity of parenteral pentamidine, some investigators have explored the use of aerosolized pentamidine (AP) as treatment for acute *P. carinii* pneumonia. Aerosolization of an active agent is appealing, since drug can be targeted to the affected organ, while systemic absorption—and thus toxicity—is minimized (29). Implicit in this approach is that AP would not be useful for treatment of disseminated disease. Pilot studies in *P. carinii* pneumonia reported favorable results with response rates of 70–100% in patients with mild to moderate pneumonitis receiving AP as either initial or salvage therapy (7,30). Subsequent prospective trials comparing AP to intravenous pentamidine found unacceptably high failure rates of 45% or greater in the AP-treated groups (31,32). Despite the few and relatively minor adverse reactions associated with AP administration—primarily cough and bronchospasm—the use of AP for treatment of *P. carinii* pneumonia cannot be advocated at this time based on the available data.

F. Other Agents

Several other agents are currently being evaluated in the treatment of *P. carinii* pneumonia. Trimetrexate, a lipid-soluble derivative of methotrexate, is 1500 times more potent that TMP in vitro as an inhibitor of protozoan dihydrofolate reductase (33). Preliminary clinical trials in patients with AIDS and *P. carinii* pneumonia revealed response rates ranging from 63 to 71% in diverse populations of patients, including those being treated for first or subsequent episodes of *P. carinii* pneumonia, those receiving salvage therapy, and those receiving trimetrexate alone or with a sulfonamide (34,35).

Despite a full course of trimetrexate therapy and good response rates, relapses of pneumocystis pneumonia occurred in up to 60% of patients within 3 months of treatment (34). Relapses were not seen in the group of patients who could tolerate combination therapy with sulfadiazine, however. Like other potent antifolates, trimetrexate may cause bone marrow suppression, and nearly 25% of patients who received trimetrexate for *P. carinii* pneumonia required dose reductions because of neutropenia or thrombocytopenia. Leucovorin administered concomitantly at 20 mg/m^2 every 6 hr may help preserve normal hematological indices. Other adverse effects of trimetrexate include hepatitis and rash.

A prospective, randomized trial comparing trimetrexate with leucovorin to TMP–SMX for moderately severe *P. carinii* pneumonia in patients with AIDS was prematurely terminated when an interim analysis revealed improved survival in patients receiving TMP–SMX (81 vs 69% survival in the trimetrexate arm; 36). Treatment failures were more often due to lack of efficacy or death among those receiving trimetrexate, whereas TMP–SMX failures were more often due to toxicity. Trimetrexate remains an investigational second-line agent and is currently available under the Treatment Investigational New Drug (IND) mechanism for patients failing or intolerant of standard therapies.

The hydroxynaphthoquinone BW 566C80 (atovaquone), a novel agent with potent anti-*P. carinii* activity in vitro and in animal models, is currently under evaluation in clinical trials and was recently made available for patients under a Treatment IND (37,38). Its mechanism of action is poorly understood, but is thought to involve inhibition of the enzyme dihydroorotate dehydrogenase, resulting in inhibition of de novo synthesis of pyrimidines (39). Because 566C80 has broad-spectrum antiprotozoan activity against *Toxoplasma gondi* and plasmodia as well as *P. carinii*, it has important potential as a therapeutic and prophylactic agent in HIV disease for a wide range of opportunistic pathogens.

In a recent, open-label trial, 27 (79%) of 34 patients with AIDS and mild to moderate *P. carinii* pneumonia were successfully treated with various doses of oral 566C80 (40). The major adverse reactions requiring discontinuation of therapy were rash and fever, which occurred in 4 (12%) patients. Other side effects seen were elevations in hepatic transaminases, neutropenia, and anemia, all of which were mild and self-limited. Concomitant administration of zidovudine or ganciclovir with 566C80 was well tolerated in those few patients taking these agents. The investigators of this study concluded that 566C80, at a dosage of 750 mg thrice daily, was safe and effective, although it has poor oral bioavailability. Altered formulations that promote gastrointestinal absorption and, presumably, enhance efficacy are currently being developed, as are formulations for intravenous use.

A large, randomized trial comparing 566C80 to TMP–SMX in over 300 patients with AIDS and mild to moderately severe *P. carinii* pneumonia was recently completed. Although inadequate responses occurred more frequently in those treated with 566C80 than in those receiving TMP–SMX (17 vs 6%), failures due to toxicity were more common among those assigned to TMP–SMX (20 vs 7%) (41). As a result, the overall success rates were similar for the two drugs—62% for 566C80 and 64% for TMP–SMX. Treatment-limiting adverse effects of 566C80 included rash, fever, hepatic enzyme abnormalities, and vomiting.

The combination of clindamycin with primaquine has also had activity in vitro and in a rat model of *P. carinii* pneumonia (42,43). Several small, open-label, nonrandomized trials have shown this combination to be safe and well tolerated in patients with AIDS-related *P. carinii* pneumonia. In patients with pneumonitis ranging from mild to severe, reported efficacy rates are 70–100% (44–48). Differing doses and routes of administration and varying patient entry criteria make direct comparisons of these trials difficult. Clindamycin, 3600 mg/day intravenously or 1800 mg/day orally in divided doses with primaquine base 30 mg/day, orally has been well tolerated (45). Skin rashes occurred in 50% of patients, but these frequently resolved, even with continued treatment (46,47). Toxic effects requiring interruption of therapy occurred in approximately 20% and included fever, rash, granulocytopenia, and methemoglobinemia (45). Pseudomembranous colitis, secondary to clindamycin, has not been reported in these series. Because of the risk of hemolysis, G6PD deficiency should be excluded before initiating primaquine. Primaquine does not exist in parenteral form.

Without prospective, randomized trials comparing clindamycin plus primaquine with standard therapy, it is difficult to assign a specific role to this combination in the treatment of *P. carinii* pneumonia. Until such data are available, clindamycin with primaquine should be reserved for patients who are intolerant of the first- and second-line agents already discussed. Several 8-aminoquinoline derivatives of primaquine (e.g., WR6026) with anti-*P. carinii* activity and potentially reduced toxicity are currently under evaluation (49).

Difluoromethylornithine (DFMO; eflornithine), a synthesis inhibitor of polyamines required for *P. carinii* growth, has been used successfully as salvage therapy in patients with pneumocystosis. Regimens reported to be effective range from 6 g/m^2 body surface area per day in three divided doses orally, to 400 mg/kg per day, administered intravenously either in four divided doses or by continuous infusion, followed by 300 mg/kg per day orally (50–53). Toxic reactions include thrombocytopenia, anemia, leukopenia, nausea, vomiting, diarrhea, local phlebitis, and hearing loss that is only partially reversible.

In a recently reported prospective, randomized trial comparing 14 days of DFMO (400 mg/kg per day by continuous intravenous infusion) to TMP–SMX in the primary treatment of *P. carinii* pneumonia, DFMO resulted in significantly more treatment failures (49% of 51 patients receiving DFMO vs 21% of 47 patients assigned to TMP–SMX; 54). Because of DFMO's inferior efficacy, this study was prematurely terminated. Significantly more patients were withdrawn from the TMP–SMX arm, however, because of drug-related toxicity (38 vs 12%), making the overall success rates comparable for the two agents in this study. The most frequently encountered dose-limiting toxic effects were nausea and rash with TMP–SMX and thrombocytopenia and anemia with DFMO. Additional studies are required to determine whether DFMO has a role as first-line therapy or whether it should be reserved for those patients who cannot tolerate or who have failed to respond to standard therapeutic regimens.

In summary, the standard treatment for *P. carinii* pneumonia is oral or intravenous TMP–SMX or intravenous pentamidine. These regimens provide equivalent efficacy and comparable frequencies of adverse effects. Because the toxicity of TMP–SMX tends to be less severe than that of pentamidine, TMP–SMX is generally the preferred first-line therapy in patients who can tolerate it. Trimethoprim–dapsone may arguably be the agent of choice in patients with mild or moderate pneumonia who can be treated orally. A diverse array of other agents are available as alternative treatments for those failing to respond to or intolerant of TMP–SMX and parenteral pentamidine. These include TMP–dapsone, trimetrexate, 566C80 (atovaquone), and clindamycin with primaquine. Aerosolized pentamidine and DFMO cannot be recommended for therapy on the basis of existing data. Clearly, there is still a need to develop novel agents with potent antipneumocystis activity and differing mechanisms of action that are convenient to administer, nontoxic, and compatible with the numerous other chemotherapeutic agents often required in the care of immunosuppressed patients.

III. Adjunctive Corticosteroids

The best predictor for survival in patients with AIDS and *P. carinii* pneumonia is the arterial oxygen status upon presentation (55,56). As oxygenation is progressively compromised, mortality from pneumocystosis rises. In nearly 300 patients with AIDS-related pneumocystis pneumonia who were studied at San Francisco General Hospital, survivors and nonsurvivors had mean admission arterial oxygen pressures on room air of 70 and 55 torr, respectively (57).

Many patients with *P. carinii* pneumonia, including those with mild disease, will experience a decline in pulmonary function in association with the institution of anti-*P. carinii* therapy. Clinically, this deterioration is characterized by worsening gas exchange and progression of radiographic infiltrates. The pathophysiology of this phenomenon, which generally occurs within the first 3–5 days of treatment, is poorly understood. Some investigators postulate that the release of intracystic proteolytic substances from dead organisms incites an intense inflammatory response in the lungs. For patients with marginal respiratory status at the outset, the consequences of this effect may be rapid progression to hypoxemic respiratory failure, adult respiratory distress syndrome, and death. Thus, therapeutic regimens for *P. carinii* infection should incorporate measures to prevent this potentially fatal decline.

A series of clinical trials involving a combined total of over 400 patients have investigated the role of adjunctive corticosteroids to prevent early deterioration in the treatment of AIDS-related *P. carinii* pneumonia (see Chap. 31). Four of the five trials demonstrated a statistically significant benefit in those who received adjunctive steroids during the initial 72 hr of antipneumocystis therapy. Upon review of these data, an expert panel issued a consensus statement recommending that corticosteroids be started within 72 hr of initiating antipneumocystis therapy in adults and children over 13 years of age with documented or suspected HIV infection and documented or suspected *P. carinii* pneumonia if moderate or severe pulmonary dysfunction is present (57). Pulmonary dysfunction was defined as *moderate or severe* if room air arterial oxygen pressure is below 70 torr or if the alveolar–arterial oxygen gradient exceeds 35 torr. The specific regimen recommended is oral prednisone at 40 mg twice daily for 5 days, then 40 mg once daily for 5 days, and then 20 mg once daily to complete a total of 21 days of steroid therapy. For patients requiring parenteral therapy, methylprednisolone at 75% of these doses is suggested.

Important questions remain concerning the use of corticosteroids for *P. carinii* pneumonia. For example, whether they confer similar benefit to immunosuppressed patients without HIV infection is unknown. The role of steroids in pediatric patients, in patients with mild pneumonitis, and as salvage therapy in patients failing standard treatment has not been carefully assessed. Although the only adverse consequences of steroids reported in these studies were mucocutaneous herpes simplex infections, oral candidiasis, and mild metabolic derangements, administering corticosteroids to patients with profoundly impaired immune function is likely to further depress host defense. Consequently, it is important to base the use of adjunctive steroid therapy on well-controlled, prospective data addressing the relative safety and efficacy in specific subgroups of patients.

IV. Prophylaxis

Prophylaxing against *P. carinii* infections presupposes the existence of clearly defined target populations, effective and available agents, and favorable risk–and cost–benefit assessments. Much information accumulated in recent years suggests that these preconditions can be met, making prophylaxis the current standard of care in many situations. Indeed, one of the most significant advances affecting the course of HIV infection has resulted from the widespread institution of prophylaxis for *P. carinii* infections.

Prophylaxis may be directed at either primary (first episode) or secondary (recurrent) disease. For HIV-infected individuals, the absolute CD4 lymphocyte count is the best identifier for those at risk of a first episode of *P. carinii* pneumonia (58,59). Data collected in a multicenter cohort study involving 1665 HIV-infected persons demonstrate that the risk of developing *P. carinii* pneumonia over a 4-year period is highest for those with CD4 cell counts below 200/mm^3 (59). For individuals with baseline CD4 counts below 200, the risk of developing *P. carinii* pneumonia after 6, 12, and 36 months was 8.4, 18.4, and 33.3%, respectively. The likelihood of contracting *P. carinii* pneumonia within 1 year was less than 5% for those with baseline counts above 200. Constitutional symptoms such as persistent fevers and oral candidiasis were also independent risk factors for the development of pneumocystosis in this study. Thus, those clinical features that serve to identify individuals with HIV infection at risk of developing a first episode of pneumocystis pneumonia include CD4 count below 200, persistent unexplained fevers, or oral thrush. Those patients who have had other AIDS-defining illnesses, such as disseminated Mycobacterium *avium* complex or cytomegalovirus end-organ disease, and those who have AIDS-related complex (ARC) are also at risk for developing *P. carinii* pneumonia.

Patients with HIV infection who have recovered from a prior episode of pneumocystosis represent another group of at-risk individuals who clearly warrant prophylaxis (i.e., secondary prophylaxis). In patients with a previous history of AIDS-related *P. carinii* pneumonia receiving zidovudine without *P. carinii* pneumonia prophylaxis, the risk of developing recurrent pneumocystosis at 6 and 12 months of follow-up was 31 and 66%, respectively (60).

Patients undergoing immunosuppressive therapy represent another population at high risk of developing *P. carinii* pneumonia. Historically, pneumocystis pneumonia was the most frequent cause of death in children with acute lymphoblastic leukemia (ALL) in remission (61). Aggressive, multiple-drug regimens and intensive radiotherapy protocols, although associated with higher tumor response rates, are also more frequently complicated by the development of *P. carinii* pneumonia. Several studies now exist establishing the safety and efficacy of primary *P. carinii* pneumonia prophylaxis in such high-risk patients. For example, in a randomized, double-blind placebo-controlled study evaluating the efficacy of TMP–SMX in pediatric ALL patients at high risk of developing *P. carinii* pneumonia, none of 80 receiving TMP–SMX versus 17 (21%) of 80 receiving placebo contracted *P. carinii* pneumonia (62). The doses used were 150 mg of trimethoprim and 750 mg of sulfamethoxazole per square meter daily, administered orally in two divided doses. A subsequent study conducted at the same institution showed that dosing could be reduced from twice daily 7 days per week to twice daily on 3 consecutive days per week with equivalent prophylactic efficacy (63). One major advantage of the less–frequent-dosing regimen is the reduced incidence of systemic fungal infections. Given these and other studies, *P. carinii* pneumonia prophylaxis administered twice daily on 3 consecutive days weekly is now considered standard practice in certain pediatric oncology populations. Breakthrough episodes of *P. carinii* pneumonia on this regimen are extremely rare.

Pneumocystis carinii pneumonia is a common problem in other clinical settings as well, such as bone marrow and solid organ transplantation, for which prophylaxis is used regularly (64). In heart–lung and lung allograft recipients, for example, the incidence of *P. carinii* pneumonia may approach 90% in the absence of routine prophylaxis (65). Patients with human T-cell lymphotropic virus type

1-related leukemias and lymphomas, and patients with lymphoreticular malignancies undergoing intensive chemotherapy (such as Promace/Cytobam) represent other groups at particularly high-risk who should also receive *P. carinii* pneumonia prophylaxis.

In summary, those patients considered at high risk of developing *P. carinii* pneumonia who are candidates for primary prophylaxis include certain oncology patients and transplant recipients undergoing intensive immunosuppressive treatment and individuals with HIV infection whose peripheral CD4 lymphocyte cell counts are below $200/mm^3$ or who have had an AIDS-defining illness, persistent unexplained fevers, or thrush. Patients in whom secondary prophylaxis is indicated are those with HIV infection and a history of microbiologically proved *P. carinii* infection.

In the setting of HIV infection, TMP–SMX and AP are now the best-studied treatments (66). Although both therapies have been demonstrated to have prophylactic efficacy, a recent prospective comparative trial in secondary prophylaxis showed TMP–SMX to be superior (23). The comparative efficacy of these agents in preventing a first episode of *P. carinii* pneumonia is currently under evaluation in a similarly designed clinical trial. Several agents other than TMP–SMX and AP are in common use for prophylaxis, including some of the same drugs discussed as therapies for *P. carinii* pneumonia (see Tables 2 and 3). Before evaluating a potential agent for prophylaxis, however, it is usually desirable to demonstrate therapeutic activity first in animal models and in human disease.

Trimethoprim–sulfamethoxazole is probably the most commonly prescribed prophylactic agent. Although several clinical trials have studied the role of this drug in preventing HIV-related infection, no single trial emerges as the ideally executed, definitive study. In one prospective unblinded trial of patients with newly diagnosed Kaposi's sarcoma, patients without a prior history of *P. carinii* pneumonia were randomly assigned either to treatment with TMP–SMX, one double-strength tablet twice daily (along with 5 mg of calcium leucovorin daily to protect against myelosuppression from trimethoprim), or to no treatment, and were followed for at least 2 years (67). Only 4 (13%) of 30 patients receiving TMP–SMX developed pneumocystosis compared with 16 (53%) of 30 on no treatment. All 4 patients who developed pneumocystis pneumonia in the treatment arm had been taken off TMP–SMX because of toxicity a mean of 4 months before the diagnosis of *P. carinii* pneumonia. Although this study was small and unblinded, the impressive difference in attack rates strongly suggested prophylactic efficacy of the drug combination. A second prospective, but uncontrolled trial, and several uncontrolled retrospective trials support the ability of TMP–SMX to prevent primary and recurrent episodes of *P. carinii* pneumonia at doses as low as one double-strength tablet on alternate days (68–70). Doses and schedules in common use for adults and children are listed in Tables 2 and 3. Although studies of chemoprophylaxis in HIV-infected children are lacking, extrapolations have

Current Regimens of Therapy

Table 2 Current Regimens for Chemoprophylaxis of *Pneumocystis carinii* Pneumonia in Adults

Drug	Dose	Route	Frequency
Conventional regimens			
Trimethoprim–sulfamethoxazole	160 mg trimethoprim + 800 mg sulfamethoxazole	po	Thrice weekly, daily or twice daily
Pentamidine isethionate	300 mg	By Respirgard II nebulizer	Monthly
Investigational regimens			
Pentamidine isethionate	60 mg	By Fisoneb nebulizer	Biweekly, after five dose/ 2-wk induction
Pentamidine isethionate	4 mg/kg	iv	Biweekly
Dapsone	50, 100, or 200 mg	po	Weekly, twice weekly, daily, or twice daily
Dapsone–pyrimethamine	50–100 mg dapsone + 25–50 mg pyrimethamine	po	Weekly, twice weekly, or daily
Pyrimethamine–sulfadoxine (Fansidar)	150 mg pyrimethamine + 500 mg sulfadoxine	po	Thrice monthly, weekly, or twice weekly
Clindamycin–primaquine	150 mg clindamycin + 15 mg primaquine base	po	qid Daily
566C80 (atovaquone)	?	po	?

Table 3 Pediatric Regimens for Treatment and Chemoprophylaxis of *Pneumocystis carinii* Pneumonia

Drug	Dose	Route	Frequency	Duration
Treatment				
Trimethoprim–sulfamethoxazole	5 mg/kg trimethoprim + 100 mg/kg sulfamethoxazole	iv	q 6 h	14–21 days
Pentamidine isethionate	4 mg/kg	iv	Daily, over 60–90 min	14–21 days
Prophylaxis				
Recommended				
Trimethoprim–sulfamethoxazole	75 mg/m^2 trimethoprim + 375 mg/m^2 sulfamethoxazole	po	Twice daily, 3 days/wk on three consecutive days (e.g., Mon, Tues, Weds)	
Alternative				
Trimethoprim–sulfamethoxazole	75 mg/m^2 trimethoprim + 375 mg/m^2 sulfamethoxazole	po	Twice daily 3 days/wk on alternate days (e.g., Mon, Weds, Fri) or twice daily 7 days/wk	
Trimethoprim–sulfamethoxazole	150 mg/m^2 trimethoprim + 750 mg/m^2 sulfamethoxazole	po	Once daily	
Pentamidine isethionate (if age ≥5 years)	300 mg	By Respirgard II nebulizer	Monthly	
Dapsone (if age ≥1 month)	1 mg/kg to a maximum of 50 mg	po	Daily	
Pentamidine isethionate	4 mg/kg	iv	q 2 or 4 wk	

been made from clinical trials of children with *P. carinii* pneumonia related to other illnesses, from the pediatric experience with these drugs in diseases other than pneumocystis pneumonia, and from trials in HIV-infected adults.

Despite encouraging results with TMP–SMX, up to 50% of patients in reported series developed adverse reactions, and as many as 17% required termination of therapy. Common dose-limiting side effects were fever, rash, nausea, vomiting, and leukopenia. In a retrospective series of 116 patients receiving reduced dosages of TMP–SMX—one double strength tablet thrice weekly on Monday, Wednesday, and Friday—no episodes of *P. carinii* pneumonia occurred during treatment, but 28% of patients experienced adverse reactions, and 13% required termination of therapy because of toxicity (69). Thus, although TMP–SMX appears to be an effective prophylactic agent in HIV-infected patients, a significant fraction of patients are unable to tolerate this drug for prolonged periods, even at reduced doses. Therefore, the need for alternative regimens with equivalent efficacy is still great.

Aerosolized pentamidine is the only other agent that has been extensively evaluated for *P. carinii* pneumonia prophylaxis. When assessing clinical trials and when prescribing AP, there are at least two factors that need to be considered: the dose of drug used, and the nebulization approach employed. Nebulizing devices differ in particle size generation and in other physical determinants of particle distribution, resulting in different concentrations of drug that actually deposit in lung parenchyma. One device should not be substituted for another unless comparative data exist on which to judge relative safety, efficacy, and the potential need for dose adjustment. Patient specific factors, such as age, degree and type of pulmonary dysfunction, and even body position during treatment, may substantially influence the adequacy of drug delivery. The risks of occupational and nosocomial exposures related to AP and the need for a properly ventilated room for drug administration are important factors to consider as well. Patients actively infected with respiratory pathogens, particularly *M. tuberculosis*, represent a potential source of transmission to other patients and staff. Aerosolized pentamidine should be deferred in such patients until they are no longer infectious.

Aerosolized pentamidine has proved to be safe and effective for primary and secondary prophylaxis in HIV-infected individuals. In a prospective, double-blind, placebo-controlled trial involving over 200 patients with CD4 lymphocyte cell counts below $200/mm^2$ and no prior history of *P. carinii* pneumonia, occurrences of pneumocystis pneumonia were 27% per year in the placebo (sodium isethionate) group and 8.6% in the AP group (300 mg pentamidine monthly by the Respirgard II nebulizer) (71). Although the major side effect—moderate to severe cough—occurred in one-third of the patients who received AP, only 3.5% of patients discontinued therapy for this reason. Additional studies have produced data supporting the efficacy of this dose and delivery system of pentamidine for both primary and secondary prophylaxis (72).

Other investigations have used varying doses of pentamidine, sometimes in association with different nebulizers. In one prospective, double-blind, placebo-controlled study of secondary prophylaxis, 162 patients were randomized to receive either pentamidine, 60 mg biweekly (after induction with five treatments over 2 weeks), or sterile water placebo (73). The nebulizer used in this trial was the Fisoneb hand-held ultrasonic nebulizer, which has different delivery characteristics than the Respirgard II. The cumulative relapse rates of *P. carinii* pneumonia by 24 weeks of follow-up were 50% for the placebo group and 9% for the pentamidine group. Adverse reactions, primarily cough and bronchospasm, occurred in one-third of patients receiving AP, but no patient required discontinuation of therapy because of side effects. A third delivery system, the Ultraneb 99 ultrasonic nebulizer, has been studied in a randomized, unblinded study of 51 patients with a history of *P. carinii* pneumonia (74). The dose employed was 4 mg/kg of pentamidine base monthly, after biweekly treatments for the first 4 weeks. Pneumocystis pneumonia relapses occurred in 61% of untreated patients, compared with 9% in those receiving AP after 8–10 months of follow-up. Only one patient discontinued therapy because of side effects.

In summary, AP, 300 mg monthly delivered by the Respirgard II, is effective primary and secondary prophylaxis. The Fisoneb and Ultraneb devices appear to be effective modes of delivery for secondary prophylaxis, but they have not yet been directly compared to the Respirgard II system. No published studies address the use of either the Fisoneb or Ultraneb systems for primary prophylaxis. Currently, only the Respirgard II system is licensed in the United States for use with pentamidine. Cough and bronchospasm are common side effects of AP. For patients with a history of bronchospasm or who develop bronchospasm or moderate to severe cough in association with AP treatments, administration of an inhaled β-agonist before AP is advisable. Because of concerns about unreliable deposition of drug in the lungs owing to inability to use the nebulizer correctly, AP is not recommended for children younger than 5 years of age (75).

Because active drug is delivered almost exclusively to the patient's lungs, AP does not afford protection against dissemination of *P. carinii*. Thus, patients receiving AP may be predisposed to develop extrapulmonary disease (76). Clinicians also need to recognize that the clinical presentation of breakthrough episodes of *P. carinii* pneumonia in patients on AP prophylaxis may be unusual with a predominance of focal or upper lobe infiltrates radiographically. Moreover, diagnosis may be more difficult to establish microscopically, even with invasive techniques (77,78).

Until recently, no direct comparative data permitted an assessment of which regimen—TMP–SMX or AP—affords superior protection. In a multicenter, prospective, unblinded study conducted by the AIDS Clinical Trials Group of the National Institutes of Health, patients who had recovered from a previous episode of *P. carinii* pneumonia were randomized to treatment with either one double-strength tablet daily of TMP–SMX or 300 mg monthly of AP by Respirgard II

(23). Patients were switched from one regimen to the other if intolerance developed to their initial treatment. Among the 310 evaluable patients, 50 recurrences of *P. carinii* pneumonia were reported: 14 in the TMP–SMX group and 36 in the AP group. The 1-year–estimated recurrence rate was 3.5% for the TMP–SMX group versus 18.5% in the AP group. Seven of the 14 recurrences among the TMP–SMX group were in patients who had switched to AP because of TMP–SMX intolerance, and all 7 had been receiving AP a minimum of 6 months: all 36 recurrences in the AP group were in patients who continued to receive AP throughout the study.

Despite the apparent superiority of TMP–SMX for efficacy, drug intolerance developed in 27% of patients assigned to TMP–SMX compared with 4% of patients on AP. Thus, although TMP–SMX was clearly shown to be superior to AP in preventing or delaying recurrent *P. carinii* pneumonia, it was less well tolerated, suggesting it may be unsuitable for long-term administration in a substantial number of patients. A multicenter comparative trial of TMP–SMX and AP primary prophylaxis is currently in progress. Although definitive recommendations about primary prophylaxis must await the results of this study, it seems reasonable to prefer TMP–SMX over AP, based on inference from experience with secondary prophylaxis.

Reported success with TMP–dapsone for treating acute *P. carinii* pneumonia led to the use of dapsone alone or in combination with other antifolates (e.g., TMP or pyrimethamine) in various schedules for *P. carinii* pneumonia prophylaxis. Dapsone doses have ranged from 50 to 200 mg, and frequency of administration has varied from once or twice weekly to daily. A number of small, uncontrolled series have suggested efficacy and safety, although breakthrough episodes of *P. carinii* pneumonia have been observed (79–84). Several large, comparative trials, one assessing dapsone for primary prophylaxis, another assessing dapsone with pyrimethamine for secondary prophylaxis, are currently in progress. Preliminary results concerning differences in frequency of *P. carinii* pneumonia, toxoplasmosis, and death bear close scrutiny so that dapsone's role can be adequately assessed.

Clindamycin with primaquine, another combination regimen with efficacy in acute *P. carinii* pneumonia, may also have a potential role in prophylaxis. Several small series suggest that oral clindamycin with primaquine may be safely administered for nearly 10 months (85,86). However, when oral clindamycin alone was compared with pyrimethamine alone as prophylaxis against toxoplasmic encephalitis in patients with HIV infection, the incidence of adverse reactions, such as diarrhea (31%) and rash (21%), was sufficiently high to warrant premature termination of the clindamycin arm of the study (87). Such results suggest that clindamycin-containing regimens may not be appropriate for long-term suppressive therapy in this patient population. Still, well-designed studies evaluating the combination of clindamycin with primaquine are needed before definitive statements can be made about tolerance and efficacy.

Other agents with theoretical potential as preventive therapy include pyrimethamine with sulfadoxine (Fansidar), intermittent parenteral pentamidine, and 566C80 (atovaquone). Although the major limitation to broader use of Fansidar is likely to be toxicity, parenteral pentamidine and 566C80 are probably safer, but may be less effective than standard regimens. The data for each of these agents, however, are now extremely limited, and their use as prophylactic therapies outside the context of research protocols cannot be supported on the basis of existing information.

In summary, TMP–SMX and AP are the agents of choice for *P. carinii* pneumonia prophylaxis in adults and children at risk for pneumocystis pneumonia who can tolerate these therapies. Trimethoprim–sulfamethoxazole has been shown to have superior efficacy for secondary prophylaxis. Results from an ongoing comparative trial will help establish whether TMP–SMX is superior to AP for primary prophylaxis as well. However, TMP–SMX is less well tolerated than AP, and nearly one-third of patients will be unable to continue TMP–SMX long-term. Other regimens, such as dapsone, dapsone with pyrimethamine, and clindamycin with primaquine, may be effective alternatives, but require more extensive evaluation. As newer anti-*P. carinii* agents become available, carefully designed clinical trials will need to address issues of efficacy and safety for both primary and secondary prophylaxis in the different populations of patients at risk of developing *P. carinii* infections.

V. Treatment and Prophylaxis in Pediatric Patients with Human Immunodeficiency Virus Infection

The principles that guide the choice of anti-pneumocystis agents for acute infection and for prophylaxis in children are, in general, no different from those applied to the care of the HIV-infected adult patient. As with adults, microbiological documentation of acute *P. carinii* pneumonia should be aggressively pursued, and presumptive diagnosis followed by empiric therapy is discouraged. Either TMP–SMX (20 mg/kg of the TMP component administered intravenously in four equally divided doses daily) or pentamidine (4 mg/kg administered daily over 60–90 min intravenously) is the preferred therapy, and treatment should be continued to complete at least a 14-, and preferably, a 21-day course (see Table 3) (88). No trials have been reported comparing pentamidine to TMP–SMX in HIV-infected children.

Little or no data exist on the safety and efficacy of many of the alternative antipneumocystis agents in children. Similarly, no controlled trials of adjunctive corticosteroids in HIV-infected children with *P. carinii* pneumonia have been reported. In the absence of such information, it is impossible to know whether extrapolating from the adult experience with alternative therapies and corticosteroids is reasonable. Well-designed prospective pediatric trials are clearly needed to evaluate the risks and benefits of these novel approaches to therapy in children.

Identifying HIV-infected infants and children at risk for *P. carinii* pneumonia and instituting effective chemoprophylaxis remains a major challenge for pediatric practitioners. Because of transplacental passage of maternal antibodies against HIV, a sizable fraction of infants with serological positivity will ultimately prove to be uninfected. Yet, distinguishing those infants who are truly infected from those with passively acquired maternal antibody may require 3–6 months. In addition, more sophisticated tests that permit easy diagnosis (such as HIV culture, p24 antigen assay, or polymerase chain reaction) are not readily available in many communities. Unfortunately, *P. carinii* pneumonia occurs most frequently in HIV-infected infants during the third through sixth months of life—often before HIV infection has been definitely diagnosed (75). Thus, the pediatric population standing to benefit the most from prophylaxis is the same group in whom the diagnosis of HIV infection may yet be uncertain.

A further complicating factor is the inability of a CD4 threshold to predict reliably an infant's risk of developing pneumocystis pneumonia. Because normal infants and young children have much higher CD4 counts than healthy adults, significant CD4 depletion and opportunistic infections may occur in children with HIV infection, despite an absolute CD4 cell count exceeding $200/mm^3$ (89–91). Given pediatric population studies and studies relating CD4 counts to the occurrence of *P. carinii* pneumonia in HIV-infected children, the CDC recommends initiating primary prophylaxis according to aged-adjusted CD4 counts: fewer than 1500 for children 1–11 months; than 750 for children 12–23 months; than 500 for children 24 months to 5 years; and than 200 for children 6 years and older (75). A CD4 percentage less than 20% at any age is also an indication for beginning prophylaxis, irrespective of the absolute CD4 count. As with adults, a prior episode of *P. carinii* pneumonia, regardless of a child's CD4 count, is an indication for lifelong secondary prophylaxis.

The currently recommended prophylactic regimen for children is TMP–SMX (75 mg TMP with 375 mg SMX per square meter twice daily) orally on 3 consecutive days weekly (75). Alternative TMP–SMX regimens and alternative agents are listed in Table 3. Aerosolized pentamidine is not advised for children younger than 5 years of age because of questions about their ability to cooperate with the procedure and uncertainty about sufficient drug delivery to the lungs. Neither TMP–SMX nor dapsone should be administered to infants younger than 1 month of age, since the potential for adverse drug effects is greater in neonates and since *P. carinii* pneumonia rarely occurs during the first month of life.

VI. Conclusion and Future Directions

Until the advent of HIV infection, *P. carinii* pneumonia was an infrequent clinical event. Within the last decade, this lung infection has become so common that clinicians in nearly every medical discipline have become increasingly familiar with its expression and treatment. With the upsurge in numbers of cases, attention has focused on developing therapeutic agents that are safer, better tolerated, and more convenient to administer than TMP–SMX and pentamidine, the current standards. A variety of compounds with differing chemical properties, mechanisms of action, and side effects are now available, but none has proved superior to the traditional first-line agents. Yet, because of the frequency of adverse effects from therapy, oftentimes requiring discontinuation of one or more agents, the need for the rapid development of safe and effective alternative drugs is still great. Compounds, such as clindamycin–primaquine, appear to have in vivo activity against *P. carinii* but need to be studied in prospective comparative trials, rigorously designed to provide definitive answers. Efforts to discover and develop promising new therapies also need to be intensified both in the academic institutions and in the pharmaceutical industry. Agents such as 566C80 (atovaquone) and the 8-aminoquinolines potentially represent important advances; their development, and that of other drugs in preclinical or early clinical studies, needs to be accelerated.

One of the most important lessons of the AIDS epidemic has been the potential for prophylaxis to profoundly alter the natural history of disease. Increased survival and reduced morbidity are, in large part, due to wide-scale institution of effective prophylactic regimens against *P. carinii* for those at risk. Chemoprophylaxis remains an imperfect art, however, with a relatively long list of agents undergoing investigation, but with relatively few having documented safety and efficacy. Current practice in both adult and pediatric sectors is based largely on extrapolation from narrowly defined populations, such as children with leukemia receiving primary prophylaxis or HIV-infected adults receiving secondary prophylaxis against *P. carinii*. Although large-scale prophylaxis studies are cumbersome and expensive, it is clear that they are required if our understanding is to advance.

Preventing and treating *P. carinii* infection encompasses more than chemotherapy alone. Immunotherapy and immunoprophylaxis, including vaccines, monoclonal antibodies, and cytokine-based therapies for *P. carinii* infection, represent important directions for future research. As further insights are gained into the basic biology of the microorganism, additional potential targets for therapeutic intervention will, we hope, be identified and exploited.

Note Added in Proof

Since the preparation of this chapter, atovaquone (formerly BW 566C80) has been licensed by the U.S. Food and Drug Administration for the treatment of mild to moderate episodes of *P. carinii* pneumonia in patients who are intolerant to TMP-SMX.

References

1. Ivady G, Paldy L, Koltay M, et al. *Pneumocystis carinii* pneumonia. Lancet 1967; 1: 616–617.
2. Western KA, Perera DR, Schultz MG. Pentamidine isethionate in the treatment of *Pneumocystis carinii* pneumonia. Ann Intern Med 1970; 73:695–702.
3. Walzer PD, Perl DP, Krogstad DJ, et al. *Pneumocystis carinii* pneumonia in the United States: epidemiologic, diagnostic, and clinical features. Ann Intern Med 1974; 80: 83–93.
4. Hughes WT, Feldman S, Chaudhary SC, et al. Comparison of pentamidine isethionate and trimethoprim–sulfamethoxazole in the treatment of *Pneumocystis carinii* pneumonia. J Pediatr 1978; 92:285–291.
5. Siegel SE, Wolff LJ, Baehner RL, et al. Treatment of *Pneumocystis carinii* pneumonitis: a comparative trial of sulfamethoxazole–trimethoprim vs pentamidine in pediatric patients with cancer. Am J Dis Child 1984; 138:1051–1054.
6. Wharton JM, Coleman DL, Wofsy CB, et al. Trimethoprim–sulfamethoxazole or pentamidine for *Pneumocystis carinii* pneumonia in the acquired immunodeficiency syndrome: a prospective randomized trial. Ann Intern Med 1986; 105:37–44.
7. Conte JE, Jr, Hollander H, Golden JA. Inhaled or reduced-dose intravenous pentamidine for *Pneumocystis carinii* pneumonia. Ann Intern Med 1987; 105:495–498.
8. Sattler FR, Cowan R, Nielsen DM, Ruskin J. Trimethoprim–sulfamethoxazole compared with pentamidine for treatment of *Pneumocystis carinii* pneumonia in the acquired immunodeficiency syndrome: a prospective, noncrossover study. Ann Intern Med 1988; 109:280–287.
9. Kovacs JA, Hiemenz JW, Macher AM, et al. *Pneumocystis carinii* pneumonia: a comparison between patients with the acquired immunodeficiency syndrome and patients with other immunodeficiencies. Ann Intern Med 1984; 100:663–671.
10. Salmeron S, Petitpretz P, Katlama C, et al. Pentamidine and pancreatitis [letter]. Ann Intern Med 1986; 105:140–141.
11. Zuger A, Wolf BZ, El-Sadr W, et al. Pentamidine-associated fatal acute pancreatitis. JAMA 1986; 256:2383–2385.
12. Hughes WT, McNabb PC, Makres TD, Feldman S. Efficacy of trimethoprim and sulfamethoxazole in the prevention and treatment of *Pneumocystis carinii* pneumonitis. Antimicrob Agents Chemother 1974; 5:289–293.
13. Rubin RH, Swartz MN. Trimethoprim–sulfamethoxazole. N Engl J Med 1980; 303: 426–432.
14. Lau WK, Young LS. Trimethoprim–sulfamethoxazole treatment of *Pneumocystis carinii* pneumonia in adults. N Engl J Med 1976; 295:716–718.
15. Winston DJ, Lau WK, Gale RP, Young LS. Trimethoprim–sulfamethoxazole for the treatment of *Pneumocystis carinii* pneumonia. Ann Intern Med 1980; 92: 762–769.
16. Sattler FR, Remington JS. Intravenous trimethoprim–sulfamethoxazole therapy for *Pneumocystis carinii* pneumonia. Am J Med 1981; 70:1215–1221.
17. Hughes WT. Trimethoprim–sulfamethoxazole therapy for *Pneumocystis carinii* pneumonitis in children. Rev Infect Dis 1982; 4:602–607.

18. Young LS. Trimethoprim–sulfamethoxazole in the treatment of adults with pneumonia due to *Pneumocystis carinii*. Rev Infect Dis 1982; 4:608–613.
19. Medina I, Mills J, Leoung G, et al. Oral therapy for *Pneumocystis carinii* pneumonia in the acquired immunodeficiency syndrome: a controlled trial of trimethoprim–sulfamethoxazole versus trimethoprim–dapsone. N Engl J Med 1990; 323:776–782.
20. Gordin FM, Simon GL, Wofsy CB, Mills J. Adverse reactions to trimethoprim–sulfamethoxazole in patients with the acquired immunodeficiency syndrome. Ann Intern Med 1984; 100:495–499.
21. Johnson MP, Goodwin SD, Shands JW. Trimethoprim–sulfamethoxazole anaphylactoid reactions in patients with AIDS: case reports and literature review. Pharmacotherapy 1990: 10:413–416.
22. Kelly JW, Dooley DP, Lattuada CP, et al. A severe, unusual reaction to trimethoprim–sulfamethoxazole in patients infected with human immunodeficiency virus. Clin Infect Dis 1992; 14:1034–1039.
23. Hardy WD, Feinberg J, Finkelstein DM, et al. A controlled trial of trimethoprim–sulfamethoxazole or aerosolized pentamidine for secondary prophylaxis of *Pneumocystis carinii* pneumonia in patients with the acquired immunodeficiency syndrome. N Engl J Med 1992; 327:1842–1848.
24. Smith RM, Iwamoto GK, Richerson HB, et al. Trimethoprim–sulfamethoxazole desensitization in the acquired immunodeficiency syndrome [letter]. Ann Intern Med 1987; 106:335.
25. Mills J, Leoung G, Medina I, et al. Dapsone treatment of *Pneumocystis carinii* pneumonia in the acquired immunodeficiency syndrome. Antimicrob Agents Chemother 1988; 32:1057–1060.
26. Safrin S, Sattler FR, Lee BL, et al. Dapsone as a single agent is suboptimal therapy for *Pneumocystis carinii* pneumonia. J AIDS 1991; 4:244–249.
27. Leoung GS, Mills J, Hopewell PC, et al. Dapsone–trimethoprim for *Pneumocystis carinii* pneumonia in the acquired immunodeficiency syndrome. Ann Intern Med 1986; 105:45–48.
28. Edelson PJ, Friedman-Kien A. Dapsone, trimethoprim–sulfamethoxazole, and the acquired immunodeficiency syndrome [letter]. Ann Intern Med 1985; 103:963.
29. Conte JE, Golden JA. Concentrations of aerosolized pentamidine in bronchoalveolar lavage, systemic absorption and excretion. Antimicrob Agents Chemother 1988; 32: 1490–1493.
30. Montgomery AB, Debs RJ, Luce JM, et al. Aerosolized pentamidine as second line therapy in patients with AIDS and *Pneumocystis carinii* pneumonia. Chest 1989; 95: 747–750.
31. Conte JE Jr, Chernoff D, Feigal DW, et al. Intravenous or inhaled pentamidine for treating *Pneumocystis carinii* pneumonia in AIDS: a randomized trial. Ann Intern Med 1990; 113:203–209.
32. Soo Hoo GW, Mohsenifar Z, Meyer RD. Inhaled or intravenous pentamidine therapy for *Pneumocystis carinii* pneumonia in AIDS: a randomized trial. Ann Intern Med 1990; 113:195–202.
33. Allegra CJ, Kovacs JA, Drake JC, et al. Activity of antifolates against *Pneumocystis carinii* dihydrofolate reductase and identification of a potent new agent. J Exp Med 1987; 165:926–931.

34. Allegra CJ, Chabner BA, Tuazon CU, et al. Trimetrexate for the treatment of *Pneumocystis carinii* pneumonia in patients with the acquired immunodeficiency syndrome. N Engl J Med 1987; 317:978–985.
35. Sattler FR, Allegra CJ, Verdegem TD, et al. Trimetrexate–leucovorin dosage evaluation study for treatment of *Pneumocystis carinii* pneumonia. J Infect Dis 1990; 161: 91–96.
36. Sattler FR, Feinberg J. New developments in the treatment of *Pneumocystis carinii* pneumonia. Chest 1992; 101:451–457.
37. Hughes WT, Gray VL, Gutteridge WE, et al. Efficacy of a hydroxynaphthoquinone, 566C80, in experimental *Pneumocystis carinii* pneumonitis. Antimicrob Agents Chemother 1990; 34:225–228.
38. Araujo FG, Huskinson J, Remington JS. Remarkable in vitro and in vivo activities of the hydroxynaphthoquinone 566C80 against tachyzoites and tissue cysts of *Toxoplasma gondii*. Antimicrob Agents Chemother 1991; 35:293–299.
39. Hammond DJ, Burchell JR, Pudney M. Inhibition of pyrimidine biosynthese de novo in *Plasmodium falciparum* by 2-(4-*t*-butylcyclohexyl)-3-hydroxy-1, 4-naphthoquinone in vitro. Mol Biochem Parasitol 1985; 14:97–109.
40. Falloon J, Kovacs J, Hughes W, et al. A preliminary evaluation of 566C80 for the treatment of pneumocystis pneumonia in patients with the acquired immunodeficiency syndrome. N Engl J Med 1991; 325:1534–1538.
41. Hughes W, Leoung G, Kramer F, et al. Comparison of atovaquone (566C80) and trimethoprim–sulfamethoxazole for the treatment of *Pneumocystis carinii* pneumonia in patients with the acquired immunodeficiency syndrome (AIDS). N Engl J Med 1993 (in press).
42. Queener SF, Bartlett MS, Richardson JD, et al. Activity of clindamycin with primaquine against *Pneumocystis carinii* in vitro and in vivo. Antimicrob Agents Chemother 1988; 32:807–813.
43. Smith JW, Studies of the susceptibility of *Pneumocystis carinii* to clindamycin/primaquine in rats. Eur J Clin Microbiol Infect Dis 1991; 10:201–203.
44. Toma E, Poisson M, Phaneuf D, et al. Clindamycin with primaquine for *Pneumocystis carinii* pneumonia. Lancet 1989; 1:1046–1048.
45. Black JR, Feinberg J, Murphy RL, et al. Clindamycin and primaquine as primary treatment for mild and moderately severe *Pneumocystis carinii* pneumonia in patients with AIDS. Eur J Clin Microbiol Infect Dis 1991; 10:204–207.
46. Ruf B, Rohde I, Pohle HD. Efficacy of clindamycin/primaquine versus trimethoprim/sulfamethoxazole in primary treatment of *Pneumocystis carinii* pneumonia. Eur J Clin Microbiol Infect Dis 1991; 10:207–210.
47. Toma E. Clindamycin/primaquine for treatment of *Pneumocystis carinii* pneumonia in AIDS. Eur J Clin Microbiol Infect Dis 1991; 10:210–213.
48. Noskin GA, Murphy RL, Black JR, et al. Salvage therapy with clindamycin/primaquine for *Pneumocystis carinii* pneumonia. Clin Infect Dis 1992; 14:183–188.
49. Bartlett MS, Queener SF, Tidwell RR, et al. 8-Aminoquinolines from Walter Reed Army Institutes for research for treatment and prophylaxis of pneumocystis pneumonia in rat models. Antimicrob Agents Chemother 1991; 35:277–282.
50. Golden JA, Sjoerdsma A, Santi DV. *Pneumocystis carinii* pneumonia treated with α-difluoromethylornithine. West J Med 1984; 141:613–623.

51. Smith D, Davies S, Nelson M, et al. *Pneumocystis carinii* pneumonia treated with eflornithine in AIDS patients resistant to conventional therapy. AIDS 1990; 4:1019–1021.
52. McLees BD, Barlow JLR, Kuzma RJ, et al. Studies on the successful eflornithine treatment of *Pneumocystis carinii* pneumonia (PCP) in AIDS patients failing conventional therapy. Abstracts of the III International Conference on AIDS 1987: Th. 4.2.
53. Paulson YJ, Gilman TM, Heseltine PNR, et al. Eflornithine treatment of refractory *Pneumocystis carinii* pneumonia in patients with acquired immunodeficiency syndrome. Chest 1992; 101:67–74.
54. Smith DE, Davies S, Smithson J, et al. Eflornithine versus co-trimoxazole in the treatment of *Pneumocystis carinii* pneumonia in patients with the acquired immunodeficiency syndrome. AIDS 1992; 6:1489–1493.
55. Brenner M, Ognibene FP, Lack EE, et al. Prognostic factors and life expectancy of patients with acquired immunodeficiency syndrome and *Pneumocystis carinii* pneumonia. Am Rev Respir Dis 1987; 136:1199–1206.
56. El-Sadr W, Simberkoff MS. Survival and prognostic factors in severe *Pneumocystis carinii* pneumonia requiring mechanical ventilation. Am Rev Respir Dis 1988; 137:1264–1267.
57. The National Institutes of Health–University of California Expert Panel. Consensus statement on the use of corticosteroids as adjunctive therapy for pneumocystis pneumonia in the acquired immunodeficiency syndrome. N Engl J Med 1990; 323:1500–1504.
58. Masur H, Ognibene FP, Yarchoan R, et al. CD4 counts as predictors of opportunistic pneumonias in human immunodeficiency virus (HIV) infection. Ann Intern Med 1989; 111:223–231.
59. Phair J, Munoz A, Detels R, et al. The risk of *Pneumocystis carinii* pneumonia among men infected with human immunodeficiency virus type 1. N Engl J Med 1990; 322:161–165.
60. Fischl MA, Parker CB, Pettinelli C, et al. A randomized controlled trial of reduced daily dose of zidovudine in patients with the acquired immunodeficiency syndrome. N Engl J Med 1990; 323:1009–1014.
61. Simone JV, Holland E, Johnson W. Fatalities during remission of childhood leukemia. Blood 1972; 39:759–770.
62. Hughes WT, Kuhn S, Chaudhary S, et al. Successful chemoprophylaxis for *Pneumocystis carinii* pneumonitis. N Engl J Med 1977; 297:1419–1426.
63. Hughes WT, Rivera GK, Schell MJ, et al. Successful intermittent chemoprophylaxis for *Pneumocystis carinii* pneumonitis. N Engl J Med 1987; 316:1627–1632.
64. Dummer JS. *Pneumocystis carinii* infections in transplant recipients. Semin Respir Infect 1990; 5:50–57.
65. Gryzan S, Paradis IL, Zeevi A, et al. Unexpected high incidence of *Pneumocystis carinii* infection after heart–lung infection transplantation. Am Rev Respir Dis 1988; 137:1268–1274.
66. Centers for Disease Control. Recommendations for prophylaxis against *Pneumocystis carinii* pneumonia for adults and adolescents infected with human immunodeficiency virus. MMWR 1992; 41(RR-4):1–11.

67. Fishl MA, Dickinson GM, La Voie L. Safety and efficacy of sulfamethoxazole and trimethoprim chemoprophylaxis for *Pneumocystis carinii* pneumonia in AIDS. JAMA 1988; 259:1185–1189.
68. Stein DS, Stevens RC, Terry D, et al. Use of low-dose trimethoprim–sulfamethoxazole thrice weekly for primary and secondary prophylaxis of *Pneumocystis carinii* pneumonia in human immunodeficiency virus-infected patients. Antimicrob Agents Chemother 1991; 35:1705–1709.
69. Ruskin J, LaRiviere M. Low-dose co-trimoxazole for prevention of *Pneumocystis carinii* pneumonia in human immunodeficiency virus disease. Lancet 1991; 337:468–471.
70. Wormser GP, Horowitz HW, Duncanson FP, et al. Low-dose intermittent trimethoprim–sulfamethoxazole for prevention of *Pneumocystis carinii* pneumonia in patients with human immunodeficiency virus infection. Arch Intern Med 1991; 151:688–692.
71. Hirschel B, Lazzarin A, Chopard P, et al. A controlled study of inhaled pentamidine for primary prevention of *Pneumocystis carinii* pneumonia. N Engl J Med 1991; 324:1079–1083.
72. Leoung GS, Feigal DW Jr, Montgomery AB, et al. Aerosolized pentamidine for prophylaxis against *Pneumocystis carinii* pneumonia: The San Francisco Community Prophylaxis Trial. N Engl J Med 1990; 323:769–775.
73. Montaner JSG, Lawson LM, Gervais A, et al. Aerosol pentamidine for secondary prophylaxis of AIDS-related *Pneumocystis carinii* pneumonia. Ann Intern Med 1991; 114:948–953.
74. Girard PM, Gaudebout C, Lottin P, et al. Prevention of *Pneumocystis carinii* pneumonia relapse by pentamidine aerosol in zidovudine-treated AIDS patients. Lancet 1989; 1:1348–1353.
75. Centers for Disease Control. Guidelines for prophylaxis against *Pneumocystis carinii* pneumonia for children infected with human immunodeficiency virus. MMWR 1991; 40(RR-2):1–13.
76. Northfelt DW, Clement MJ, Safrin S. Extrapulmonary pneumocystosis: clinical features in human immunodeficiency virus infection. Medicine 1990; 69:392–398.
77. Jules-Elysee KM, Stover DE, Zaman MB, et al. Aerosolized pentamidine effect on diagnosis and presentation of *Pneumocystis carinii* pneumonia. Ann Intern Med 1990; 112:750–757.
78. Levine SJ, Masur H, Gill VJ, et al. Effect of aerosolized pentamidine prophylaxis on the diagnosis of *Pneumocystis carinii* pneumonia by induced sputum examination in patients infected with the human immunodeficiency virus. Am Rev Respir Dis 1991; 144:760–764.
79. Hughes WT, Kennedy W, Dugdale M, et al. Prevention of *Pneumocystis carinii* pneumonia in AIDS patients with weekly dapsone [letter]. Lancet 1990; 336:1066.
80. Kemper CA, Tucker RM, Lang OS, et al. Low-dose dapsone prophylaxis of *Pneumocystis carinii* pneumonia in AIDS and AIDS-related complex. AIDS 1990; 4:1145–1148.
81. Lavelle J, Falloon J, Morgan A, et al. Weekly dapsone and dapsone/pyrimethamine for pneumocystis pneumonia prophylaxis. Abstracts of the VII International Conference on AIDS 1991:WB 2207.
82. Giovanni P, Crisalli MP, Guida B, et al. Dapsone in the prophylaxis of *Pneumocystis*

carinii pneumonia. Abstracts of the VII International Conference on AIDS 1991: WB 2181.
83. Cruciani M, Danzi MC, Di Perri G, et al. Dapsone in secondary prophylaxis of PCP. Abstracts of the VII International Conference on AIDS 1991:WB 2208.
84. Clotet B, Sirera G, Romeu J, et al. Twice-weekly dapsone–pyrimethamine for preventing primary and secondary *Pneumocystis carinii* pneumonia (PCP): its role in prevention of cerebral toxoplasmosis. Abstracts of the VII International Conference on AIDS 1991:WB 2185.
85. Kay R, DuBois RE. Clindamycin/primaquine therapy and secondary prophylaxis against *Pneumocystis carinii* pneumonia in patients with AIDS. South Med J 1990; 83:403–404.
86. Girard P-M, Lepretre A, Detruchis P, et al. Failure of pyrimethamine–clindamycin combination for prophylaxis of *Pneumocystis carinii* pneumonia [letter]. Lancet 1989; 1:1459.
87. Jacobson MA, Child C, Matts JP, et al. Toxicity of clindamycin as prophylaxis for AIDS-associated toxoplasmic encephalitis. Lancet 1992; 339:333–334.
88. Falloon J, Eddy T, Wiener L, et al. Human immunodeficiency virus in children. J Pediatr 1989; 114:1–30.
89. Leibovitz E, Rigaud M, Pollack H, et al. *Pneumocystis carinii* pneumonia in infants infected with the human immunodeficiency virus with more than 450 CD4 T lymphocytes per cubic millimeter. N Engl J Med 1990; 323:531–533.
90. Connor E, Bagarazzi M, McSherry G, et al. Clinical and laboratory correlates of *Pneumocystis carinii* pneumonia in children infected with HIV. JAMA 1991; 265:1693–1697.
91. Kovacs A, Frederick T, Church J, et al. CD4 T-lymphocyte counts and *Pneumocystis carinii* pneumonia in pediatric HIV infection. JAMA 1991; 265:1698–1703.

23

Pharmacokinetic and Pharmacodynamic Considerations for Drug Dosing in the Treatment of *Pneumocystis carinii* Pneumonia

FRED R. SATTLER and ROGER W. JELLIFFE

University of Southern California School of Medicine
and Los Angeles County–University of Southern California Medical Center
Los Angeles, California

I. Introduction

It is unfortunate that more than 10 years into the acquired immunodeficiency syndrome (AIDS) epidemic there is little information from controlled studies on the appropriate dose or duration of treatment for *Pneumocystis carinii* pneumonia. What is certain is that therapies currently licensed for treatment of *P. carinii* pneumonia, namely, trimethoprim–sulfamethoxazole and parenteral pentamidine, are associated with adverse drug effects in most patients with AIDS. These toxic reactions often cause appreciable morbidity and may occasionally contribute to mortality. Whether some or all of these adverse affects are related to dose is unknown.

In attempt to reduce drug-related side effects, some practitioners prescribe other yet invalidated therapies, such as trimethoprim plus dapsone or clindamycin plus primaquine. These therapies are attractive considerations for patients who are intolerant of existing therapies, or for initial therapy, based on a belief that the combinations are less toxic than and equally as effective as licensed therapies. However, the relative efficacy and frequency of adverse events of both the licensed and newer-prescribed therapies for AIDS-related *P. carinii* pneumonia remain unknown. Thus, selection of therapies for treatment of *P. carinii* pneumonia is invariably determined by physicians' preference, patients' perceptions, and patients' history of previous intolerance to specific or related therapies.

Over the last few years, information has been slowly emerging that sheds light on the relation of dose to outcome (toxicity and efficacy) and on the potential value of pharmacokinetic monitoring and dosage modifications to achieve targeted serum concentrations to optimize therapy. In this chapter, we will review recent studies relating dose and drug concentrations to adverse effects and efficacy.

II. Trimethoprim–Sulfamethoxazole

Intravenous trimethoprim–sulfamethoxazole (TMP–SMX) is commonly the first therapy selected by practitioners for treatment of *P. carinii* pneumonia. This preference is based, in part, on availability of an oral formulation that can be prescribed once patients are improved and ready for discharge from the hospital. However, the frequency and severity of adverse drug effects make it difficult to complete a full course of treatment except in a few patients, since these toxic effects are often treatment-terminating (1–4). The ideal dose of TMP–SMX is that which produces the highest success rate, with the least toxicity.

A. Clinical Studies

The dose of trimethoprim–sulfamethoxazole recommended and prescribed for treatment of *P. carinii* pneumonia has been 15–20 mg/kg per day of trimethoprim with 75–100 mg/kg per day sulfamethoxazole. There are no controlled studies documenting whether either is the optimal dose for efficacy or toxicity. In one trial involving a noncrossover design, surviving patients received a full 3-week course of therapy with TMP–SMX (5). This study provided a reasonably accurate estimate of the toxic effects associated with TMP–SMX, since patients did not receive other therapies for *P. carinii* pneumonia. Thirty-two (89%) of 36 subjects randomized to TMP–SMX experienced an average of 2.3 side effects (Table 1). It is probable that such toxic drug effects compromise the effectiveness of treatment. Thus, it would be highly desirable to develop strategies to reduce the frequency of such effects.

The fact that hematological toxic reactions and possibly other adverse effects of antifolate drugs (such as TMP–SMX and trimetrexate) are dose-dependent (6) provided the rationale for the first study of pharmacokinetic monitoring and dosage modification to achieve targeted concentrations (5). In that study, dosage modifications were made in an ad hoc manner to maintain serum trimethoprim (TMP) concentrations in the 5–8 μg/mL range. These values were chosen, based on two observations. First, treatment failures were reported to be associated with TMP levels below 5 μg/mL in non-AIDS patients with *P. carinii* pneumonia (7). Second, TMP levels of 20–30 μg/mL had been detected in some patients

Table 1 Adverse Drug Effects Occurring in 36 Patients Treated with TMP–SMX for 3 Weeks

Effects	No. patients (%)
Clinical	
Drug-induced fever[a]	28 (78)
Generalized rash	16 (44)
Nausea or vomiting	9 (25)
Laboratory	
Neutropenia (or >25% decline in WBC)	26 (72)
Anemia (Hgb ↓ >3 g/dL)	14 (39)
ALT ↑ > 2× baseline	8 (22)
Azotemia[b]	5 (14)
Thrombocytopenia (↓ >25,000/mm^3)	1 (03)

[a]Temperature >100°F without apparent cause and occurring after at least 36 h without fever during treatment with TMP–SMX.
[b]Absolute increase in serum creatinine of >0.5 mg/dL if the baseline value was < 2.0 mg/dL or an absolute increase of 1.5 mg/dL if the baseline value was > 2.0 mg/dL.
Source: Ref. 5.

experiencing severe myelosuppression during therapy of *P. carinii* pneumonia in the second and third week of therapy with the standard dose of 20 mg/kg per day of TMP and 100 mg/kg per day of SMX (Sattler FR, personal observations). However, neutrophil counts increased after the dose of TMP–SMX was reduced and serum levels declined.

By using the targeted concentrations of 5–8 μg/mL for TMP, the dose was modified 36 times in 25 of the 36 patients. With this strategy, the 31 surviving patients assigned to receive TMP–SMX were able to tolerate a 3-week course of therapy with the combination. It could be argued that the fortitude of the investigators in treating through toxic reactions was as important as monitoring serum concentrations and making dose modifications in not having to switch patients to alternative therapy. What was undeniable was that the final average dose of the TMP component was 12 mg/kg per day (well below the "accepted" standard dose), and yet 31 (86%) of the 36 patients were cured of that episode of *P. carinii* pneumonia. The excellent survival results were not anticipated, since the median baseline $(A-a)Do_2$ of the study subjects was 44 mmHg, suggesting that from 7 to 11 patients in the cohort of 36 would have been expected to die, based on the severity of their infection at the outset of treatment (8).

Despite these favorable results, the study was limited by the fact that the comparative treatment arm involved patients who received pentamidine, rather than a group receiving standard doses of TMP–SMX without adaptive control.

Although there was no treatment-terminating toxicity with TMP–SMX, adverse effects still occurred in 89% of patients. The results are consistent with the possibility that adaptive control may have reduced the severity, although not necessarily the frequency of adverse drug effects and, therefore, may have contributed to the better-than-expected efficacy outcome.

More recently, a second study was conducted to determine whether monitoring "trough" serum levels of TMP, SMX, and the N-acetyl metabolite of SMX on treatment days 5, 10, 15, and 21 in patients receiving therapy with TMP–SMX for *P. carinii* pneumonia affected outcome (9). This study was better-designed since half the patients had their dose adjusted to achieve targeted concentrations of SMX in the range of 150–200 µg/mL, and in the other half, the dose was not modified. However, the initial dose was 20 mg/kg per day for the first 48 hr and was reduced to 15 mg/kg per day after the first 48 hr in both groups. Of 38 patients enrolled, only 6 of 19 undergoing adaptive control and 8 of 19 in the control group were able to complete a full 3-week course of therapy. Treatment was terminated in most cases because of rash, nausea, and vomiting. The SMX, TMP, and SMX–acetyl concentrations in the group assigned to adaptive control were 158 ± 53, 5.4 ± 2.3, and 20 ± 8, respectively, compared with similar values of 144 ± 62, 5.1 ± 1.7, and 20 ± 13, respectively, in the control group. In the group having dose modifications, concentrations of SMX were similar on treatment days 5, 10, 15, and 21 (157 ± 47, 160 ± 41, 158 ± 57, and 157 ± 95, respectively). Moreover, concentrations of all three drugs were similar, regardless of whether patients were able to tolerate and complete therapy. In addition, there was no difference in hematological or liver test abnormalities between the groups. The study was stopped because of the high rate of dropouts. The authors concluded that drug toxicity did not appear to correlate with serum drug concentrations, and monitoring with dose modifications did not improve efficacy or reduce the incidence of side effects. It is also possible that the 25% reduction in dosage after 48 hr may have attenuated any benefits of adaptive control.

B. Pharmacokinetic Studies

The ideal trial design would be one in which patients are initially treated with 20 mg/kg per day of the TMP component of TMP–SMX; then half of the patients are randomized to receive dosing by adaptive control to achieve targeted serum concentrations, and the remainder continue to receive the full dose. In preparation for such a study, we developed a pharmacokinetic population model based on 179 TMP serum concentrations obtained from the 36 patients treated in the first study just described (5). Trough and peak samples had been collected 30 min before and 90 min after dose 5, again on day 5, and following four or five doses after each dosage adjustment to achieve targeted concentrations of 5–8 µg/mL. All samples were assayed for both TMP and SMX concentrations by high-performance liquid chromatography.

The time–concentration data were analyzed by a nonparametric EM population pharmacokinetic modeling program (10–12) which has been added to the current USC*PACK PC clinical software (13). The model employed has a V_d (liters/kg), but breaks up the K_{el} into a nonrenal component (K intercept [K_{int}]) and an excretory component (K_{slope}), which is multiplied by creatinine clearance. Thus, the overall K_{el} can vary with changes in renal function from dose to dose, whereas the parameters K_{int} and K_{slope} usually remain constant throughout short-term treatment. Thus, unlike the Sawchuk–Zaske linear regression approach to modeling (14), the K_{slope} method is usually able to use the information of all drug concentrations obtained during the entire course of therapy, even when there is changing excretory function. By contrast, most other approaches are limited by the necessity to use only the most recent data set, and the patient needs to be in steady state before the analysis.

The following population parameter values were obtained for TMP. The median V_d was 0.8016 ± 0.6415 liters/kg and median K_{slope} was 0.0010067 ± 0.00136 (hr[mL/min per 1.73 m²])$^{-1}$. The K_{int} was set and fixed at 0.01155 ± 0.01155 hr^{-1}. The correlation between V_d and K_{slope}, analogous to the covariance between the parameters, was −0.36664. With these parameter values for a hypothetical patient (e.g., one who is 40 years old, 69-in. [172.5-cm] tall, weighs 60 kg, has a muscle mass 85% of normal, and serum creatinine level of 1.15 mg/dL), the model predicts that a loading dose of 508 mg of TMP should be followed by 228 mg every 8 hr (each dose to be infused over 1.5 hr) to achieve a "true" peak (immediately after the completion of the infusion) serum concentration of 10 µ/dL and a trough of 6.16 µg/dL. For that patient, the maintenance dose would be 3.8 mg/kg every 8 hr (12.4 mg/kg per day) and the median serum half-life of TMP would be 9.31 hr.

C. Dosing in Renal Failure

Given existing data, we would advise that doses of intravenous TMP–SMX be chosen to achieve true peak concentrations (level at the completion of the infusion) of 8–10 µg/mL and trough concentrations of 5–7 µg/mL. From the model described earlier, we developed an algorithm to achieve these serum concentrations during treatment for an average male AIDS patient who was 35 years old, 69-in. [172.5-cm] tall, weighed 60 kg, and whose muscle mass was 85% of normal (Table 2).

D. Conclusions

Results from the two pharmacokinetic monitoring–dose-modifying studies are inconclusive. However, the outcome of the first trial suggests that 15 mg/kg per day (TMP component) of TMP–SMX provides effective therapy, even for severe episodes of *P. carinii* pneumonia. Unfortunately, the design does not permit a definitive statement to be made about whether, in fact, the lower dose results in less

Table 2 Dosing of TMP–SMX for Patients with Renal Impairment

Serum creatinine (mg/dL)	Cl_{cr} (mL/min)	Loading dose (mg)	Maintenance dose (mg)	Dose interval (h)	Maintenance dose (mg/kg per day)	Peak concentration (µg/mL)	Trough concentration (µg/mL)
0.7	109	525	275	6	18.32	10.1	5.9
1.0	76	525	250	8	12.51	9.8	5.5
1.5	50	500	200	8	10.00	10.1	6.8
2.0	37	500	225	12	7.50	10.2	6.1
2.5	29	500	200	12	6.66	10.3	6.8
3.0	24	500	175	12	5.83	10.2	7.1
5.0	13	500	225	24	3.75	10.2	5.9
8.0	7	500	175	24	2.92	10.0	6.6
10.0	5	500	150	24	2.50	9.7	6.6

drug toxicity or whether even lower doses could be equally effective and potentially more tolerable. One interpretation of the results of the second trial is that if the dose of TMP–SMX is reduced from 20 to 15 mg/kg per day after 48 hr, monitoring serum drug levels and dose modification provide little benefit, as long as renal function remains relatively normal. Regardless, it is unlikely that additional studies will be conducted to compare the standard "high" dose of 20 mg/kg per day without adaptive control versus a strategy to achieve targeted peak-and-trough serum concentrations of 10 and 6 μ/mL, since many physicians at centers with large numbers of patients with AIDS-related *P. carinii* pneumonia now routinely treat patients with 15 mg/kg per day and, importantly, serum TMP and SMX assays are not commercially available in most cities. Therefore, although this treatment would be ideally suited for therapeutic drug monitoring and adaptive control of the dosage regimen, existing data and practical constraints seem to favor empiric selection of the 15 mg/kg per day. Treatment regimens adjusted for body weight and renal function (as exemplified in Table 2) would provide more precise therapy, and if serum assays for TMP were available, even greater precision could be obtained.

III. Pentamidine

Intravenous pentamidine is frequently reserved for patients intolerant to TMP–SMX, since there is no oral formulation, and some of the adverse effects associated with this agent may be life-threatening. Nephrotoxicity and hypoglycemia, the two most serious toxic effects attributable to parenteral pentamidine, appear to be dose-related, since the relative risk for these adverse reactions is significantly greater for patients who have received a cumulative dose of more than 4 g, especially for patients receiving more than 2-weeks of therapy (15). It would be desirable, therefore, to treat patients with lower systemic doses. However, there are uncertainties about whether 3 mg/kg per day, which has been advocated recently, is as effective as the standard dose of 4 mg/kg per day or whether aerosol therapy is as effective as parenteral treatment.

A. Clinical Studies

1. Parenteral Therapy

There have been several controlled trials using lower doses of parenteral pentamidine. In the noncrossover trial described earlier, in which patients were prospectively randomized to receive either TMP–SMX or parenteral (intravenous or intramuscular) pentamidine, the initial dose of pentamidine was 4 mg/kg per day intravenously (5). The study was designed so that the dose was empirically reduced by 30–50% when patients developed serious adverse effects, generally an absolute increase in the serum creatinine of at least 1 mg/dL. Patients were allowed to be switched to intramuscular therapy once they were improved and were discharged home to complete a 21-day course. Of 33 patients assigned to receive pentamidine, only 2 had their dose reduced because of toxic effects in the first week, 6 in the second week, and none were reduced in the third week of therapy. The final intravenous dosage was 3.8 ± 0.6 mg/kg per day (average duration was 15 ± 7.0 days), and intramuscular dosage 3.1 ± 0.6 mg/kg per day (average duration was 1.7 ± 3.5 days). Since most patients received the bulk of their treatment intravenously, the average reduction in dose was relatively minor. Although improvement in blood gas measurements occurred more rapidly and survival was greater for the 36 patients assigned to TMP–SMX ($p < 0.05$ for both comparisons), this difference was not likely to be due to the reductions in the dose of pentamidine. In fact, only one of the eight patients in the pentamidine group who died had his dose reduced.

Of import, 31 (94%) of the patients assigned to receive pentamidine experienced adverse effects (Table 3). These patients experienced on average 2.7 different toxic reactions. The most frequent serious adverse effects were nephrotoxicity in 21 (64%), hypotension in 9 (27%), and hypoglycemia in 6 (18%). In 1 patient, hypoglycemia occurred precipitously during the third week and was fatal (glucose concentrations in venous and capillary blood were not detectable).

Table 3 Adverse Effects Associated with Parenteral Pentamidine

Effects	No. patients (%)
Clinical	
Drug-induced fever	27 (82)
Hypotension (systolic < 80 mmHg)	9 (27)
Nausea or vomiting	8 (24)
Rash	5 (15)
Laboratory	
Azotemia[a]	21 (64)
Neutropenia	16 (47)
Anemia	8 (24)
Hypoglycemia	7 (21)
Thrombocytopenia (glucose < 70 mg/d)	6 (18)
ALT > 2× baseline	5 (15)
Hypocalcemia	1 (3)

[a]The average absolute increase in serum creatinine was 1.6 ± 1.1 mg/dL and four patients had increases to > 4.0 mg/dL.
Source: Ref. 5.

Because of the noncrossover nature of the study design, all survivors received a full 3-week course of therapy. This most likely amplified the frequency and severity of adverse events attributable to pentamidine, compared with standard practice in which patients are often switched to alternative therapies after the first sign of toxicity. Moreover, it is possible that these adverse effects contributed to the less favorable outcome of individuals randomized to receive pentamidine, compared with those treated with TMP–SMX.

In a study comparing aerosol treatment versus intravenous therapy with 3 mg/kg per day in patients with initial values of Pao_2 greater than 55 mmHg, eight (92%) of nine receiving parenteral therapy responded; the ninth patient improved, but had therapy changed to TMP plus dapsone when his neutrophil cell count declined to 630/mm^3 (16). In a second study conducted at the same institution and of similar design, only 4 (19%) of 22 patients randomized to 3 mg/kg per day failed to respond (17). Although response rates appeared favorable, these results with the lower dose may not be generalizable to sicker patients with more severe hypoxemia. A controlled trial is needed to determine whether this dose is as effective and safer than the standard dose of 4 mg/kg per day.

2. Aerosolized Pentamidine

In attempt to reduce systemic toxicity, it was hypothesized that pentamidine could be delivered directly to the alveoli, the putative site of infection with *P. carinii*. This should result in high concentrations of drug in the lung with minimal systemic absorption. In one study testing the Ultra Vent nebulizer to deliver pentamidine to patients with *P. carinii* pneumonia, two to four consecutive 15-mL bronchoalveolar lavage aliquots were collected during the same bronchoscopy 1–15 days after the start of aerosol therapy (16). Lavage concentrations of pentamidine ranged from 16.8 ± 7.3 to 149.7 ± 38.2 ng/mL in patients receiving aerosol pentamidine, compared with 3.4 ± 0.2–10.9 ± 2.9 ng/mL for patients treated with intravenous pentamidine. By contrast, maximum plasma concentrations ranged from 6.1 to 79 ng/mL in the aerosol treatment group compared with values of 164–1360 ng/mL in the parenteral treatment group.

In a multicenter investigation (18), 364 patients with initial room air $(A-a)Do_2$ less than 55 mmHg were randomized to receive either 600 mg of aerosolized pentamidine once daily by the Respirgard II jet nebulizer or TMP–SMX at 15 mg/kg per day (TMP). As expected, treatment-terminating toxicity occurred significantly more often with TMP–SMX. However, Pao_2 and chest radiographs improved significantly faster with TMP–SMX, and there were significantly fewer overt efficacy failures with TMP–SMX. This study does not address the relative efficacy of aerosol versus parenteral pentamidine, since it was designed to test therapies of mild to moderate severity in which patients could continue to receive convenient therapies (i.e., aerosol pentamidine or oral TMP–

SMX) out of the hospital once they were improved. However, it does raise concern that drug deposition may have been suboptimal with aerosol delivery of pentamidine, although the alternative explanation is that pentamidine per se is inherently less effective than TMP–SMX.

In two smaller studies using the same nebulizer system, outcome with aerosolized therapy was compared with intravenous pentamidine (17,19). In the first trial, 45 patients with baseline room air PaO_2 greater than 55 torr were randomized to receive 600 mg of aerosolized pentamidine daily or 3 mg/kg per day of intravenous pentamidine for 2–3 weeks (17). Although initial failure rates were similar (12 vs 19%), recrudescence of symptoms (35 vs 0%) and relapse (24 vs 0%) were significantly more common with aerosolized pentamidine ($p < 0.05$ for both). In the second study, only 6 of 11 patients randomized to receive inhaled pentamidine (8 mg/kg per day by Respirgard II) responded, whereas all 10 assigned to the parenteral formulation responded ($p = 0.02$) (19). Nonresponders to inhaled pentamidine had lower mean baseline PaO_2 compared with responders (60 vs 81 torr; $p = 0.005$).

Taken together, these studies suggest that aerosol pentamidine causes less systemic toxicity than TMP–SMX or parenteral pentamidine. However, aerosol treatment may not be effective in areas of the lung with extensive airspace consolidation, which could predispose to early relapse. Moreover, in sicker patients with higher minute ventilation or in those with shallow, rapid respirations, peripheral alveolar deposition may be suboptimal, thereby predisposing these individuals to failure.

B. Pharmacokinetic Studies

The pharmacokinetics of intravenous pentamidine using a liquid chromatographic assay was determined in six AIDS patients with normal renal function after a 4 mg/kg single infusion of the drug (20). The mean peak concentration was 612 ± 371 ng/mL with concentrations falling below 25 mg/mL after 8 hr. Drug was eliminated from blood biexponentially. With an open two-compartment model, the plasma clearance was 248 ± 91 liters /hr, terminal elimination half-life was 6.40 ± 1.32 hr, and apparent volume of distribution at steady state was 821 ± 535 liters. Less than 2.5% of the administered dose was detected in the urine after 24 hr. No metabolites were detected. Although the molecular weight of 593 is in the range of drugs eliminated in the bile, the hydrophilic nature of its molecular structure suggests that pentamidine should be excreted in the urine. Take together with the large volume of distribution and low urinary concentrations, this suggests that the drug is avidly bound to tissues and released slowly in the urine.

C. Renal Failure

In ten dogs that had their ureters ligated to induce renal failure, 6.5 mg/kg infusions of pentamidine before and after surgery produced peak serum concentrations of 867 versus 780 ng/mL, which declined at 6 hr to 30 versus 28 ng/mL, respectively (21). Total clearance was also little affected by the surgery (46.7 vs 40.0 mL min^{-1} kg^{-1}). The kinetic parameters in two controls and two dogs with azotemia who received 14 daily infusions of pentamidine did not differ significantly after the first and the last dose. These data provide further evidence that renal clearance of pentamidine accounts for a only a small portion of total body clearance, at best.

In 5 AIDS patients with normal kidney function and 13 with varying degrees of renal impairment, there was no relation between elimination half-life or plasma clearance of pentamidine and renal function (22). However, the number of prior doses and the elimination half-life estimated from the terminal slope were related ($r = 0.81$, $p = 0.025$) which suggested that the chromatography assay used was not sensitive enough to determine the true terminal elimination half-life. In addition, trough concentrations ranged from 4.3 to 67.5 ng/mL in patients who had received prior doses, which suggested that drug accumulation occurs with multiple dosing and existing models probably did not adequately describe the probable multicompartment pharmacokinetic behavior of pentamidine.

In the most recently reported study, the pharmacokinetics of intravenous pentamidine at 3 mg/kg per day were determined in ten patients with acute *P. carinii* pneumonia and normal renal function and in a second group of nine volunteers without *P. carinii* pneumonia who were receiving hemodialysis (23). The mean peak plasma concentrations, plasma clearance, and elimination half-life were 249 ± 80 and 227 ± 110 ng/mL, 268 ± 70 and 329 ± 58 liter/hr, and 29 ± 25 and 118 ± 119 hr, respectively. The concentration versus time data were best described by a three-compartment model. In the group with *P. carinii* pneumonia, trough concentrations increased progressively with time ($r = 0.91$, $p = 0.001$), without achieving steady state, and the renal/plasma clearance ratio was 2.1 ± 0.01%. In a third group of five patients with normal or mildly abnormal renal function who were being treated for *P. carinii* pneumonia, the elimination half-life was 12 ± 2.3 days after the last dose of pentamidine. These results indicate that the true elimination half-life of pentamidine is actually quite long, and that drug accumulation occurs even with daily dosing in patients with normal renal function. The investigators concluded that dose adjustment for pentamidine is unnecessary for patients with impaired renal function or patients receiving hemodialysis.

D. Conclusions

That the relative risk for nephrotoxicity and hypoglycemia is increased significantly for patients receiving a total dose of more than 4 g and after more than 2 weeks of therapy suggests that some adverse effects with pentamidine are dose-dependent. The pharmacokinetic data indicate that serum and presumably tissue concentrations of pentamidine accumulate with multiple dosing. Thus, it is important that the pharmacokinetic behavior of the drug be modeled in a manner that would lead to a rational dosage regimen to achieve selected therapeutic goals. It is likely that the dose of pentamidine could be reduced after an initial treatment period to maintain targeted concentrations and, thereby, reduce the total cumulative dose and risk of toxicity. However, we believe that there is currently insufficient evidence of the efficacy of low doses of pentamidine to warrant an empiric dosage of 3 mg/kg per day as standard therapy for *P. carinii* pneumonia. Further controlled studies need to be conducted to test the efficacy and safety of lower doses in more severely hypoxemic patients and to test the usefulness of adaptive control and individualized dosage regimens to achieve targeted concentrations, especially with multicompartmental models.

Aerosolized pentamidine has considerable appeal because of its markedly lower risk for producing systemic toxicity. However, inadequate regional alveolar deposition may occur in patients with rapid shallow breathing or with considerable air space consolidation. Thus, this form of therapy is probably best suited for patients with mild *P. carinii* pneumonia who cannot tolerate other treatments.

IV. Trimethoprim–Dapsone

Of therapies in widespread use for treatment of *P. carinii* pneumonia, the pharmacokinetic and pharmacodynamic considerations should affect the use of TMP plus dapsone perhaps more than any of the other therapies for this infection. Several studies have shown the potential of TMP and dapsone to interact with each other and with other agents.

A. Clinical Studies

In a double-blind trial, 60 patients with initial baseline Pao$_2$ greater than 60 torr were randomly assigned to receive 20 mg/kg of trimethoprim plus 100 mg of dapsone per day or oral TMP–SMX at 20 mg/kg per day (TMP component) for 3 weeks (24). Treatment efficacy was similar in the two groups, although the sample size was too small to determine any relevant difference in efficacy between the two therapies. Treatment-terminating drug toxicities were restricted to laboratory abnormalities and occurred in 17 patients (57%) in the TMP–SMX arm compared with 9 (30%) in the trimethoprim–dapsone arm ($p < 0.025$). Neutrophil counts declined to fewer than 750/mm^3 and liver transaminase levels rose to more than five times normal more often in patients treated with TMP–SMX. By contrast, clinical toxic reactions of intolerable rash and vomiting were similar in both groups.

However, all patients treated with the combination of TMP and dapsone developed methemoglobinemia, although the concentration exceeded 20% in only one individual. This is potentially the most serious complication of therapy, and it is most likely attributable to the sulfone structure of dapsone. Indeed, in a study of dapsone therapy alone, at 200 mg once daily, for patients with mild episodes of *P. carinii* pneumonia, methemoglobinemia was severe and contributed to an unacceptable failure rate (25). The study was terminated after seven patients had been enrolled because of two deaths and five failures. Treatment was terminated in four patients because of methemoglobinemia (9.5–17.4%) and respiratory distress, and none of the seven patients were able to successfully complete a full course of therapy with dapsone. It is possible that 200 mg was an excessive dose for AIDS patients, although doses of 300–400 mg/day are commonly prescribed for patients with leprosy and dermatitis herpetiformis without serious complications. Alternatively, patients with *P. carinii* pneumonia receiving 200 mg may have differed appreciably from the large number of patients who have been treated with TMP plus 100 mg of dapsone daily and in whom the combination is reasonably well tolerated (24). It is clear, however, that studies to determine the maximal tolerable dose of dapsone in patients at risk for *P. carinii* pneumonia, namely those with low CD4 lymphocyte counts, would provide valuable information in designing and testing regimens that contain this drug.

B. Pharmacokinetic and Interaction Studies

Pharmacokinetic studies of patients receiving TMP–SMX or trimethoprim plus dapsone, just discussed (26) and of 18 additional subjects with *P. carinii* pneumonia who were treated only with 100 mg/day of dapsone (27) have shown that there is a drug interaction between trimethoprim and dapsone. Peak serum concentrations of dapsone were 40% higher on treatment day 7 during concurrent therapy with trimethoprim than with dapsone alone (2.1 vs 1.5 μg/mL). Similarly, monoacetyl-dapsone, a major metabolite of dapsone, was 38% higher at the same time (1.2 vs 0.87 μg/mL). In addition, concentrations of trimethoprim on day 7 of therapy were 48% higher during concurrent therapy with dapsone than with SMX (18.4 vs 12.4 μg/mL). Both interactions reached statistical significance ($p < 0.05$). Thus, drug concentrations of both trimethoprim and dapsone are higher when the two agents are used together, compared with their use alone or with other antifolate compounds. The results suggest that the two drugs may be competing for sites of metabolism common to both drugs.

Other interactions may occur with dapsone. A recent investigation in which 66 patients with fewer than 200 CD4 lymphocytes were enrolled in the dideoxyinosine (DDI) expanded access program revealed that 11 of 28 patients who had been receiving prophylaxis for *P. carinii* pneumonia with 25 mg of dapsone four times daily developed *P. carinii* pneumonia within 10–130 days (mean of 66 days) after beginning treatment with DDI (28). By contrast, none of 17 patients receiving prophylaxis with TMP–SMX and only one of 12 receiving 300 mg of aerosolized pentamidine monthly developed *P. carinii* pneumonia. The most likely explanation for the high rate of breakthroughs of pneumocystis pneumonia in patients receiving both dapsone and DDI involves the buffer in the DDI sachet. The buffer contains citrate-phosphate to neutralize or alkalinize gastric contents, which is necessary for the absorption of DDI at its optimal pH of 7–8. However, in humans, dapsone is virtually insoluble at neutral or alkaline pH, but will completely dissolve in 100 mL of acidic gastric acid fluid. Thus, it is possible that the citrate-phosphate buffer in the sachet impaired the absorption of dapsone in these patients, resulting in the "apparent" failure of this drug to prevent patients from developing *P. carinii* pneumonia. It is unknown whether administering dapsone several hours before DDI, which is generally given twice daily, will overcome the problem. Some patients with AIDS have hypochlorhydria or even achlorhydria, and ingestion of the buffered medication 12–16 hr earlier may be sufficient to maintain a neutral or alkaline pH in the stomach before the next dose. If this were true, an altered dosing schedule would not overcome the problem.

C. Dosing in Renal Failure

Because of the bidirectional interference in clearance when both agents are used together and the absence of pharmacokinetic data for the combination in patients with renal impairment, little can be said about dosing for patients with diminished kidney function. However, both drugs have appreciable hepatic metabolism and extrarenal clearance. It is unlikely, therefore, that dosage modifications would be necessary for creatinine clearances above 30 mL/min. When the clearance is below 30 mL/min, the authors would empirically reduce the dose by 50% after 2–3 days of therapy. When the clearance is less than 5–10 mL/min, other therapies should be considered, since several of the metabolites excreted by the kidneys could accumulate to potentially toxic levels. If assays for these drugs were available to practitioners, serum concentrations could be monitored and dosages modified to achieve targeted levels, which would likely enable the drug combination to be used in patients with severe renal impairment.

D. Conclusions

The first study suggests that laboratory abnormalities occur less often with the combination of trimethoprim plus dapsone than with TMP–SMX, although clinical side effects are similar with the two therapies. Unfortunately, the trial did not establish whether trimethoprim–dapsone is of comparable efficacy to TMP–SMX because of the relatively small study population. Regardless, that trimethoprim–dapsone is associated with fewer episodes of toxicity makes this an attractive therapy.

Results of the pharmacokinetic study suggested that potentially effective treatment with the combination could be achieved with doses of trimethoprim lower than generally used with SMX, since there is a bidirectional interference in the clearance of both trimethoprim and dapsone when the two drugs are administered together. By extrapolation from observations with TMP–SMX that were discussed earlier, the dose of trimethoprim most likely need not exceed 15 mg/kg per day for patients with normal renal function. Because of the interaction with dapsone, it is conceivable that doses of trimethoprim in the 10–12 mg/kg per day range could be equally effective in combination with dapsone and might reduce the potential for adverse drug effects. Whether dapsone at a dosage of 100 mg daily, which was suboptimal for monotherapy of *P. carinii* pneumonia in one study (27), is the best dose for combination with trimethoprim is unclear. Only dose-ranging studies will answer these important questions. In addition, treatment with DDI should be suspended during therapies involving dapsone for *P. carinii* pneumonia until the interaction of the two agents is better delineated.

V. Clindamycin–Primaquine

A. Clinical Trials

The combination of clindamycin and the antimalarial drug primaquine has shown considerable promise for treatment of *P. carinii* pneumonia in uncontrolled studies (29). In one trial, 22 previously untreated patients with mild episodes of pneumocystis pneumonia received 900 mg, followed by 450 mg orally every 6 hr for 11 days, together with 30 mg of primaquine base orally once daily for 3 weeks. Twenty (91%) of these patients improved by day 7 of treatment; two failed and were switched to other therapies (30). Generalized rash was the most common adverse effect and occurred in 15 (68%) cases, but required treatment cessation in only three patients. Mild diarrhea occurred in one case. The trial was extended to evaluate oral clindamycin (450 mg three times daily) and the same dose of primaquine in 46 patients who had baseline $(A-a)Do_2$ less than 40 torr. Of the first 14 patients treated with all-oral therapy, 13 (93%) responded. Generalized rash occurred in 7 (54%) but was not treatment-limiting.

B. Conclusions

In these two studies, the combination of clindamycin plus primaquine appeared to be highly effective and, in fact, the therapy is being widely prescribed for *P. carinii* pneumonia. A generalized morbilliform rash was the most common adverse effect and occurred in most patients. Whether this side effect is related to dose is unknown.

Since neither agent alone has activity against *P. carinii* in the cortisone-treated rat (29), it is imperative to emphasize that monotherapy with either agent should not be prescribed for patients with *P. carinii* pneumonia. In addition, since there is currently no parenteral form of primaquine, the combination probably would not be suitable for patients in whom absorption of primaquine might be impaired (e.g., those with ileus or with upper bowel diarrhea).

VI. Experimental Therapies

Several promising experimental therapies are undergoing fast-track development. However, each has certain pharmacological limitations that could restrict their clinical usefulness.

A. Atovaquone

Atovaquone (BW 566C80) is a hydroxynaphthoquinone, originally developed in England as an antimalarial compound. It inhibits the mitochondrial electron transport that is necessary for the biosynthesis of pyrimidines in protozoa. In the steroid-suppressed rat, which has been highly predictive of the effectiveness of antipneumocystis pneumonia therapies in humans, atovaquone is not only curative at low doses, but relapse does not occur after treatment is stopped. This suggests that, unlike other agents, atovaquone may be "cidal" for *P. carinii* (31). Several of its pharmacokinetic properties are unique, including a terminal serum half-life of approximately 50 hr (32) and a bioavailability that increases appreciably with food. In fact, serum concentrations are two- to threefold higher after a fatty meal. Although results of atovaquone versus TMP–SMX in a multicenter, prospective controlled study appeared promising, patients with diarrhea had impaired absorption of this agent and a significantly higher failure rate (33). Thus, a better formulation should be developed for this agent to be fully effective.

B. Walter Reed Compound 6026

Water Reed (WR) compound 6026 is an 8-aminoquinoline that was developed by the military and used to treat leishmaniasis in Africa, with a good safety profile. The agent also appears to have excellent activity for treatment of *P. carinii* pneumonia in the rat model (34). In Phase I clinical testing in the United States, methemoglobinemia appeared to be a dose-related consequence of treatment with WR 6026, and concentrations of methemoglobin up to 6.9% were detected in normal volunteers treated with doses of 60 mg/day (35). Thus, dose evaluation studies need to be done to determine the magnitude of this effect in immunodeficient patients with decreased bone marrow reserve before the agent is tested in hypoxemic patients with *P. carinii* pneumonia.

VII. Summary

It is apparent from the studies reviewed that a body of data already exists to support the notion that for specific therapies of *P. carinii*, investigation of dose, serum concentrations, and pharmacodynamics are necessary for this concept to be fully applied to improve both efficacy and safety for all treatments of *P. carinii* pneumonia.

References

1. Kovacks JA, Hiemenz JW, Macher AM, Stover D, Murray HW, Shelhamer J, Lane HC, Urmacher C, Honig C, Longlo DL, Parker MM, Natanson C, Parrillo JE, Fauci AS, Pizzo PA, Masur H. *Pneumocystis carinii* pneumonia: a comparison between patients with the acquired immunodeficiency syndrome and patients with other immunodeficiencies. Ann Intern Med 1984; 100:663–671.
2. Wharton JM, Coleman DL, Wofsy CB, Luce JM, Blumenfield W, Hadly WK, Ingram-Drake L, Volberding PA, Hopewell PC. Trimethoprim–sulfamethoxazole or pentamidine for *Pneumocystis carinii* pneumonia in the acquired immunodeficiency syndrome: a prospective randomized trial. Ann Intern Med 1986; 105:37–44.
3. Jaffe HS, Abrams DI, Ammann AJ, Lewis BJ, Golden JA. Complications of co-trimoxazole in treatment of AIDS-associated *Pneumocystis carinii* pneumonia in homosexual men. Lancet 1983; 2:1109–1111.
4. Gordin FM, Simon GL, Wofsy CB, Mills J. Adverse reactions to trimethoprim–sulfamethoxazole in patients with the acquired immunodeficiency syndrome. Ann Intern Med 1984; 100:495–499.
5. Sattler FR, Cowan R, Nielsen DM, Ruskin J. Trimethoprim–sulfamethoxazole compared with pentamidine for treatment of *Pneumocystis carinii* pneumonia in the acquired immunodeficiency syndrome: a prospective, noncrossover study. Ann Intern Med 1988; 109:280–287.
6. Sattler FR, Allegra CJ, Verdegem TD, Akil B, Tuazon CU, Hughlett C, Ogata-Araki D, Feinberg J, Shelhamer J, Lane HC, Davis R, Boylen CT, Leedom JM, Masur H. Trimetrexate–leucovorin dosage evaluation study for treatment of *Pneumocystis carinii* pneumonia. J Infect Dis 1990; 161:91–96.
7. Miser JS, Savitch, Bleyer WA. Management of *Pneumocystis carinii* pneumonia [letter]. N Engl J Med 1977; 296:47.
8. Brenner M, Ognibene FP, Lack EE, Simmons JT, Suffredini AF, Lane HC, Fauci AS, Parrillo JE, Shelhamer JH, Masur H. Prognostic factors and life expectancy of patients with the acquired immunodeficiency syndrome and *Pneumocystis carinii* pneumonia. Am Rev Respir Dis 1987; 136:1199–1206.
9. Joos B, Blase JP, Chave JP, Opravil M, Luthy L. Monitoring of trimethoprim/sulfamethoxazole serum concentrations during high-dose therapy of *Pneumocystis carinii* pneumonia in human immunodeficiency virus-infected patients [abstract]. Prog Abstr 31st Intersci Conf Antimicrob Agents Chemother 1991; 228:136.
10. Schumitzky A. Nonparametric EM algorithms for estimating prior distributions. Technical report 90-2, USC Laboratory of Applied Pharmacokinetics. Appl Math Comput (in press).
11. Jelliffe R, Schumitzky A, Gomis P. A population model of gentamicin made with a new nonparametric EM (NPEM) algorithm. Technical report 90-4, USC Laboratory of Applied Pharmacokinetics. Clin Pharmacol Ther (submitted).
12. Dodge W, Jelliffe R, Richardson CJ, McCleery R, Hokanson J, Snodgrass W. Gentamicin population pharmacokinetic models for low birth weight infants using a new nonparametric method. Clin Pharmacol Ther 1991; 50:25–31.
13. Jelliffe R, D'Argenio D, Shumitzky A, Hu L, Liu M. The USC*PACK PC programs

for planning, monitoring, and adjusting drug dosage regimens. Proc 23rd Annu Meet Assoc Adv Med Instrum, Washington DC, May 14–18, 1988:51.
14. Sawchuk R, Zaske D. Pharmacokinetics of dosing regimens which utilize multiple intravenous infusions: gentamicin in burn patients. J Pharmacokinet Biopharm 1976; 4:183–195.
15. Waskin H, Stehr-Green J, Helmick CG, Sattler FR. Risk factors for hypoglycemia associated with pentamidine therapy of pneumocystis pneumonia. JAMA 1988; 260:345–347.
16. Conte JE Jr, Hollander H, Golden JA. Inhaled or reduced-dose intravenous pentamidine for *Pneumocystis carinii* pneumonia. A pilot study. Ann Intern Med 1987; 107:495–498.
17. Conte JE, Chernoff D, Feigal DW, Joseph P, McDonald C, Golden JA. Intravenous or inhaled pentamidine for treating *Pneumocystis carinii* pneumonia in AIDS. A randomized trial. Ann Intern Med 1990; 113:203–209.
18. Montgomery AB, Edison RE, Sattler F, Hopewell P, Mason G, Feigal D, the Aerosolized Pentamidine Study Group. Aerosolized pentamidine versus trimethoprim/sulfamethoxazole for acute *Pneumocystis carinii* pneumonia [abstract]. Proc VI Int Conf AIDS 1990; 6:220, ThB 395.
19. Soo Hoo GW, Mohsenifar Z, Meyer RD. Inhaled or intravenous pentamidine therapy for *Pneumocystis carinii* pneumonia in AIDS. A randomized trial. Ann Intern Med 1990; 113:195–202.
20. Conte JE, Upton RA, Phelp RT, Wofsy CB, Zurlinden E, Lin ET. Use of a specific and sensitive assay to determine pentamidine pharmacokinetics in patients with AIDS. J Infect Dis 1986; 154:923–929.
21. Navin TR, Dickinson CM, Adams SR, Mayersohn M, Juranek DD. Effect of azotemia in dogs on the pharmacokinetics of pentamidine. J Infect Dis 1987; 155:1020–1026.
22. Conte JE, Upton RA, Lin ET. Pentamidine pharmacokinetics in patients with AIDS with impaired renal function. J Infect Dis 1987; 156:885–890.
23. Conte JE Jr. Pharmacokinetics of intravenous pentamidine in patients with normal renal function or receiving hemodialysis. J Infect Dis 1991; 163:169–175.
24. Medina I, Mills J, Leoung G, et al. Oral therapy for *Pneumocystis carinii* pneumonia in the acquired immunodeficiency syndrome. A controlled trial of trimethoprim–sulfamethoxazole versus trimethoprim–dapsone. N Engl J Med 1990; 323:776–782.
25. Safrin S, Sattler FR, Lee BL, et al. Dapsone as a single agent is suboptimal therapy for *Pneumocystis carinii* pneumonia. J AIDS 1991; 4:244–249.
26. Lee BL, Medina I, Benowitz NL, Jacob P, Wofsy CB, Mills J. Dapsone, trimethoprim, and sulfamethoxazole plasma levels during treatment of *Pneumocystis carinii* pneumonia in patients with the acquired immunodeficiency syndrome (AIDS). Evidence of drug interactions. Ann Intern Med 1989; 110:606–611.
27. Mills J, Leoung G, Medina I, Hopewell PC, Hughes WT, Wofsy C. Dapsone treatment of *Pneumocystis carinii* pneumonia in the acquired immunodeficiency syndrome. Antimicrob Agents Chemother 1988; 32:1057–1060.
28. Metroka CE, McMechan MF, Andrada R, Laubenstein LJ, Jacobus DP. Failure of prophylaxis with dapsone in patients taking dideoxyinosine. N Engl J Med 1991; 325:737.

29. Queener SF, Bartlett MS, Richardson JD, Durkin MM, Jay MA, Smith JW. Activity of clindamycin with primaquine against *Pneumocystis carinii* in vitro and in vivo. Antimicrob Agents Chemother 1988; 32:807–813.
30. Black JR, Feinberg J, Murphy R, Fass RJ, Carey J, Sattler, FR. Clindamycin and primaquine as primary treatment for mild and moderately severe *Pneumocystis carinii* pneumonia in patients with AIDS. Eur J Clin Microbiol Infect Dis 1991; 10: 204–207.
31. Hughes WT, Gray VL, Gutteridge WE, Latter VS, Pudney M. Efficacy of a hydroxynaphthoquinone, 566C80, in experimental *Pneumocystis carinii* pneumonia. Antimicrob Agents Chemother 1990; 34:225–228.
32. Hughes WT, Kennedy W, Shenep JL, et al. Safety and pharmacokinetics of 566C80, a hydroxynapthoquinone with anti-*Pneumocystis carinii* activity: a Phase I study in HIV infected men. J Infect Dis 1991; 163:843–848.
33. Hughes W, Leoung G, Kramer F, Bozzette S, Frame P, Clumeck N, Masur H, Sattler F. Comparison of 556C80 and trimethoprim–sulfamethoxazole for treatment of *P. carinii* pneumonia [abstract]. Proc VIII Int Conf AIDS/III STD World Congr, Amsterdam, Netherlands, July, 1992; WeB 1019.
34. Bartlett MS, Queener SF, Tidwell RR, Milhous WK, Berman JD, Ellis WY. 8-Aminoquinolines from Walter Reed Army Institute for Research for treatment and prophylaxis of pneumocystic pneumonia in rat models. Antimicrob Agents Chemother 1991; 35:277–282.
35. Petty BG, Cornhauser DM, Shapiro TB. Multiple-dose pharmacokinetics, safety and tolerance of WR 6026 HCl in healthy subjects. Final report, task order 10, Contract No. DAMD17-85-C5133, 31 March 1990.

24

Development of Models and Their Use to Discover New Drugs for Therapy and Prophylaxis of *Pneumocystis carinii* Pneumonia

JAMES W. SMITH, MARILYN S. BARTLETT, and SHERRY F. QUEENER

Indiana University School of Medicine
Indianapolis, Indiana

I. Introduction

Pneumocystis carinii was considered to be a protozoan by many early researchers (1,2), and drugs with known antiprotozoal activity were tested for treatment of the pneumonia it caused. Pentamidine isethionate was the only recommended therapeutic agent, in spite of its significant side effects, until Hughes et al. (3), using the immunosuppressed rat model (4) found the first effective alternative, trimethoprim plus sulfamethoxazole. The combination could be used for prophylaxis in high-risk patients, and clinical cases become infrequent. With the onset of the AIDS epidemic in which *P. carinii* pneumonia was very frequent, it was noted that trimethoprim–sulfamethoxazole caused serious reactions, requiring cessation of therapy in many AIDS patients, thereby precluding widespread use of the combination for prophylaxis. Less toxic, yet more effective agents were needed. To screen numerous compounds for possible effectiveness, better models were required.

Several models have been developed or improved to test compounds for efficacy. The culture model employing feeder cells and measuring inhibition of proliferation of *P. carinii* trophic forms has been used extensively at Indiana University. Inhibition of labeled *para*-aminobenzoic acid (PABA) incorporation as a measure of activity of folate pathway antagonists has been used by Kovacs et al. (5) and Comley et al. (6). Direct evaluation of dihydrofolate reductase inhibitors by assay with enzyme extracted from *P. carinii* has been used by Queener (7). Animal models continue to be used for selection and evaluation of compounds. In this chapter we describe in some detail the cell culture method that has been used to identify potentially effective antipneumocystis compounds and list some of the other uses of organisms obtained from culture. In addition, other in vitro methods for drug evaluation are described, and both latent-infection rat models and transtracheally inoculated animal models are outlined.

II. Culture Method

The feeder cell culture method developed in our laboratory has been used both to evaluate compounds for antipneumocystis activity and to provide organisms for biochemical, molecular biological, and electron microscopic studies. Cultures have used human embryonic lung fibroblasts, WI-38, MRC-5, or HEL cells (8,9) in flasks, tissue culture plates, or in suspension cultures employing "spinner flasks" with microcarriers (10). *Pneumocystis carinii* from infected rat lung is the only source of *P. carinii* to reliably proliferate in the system described. During an outbreak of *P. carinii* pneumonia (11) when many biopsy specimens of human lung infected with *P. carinii* were cultured, all were unsuccessful (9). Recently, we developed a transtracheally inoculated mouse model that has provided very heavily infected lung from which to prepare inocula. Cultures using the mouse organisms likewise have been unsuccessful (9), as have cultures of *P. carinii* from infected ferret lung. Jackson et al. reported there was proliferation of *P. carinii* from rat lung in cultures employing human embryonic lung fibroblasts, MRC-5, but not WI-38 VA13. Cultures were sampled over 8 days, similarly to our method. Yields reported were comparable with those we have reported for MRC-5, WI-38, and HEL cells. Our tests of WI-38 VA13 agreed with those of Jackson, indicating little or no proliferation. Jackson did not evaluate WI-38 or HEL cells (12).

Initially, when latently infected rat lungs were used for inocula for culture, we found great variability in proliferation among cultures. This inconsistency may result from variability of strains of *P. carinii* or from other undefined factors. Since we have been using *P. carinii* from transtracheally inoculated rats, culture results have been more consistent, perhaps related to the strain of *P. carinii* used. Cultures using organisms from lungs of transtracheally inoculated rats regularly show a three- to tenfold increase in numbers of trophozoites over 7–10 days, at which time proliferation ceases.

Cultures provide a source of organisms with few contaminating host cells or attached host material. Cultures have provided organisms for characterization of the β-tubulin gene (13), study of components of the surface glycoprotein (14), and studies of binding sites including fibronectin (15) and mannose-specific receptor of surfactant protein A (16). Electron microscopic studies using organisms from culture have helped in development of improved fixation that allows better definition of organelles (17), shows cell organism associations (18), and demonstrates drug effects on ultrastructure for investigating mechanisms of drug action (19). Spinner cultures using cells sheeted on Cytodex beads in suspension have allowed sequential sampling over time for study of attachment, metabolism, and drug effects, as well as for provision of large numbers (10^8–10^9) of relatively pure organisms (10).

III. Culture Screen

Use of the culture screen to select agents for trial in animals has been described (8). Briefly, monolayers of WI-38, MRC-5, or HEL cells are sheeted to confluency and then inoculated with *P. carinii* trophozoite forms obtained from infected rat lungs. We have shown that trophozoite forms are required for proliferation with this system (20). Inoculum is prepared by grinding heavily infected rat lung in a Ten Broeck grinder and centrifuging slowly ($200\times$ g) to settle lung material. Organisms in the supernate are counted using Giemsa stain. Viability is assessed with fluorescein diacetate and ethidium bromide, as described by Jackson et al. (21) and adapted for *P. carinii* by Bartlett et al. (22). Fluorescein diacetate is metabolized by viable organisms to fluorescein, which fluoresces green, whereas ethidium bromide binds to nucleic acid of dead organisms and fluoresces red. Organisms in inocula are counted and the number of viable organisms in the inoculum is adjusted to provide approximately 7×10^5 viable organisms per plate well (1 mL). The size of inoculum is crucial for culture success.

Culture plates include four wells for each parameter, for each time point, and always incorporate both untreated control wells and either trimethoprim–sulfamethoxazole- or pentamidine-treated control wells. Plates are incubated at 38°C in an atmosphere of 5–10% CO_2, 5% O_2, with the balance N_2. Samples are taken on days 1, 3, 5, 7, and 10. After gentle agitation to suspend organisms that have settled or are loosely attached to cells, 10-µL samples are removed and placed on 1-cm² areas on slides. Slides are evaluated for numbers of *P. carinii* trophozoites, cysts, and contaminating feeder cells by microscopic examination of Giemsa-stained samples, and for *P. carinii* antigen by enzyme-linked immunosorbent assay (ELISA) (23) using convalescent rat anti-*P. carinii* polyvalent antisera. We have shown that numbers of organisms in Giemsa stain correlate with numbers in fluorescein diacetate viability stain (22). A photomicrograph of Giemsa-stained *P. carinii* trophozoites from culture supernate is shown in Figure 1.

Growth curves are plotted for the untreated and drug-treated culture wells so that numbers of organisms in drug-treated wells can be compared with numbers in

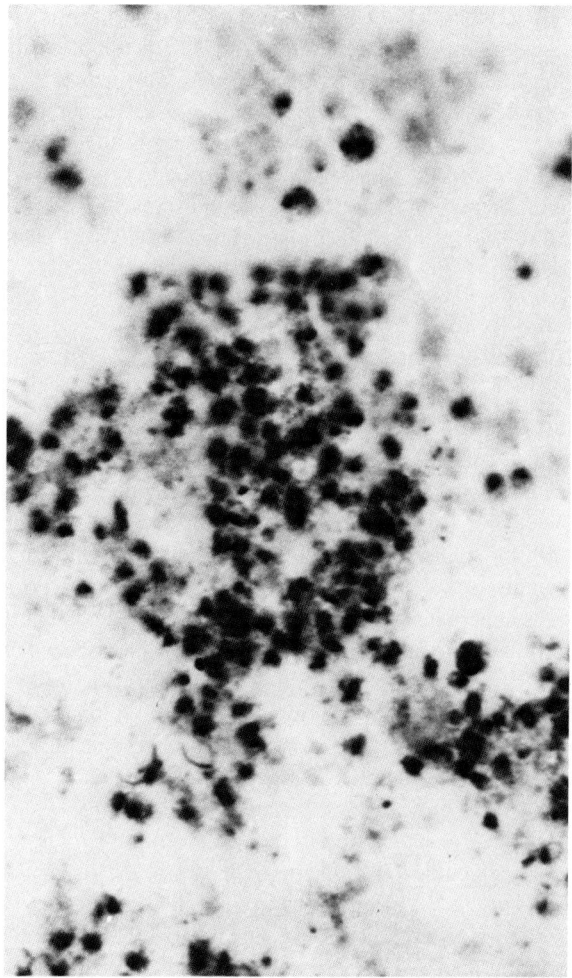

Figure 1 Giemsa-stained clump of trophozoites of *P. carinii* in supernate from culture with HEL cells (original magnification 1250×).

the untreated wells. For a culture to be evaluated, untreated wells must show at least threefold proliferation. These comparisons allow assessment of activity of the trial drugs. We have also developed an ELISA system to quantitate antigens of *P. carinii* in culture supernates. The antisera is from transtracheally inoculated rats, immunosuppressed with dexamethasone, that develop severe *P. carinii* pneumonia in 4 weeks, at which time immunosuppression is stopped. Antisera is obtained 6–8 weeks later.

A sample growth curve showing *P. carinii* growth inhibition by primaquine and WRAIR compound BH58522 is shown in Figure 2. Proliferation of *P. carinii* over 7 days was demonstrated both by the ELISA (absorbance units) on days 1, 3, 5, and 7, and by direct counts of number of organisms detected with Giemsa stain of measured samples on day 7. On day 7, untreated control culture wells had absorbance of 0.55 and an average of eight organisms per 1000 × field, as compared with culture wells treated with primaquine at 1.0 µg/mL, which had absorbance of 0.1 and fewer than one organism per 1000 × field. The other drug tested, BH58522, gave a dose–response curve, with the concentration of 1.0 µg/mL being very inhibitory (absorbance <0.2), and the concentration of 0.1 µg/mL being similar to the untreated control. The excellent correlation between Giemsa-stain counts and ELISA is shown by the representative graph of correlation in Figure 3. The reproducibility of the method and similarity of growth curves is demonstrated in Figure 4, a composite of culture studies showing both Giemsa counts and ELISA values.

Cell monolayers are examined by phase microscopy for alterations of morphology. Detection of direct drug toxicity (rounding or sloughing of cells)

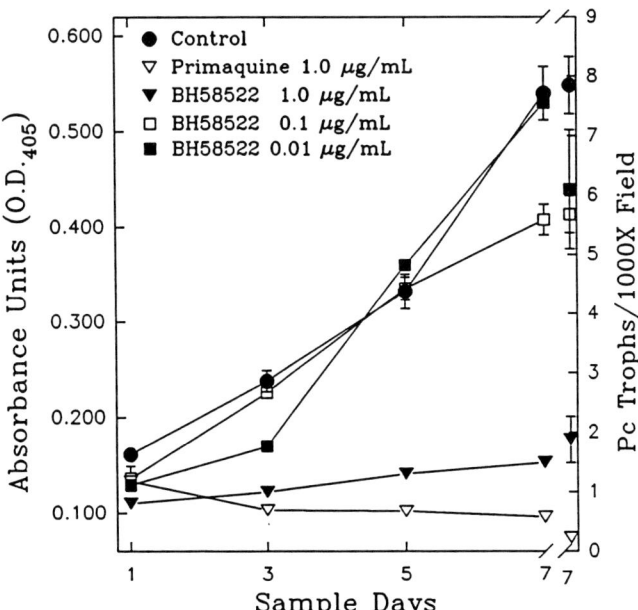

Figure 2 Growth curve of primaquine and dose response curves of compound BH 58522 plotted using data from ELISA antigen detection for 7 days and including day 7 Giemsa-stain counts.

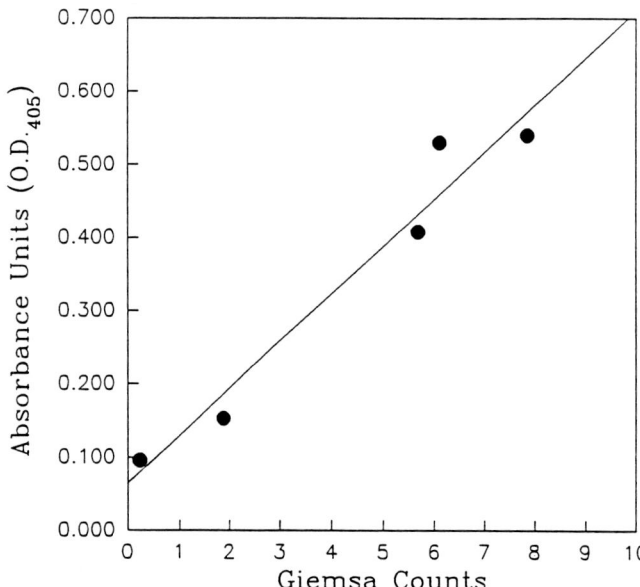

Figure 3 Correlation of day 7 ELISA values and Giemsa counts for compound BH 58522.

precludes evaluation for drug effects on *P. carinii*. With intact adherent monolayers of normal morphology, it is assumed that effects of drugs are by their action against *P. carinii*, rather than damage to feeder cell monolayers.

The culture system for *P. carinii* is crude and expensive compared with most culture systems used for susceptibility testing of bacteria and fungi, but susceptibility testing employing tissue culture has been used for other organisms (24). It has proved useful for selection of compounds to progress to testing in animals (25–28).

The advantages of the culture screen include rapid assessment of drugs (10 days vs 2 months for rat models) at relatively low cost. Time for culture evaluation as compared with animal evaluation is shown in Figure 5. Moreover, high concentrations that could not be tolerated in vivo may be tested in this system. Activity at a high dose may suggest that related compounds should be tested. The in vitro system also affords the ability to test combinations of drugs rapidly and inexpensively. Since we have ben using culture inocula of *P. carinii* from transtracheally inoculated virus-free rats raised in microisolator cages, we have had little problem with microbial contamination of cultures.

Disadvantages are several. If a drug must be metabolized to an active form, its effectiveness may be missed in all in vitro systems. Conversely, drugs that are rapidly inactivated in animals, but not in culture may appear active in culture,

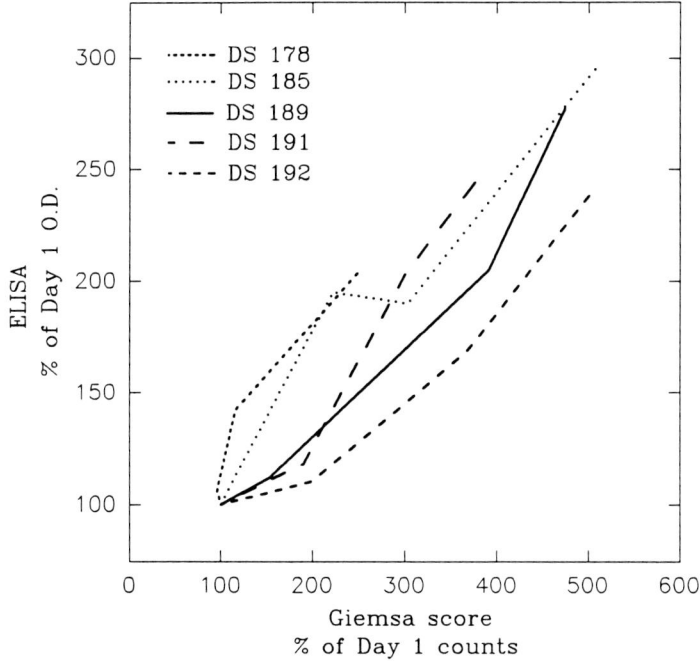

Figure 4 Giemsa counts and ELISA data for five drugs labeled DS 178, 185, 189, 191, and 192 are shown. Growth curves are similar. Data are for both ELISA and Giemsa counts.

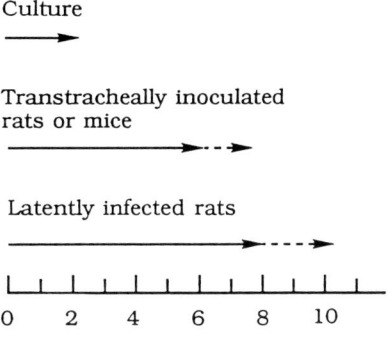

Figure 5 Time required for evaluation of drug effects on *P. carinii*.

but not in animals. Drugs that deteriorate in culture medium may not appear effective because drug is added only once, at the beginning of the test. The same drug might be effective in an animal model in which the drug is administered frequently. Occasionally, drugs are effective in culture, but do not prove effective in animal models. An example of such a drug is chloroquine, which is effective in culture at 10 µg/mL but not effective in rats at 20 mg/kg. A pharmacological explanation for this discrepancy is hypothesized, but has not been proved.

In vitro activity of related compounds may not always correlate with relative efficacy in animal models for a variety of reasons, including those just outlined. Nevertheless, we have observed close correlation with some classes of compounds. For example, the 8-aminoquinoline that was most active in culture (WR242511) was also most active in the animal model (25). Conversely, for the diamidines, although culture showed activity of compounds that were active in rats, it did not predict relative efficacy of these compounds in animals. Because the culture system has suggested numerous drugs for testing in animals, we have not tested culture-negative compounds, except in one instance. Isoprinosine was negative in culture and was also tested in rats where it showed no activity.

In spite of shortcomings, but considering the thousands of potentially effective compounds, initial screening of drugs with the culture model has allowed us to focus on those with demonstrated activity against *P. carinii*. With this short-term culture system we have screened over 300 compounds in culture, many of which were subsequently confirmed to be effective in animal models. For example, culture demonstrated inhibition of growth of *P. carinii* by trimetrexate (29), piritrexim (29), 9-deazainosine (28), primaquine (26), the 8-aminoquinolines, WR 6026, WR 238605, and WR 242511 from Walter Reed Army Institute for Research (25), BW 566C80, and analogues of pentamidine.

IV. In Vitro Evaluations of Folate Pathway Antagonists

The [^{3}H]PABA incorporation method has evaluated several compounds (6). All of these compounds are also active in the short-term culture method, as reported in the foregoing.

The enzyme assay developed by Queener (7) has been used to evaluate almost 800 folate inhibitors and has discovered 31 compounds with significant activity against *P. carinii* dihydrofolate reductase. These compounds are currently being tested in culture and animal models.

V. Animal Models

Models include both latently infected rats and transtracheally inoculated rats. All early work with *P. carinii* used the latent-infection model described by Weller (2) and Frenkel (4) in which rats, immunocompromised with adrenal corticosteroids, developed *P. carinii* pneumonia through activation of latent infections. Frenkel showed that rats became infected with *P. carinii* when housed with immunocompromised rats with *P. carinii* pneumonia. Hendley (30) showed that infection could be enhanced by increasing immunosuppression with a low-protein diet.

Models using latently infected rats have been used extensively to evaluate drug efficacy. Hughes showed that trimethoprim–sulfamethoxazole was effective both for prophylaxis and therapy (3). He also used the rat model to show effectiveness of dapsone (31), BW 566C80 (32), and the combination of macrolides and sulfamethoxazole (33). The following compounds were also shown effective in similar models: tetroxoprim (34), trimetrexate (35), clindamycin plus primaquine, trimetrexate and piritrexim, (26,29), 9-deazainosine (28), β1-3-glucan inhibitors (36), antitrypanosomal agents (37), and aerosolized pentamidine (38).

The latent-infection model, although widely used, has several disadvantages. One disadvantage is that there is no standard latently infected rat model. Rats used for evaluation of drugs have been from a variety of suppliers and most have been infected with a variety of other organisms. Weight and sex of animals have varied as have diet and method of immunosuppression. Problems in comparing results are most obvious in the differences in severity of infection detected. Other variables include methods for evaluating the degree of infection, numbers of animals per group, and times of evaluation.

Hayes et al. (39) used dexamethasone at 2.0 mg/liter in water, had three nonimmunosuppressed and six immunosuppressed rats per group, and evaluated *P. carinii* infection by immune-specific staining of cysts. They found that nonimmunosuppressed rats had mild infection, defined as 11–1100 cysts per sample, and immunosuppressed rats had heavy infection, defined as 10,000 cysts per sample only after 10 weeks. He stated, "A somewhat variable level of infection was observed in the treated groups (a reflection of the unpredictability of the immunosuppressed latent rat model), but there was a general increase in infection with time."

Eisen (40) used 35 rats, 5 per group, with one group given nothing and the others immunosuppressed with cortisone acetate, 50 mg/mL twice a week. All but one immunosuppressed group of 5 were also given intranasal inoculations. Of the 30 immunosuppressed rats, 26 lived to be evaluated, and 2 had detectible cysts in lungs. The author states, "The prevalence and intensity of *P. carinii* in lungs of cortisonized rats were far lower than reported in previous experiments (e.g., Frenkel et al., 1966)."

Hendley (30) and Frenkel (4) both pointed out the importance of spread from infected to uninfected animals in open cages. Hendley reported that isolated steroid-treated rats failed to develop *P. carinii*, but four steroid-treated animals housed with infected animals became infected.

D'Antonio et al. (41) reported a careful study employing 106 rats. Animals were immunosuppressed with dexamethasone and either treated with trimethoprim plus sulfamethoxazole alone or with folinic acid. In the control group of ten rats given immunosuppression only, five rats (50%) had detectible infection when sacrificed at 8 weeks.

Because of this variation in severity of infection from animal to animal in the latently infected rat model, our laboratory studied ways to minimize the differences. It was observed that the severity of infection correlated with weight loss (42), such that the animals losing the most weight had the most severe infection. Selecting rats for drug treatment so that study groups had similar mean weights helped compensate for the variability from animal to animal. With the latent model, most *P. carinii* workers are well aware of the problem of differences in severity of *P. carinii* infection in rats and house newly acquired animals in the same room with infected animals to assure that all become infected. Animals as received from suppliers whose colonies contain latent *P. carinii* infections may have only a small percentage of animals with latent infection. For new workers or those who cannot afford to keep large numbers of *P. carinii*-infected animals on hand, there may be difficulty in reproducibly developing infections. Colonies with latent *P. carinii* infection are usually not virus-free and may have other potentially pathogenic microorganisms, such as bacteria, viruses, and fungi that rapidly proliferate when the animals are immunosuppressed.

The variability in severity of *P. carinii* infection among latently infected animals makes drug effects more difficult to assess; in addition, other infecting organisms may lead to loss of animals before evaluation times. Both of these problems have been partially solved by use of virus-free rats that are transtracheally inoculated with *P. carinii* (43). The inoculated rats have infections of uniform severity, and time for development of heavy infections is less than for the latently infected model because animals start with a larger number of organisms. In addition, fewer animals are lost to infections by contaminating organisms. The inoculated rat model precludes the necessity of maintaining large rat colonies and allows use of virus free rats as required by many animal facilities.

The inoculated rat model was used to evaluate 8-aminoquinolines by Bartlett et al. and compared with a latent-infected rat model for evaluation of the same compounds by Tidwell (25). Data for both rat models testing WR 6026, WR 238605, and WR 242511 are shown in Table 1. In both models the three 8-aminoquinolines inhibited *P. carinii* such that infectivity scores were markedly reduced compared with untreated controls. Although the models and methods used for their evaluation were different, both showed that the compounds were very effective in inhibiting *P. carinii*.

In collaboration with Dr. Jay Fishman we developed the transtracheally inoculated rat model in 1987 and, in ensuing years, have found the model consistent and reproducible. Scores for Giemsa-stained samples for ten of our first studies are shown in Table 2. In controls the scores for the ten studies ranged

Use of Models in New Drugs Development

Table 1 IU/UNC Correlation: Comparative Study IU, Indianapolis, and UNC, Chapel Hill[a]

Drug/dose	IU mean score[b]	UNC mean score[b]	UNC rats/score					IU rats/score				
			0.5	1	2	3	4	≤0.5	1	2	3	4
238605 4 mg/kg	0.0	0.9	4	5	1	0	0	10	0	0	0	0
242511 2 mg/kg	0.0	0.6	9	1	0	0	0	10	0	0	0	0
6026 2 mg/kg	0.4	0.7	6	4	0	0	0	9	0	1	0	0
Untreated	3.4	3.0	0	0	1	8	1	0	0	1	5	4

Comparison of IU, Indianapolis, and UNC, Chapel Hill, scoring methods

IU Indianapolis	UNC Chapel Hill	
Counts numbers of organisms, both trophozoites and cysts, in impression smears of lung and after counting between 10 and 50 1000× fields arrives at score	Evaluates involvement of lung by examining silver-stained sections and determining percentage of lung involved	
No organisms in 50 fields = 0	No score of zero (whole lung required)	
1 or 2 organisms in 50 fields = 0.5	<10 cysts in 2 sections	= 0.5
1 organism in 10 field = 1.0	<5% lung involved (scattered cysts)	= 1.0
2–9 organisms in 10 fields = 2.0	10–25% lung involved (limited focal)	= 2.0
1–10 organisms per field = 3.0	26–50% lung involved	= 3.0
11–100 organisms per field = 4.0	>50% lung involved	= 4.0
>100 per field = 5.0		

[a]IU, Indiana University; UNC, University of North Carolina.
[b]Silver scores.

from 3.2 to 4.8, with a mean and standard error of 4.1 ± 0.4, a very close range. Likewise, the trimethoprim plus sulfamethoxazole treatment animals had similar scores. The mean and standard error was 0.58 ± 0.3, a close range.

Rats inoculated with *P. carinii* are now being used in several centers. The transtracheally inoculated model has been modified and used for drug evaluation by Boylan and Current (44–46), with consistently infected immunosuppressed control animals, but not uninoculated control animals.

A. Inoculated Rat Model

The inoculated rat model at Indiana University uses 120- to 140-g female Sprague–Dawley or Lewis rats from Harlan Sprague–Dawley colony 202, Indianapolis,

Table 2 Giemsa-Stain Mean Score ± Standard Error: Early Studies with Inoculated Rats

Study no.	Untreated control	Trimethoprim–sulfomethexozole-treated (50/250 mg/kg per day)
1	4.4 ± 0.2	0.6 ± 0.1
2	4.0 ± 0.3	0.6 ± 0.1
3	4.8 ± 0.1	0.1 ± 0.0
4	4.2 ± 0.2	0.8 ± 0.2
5	4.4 ± 0.3	0.3 ± 0.1
6	3.2 ± 0.7	0.4 ± 0.2
7	4.2 ± 0.1	0.5 ± 0.4
8	4.3 ± 0.2	1.4 ± 0.3
9	3.8 ± 0.3	0.6 ± 0.3
10	4.6 ± 0.1	1.1 ± 0.5

Indiana, which provides virus-free rats. Rats are immunosuppressed with dexamethasone at 0.36 mg/kg per day administered in drinking water for at least 4 days or until lymphocytes are depleted by 50%, or with methyl prednisolone at 20–40 mg/kg administered subcutaneously once a week. Animals are anesthetized by intramuscular injection with 0.2 mL ketamine "cocktail" composed of ketamine hydrochloride, 80 mg/mL, atropine, 0.38 mg/mL, and acepromazine, 1.76 mg/mL. A small (1-cm) midline neck incision is made and with blunt dissection the tracheal rings are exposed. A 0.2-mL aliquot of supernate from ground rat lung containing about 10^6 trophozoites is injected directly into the trachea followed by 0.4 mL of air. The wound is closed with a clip. Animals will be sufficiently infected in 3–4 weeks to begin therapy studies. Untreated animals will progress to very heavy infections in the additional 2–3 weeks required for therapy of the other rats. To assess levels of infection in control and drug-treated rats, impression smears are prepared from representative lung samples. Smears are stained with both Giemsa and modified methenamine silver nitrate stain and examined by three microscopists. Smears are blinded and scored by the three observers on a scale of 0–5, according to the scheme outlined in Table 1. Scores of Giemsa-stained samples from heavily infected animals are always higher than scores of silver-stained samples because of the large number of trophozoite forms. Conversely, lightly infected animals may have higher silver scores than Giemsa scores because the cyst wall stain makes rare cyst forms more easily detected and also detects empty cysts. Since the two stains have different optimal detection capabilities, we use both for evaluation of all animal samples. Inoculum for the rats is prepared as described for the culture model, and the numbers of trophozoites adjusted so that there are about 10^6 in 0.2 mL. Rat lung, which is frozen slowly and stored at $-80°$ to $-195°C$, may be used for preparation of inocula, allowing flexibility in use of rats for drug testing. For all drug testing, animals are used in groups of ten.

The inoculated rat model has also been used to test drugs for prophylaxis and for intermittent prophylaxis (27). Again, immunocompromised rats are infected by transtracheal inoculation as described earlier, but the drug administration is begun immediately and continued for 6 weeks, at which time animals are sacrificed. This model has been shown to give results comparable with the prophylaxis studies done with latently infected rats.

Data for prophylaxis studies using transtracheally inoculated rats are shown in Table 3, which shows infectivity scores for rats given clindamycin plus primaquine for prophylaxis. A study with latently infected rats showed reduction of *P. carinii*. In the inoculated rat model the same drug doses given prophylactically reduced scores to the same level, but the untreated control rats had much greater severity of infection, 4.4 ± 0.3.

An ideal therapy will eradicate *P. carinii*. If infection is only suppressed or if resistance develops, relapse will occur when therapy is stopped. One of the problems with trimetrexate for therapy in humans was the high rate of relapse (47). Drugs that initially appear effective only to have unacceptable degrees of relapse are not as useful for therapy and might be given lower priority for evaluation in drug trials if the propensity for relapse were recognized. Transtracheally inoculated rats may be used to test for relapse to drug therapy. To our knowledge, this is the only published relapse model. Hughes (48) described use of trimethoprim–sulfamethoxazole (TMP–SMX) at 50/250 mg/kg per day to treat latently infected rats for 2, 4, or 6 weeks, then placed animals in isolator cages and began immunosuppression with dexamethasone. Most animals developed *P. carinii* infection, regardless of the length of TMP–SMX administration. Unfortunately, there were no known *P. carinii*-negative animals in isolator cages to prove that the isolation procedures were adequate. The lack of effectiveness in this study by Hughes may have been because latent organisms are not very susceptible to killing by TMP–SMX or because animals became reinfected even though they were housed in isolator cages.

The relapse model we use requires 20 rats for each test parameter. At the conclusion of the treatment period, half of the rats in each group are sacrificed and evaluated for effectiveness of the trial drugs for therapy. The second half of each group is moved to individual isolator cages and continued on immunosuppression for an additional 4–6 weeks and then evaluated for *P. carinii* infection. Animals that receive therapy that eliminates *P. carinii* organisms will remain free of *P. carinii* after the period of additional immunosuppression. In contrast, animals receiving therapy that has only suppressed the infection, or animals in which resistance has developed, will show moderate or severe *P. carinii* pneumonia after the additional period of immunosuppression. It is critical to house animals in strict

Table 3 Prophylaxis Models

	Latent rat model			Inoculated rat model	
Regimen	Giemsa score ± SEM	Silver score ± SEM	Regimen	Giemsa score ± SEM	Silver score ± SEM
Untreated	2.6 ± 0.2	3.3 ± 0.1	Untreated	4.4 ± 0.3	3.9 ± 0.1
Clindamycin 50/primaquine 0.2 mg/kg per day	1.8 ± 0.1	2.2 ± 0.2	Clindamycin 225/primaquine 0.57 mg/kg per day	1.4 ± 0.4	1.8 ± 0.3
			Trimethoprim 50/sulfamethoxazole 250 50/250 mg/kg per day	0.07 ± 0.1	0.1 ± 0.1

isolation for relapse studies, as it is well documented that infection is spread by the airborne route (4). Two sets of controls are necessary for the study of drug relapse. The initial untreated controls must be sacrificed with the initial therapy study animals to establish the degree of infection produced by the inoculum. (They would die of infection if not sacrificed at this time.) A second set of immunosuppressed uninoculated controls are placed in individual isolator cages at the start of the relapse phase to assure that the isolation procedure is effective. If these animals remain free of *P. carinii* infection after the immunosuppressive period, any infection in the study animals can be ascribed to relapse, rather than to reinfection. Animals receiving immunosuppression for the long period required for relapse evaluation are extremely fragile and often die from the effects of the immunosuppression. Data from a relapse study are shown in Table 4, which shows, for example, that seven of eight animals treated with WR 238605 at 4 mg/kg per day for 3 weeks did not relapse when placed in isolation and continued on immunosuppression. The fact that one in nine animals was infected at the conclusion of therapy is consistent with a relapse rate of one in eight after the additional period of immunosuppression. Animals treated with trimethoprim–sulfamethoxazole had a similar response to initial therapy, with 3 of 11 being infected at the end of treatment. Only four animals survived the continued immunosuppression and of these three were infected.

In a second study of relapse with trimethoprin–sulfamethoxazole, 15 transtracheally inoculated immunosuppressed rats were treated with TMP–SMX 50/250 mg/kg per day, given in drinking water for 3 weeks. At the end of treatment, 5 animals were sacrificed and evaluated for infection; of these, 3 had rare organisms, whereas untreated controls were heavily infected. Of the 8 animals that survived the 4 weeks of continued immunosuppression without therapy, 6 had no infection and 2 had low levels of infection.

As with other antimicrobials, dosage may be important in determining whether relapse will occur. Higher doses than those tested might eliminate the rare surviving organisms and prevent relapse.

B. Inoculated Mouse Model

We have recently developed a transtracheally inoculated mouse model (49). Mice are useful for testing drugs that are in short supply, as less drug is required. Mice may be housed in larger numbers per cage, decreasing costs for animal maintenance. Immunosuppressed BALB/c mice are transtracheally inoculated with infected mouse lung in the same fashion as described for rats. The model has been used to evaluate drugs and has given results similar to those of the rat model for the limited number of the drugs evaluated. Data comparing a mouse model drug evaluation with a rat model drug evaluation are shown in Table 5.

For the inoculated mouse model, female 18- to 22-g BALB/c mice are

Table 4 Relapse Model Evaluation of 8-Aminoquinoline WR 6026, WR 238605, and Clindamycin Plus Primaquine

Drug dose	Initial treatment score		Number infected of total		Relapse score		Number infected of total	
	Giemsa	Silver	Giemsa	Silver	Giemsa	Silver	Giemsa	Silver
WR 6026 2 mg/kg per day	0.1	0.4	1/12	5/12	3.3	3.3	11/11	3/10
WR 238605 4 mg/kg per day	0.0	0.0	0/9	1/9	0.1	0.3	1/8	1/8
Clindamycin 225 mg/kg per day + primaquine 2 mg/kg per day	0.6	1.0	5/7	5/7	4.3	3.8	3/3	3/3
Trimethoprim 50 mg/kg per day + sulfamethoxazole 250 mg/kg per day	0.2	0.3	2/11	3/11	0.3	0.8	3/4	3/4
Untreated initial	4.3	3.4	6/6	6/6				
Sentinels control	0	0	0/5	0/5				

Numbers of rats surviving the additional 4 weeks of imunosuppression were low. Animals that died during the relapse period did not die of *P. carinii* infection (many were not infected), but could not be included in evaluation because they might have relapsed by the end of the period.

Table 5 Infectivity Scores of Transtracheally Inoculated Rats and Mice Treated with Known Antipneumocystis Therapies Clindamycin–Primaquine and Trimethoprim–Sulfamethoxazole

Treatment[a] (mg/kg per day)	Mouse mean score		Rat mean score	
	Giemsa score	Silver score	Giemsa score	Silver score
Clindamycin 225 ($n = 1$)	4.4 ± 0.2 ($n = 1$)	3.4 ± 0.2	4.4 ± 0.2 ($n = 1$)	3.8 ± 0.1
Primaquine 2.0 ($n = 1$)	4.4 ± 0.2 ($n = 1$)	3.4 ± 0.1	4.3 ± 0.3 ($n = 1$)	3.4 ± 0.3
Clindamycin 225 + primaquine 2.0 ($n = 1$)	2.1 ± 0.7 ($n = 1$)	1.9 ± 0.6	2.8 ± 0.4 ($n = 1$)	3.0 ± 0.3
Trimethoprim 50/ sulfamethoxazole 250 ($n = 5$)	0.1 ± 0.1 ($n = 5$)	0.1 ± 0.1	0.5 ± 0.1 ($n = 7$)	0.4 ± 0.1
Untreated ($n = 7$)	4.0 ± 0.2 ($n = 7$)	3.3 ± 0.1	4.2 ± 0.2 ($n = 7$)	3.8 ± 0.1

[a]n = number of studies.

immunosuppressed with dexamethasone at 1.2 mg/kg per day for 10–11 days before inoculation with 0.05 mL suspension of *P. carinii* organisms from an infected mouse lung, prepared as described for rats. Mice are anesthetized with 50 μL per mouse of ketamine cocktail, described earlier. Mice develop moderate infection in 3–4 weeks, at which time therapy may be started. Just as for rats, the untreated control animals will have very heavy infections after the additional 2–3 weeks of treatment of the other animals.

Mice differ from rats in the appearance of the organisms in impression smears of lungs. In mice, *P. carinii* organisms are in massive clumps, whereas, in rats, the organisms are more uniformly dispersed. In examining mouse lung impression smears microscopically, it is best to use lower-power objectives (50× oil-immersion) and look at several fields, because the clumping makes distribution less uniform than for rats. Photomicrographs of a heavily infected rat lung impression smear and a heavily infected mouse lung impression smear are shown in Figure 6.

An animal model for drug evaluation that is not dependent on immunosuppression by adrenal corticosteroids is useful for study of drugs that are immune modulators. The use of monoclonal antibodies to suppress specific lymphocyte populations shows promise for developing such models. In a mouse model, described by Shellito et al. (50), mice were immunosuppressed by using monoclonal antibody from clone GK1.5 against the L3T4 lymphocyte marker (51). These animals developed *P. carinii* infection, but the model was not used for drug

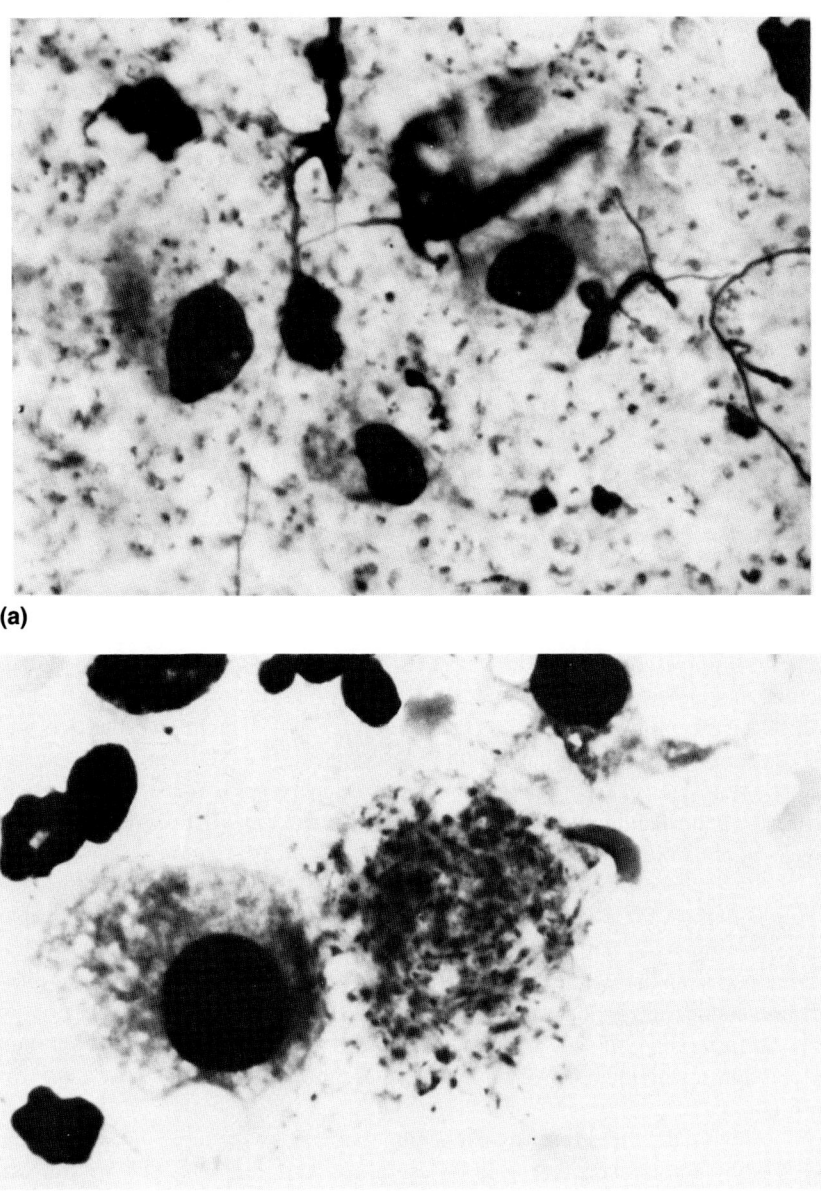

Figure 6 Giemsa-stained impression smears of *P. carinii*-infected rat and mouse lungs. (a) Infected rat lung has *P. carinii* trophic forms distributed throughout. (b) Infected mouse lung has clumps of trophic forms (original magnifications 1250×).

testing. We are currently evaluating this antibody model for drug testing, and it shows promise. The costs of producing monoclonal antibody in ascites of nude mice and its subsequent concentration and standardization are significant, precluding the routine use of this model.

C. Technical Difficulties with Animal Models

There are inherent problems with all animal testing as well as culture testing for selection of drugs for treatment of *P. carinii* pneumonia in humans. Finding the appropriate dose and route of administration is a major problem in designing successful drug evaluation studies in animals. Often drugs submitted for testing are nearly insoluble and require vehicles that may be toxic in themselves (e.g., dimethyl sulfoxide) or that may inactivate the test compound. Drugs given in suspension by subcutaneous injection may be poorly absorbed and may appear ineffective because they never reach the site of infection. Suspensions of compounds are difficult to administer. If they cannot be given by injection because of toxicity or poor absorption, the alternative route is oral, requiring gavage. If a drug has a relatively short half-life, treatment must be frequent. Even daily gavage can be detrimental to the fragile immunosuppressed animals. Daily gavaging, even with the most experienced animal handlers, causes irritation of the esophagus and minute abrasions that may make the animal refuse to eat or drink or may cause development of bacteremia from oral bacteria. We have found that rats or mice gavaged daily for 2 weeks or longer often lose weight and die. Necropsy samples of liver, kidney, and lung have shown death resulted from bacterial infection, usually with streptococci or staphylococci. Long-term treatments need to be as gentle as possible. Administration of drug in drinking water is preferred if the drug is soluble and stable, as it assures constant blood and tissue levels. Once- or twice-a-day administration of a rapidly cleared or inactivated drug may provide insufficient tissue levels. It would be ideal if pharmacokinetic and stability data for the appropriate animal species were available for each drug; however, it would be extremely costly.

Although effectiveness in rats has been a useful predictor for efficacy in humans, the numbers of compounds tested in humans remain small. There may be significant differences in susceptibility of organisms that normally inhabit rats, mice, and humans, but to date, none have been observed.

VI. Conclusions

Both culture and animal models are important for detection of effective drugs to test *P. carinii*. The culture model allows rapid screening of many compounds. From these culture studies, available pharmacokinetic data, and the potential of the compound to be rapidly developed for clinical use, compounds are selected for animal studies. Initial animal studies use the highest-tolerated doses to determine definitively if there is any activity. If there is good activity, dose-ranging studies are performed to establish lowest-effective doses. Subsequently, prophylaxis and relapse studies can be performed if indicated.

Promising compounds already in use in humans for treatment of other infectious agents or for other conditions allow more rapid succession to clinical trials. In all cases, finding promising compounds with in vitro or in vivo models is just the beginning of the long and arduous task of moving the compounds on to clinical trials.

Acknowledgment

Drug studies and model development reported in this chapter were supported in part by National Institutes of Health Contracts N01-AI-52543, N01-AI-72647, and PHS U01-AI-25859. We wish to thank Drs. Jay Fishman and Richard Tidwell for their assistance in model development and comparisons.

References

1. Jirovek O, Vanek J. Morphology of *Pneumocystis carinii* and pathogenesis of *Pneumocystis carinii* pneumonia. Zentralbl Allg Pathol 1954; 92:424–427.
2. Weller R. Zur erzeugung von pneumocystosen im tierversuch. Z Kinderheilkd 1955; 76:366.
3. Hughes WT, McNabb PC, Makres TD, Feldman S. Efficacy of trimethoprim and sulfamethoxazole in the prevention and treatment of *Pneumocystis carinii* pneumonitis. Antimicrob Agent Chemother 1974; 5:289–293.
4. Frenkel JK, Good JT, Shultz JA. Latent pneumocystis infection of rats, relapse and chemotherapy. Lab Invest 1966; 15:1559–1577.
5. Kovacs JA, Allegra CJ, Beaver J, Boarman D, Lewis M, Parrillo JE, Chabner B, Masur H. Characterization of de novo folate synthesis in *Pneumocystis carinii* and *Toxoplasma gondii*: potential for screening therapeutic agents. Antimicrob Agent Chemother 1989; 160:312–320.
6. Comley JC, Mullin RJ, Wolfe LA, Hanlon MH, Ferone R. Microculture screening assay for primary in vitro evaluation of drugs against *Pneumocystis carinii*. Antimicrob Agent Chemother 1991; 35:1965–1974.
7. Queener SF, Broughton MC. *Pneumocystis carinii* dihydrofolate reductase used to screen anti-pneumocystis drugs. Antimicrob Agent Chemother 1991; 35:1348.
8. Bartlett MS, Eichholtz R, Smith JW. Antimicrobial susceptibility of *Pneumocystis carinii* in culture. Diagn Microbiol Infect Dis 1985; 3:381–387.
9. Hughes WT, Armstrong M, Bartlett M, Blumenfeld W, Cushion M, Kalica A, Kovacs J, Laughon B, Martin W, Pesanti E, Richards F, Rose R, Sloande E, Walzer P. The challenge of pneumocystis culture. J AIDS 1992; (in press).

10. Durkin MM, Shaw MM, Bartlett MS, Smith JW. Culture and filtration methods for obtaining *Pneumocystis carinii* trophozoites and cysts. J Protozool 1991; 38:210S–212S.
11. Ruebush TK, Weinstein RA, Baehner RL, Wolff D, Bartlett M, Gonzales-Crussi F, Sulzer AJ, Schultz MG. An outbreak of pneumocystis pneumonia in children with acute lymphocytic leukemia. Am J Dis Child 1978; 132:143–148.
12. Jackson HC, Hancock V, Ehahi N. Analysis of the dynamics of *Pneumocystis carinii* in vitro. J Protozool 1991; 38:93S–95S.
13. Edlind TD, Bartlett MS, Smith JW. Characterization of the β-tubulin gene of *Pneumocystis carinii*. J Protozool 1991; 38:62S–63S.
14. Paulsrud JR, Queener SF, Bartlett MS, Smith JW. Isolation and characterization of rat lung *Pneumocystis carinii* gp120. J Protozool 1991; 38:10S–11S.
15. Pottratz ST, Paulsrud J, Smith JW, Martin WJ II. *Pneumocystis carinii* attachment to cultured lung cells by pneumocystis gp120, a fibronectin binding protein. J Clin Invest 1991; 88:403–407.
16. Zimmerman PE, Volker DR, McCormack FX, Paulsrud JR, Martin WJ II. 120-kd glycoprotein of *Pneumocystis carinii* is a ligand for surfactant protein A. J Clin Invest 1992; 89:143–149.
17. Goheen MP, Blumersine R, Bartlett MS, Hull MT, Smith JW, Improved intracellular morphology of *Pneumocystis carinii* from rat lung by postfixation with a mixture of potassium ferrocyanine and osmium tetroxide. Biotech Histochem 1992; 67:140–148.
18. Bartlett MS, Goheen MP, Queener SF, Durkin MM, Shaw MM, Smith JW. Close association of *Pneumocystis carinii* trophic forms with culture cells as shown by immune staining and electron microscopy. 40 Annu Meet Am Soc Trop Med Hyg 1991; p 233, abstr 345.
19. Goheen MP, Bartlett MS, Smith JW. The effect of primaquine on the ultrastructural morphology of *Pneumocystis carinii*. J Protozool 1991; 38:164S–165S.
20. Bartlett MS, Medley S, Durkin M, Piskura P, Smith JW. Proliferation of trophozoite forms of *Pneumocystis carinii* in WI-38 cell culture. Am Soc Trop Med Hyg Dec 1984; abstr 175.
21. Jackson PR, Pappas MG, Hansen BD. Fluorogenic substrate detection of viable intracellular and extracellular pathogenic protozoa. Science 1985; 277:435–438.
22. Bartlett MS, Durkin MM, Piskura J, Smith JW. Use of fluorescent staining to evaluate viability of *Pneumocystis carinii* from culture. In: Abstr. 24th Intersci Conf Antimicrob Agents Chemother October 1984; abstr 619.
23. Durkin MM, Bartlett MS, Queener SF, Shaw MM, Lee CH, Smith JW. An enzyme-linked immunosorbent assay for enumeration of *Pneumocystis carinii* in vitro and in vivo. J Clin Microbiol 1992; 30:3258–3262.
24. Derouin F, Chastang C. Enzyme immunoassay to assess effect of antimicrobial agents of *Toxoplasma gondii* in tissue culture. Antimicrob Agent Chemother 1988; 32:303–307.
25. Bartlett MS, Queener SF, Tidwell RR, Milhous WK, Berman JD, Ellis WY, Smith JW. 8-Aminoquinolines from Walter Reed Army Institute for Research for treatment and prophylaxis of *Pneumocystis carinii* pneumonia in rat models. Antimicrob Agents Chemother 1991; 35:277–282.

26. Queener SF, Bartlett MS, Jay MA, Durkin MM, Smith JW. Activity of clindamycin with primaquine against *Pneumocystis carinii* in vitro and in vivo. Antimicrob Agents Chemother 1988; 32:807–813.
27. Queener SF, Dean RA, Bartlett MS, Milhous WK, Berman JD, Ellis WY, Smith JW. Efficacy of intermittent dosage of 8-aminoquinolines for therapy or prophylaxis of pneumocystis pneumonia in rats. J Infect Dis 1992; 165;764–768.
28. Smith JW, Bartlett MS, Queener SF, Durkin MM, Jay MA, Hull MT, Klein RS, Marr JJ. Therapy of *Pneumocystis carinii* pneumonia with 9-deazainosine in rats. Diagn Microbiol Infect Dis 1987; 7:113–118.
29. Queener SF, Bartlett MS, Smith JS. Activity of lipid-soluble inhibitors of dihydrofolate reductase against *Pneumocystis carinii* in culture. Antimicrob Agents Chemother 1987; 32:802–813.
30. Hendley JW, Weller TW. Activation and transmission in rats of infection with pneumocystis. Proc Soc Exp Biol Med 1971; 137:1401–1404.
31. Hughes WT, Smith B. Efficacy of diaminodiphenylsulfone and other drugs in murine *Pneumocystis carinii* pneumonitis. Antimicrob Agents Chemother 1984; 25: 436–440.
32. Hughes WT, Gray VL, Gutteridge WE, Latter VS, Pudney M. Efficacy of a hydroxynaphthoquinone, 56680C, in experimental *Pneumocystis carinii* pneumonitis. Antimicrob Agents Chemother 1990; 34:225–228.
33. Hughes WT. Macrolide-antifol synergism in anti-*Pneumocystis carinii* therapeutics. J Protozool 1991; 38:160S.
34. Hussain Z, Carlson ML, Crain JD, Lannigan R. Efficacy of tetroxoprim/sulfadiazine in the treatment of *Pneumocystis carinii* pneumonia in rats. J Antimicrob Agents Chemother 1988; 15:575–578.
35. Kovacs JA, Allegra CJ, Kennedy S, Swan JC, Drake J, Parrillo JE, Chabner B, Masur H. Efficacy of trimetrexate, a potent lipid-soluble antifolate, in the treatment of rodent *Pneumocystis carinii* pneumonia. Am J Trop Med Hyg 1988; 39:491–496.
36. Schmatz DM, Romanchek MA, Pittarelli LA, Schwartz RE, Fromtling RA, Nollstadt KH, Vanmiddlesworth FL, Wilson KE, Turner MJ. Treatment of *Pneumocystis carinii* pneumonia with 1,3-β-glucan synthesis inhibitors. Proc Natl Acad Sci USA 1990; 87: 5950–5954.
37. Walzer PD, Kim CK, Foy J, Linke MH, Cushion MT. Cationic antitrypanosomal and other antimicrobial agents in therapy of experimental *Pneumocystis carinii* pneumonia. Antimicrob Agents Chemother 1988; 32:896–905.
38. Debs RF, Blumenfeld W, Brunette EN, Straubonger RM, Montgomery AB, Lin W, Agabian N, Papahadjopoulos D. Successful treatment with aerosolized pentamidine of *Pneumocystis carinii* pneumonia in rats. Antimicrob Agents Chemother 1987; 31: 37–41.
39. Hayes DJ, Stubberfield CR, McBride JD, Wilson DL. Alterations in cysteine proteinase content of rat lung associated with development of *Pneumocystis carinii* infection. Infect Immun 1991; 59:3581–3588.
40. Eisen S, Decreased yield of *Pneumocystis carinii* from cortisonized rats. J Parasitol 1989; 75:82–85.
41. D'Antonio RG, Johnson DB, Winn RE, VanDellen AF, Evans ME. Effect of folinic

acid on the capacity of trimethoprim–sulfamethoxazole to prevent and treat *Pneumocystis carinii* pneumonia in rats. Antimicrob Agents Chemother 1986; 29:327–329.

42. Bartlett MS, Queener SF, Jay MA, Durkin MM, Smith JW. An improved rat model for studying *Pneumocystis carinii* pneumonia. J Clin Microbiol 1987; 25:480–484.

43. Bartlett MS, Fishman JA, Durkin MM, Queener SF, Smith JW. *Pneumocystis carinii*: improved models to study efficacy of drugs for treatment or prophylaxis of pneumocystis pneumonia in the rat (*Rattus* spp). Exp Parasitol 1990; 70:100–106.

44. Boylan CJ, Current WL, An improved rat model of *Pneumocystis carinii* pneumonia: induced infections in pneumocystis-free animals. J Protozool 1991; 38:138S–140S.

45. Boylan CJ, Current WL. Improved rat model of *Pneumocystis carinii* pneumonia: induced laboratory infections in pneumocystis-free animals. Infect Immun 1992; 60:1589–1597.

46. Current WL, Boylan CJ. Anti-pneumocystis activity of antifungal compounds cilofungin and echinocandin B. In Abstr 30th Intersci Conf Antimicrob Agents Chemother 1990. 229, abstr 858.

47. Allegra CJ, Chabner BA, Tuazon CU, Ogata-Arakaki D, Baird B, Drake JC, Masur H. Treatment of *Pneumocystis carinii* pneumonia with trimetrexate in acquired immunodeficiency syndrome (AIDS). Semin Oncol 1988; 15:46–49.

48. Hughes WT. Limited effect of trimethoprim–sulfamethoxazole prophylaxis on *Pneumocystis carinii*. Antimicrob Agents Chemother 1979; 16:333–335.

49. Bartlett MS, Queener SF, Durkin MM, Shaw MM, Smith JW. Inoculated mouse model of *Pneumocystis carinii* infection. Diagn Microbiol Infect Dis 1992; 15:129–134.

50. Shellito J, Suzara VV, Blumenfeld W, Beck JM, Steger HJ, Emak TH. A new model of *Pneumocystis carinii* infection in mice selectively depleted of helper T lymphocytes. J Clin Invest 1990; 85:1686–1693.

51. Dialynas DP, Wilde DB, Marrack P, Pierres A, Wall KA, Havran W, Otten G, Loken MR, Pierres M, Kappler F, Fitch FW. Characterization of the murine antigenic determinant, designated L3T4a, recognized by monoclonal antibody GK1.5: expression of L3T4a by functional T cell clones appears to correlate primarily with class II MHC antigen reactivity. Immunol Rev 1983; 74:29–55.

25

Development of New Anti–*Pneumocystis carinii* Drugs
Cumulative Experience at a Single Institution

PETER D. WALZER

Cincinnati Veterans Affairs Medical Center
and University of Cincinnati College of Medicine
Cincinnati, Ohio

I. Introduction

The acquired immunodeficiency syndrome (AIDS) epidemic has demonstrated the limitations of currently available anti-*Pneumocystis carinii* drugs and the need to develop new forms of therapy. Yet, drug research has been severely hampered by the lack of a reliable in vitro culture system, which has forced most studies to be conducted in animal models. Rats administered corticosteroids for about 8 weeks develop pneumocystosis with histological features virtually identical with those of the human disease. Drugs that are active against rat *P. carinii* in this model have usually shown activity against human *P. carinii*.

Interest in developing new anti-*P. carinii* drugs has arisen not only among pharmaceutical firms, but also among investigators through government-sponsored grants or contracts. Information about *P. carinii* drug testing is limited because only compounds that show activity tend to be published. Since 1984, my colleagues and I at the University of Cincinnati have been awarded a National Institutes of Health (NIH) contract to evaluate new anti-*P. carinii* drugs. This has provided us with a wealth of experience that we felt might be useful to other investigators. In this chapter, I present a brief literature review of *P. carinii* drug testing and a more detailed description of our in vivo and in vitro studies over an 8-year period.

II. Review of the Literature

A. Animal Models

The feasibility of using the immunosuppressed rat model to test anti-*P. carinii* drugs was first demonstrated in the 1960s (1), but systematic use of this system did not begin until the 1970s (2–4). Over the past two decades, the following compounds have been shown to have activity against *P. carinii* in this animal model: antifolate drugs (alone or in combination) including dihydrofolate reductase (DHFR) inhibitors, sulfonamides, sulfones, and sulfonylureas (1,2,4–16); sulfonamides in combination with other drugs (e.g., macrolides) (17); diamidines and related cationic compounds (18–22); 8-aminoquinolones, alone or in combination with other agents (23,24); purine nucleosides (14,25; Bernard E, Armstrong D, personal communication); polyamine inhibitors (26,27); nitrofurans (28); β-glucan inhibitors (29–31); hydroxynaphthoquinoes (32); fluoroquinolones (33); iron chelators (27); immunological agents (antibodies, cytokines) (34,35).

Although the rat model has been very valuable in developing clinically useful anti-*P. carinii* drugs, it is cumbersome, time-consuming, and labor-intensive. Large amounts of the drugs are needed for testing, and only a few compounds can be evaluated in a given experiment. Over the years, several factors have arisen that have influenced the rat model for testing antipneumocystis drugs, and these must be considered by anyone who wishes to enter this field.

Source of Rats and Pneumocystis carinii

Investigators traditionally used Sprague–Dawley rats obtained from commercial breeders. These animals were raised in a conventional room and were latently infected with *P. carinii* and rodent viruses (virus-positive) through the environment. The administration of corticosteroids resulted in the development of pneumocystosis by reactivation of this latent infection.

In an attempt to improve the quality of rats used in research, breeders gradually developed colonies free of rodent viruses. Similarly, some research institutions developed regulations stipulating that only virus-negative rats could be used in their facilities. When these animals were immunosuppressed, they were found to be free of latent *P. carinii* infection, as judged by their failure to develop pneumocystosis (36). However, the disease could be produced in immunosuppressed rats by intratracheal inoculation (37,38). This led to efforts to develop those rats as an experimental model of pneumocystosis. Proponents emphasized that intratracheal inoculation involved a shorter time of immunosuppression and resulted in less variability in the extent of *P. carinii* pneumonia among individual animals.

Although some workers now use virus-negative rats for their *P. carinii* studies, most investigators (including this author) continue to favor virus-positive rats. A major reason for this is that the virus-positive animals rely on naturally acquired *P. carinii* infection and, thus, more closely mimic the condition in humans. These rats are also easier to use. Intratracheal inoculation is an invasive procedure, requiring technician time and training. Success in establishing pneumocystosis by intratracheal inoculation has varied among different laboratories, and the level of infection that can be achieved appears to be no higher than that achieved in virus-positive rats by simple immunosuppression.

The choice of an animal model for *P. carinii* studies may be influenced by factors beyond the control of the investigator. Virus-positive rats can be readily obtained from several commercial breeders who had stated that they are committed to supplying these animals for the foreseeable future; yet, if these vendors stop production, virus-negative animals will be more widely used. Other factors include institutional regulations, strain variation, and the influence of procedures, such as serial passage of *P. carinii* in rats on organism virulence.

Animal Housing and Associated Microbial Flora

The immunosuppressive regimen used to provide pneumocystosis puts the rats at risk of other opportunistic infections, regardless of which rats are used. The occurrence of infection with bacteria or fungi can shorten the life span of the rats and possibly influence the effects of the drugs being tested. This has emphasized the need for strict measures to house and handle the animals.

Experimental Design

Two types of studies have been used to test anti-*P. carinii* drugs. In treatment experiments, the rats are immunosuppressed to induce the development of pneumocystosis; the drugs are then given for 2–3 weeks and evaluated for their effects on the disease. In prophylaxis studies, the drugs are given throughout the period of immunosuppression. These protocols differ in purpose, in sensitivity in detecting antipneumocystis activity, in the amount of drugs needed, and in the risk of causing adverse effects. Such differences must be taken into account in designing experiments.

Drug Administration

Drugs have been given by a variety of oral and parenteral routes, and differences in administration may influence their anti-*P. carinii* activity. For example, a compound given as a single dose by oral gavage will have different pharmacokinetics than the same dose of the compound given in the food or drinking water. With newly synthesized drugs, selection of the route of administration may be a matter of trial and error.

Assessment of Drug Efficacy

Most investigators have evaluated drug efficacy by examining the effects of these agents on the extent of *P. carinii* pneumonia, rather than on animal survival. This has been done because the rats may die from causes (e.g., other opportunistic infections, drug toxicity) unrelated to *P. carinii*. The principal methods of determining the extent of pneumocystosis have been histological examination and organism quantitation in lung homogenates. Since these techniques varied among investigators, it has not been possible to compare the results of one study directly with those of another.

B. In Vitro Studies

The current status of *P. carinii* cultivation in vitro has been described in detail in Chapter 1. Limited (up to about tenfold) propagation of rat-derived *P. carinii* has been achieved in several different cell lines and in axenic media, but the organism eventually dies. Attempts to cultivate human-derived *P. carinii* have been unsuccessful. No standards have been established for inoculum preparation, organism quantitation, or determining viability. This has led to problems in data interpretation and reproducibility among different laboratories.

Several studies have demonstrated that drugs that are used in the clinical treatment of pneumocystosis inhibit organism replication in vitro (39–42). However, what these compounds really seem to be doing is speeding up the *P. carinii* dying process. Data interpretation is further complicated in monolayer systems for which it is difficult to determine whether antimicrobial agents work directly on *P. carinii* or through their effects on the mammalian cells. These factors, coupled with the problems of standardization and reproducibility in culture, as described earlier, have generated little confidence among investigators that currently available in vitro systems can reliably predict the activity of drugs against *P. carinii* in vivo.

Alternative approaches have involved examining the effects of drugs on rat *P. carinii* enzymes or metabolism (43–49). The use of native or recombinant enzymes (e.g., dihydrofolate reductase) permits drugs to be directly compared for their activity (43–45). An assay, which is based on uptake of radiolabeled *para*-aminobenzoic acid (PABA) by metabolically active organisms, is being used by some pharmaceutical firms to investigate new compounds (49). Overall, these systems appear to offer more promise than culture for studying antipneumocystis drugs; yet, further studies are needed to determine whether any of these approaches will gain widespread acceptance.

III. The University of Cincinnati Experience

A. Animal Models

Experimental Protocol

From 1984 to 1991, the same basic experimental protocol was used. The animal model used in these studies was based on the use of virus-positive rats and has been described in detail previously (48,49). Drugs were obtained from commercial sources, individual investigators, pharmaceutical firms, or through the Developmental Therapeutics Branch, Division of AIDS, NIAID, NIH. Sprague–Dawley rats weighing 200–250 g, obtained from Harlan Industries (Madison, Wisconsin) were used for most of the experiments. When this colony was discontinued in favor of production of virus-negative rats, we obtained virus-positive Sprague–Dawley animals from Sasco, Inc. (St. Louis, Missouri). No differences were noted in the severity of pneumocystosis induced by immunosuppression between these groups of animals.

Upon arrival at our animal facility, the rats were housed in a conventional colony room, ate regular food, and drank plain tap water for a 1–2 week period of acclimation. They were then administered a corticosteroid, a low (8%)-protein diet (Bioserv, Frenchtown, New Jersey), and an antibiotic (e.g., tetracycline, ampicillin, or cephradine, 1 mg/mL) in the drinking water to induce the development of *P. carinii* pneumonia. The corticosteroid preparation in the early years was cortisone acetate (Cortone, Merck, Sharp, and Dohme, Rahway, New Jersey), 25 mg injected subcutaneously (sc) twice weekly; this was later switched to methylprednisolone acetate (Depo-Medrol, The Upjohn, Co., Kalamazoo, Michigan), 4 mg injected sc once weekly. There was no change in the level of immunosuppression or pneumocystosis.

A typical experiment involved about 200 rats and 8–10 weeks of immunosuppression. The rats were weighed at regular intervals, and a few animals were sacrificed, and their lungs were examined to check the development of *P. carinii* pneumonia. By 5–7 weeks, when the infection had become moderately severe, the animals were randomly divided into treatment and control groups of 15–20 rats each. Candidate anti-*P. carinii* drugs were administered parenterally or by oral gavage in single or divided doses for 3 weeks; doses were calculated on a milligram per kilogram basis and usually were not changed throughout the period of administration. We have favored oral gavage over giving the drugs in food or drinking water because the dose can be more accurately controlled. We use a soft rubber tube for the gavage and have not encountered esophageal or gastric problems in the animals. Control rats were either given a placebo (e.g., vehicle to dissolve the test drugs) or no therapy; no differences were noted in the extent of pneumocystosis in these groups. At the end of the treatment period, the animals were sacrificed by an overdose of halothane anesthesia.

The immunosuppressive regimen resulted in weight loss, debilitation, and infection with other opportunistic pathogens. Typically, about 15–20% of the rats died or became so ill early in the study that they were deemed unsuitable for drug testing; additional animals died during the last 3 weeks of the study. The early deaths were usually attributed to other opportunistic infections, whereas deaths during the treatment portion were caused by a variety of factors (e.g., infection, drug toxicity) that could not be ascertained with certainty.

Procedures used to prevent the development of opportunistic infections included restricted access to the rats, specially designated personnel, gowns, gloves, masks, strict hygiene, and sanitation. Although these measures were helpful, the frequency and severity of infections sometimes varied for reasons that were not readily apparent or within our control. When the problem was confined to a few rats, drug testing was uninterrupted; however, infection involving a large segment of the colony precluded the evaluation of any compounds. Offending microbes included gram-positive and gram-negative bacteria, rodent viruses, and fungi. *Aspergillus* sp. was particularly troublesome during times of building construction or renovation, when it was found in the air system; the organism was also occasionally found in the food and bedding.

In 1991, a Biobubble (CSA Fluid Dynamics, Fort Collins, Colorado) was constructed in our animal facility to house the rats. This is a plastic unit, fitted to the size of any room, that has laminar air flow and a high-efficiency particulate air (HEPA) filter. The rats were housed in microisolator cages within the Biobubble and given autoclaved or irradiated food, water, and bedding; the other protective measures described earlier were continued. The same immunosuppressive regimen was used as in previous years, except for the following: the low-protein food pellets lost their shape and consistency with autoclaving, so a regular diet was substituted; lighter-weight (150–200 g) rats were used to increase the effects of the methylprednisolone, as compensation for the loss of immunosuppressive properties of the low-protein diet.

Rats housed in the Biobubble developed pneumocystosis and responded to anti-*P. carinii* drugs in a manner similar to animals housed in the conventional colony. The major difference was a marked reduction in the frequency and severity of other opportunistic infections, which enabled us to study more anti-*P. carinii* drugs in a given experiment. This finding also suggested that animal-housing and animal-handling conditions are more important in determining susceptibility to opportunistic infections than the question of whether the rats are virus-negative or virus-positive.

Evaluation of Drug Efficacy

These procedures, which were described in our earlier studies (13,22,40,51), were based on analysis of the severity of *P. carinii* pneumonia in the lungs, rather than on animal survival. In general, rats had to receive anti-*P. carinii* drugs for 10 days or more to be included in the data analysis, because it took this long to observe a therapeutic effect on microscopic examination of the lungs. This approach allowed evaluation of drugs in a consistent manner. The protocol was altered when we were interested in the early effects of drugs, or when we wished to determine whether compounds, which were highly toxic or in short supply, had any anti-*P. carinii* activity.

At death or sacrifice, the left lung of each rat was removed, infused with 4%

formaldehyde through the bronchus until fully expanded, and fixed. Three horizontal sections (one each from the upper, middle, and lower portions) of the lung were stained with hematoxylin–eosin (H&E) and Grocott's methenamine silver. The lung sections were coded and read in a blinded manner by an experienced pathologist. The following scoring system was used to assess the severity of pneumcystosis, based on the proportion of alveolar involvement: 0+, no *P. carinii* pneumonia found; 0.5+, minimal (<1% alveoli involved); 1+, light (1–25% alveoli); 2+, moderate (25–50% alveoli); 3+, severe (50–75% alveoli); 4+, very severe (>75% alveoli).

The right lung, which was used for organism quantitation, was weighed and homogenized in a Stomacher (Tekmar, Cincinnati, Ohio). Erythrocytes were lysed with ammonium chloride, the material was washed with phosphate-buffered saline (PBS), centrifuged, and resuspended in PBS. Three 0.01-mL drops, each covering an area of 1 cm^2, were placed on a glass slide and air-dried. The slides were then stained with cresyl echt violet (CEV), which selectively stains *P. carinii* cysts, and with Diff-Quik, a rapid variant of the Wright–Giemsa stain, which stains the nuclei of all developmental stages. The slides were coded, read blindly, and the number of cysts and nuclei per oil immersion field (OIF) was determined by randomly scanning 30 OIF (ten per drop). The number of cysts or nuclei per lung was calculated according to a formula, based on the dimensions of the microscope lens. The lower limit of detection was about 1.1×10^5 organisms per lung.

The histological scoring system and quantitation of *P. carinii* cysts and nuclei showed a high degree of correlation (50,51). Histological examination and cyst quantitation were performed as part of the routine drug evaluation, whereas nucleus quantitation, which was more difficult and required greater expertise, was performed on a selective basis. Typically, control rats receiving steroids (C/S), but no anti-*P. carinii* drugs, exhibited histological scores of 3–4+, cyst counts of 10^8–10^9 per lung, and nucleus counts that were about tenfold higher; this pattern remained quite constant over the years. Lung weight and lung weight/body weight ratio also reflected the extent of pneumocystosis, but were not routinely used to assess therapy.

Drug efficacy was determined by comparing the severity of *P. carinii* pneumonia in the rat groups that received the test compounds with that in the control group in the same experiment. As seen in Figure 1, the drugs showed a similar pattern of activity against *P. carinii* by lung histological examination and organism quantitations. However, data analysis was complicated by several factors. The histological scores and cyst and nucleus counts usually did not follow a pattern of normal distribution. The histological scoring and organism-quantitation techniques also were not sensitive in identifying and quantitating low levels of infection; thus, with highly active drugs such as trimethoprim–sulfamethoxazole (TMP–SMX), the values were clustered at the lower limit of detection (i.e., histological scores of 0+ or organism counts of 1.1×10^5 per lung). In other cases, an overlap in the range of histological scores and *P. carinii* counts among the

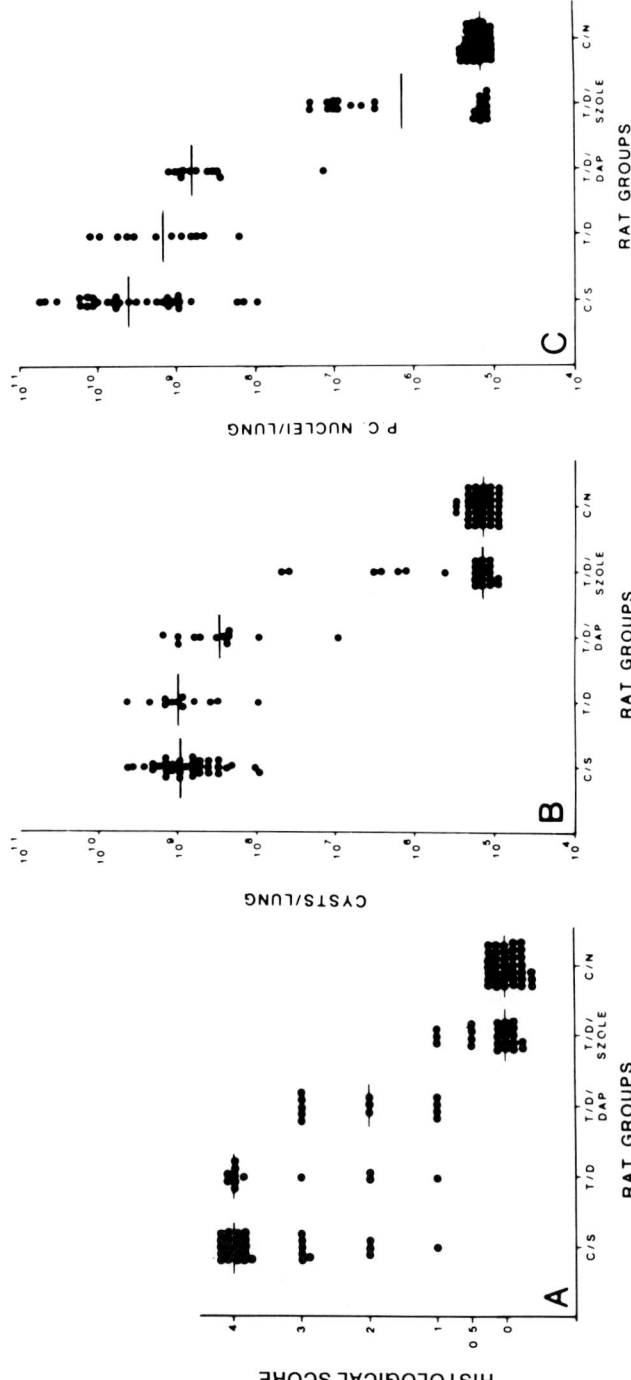

Figure 1 Assessment of therapy of pneumocystosis in different rat groups by (A) histological score; (B) number of *P. carinii* cysts; and (C) number of *P. carinii* nuclei. C/S; corticosteroid controls; T/D, trimethoprim–diaveridine treatment; T/D/DAP, trimethoprim–diaveridine–dapsone treatment; T/D/SZOLE, trimethoprim–diaveridine–sulfamethoxazole treatment; C/N, normal controls. Horizontal bars represent median values. The data compare drugs that have little or no anti-*P. carinii* activity (T/D), moderate activity (T/D/DAP), or a high degree of activity (T/D/SZOLE). (Adapted from Ref. 51.)

control and drug treatment groups sometimes occurred when there was a wide distribution of values. For these reasons, nonparametric techniques were used when statistical analysis was needed.

Drug Prophylaxis

Studies of the ability of drugs to prevent the development of pneumocystosis were performed infrequently and followed the same basic protocol used in the treatment experiments. The major difference was that the candidate anti-*P. carinii* compounds were administered throughout the period of immunosuppression. Assessment of drug efficacy was the same as in the therapy studies.

Classification of Antipneumocystis Activity

As mentioned previously, the lack of standardized methods of evaluating drug efficacy has prevented the direct comparison of studies by different investigators. We wished to develop a simple, reproducible system of classifying the activity of anti-*P. carinii* drugs that would overcome this problem. We have recently published a study describing such a system (52), which forms the basis for much of the information presented here. One goal of this system was to express the antipneumocystis activity of drugs in a quantitative manner (i.e., on the basis of the magnitude of reduction in organism burden). The other goal was to have the capability of comparing the activity of drugs investigated in different studies performed at different times. Given the consistent level of infection and results with compounds, such as TMP–SMX, in the animal model, we felt that both goals could be met by comparing *P. carinii* cyst or nucleus counts of the drug treatment groups with those of the C/S group in the same experiment. Such an approach allowed the activity of each candidate compound to be expressed in relation to its own control. Median counts were used, rather than mean counts, because they more accurately represented skewed data. The median cyst or nucleus count of the C/S group was divided by the median cyst or nucleus count of each drug treatment group, and the ratio was used as an indicator of anti-*P. carinii* activity. Thus, if the median cyst count of the C/S group was 8×10^8 per lung and the media cyst count of the drug treatment group was 2×10^6 per lung, the ratio of 400 signified a 400-fold reduction.

The following categories of activity were established, based on the fall in median *P. carinii* cyst or nucleus counts: inactive, less than 5-fold reduction; slight activity, 5- to 9-fold reduction; moderate activity, 10- to 99-fold reduction; marked activity, 100- to 999-fold reduction; very marked activity, 1000-fold reduction, or more. This system was chosen to mimic quantitative bacterial or fungal cultures, with each category representing about a logarithm difference in organism burden.

The criteria used to establish some of the categories were influenced by features of the experimental test system. For example, the fivefold decline in cyst or nucleus count was chosen as the threshold for drug efficacy to provide clear evidence of activity; several compounds resulted in slight changes in the organism burden that were inconsistent and, hence, difficult to interpret. The 1000 or more fall in organism count was chosen as the category of maximal drug activity, based on the usual median cyst count in the C/S group of at least 10^8 per lung and the detection limit of 1.1×10^5 per lung. Since compounds showing this activity usually reduced the cyst count to 1.1×10^5 per lung, it was not possible to determine whether different ratios (e.g., 8000 vs 4000) represented true differences in drug efficacy, or simply reflected higher cyst counts in the C/S groups. In the cases where the media cyst count in the C/S group was 10^7–10^8 per lung, drugs that lowered the cyst count to 1.1×10^5 per lung were classified as showing very marked activity.

Analysis of drug efficacy by nucleus quantitation raised the issue of establishing an additional antipneumocystis activity category because of the higher media nucleus counts in the C/S group (10^8–10^9 per lung). However, this was felt to be unnecessary because fewer studies using nucleus quantitation were performed.

Over the 8-year period, 38 experiments were conducted, which included 36 treatment studies, 2 prophylaxis experiments, and 1 combined treatment and prophylaxis study. The data base was composed of the following: (1) Two hundred seventy-three drug dose groups, consisting of 4143 rats; these groups included drugs tested individually or in combination at one or more doses. (2) Thirty-eight C/S groups consisting of 701 animals. (3) Thirty-six control normal (C/N) groups composed of 241 rats that ate a normal diet, drank plain tap water, and received no medications.

Drugs Tested in the Therapy of Pneumocystosis

The drugs that have been studied in the treatment of *P. carinii* pneumonia in the rat model are listed in Table 1. Most of the agents are listed by their generic name. A few compounds are listed by their general class (e.g., purine nucleoside 1, guanylhydrazone A1) to protect the confidentiality of proprietary information. Some drugs were tested at one dose, whereas others were tested at several doses; in the latter circumstance, the range of doses has been given.

Classification of Therapeutic Activity by Cyst Counts

The classification of drugs in the treatment of pneumocystosis by the reduction of cyst counts is described in Table 2. The ratios listed here signify the maximal activity of each drug or combination of drugs. Sulfonamides were among the most active anti-*P. carinii* drugs tested. Sulfadoxine, sulfadiazine, and SMX repeatedly showed marked or very marked activity in experiments performed months or years apart. The sulfone, dapsone, was studied in a more limited manner and produced somewhat less consistent results. In early studies, the highest dose of dapsone (125 mg/kg per day) exhibited only moderate anti-*P. carinii* activity; however, in later experiments, this dose showed very marked activity. The sulfonamides and sulfones caused few adverse effects in the rats.

Table 1 Drugs Evaluated in the Treatment of *Pneumocystis carinii* Pneumonia

Drug	Dosage regimen[a,b] (mg/kg per day)
Antibiotics	
Ampicillin	150 im
Chloramphenicol	20 im–40 po
Ciprofloxacin	100 po
Erythromycin	25 im–400 po
Gentamicin	10 im
Imipenem	100 im
Rifabutin	100 po–200 po
Spectinomycin	100 im
Antifungal agents	
Amphotericin B	6 sc
Flucytosine	150 po
Griseofulvin	100 po–300 po
Miconazole	100 sc
Antiviral agents	
Acyclovir	100 im
Amantadine	50 po–100 po
AZT	15 po–100
DDI	500 po
Isoprinosine	250 po–500 po
Purine nucleosides	
9-Deazainosine	7.5 sc–50 ip 5 d/wk
Purine nucleoside 1	15 sc–50 ip
Purine nucleoside 2	25 ip
Purine nucleoside 3	25 ip
Purine nucleoside 4	25 ip
Purine nucleoside 5	20 ip
Sulfonamides/sulfones	
Dapsone	5 po–125 po
Sulfadiazine	250 po–500 po
Sulfadoxine	250 po
Sulfamethoxazole	0.3 po–250 po
DHFR Inhibitors	
Diaveridine	100 po
Pyrimethamine	3 po–18.75 po
Trimethoprim	3 po–100 po
DHFR inhibitor 2 (BL-1033)	10 po–30 po
DHFR inhibitor 3 (BL-1034 or Ro 11-8958)	10 po–100 po
DHFR inhibitor 4 (BL-1035)	10 sc–30 sc
DHFR inhibitor 5 (Tetroxoprim)	50 po
Nitrofurans/nitroimidazoles	
Benznidazole	20 po
Furazolidone	50 po–200 po

Table 1 (Continued)

Drug	Dosage regimen[a,b] (mg/kg per day)
Nitrofurans/nitroimidazoles (Continued)	
Metronidazole	100 sc–600 po
Nifurtimox	50 po–400 po
Nitrofurantoin	100 po–200 po
Nitromidazole 1	12.5 im–100 im
Nitromidazole 2	12.5 im–100 im
Thiahendazole	100 po–200 po
Diamidines	
Amicarbalide	1.5 sc–10 sc 3d–7d/wk
Dimethylstilbamidine (*cis*)	4 sc 3d/wk
Dimethylstilbamidine (*trans*)	4 sc 3d/wk
Diminazine	2.5 sc–20 sc
Ethidium bromide	0.5 ip–3 im 3d–7d/wk
Guanylhydrazone	25 sc–75 im 3d–7d/wk
Guanylhydrazone A1	5 sc–10 sc 3d–5d/wk
Guanylhydrazone A2	2.5 sc–10 sc 3d–5d/wk
Guanylhydrazone A3	3 sc–10 sc 3d–5d/wk
Guanylhydrazone B1	0.5 sc–30 po
Guanylhydrazone B2	0.5 sc–30 po
Guanylhydrazone B3	3 sc
Guanylhydrazone B4	0.5 sc–3 sc
Guanylhydrazone B5	0.5 sc–3 sc
Imidocarb	2.5 sc–25 sc
Isometamidium	0.5 im–3 im 3d–7d/wk
Pentamidine	10 im–20 im 3d/wk
Propamidine	5 im–10 im 3d/wk
Arsenicals/antimonials	
Arsenical 1	1 sc–2 sc
Arsenical 2	2 sc
Arsenical 3	1 sc–2 sc
Arsenical 4	5 sc
Arsenical 5	2.5 sc–5 sc
Arsenical 6	15 sc 5d/wk
Arsenical 7	10 sc 5d/wk
Astiban	10 im 2d/wk
Melarsoprol	10 ip 3d/wk
Pentostam	10 im
Other antiparasitic drugs	
Amprolium	50 po
Bithionol	50 po
Chlorpromazine	10 po–20 po
Dehydroemetine	1 im–5 im

Table 1 (Continued)

Drug	Dosage regimen[a,b] (mg/kg per day)
Other antiparasitic drugs (Continued)	
Diethylcarbamazine	100 po
DFMO	2%–4% solution in drinking water
Furamide	300 po
MDL 27695	3 im; 15 sc 3d–7d/wk
Monensin	5 po 10 mg/kg/d po
Praziquantel	100 po
Quinacrine	6 po
Quinidine	25 po
Quinine	25 po
Combinations	
Amphotericin B + flucytosine	12 sc + 300 po
Anepbotericin B + miconazole	6 sc + 100 sc
DFMO + diminazine	2–4% solution + 2.5–5 sc
DFMO + pentamidine	2–4% solution + 10 im 3d/wk
DFMO + MDL 27695	1–2% solution + 3–7.5 im
Flucytosine + miconazole	150 po + 100 sc
Dapsone + trimethoprim	15–25 po + 20–100 po
Dapsone + diaveridine	15–25 po + 20–100 po
Dapsone + pyrimethamine	25–250 po + 3–9 po
Dapsone + DHFR inhibitor 3	25 po + 20–100 po
Quinine + clindamycin	25 po + 400 po
Sulfadiazine + diaveridine	250–500 po + 50–100 po
Sulfadiazine + pyrimethamine	250 po + 3–9 po
Sulfadiazine + trimethoprim	250–500 po + 50–100 po
Sulfadoxine + diaveridine	250 po + 50 po
Sulfadoxine + pyrimethamine	250 po + 3–9 po
Sulfadoxine + trimethoprim	250 po + 50 po
Sulfamethoxazole + diaveridine	250–500 po + 50–100 po
Sulfamethoxazole + pyrimethamine	62.5–500 po + 3–18.75 po
Sulfamethoxazole + trimethoprim	3–500 po + 0.6–100 po
Sulfamethoxazole + trimethoprim + AZT	62.5 po + 12.5 po + 15–100 po
Sulfamethoxazole + DHFR inhibitor 1	500 po + 100 im
Sulfamethoxazole + DHFR inhibitor 3	3 po + 20–100 po
Sulfamethoxazole + DHFR inhibitor 4	3 po + 20 po
Sulfamethoxazole + DHFR inhibitor 5	3 po + 50 po

[a]Dose in milligrams per kilogram per day unless otherwise stated.
[b]Rats receiving regimens containing pyrimethamine were also given folinic acid 7–15 mg/kg sc.
Source: Ref. 52.

Table 2 Classification of Drugs in the Treatment of *Pneumocystis carinii* Pneumonia by Cyst Counts

Drug	Ratio
Very marked activity (≥1000× reduction)	
Dapsone	638[a]
Dapsone + DHFR inhibitor 3	2246
Sulfadiazine	1200
Sulfadiazine + diaveridine	3600
Sulfadiazine + trimethoprim	5300
Sulfadoxine + diaveridine	2600
Sulfadoxine + pyrimethamine	4800
Sulfamethoxazole	6300
Sulfamethoxazole + AZT	2400
Sulfamethoxazole + diaveridine	7890
Sulfamethoxazole + pyrimethamine	7890
Sulfamethoxazole + trimethoprim	7890
Sulfamethoxazole + trimethoprim + AZT	1700
Sulfamethoxazole + DHFR inhibitor 1	7900
Sulfamethoxazole + DHFR inhibitor 3	1280
Guanylhydrazone B1	1280
Guanylhydrazone B4	1280
Marked activity (100–999× reduction)	
Dapsone + diaveridine	154
Dapsone + trimethoprim	213
9-Deazainosine	197
Diminazine	143
Guanylhydrazone A2	125
Imidocarb	450
Quinapyramine	806
Sulfadiazine + pyrimethamine	538
Sulfadoxine	789
Sulfadoxine + trimethoprim	278
Moderate activity (10–99 reduction)	
Amicarbalide	94
Dapsone + pyrimethamine	60
Dehydroemetine	14
Furazolidone	45
Isometamidium	30
Pentamidine	96
Pentamidine + DFMO	10
Propamidine	26
Guanylhydrazone B2	91
Guanylhydrazone B5	91
Sulfamethoxazole + DHFR inhibitor 5	14

Table 2 (Continued)

Drug	Ratio
Slight activity (5–9 reduction)	
Amantadine	5
Dimethylstilbamidine (*cis*)	6
Diminazine + DFMO	6
Metronidazole	5
Nitrofurantoin	5
Purine nucleoside 1	9
Purine nucleoside 2	7
DHFR inhibitor 5	8
Sulfamethoxazole + DHFR inhibitor 4	9
No activity (<5× reduction)	
Acyclovir	3
Amphotericin B	<1
Amphotericin B + flucytosine	<1
Amphotericin B + miconazole	<1
Ampicillin	<1
Amprolium	1
Astiban	2
AZT	3
Benznidazole	1
Bithionol	1
Chloramphenicol	<1
Chlorpromazine	<1
Ciprofloxacin	<1
DDI	<1
DFMO	3
DFMO + MDL 27695	3
Diaveridine	3
Diethylcarbamazine	1
Dimethylstilbamidine (*trans*)	1
Erythromycin	2
Ethidium bromide	1
Flucytosine	<1
Furamide	<1
Gentamicin	2
Griseofulvin	2
Guanylhydrazone	3
Guanylhydrazone A1	2
Guanylhydrazone A3	3
Imipenem	<1
Isoprinosine	1
Melarsoprol	<1

Table 2 (Continued)

Drug	Ratio
No activity (<5× reduction) (Continued)	
Miconazole	1
Miconazole + flucytosine	<1
Monensin	<1
Nifurtimox	3
Ornidazole	<1
Pentostam	<1
Praziquantel	3
Pyrimethamine	4
Quinacrine	1
Quinidine	<1
Quininine	<1
Quinine + clindamycin	3
Rifabutin	1
Spectinomycin	1
Spiramycin	1
Thiabendazole	<1
Trimethoprim	<1
Arsenical 1	<1
Arsenical 2	<1
Arsenical 3	1
Arsenical 4	<1
Arsenical 5	1
Arsenical 6	1
Arsenical 7	<1
DHFR inhibitor 2	1
DHFR inhibitor 3	1
DHFR inhibitor 4	4
Guanylhydrazone B3	1
MDL 27695	<1
Nitromidazole 1	<1
Nitromidazole 2	<1
Purine nucleoside 3	1
Purine nucleoside 4	4
Purine nucleoside 5	2

[a]Median cyst count in control steroid group was 10^7–10^8 per lung.
Source: Ref. 52.

The most detailed studies of drug efficacy were performed with SMX. The standard dose of this compound used in studies of experimental pneumocystosis is 250 mg/kg per day (2,4). Doses of 60–500 mg/kg per day, all showed very marked antipneumocystis activity; thus, there was no way to establish a dose–response curve (13). More recent experiments used SMX regimens of 0.3–15 mg/kg per day and a dose–response effect was found (14).

The DHFR inhibitors used alone were ineffective in the treatment of pneumocystosis. Although these agents were tested in a variety of combinations with sulfonamides and dapsone, no evidence of synergy was found. The classification of activity of many of these drug combinations listed in Table 2 represents the activity of the sulfonamide or sulfone component. These experiments had been performed using the higher (≥ 60 mg/kg per day) doses of these compounds, as described earlier. However, more recently, when DHFR inhibitors were used in combination with 3 mg/kg per day SMX, synergistic effects were found (53). Experiments were performed comparing the following DHFR inhibitors administered alone and in combination with SMX: TMP; BL-1034 (also known as DHFR Inhibitor 3 or Ro 11-8958), a related compound with attractive pharmacokinetic properties; diaveridine, a commonly used veterinary preparation; and pyrimethamine. As seen in Figure 2, TMP, BL-1034, and diaveridine exhibited similar, dose-related synergistic effects with SMX; pyrimethamine was less active.

Similar experiments were performed with dapsone (53). These same DHFR inhibitors were compared alone and in combination with 25 mg/kg per day dapsone (Fig. 3). BL-1034 combined with dapsone lowered the median cyst count about 1000-fold, whereas TMP and diaveridine lowered the count by 100-fold. Pyrimethamine was even less active.

Toxicity of the DHFR inhibitors varied among the individual agents. Trimethoprim and diaveridine were well tolerated by the rats, whereas pyrimethamine and trimetrexate caused bone marrow suppression and other adverse reactions. The administration of folinic acid was helpful in protecting against the toxicity of the DHFR inhibitors and did not interfere with efficacy.

These data demonstrate that the rat model can be used to compare DHFR inhibitors if they are used in combination with the appropriate dose of sulfonamide or sulfone. The reasons for the lack of efficacy of DHFR inhibitors used alone are unclear, although several mechanisms (e.g., short half-life, high serum thymidine levels) have been proposed (14). The major application of these studies is that they might lead to more potent, less toxic antifolate drugs in humans. Most clinical treatment trials of pneumocystosis have used fixed doses of DHFR inhibitors and sulfomamides (e.g., TMP–SMX) that have been selected on an empiric basis. Little is known about issues such as the contribution of the DHFR inhibitor to the regimen; the effectiveness of different DHFR inhibitors; the antipneumocystis activity of different sulfonamides and sulfones; the optimal doses of these drug combinations.

The diamidines and related cationic compounds constituted the other major

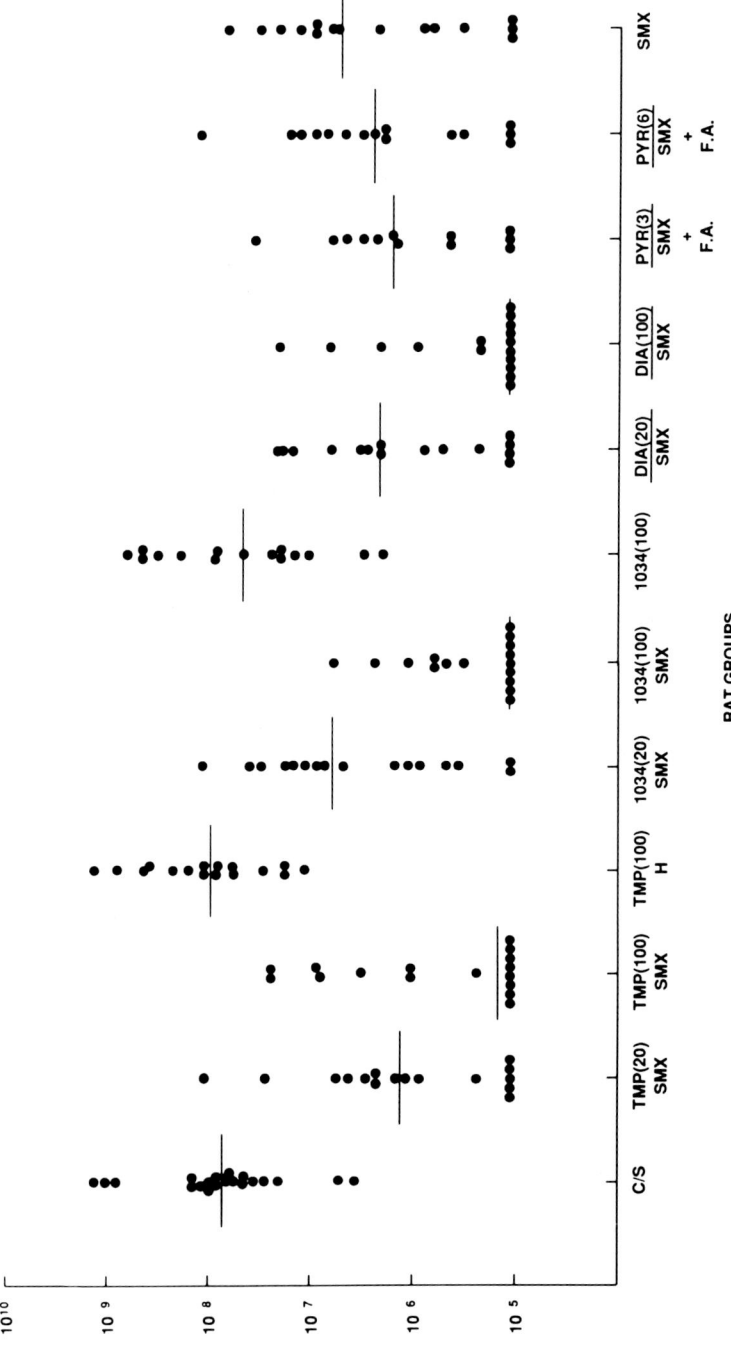

Figure 2 Assessment of the treatment of pneumocystosis in different rat groups by quantitation of *P. carinii* cysts in lung homogenates; C/S, control steroids. Dose of drugs in mg/kg/d given in parentheses. SMX, sulfamethoxazole 3 mg/kg/day; TMP, trimethoprim; 1034, DHFR inhibitor; DIA, diaveridine; PYR, pyrimethamine; FA, folinic acid. Horizontal bars represent median values. (Adapted from Ref. 53.)

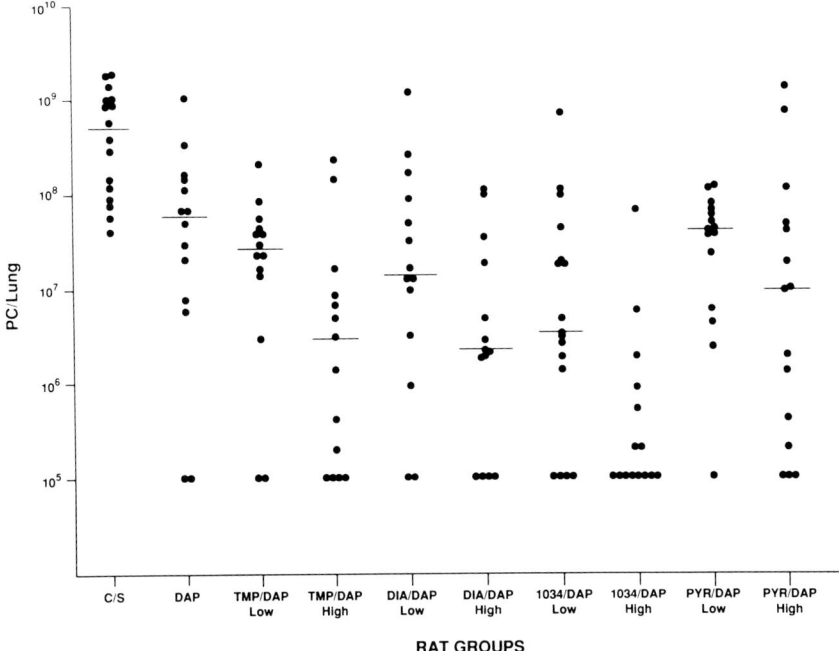

Figure 3 Assessment of the treatment of pneumocystosis in different rat groups by quantitation of *P. carinii* cysts in lung homogenates. Abbreviations as in Figure 2. DAP, dapsone 25 mg/kg per day; TMP low, 20 mg/kg per day; TMP high, 100 mg/kg per day; DIA low, 20 mg/kg per day; DIA high, 100 mg/kg per day; 1034 low, 20 mg/kg per day; 1034 high, 100 mg/kg per day; PYR, 3 mg/kg per day; PYR high, 6 mg/kg per day. Horizontal bars represent median values. (Adapted from Ref. 53.)

group of highly active antipneumocystis drugs (22,54). In contrast with the sulfonamides, these agents demonstrated a hierarchy of anti-*P. carinii* activity. The most active drugs included selected guanylhydrazone derivatives; diminazine, a diamidine; imidocarb, a carbanilide; and quinapyramine, an aminoquinaldine. The guanylhydrazone A compounds were synthesized according to procedures of Ulrich et al. (55), whereas the guanylhydrazone B derivatives were prepared by Dr. Richard Sundberg, University of Virginia (56). Pentamidine and five other compounds exhibited moderate activity. The *cis*-form of dimethylstilbamidine was slightly active, whereas the *trans*-form of this compound and several other drugs showed no activity.

The diamidine derivatives, which were originally developed as antitrypanosomal agents, presented problems of toxicity, product formulation, and limited supplies. These agents frequently caused serious averse reactions at doses only slightly higher than those found to show activity against *P. carinii*. Some compounds had been prepared many years ago, so there was little current information about their antimicrobial or pharmacological properties. Other drugs represented newly synthesized compounds and were available in small amounts; since nothing was known about what dose or form of these preparations would be best for oral or parenteral administration, drug testing was largely a matter of trial and error. Despite these limitations, the diamidine derivatives were among the most potent anti-*P. carinii* drugs (on a milligram per kilogram basis) tested in our animal model.

The diamidine derivatives are discussed in detail in Chapter 26. By contrast, there has been little investigation of the guanylhydrazones as antipneumocystis drugs. The availability of structure–activity information about the effects of guanylhydrazones in trypanosomes (56) should be helpful in studying their effectiveness against *P. carinii*.

Six purine nucleoside derivatives were studied. These compounds were initially synthesized by Dr. Robert Klein and Dr. Brian Otter, Montefiore Medical Center, and later obtained through the NIH AIDS Developmental Therapeutics Branch. Synthesis of purine nucleosides is very difficult, and only two compounds, 9-deazainosine and purine nucleoside 1, were available in sufficient quantities for testing at more than one dose. 9-Deazainosine showed marked anti-*P. carinii* activity (14) and purine nucleosides 1 and 2 showed slight activity. These results, and the lack of serious systemic toxicity, suggested that the purine nucleosides are worthy of further investigation as antipneumocystis drugs.

A variety of nitrofuran and nitroimidazole derivatives were evaluated (28). The most effective drug was furazolidone, which demonstrated moderate anti-*P. carinii* activity on repeated occasions over a dose range of 50–200 mg/kg per day. Nitrofurantoin and metronidazole showed slight activity at high doses, but this effect was not consistent and could not be improved by manipulations such as changes in the preparation, dose, or route of administration. None of the other compounds exhibited any activity against *P. carinii*.

The doses of furazolidone used in the rat model were far higher than the doses of the drug used in humans; thus, it is unlikely that furazolidone will ever be studied in clinical trials. However, since thousands of nitrofuran derivatives have been synthesized, some of these agents might have greater potency.

Many antiparasitic agents were tested, but the results were generally disappointing. The polyamine inhibitors, eflornithine (2-difluoromethylornithine; DFMO) and MD 27695, obtained from Dr. Peter McCann, Merrell-Dow (Cincinnati, Ohio), were administered alone and in combination with other agents, but showed little anti-*P. carinii* activity; DFMO was tolerated poorly by the rats (22). Similar data were obtained with arsenical derivatives synthesized by Dr. Ernst Friedheim, Rockefeller University, and antimonials. Dehydroemetine, a toxic antiamebic drug obtained from the Centers for Disease Control (Atlanta, Georgia), exhibited moderate activity at the 5-mg/kg per day dose in one experiment, but no activity at 1 mg/kg per day in another experiment; further studies of this compound would be of interest.

Antifungal drugs, administered alone or in combination, were ineffective in the therapy of pneomocystosis. Similar results were found with a series of antibiotics. We were especially interested in studying erythromycin because of anecdotal reports of its activity against *P. carinii* in humans; however, our analysis of several different preparations and doses of this agent was disappointing.

Of the antiviral agents studied, amantadine showed slight anti-*P. carinii* activity, but the dose had to be reduced from 100 to 50 mg/kg daily because of side effects in the rats (14). The anti-HIV compounds, zidovudine (azidothymidine; AZT), didanosine (dideoxyinosine; DDI), and the combination product Isoprinosine (dimepranol–inosine), were active. Zidovudine also had no influence on the antipneumocystis activity of TMP–SMX (14). Zidovudine is commonly administered to HIV patients with drugs, such as TMP–SMX, that prevent the development of opportunistic infections. Data obtained in the rat model suggest this can be done without loss of effectiveness.

Classification of Therapeutic Activity by Nucleus Counts

These data have been summarized in Table 3. In general, the pattern of antipneumocystis drug activity, as judged by nucleus counts, was similar to that determined by cyst counts; sulfonamides and diamidines were the most active groups of compounds. The major difference was in the magnitude of the changes with nucleus counts. Drugs that lowered the cyst count by 1000–10,000 frequently lowered the nuclei count by more than 10,000. This probably reflected that nucleus counts were usually tenfold higher than the cyst counts; however, a greater sensitivity of *P. carinii* nuclei than cysts to some drugs could not be ruled out. The practical result of classifying drugs on the basis of changes in the nucleus counts was to increase the level of activity of some agents (e.g., pentamidine, amicarbalide).

Prophylaxis Studies

Only three experiments were performed investigating the efficacy of antimicrobial drugs in the prevention of pneumocystosis. The compounds used in these studies and classification of their anti-*P. carinii* activity are presented in Tables 4 and 5, respectively. Most of the attention was devoted to antifolate drugs. Sulfamethoxazole was highly effective as a prophylactic agent when administered alone over a broad dose range, as judged by the reduction in cyst counts. No evidence of synergy was found when the DHFR inhibitors were combined with SMX. pyrimethamine and TMP both exhibited anti*P. carinii* activity when used alone in one experiment, but this effect could not be reproduced in another experiment.

Of the other drugs tested, diminazene showed activity at a dose of 5 mg/kg

Table 3 Classification of Drugs in the Treatment of *Pneumocystis carinii* Pneumonia by Nucleus Counts

Drug	Ratio
Very marked activity ($\geq 1000\times$ reduction)	
Dapsone	2,000
Dapsone + pyrimethamine	2,000
Imidocarb	3,600
Pentamidine	25,000
Quinapyramine	30,000
Sulfadiazine	9,300
Sulfadiazine + diaveridine	9,300
Sulfadiazine + pyrimethamine	73,000
Sulfadiazine + trimethoprim	9,300
Sulfadoxine	25,000
Sulfadoxine + pyrimethamine	73,000
Sulfamethoxazole	15,000
Sulfamethoxazole + diaveridine	3,270
Sulfamethoxazole + pyrimethamine	73,000
Sulfamethoxazole + trimethoprim	15,000
Sulfamethoxazole + DHFR inhibitor 1	2,700
Marked activity (100–999$\times$ reduction)	
Amicarbalide	491
Diminazine	714
Sulfadoxine + trimethoprim	884
Moderate activity (10–99$\times$ reduction)	
Isometamidium	37
Pyrimethamine	10
Slight activity (5–9$\times$ reduction)	
Dapsone + diaveridine	5
Dapsone + trimethoprim	5
DFMO	7
DFMO + diminazine	6
DFMO + pentamidine	9
Guanylhydrazone	8
No activity (<5$\times$ reduction)	
Ampicillin	<1
Astiban	2
Chloramphenicol	<1
Dehydroemetine	3
Diaveridine	<1
Ethidium bromide	3
Gentamicin	<1
Pentostam	1
Spectinomycin	<1
Spiramycin	1
Trimethoprim	<1

Source: Ref. 52.

Table 4 Drugs Evaluated in the Prevention of *Pneumocystis carinii* Pneumonia[a]

Drug	Dosage regimen (mg/kg per day)
Diminazine	1 sc–5 sc 3d–7d/wk
Furazolidone	50 po 5d/wk
Pentamidine	5 sc 2d/wk
Pyrimethamine	3–4.5 po
Sulfamethoxazole	3–60 po
Trimetrexate	3–4.5 sc
Trimethoprim	3–50 po
Sulfamethoxazole + pyrimethamine	15 po + 3 po
Sulfamethoxazole + trimetrexate	15 po + 3 po
Sulfamethoxazole + trimethoprim	3–15 po + 0.6–3 po

[a]Rats administered regimens containing pyrimethamine and trimetrexate were also given folinic acid 7–15 mg/day sc.
Source: Ref. 52.

Table 5 Classification of Drugs in the Prevention of *Pneumocystis carinii* Pneumonia by Cyst Counts

Drug	Ratio
Very marked activity (≥1000 × reduction)	
Sulfamethoxazole	6300
Sulfamethoxazole + pyrimethamine	6300
Sulfamethoxazole + trimetrexate	6300
Sulfamethoxazole + trimethoprim	6300
Marked activity (100–999 × reduction)	
Pyrimethamine	168
Moderate activity (10–99 × reduction)	
Diminazene	23
Trimethoprim	16
Slight activity (5–9 × reduction)	
Pentamidine	5
No activity (<5 × reduction)	
Furazolidone	1
Trimetrexate	1

Source: Ref. 52.

daily sc, but not when given less frequently or at a lower dose. Pentamidine and furazolidone were tested at only one dose.

Critique of the Classification System

Overall, the data suggest that the classification system is a simple, quantitative, and reproducible method of expressing and comparing the activity of antipneumocystis drugs. The system was modeled after the approach used for quantitative microbial cultures and provided clear categories of anti-*P. carinii* activity that followed a logarithmic scale. Classes of drugs as well as individual members of a drug class could be distinguished from each other, and studies of dose–response curves were enhanced. *Pneumocystis carinii* cyst and nucleus counts showed a similar pattern of response with therapy, although there were differences in the magnitude of this response. We believe that cyst quantitation can be used to screen most drugs for antipneumocystis activity; yet, with compounds (e.g., β-glucan inhibitors) that act on selective developmental stages of *P. carinii* (30,31), both cyst and nucleus counts are needed to obtain a complete picture of drug effects on the organism.

The classification system presented challenges for data analysis at both ends of the spectrum of drug activity. The long list of agents classified as inactive suggested that the level of reduction in *P. carinii* cyst or nucleus counts established for minimal activity was effective in screening out the minor effects of drugs. We feel that the benefits of this standard far outweighed any loss of sensitivity. Quantitative differences in the reduction in cyst or nucleus counts among drugs classified as very markedly active could not be accurately interpreted because of the inability of our system to detect fewer than 1.1×10^5 organisms per lung. This emphasized the need for more sensitive techniques to quantitate low levels of infection.

B. In Vitro Studies

The in vitro studies have been conducted mainly under the direction of Dr. Melanie Cushion. Our attempts over the years to develop *P. carinii* culture systems to study the effects of antimicrobial drugs followed a similar pattern: initial promising results, which raised our hopes, followed by inconsistent results or technical problems, which led to frustration. Our initial efforts focused on extending the data we obtained in tissue culture (40). The basic system involved rat *P. carinii* grown on A549 cells in multiwell plates. The cultures were inoculated with 1–2×10^7 *P. carinii* nuclei from infected rat lung homogenates. Each drug was usually tested at concentrations of 1 μg/mL and 0.1 μ/mL. The entire contents of three wells were harvested for each drug dose at days 1, 3, 5, and 7 of culture. *Pneumocystis carinii* organisms were counted in each well, and the result was expressed as the mean ± SEM. Drug activity was calculated on the basis of peak organism counts in the treated and control cultures and expressed as the percentage inhibition, as outlined in Table 6. Propagation of *P. carinii* was quite modest (three- to fivefold) in these studies, but it did permit analysis of the drugs.

Representative experiments are presented in Table 6. In the first study, pentamidine was compared with diminazene, quinapyramine, and propamidine. As can be seen, all drugs inhibited *P. carinii* growth in a similar manner. In a second experiment, guanylhydrazone was compared with three derivatives (gua-

Table 6 Evaluation of Antimicrobial Drugs on *Pneumocystis carinii* (Pc) Replication In Vitro

Experiment	Drug	Concentration (μg/mL)	Activity[a] (% inhibition)
1	Pentamidine	1	46
	Pentamidine	0.1	56
	Diminazene	1	56
	Quinapyramine	1	51
	Propamidine	1	67
2	Guanylhydrazone A1	1	81
	Guanylhydrazone A1	0.1	71
	Guanylhydrazone A3	1	82
	Guanylhydrazone A3	0.1	85
	Guanylhydrazone A2	1	79
	Guanylhydrazone A2	0.1	80
	Guanylhydrazone	1	75
	Guanylhydrazone	0.1	78
	Imidocarb	1	78
	Imidocarb	0.1	74
	Primaquine	1	59
	Primaquine	0.1	74
3	Pentamidine	1	79
	Pentamidine	0.1	59
	Diminazene A	1	61
	Diminazene A	0.1	72
	Amicarbalide	1	50
	Amicarbalide	0.1	75
	Isometamidium	1	35
	Isometamidium	0.1	77
	Ethidium	0.1	84
	Diminazene B	1	75
	Diminazene B	0.1	77

[a] $\% \text{ Inhibition} = \dfrac{\text{Peak Pc no. (control)} - \text{Peak Pc no. (treated)}}{\text{Peak Pc no. (control)}} \times 100$

nylhydrazone A1–A3) that had been used in the rat studies. Imidocarb and a structurally unrelated drug, primaquine, were also evaluated. As can be seen, the anti-*P. carinii* activity of these agents was quite similar. A consistent dose–response effect was not observed. In a third experiment, pentamidine was compared with closely related drugs. Diminazene was run twice (diminazene A, diminazene B) as an internal control. Pentamidine, diminazene, amicarbalide, isometamidium, and ethidium, all inhibited *P. carinii* growth in a manner similar to that found for the drugs reported earlier. Again, no dose–response effect was apparent.

Overall, the data suggested a general inhibitory effect of these compounds on *P. carinii* in vitro growth. Many of these agents also showed antipneumocystis activity in the rat model. That the results appeared to be reproducible was also encouraging. However, we had several major concerns: (1) The very modest growth of *P. carinii* made it difficult to detect real differences between compounds. (2) We were unable to show any differences in these agents based on structure or dose, whereas such differences were apparent in the rat model. (3) The results we obtained from the in vitro system in these experiments would not be helpful in predicting which compounds might be active in vivo. As time went on, we became more and more frustrated with the tissue culture system for studying antimicrobial drugs. Problems included high labor intensity, contamination by bacteria or fungi (probably present in the lung inoculum), and inconsistent results. Technicians varied considerably in their success in operating the system; the time-consuming and tedious nature of the work also led to a high degree of "burn-out." Thus, we ultimately came to the conclusion that tissue culture was of little value as a tool for drug screening.

In light of the ribosomal RNA data suggesting *P. carinii* is a fungus, we then began exploring the organism's growth in fungal media (57). The *P. carinii* inoculum was added to an experimental liquid medium in 25-mL flasks and sampled at different time points over a 1–2 week period. A variety of media, supplements, and environmental conditions were explored. Optimal *P. carinii* growth occurred in a medium of 1% Neopeptone and 0.2% *N*-acetylglucosamine, pH 4.0, at 37°C. In direct comparison experiments, propagation of *P. carinii* in the axenic medium was equal to or greater than than in tissue culture with A549 cells. The axenic system was then used to test antimicrobial drugs. The culture was inoculated with 10^7– 10^8 organisms per milliliter and sampled on different days. Drugs (e.g., pentamidine) that were active in the rat model inhibited *P. carinii* replication in a manner similar to that in tissue culture.

In metabolic studies, ^{3}H-labeled thymidine, uracil, methionine, and *N*-acetylglucosamine were added to the axenic medium, and uptake by *P. carinii* was examined at different times (57). Uptake of these labeled compounds occurred with live, but not dead (autoclaved), *P. carinii*; peak uptake in these experiments was at 12 hr. Further studies of incorporation of a metabolic label were conducted with [^{35}S]methionine. Autoradiographs demonstrated protein bands that stained with monoclonal and polyclonal antibodies specific for *P. carinii* antigens.

We then extended this work in an attempt to use the uptake of radiolabeled compounds by *P. carinii* as a method of evaluating the effects of antimicrobial drugs. Preliminary studies established the following points: [^{3}H]hypoxanthine was superior to other radiolabeled compounds for this purpose; the number of *P. carinii* (10^9–10^{10}/mL) needed to achieve peak uptake of [^{3}H]hypoxanthine differed from the number (10^7–10^8/mL) needed to achieve peak replication; 48 hr appeared to be the best time to study uptake and propagation.

Two experiments illustrating the effects of drugs on *P. carinii* replication and uptake of [^{3}H]hypoxanthine are presented in Table 7. In experiment 1, dose-related anti-*P. carinii* activity was detected by both methods with diamidines (pentamidine, quinapyramine) and polyamine inhibitors (DFMO, MDL 27,605). 9-Deazainosine (9 DI) also exhibited dose-related activity but purine nucleoside 1 was less active. Primaquine showed activity only at the higher dose, whereas inconsistent results were obtained with furazolidone. Chloramphenicol and quinine, which were ineffective against *P. carinii* in the rat model, showed activity in vitro. In experiment 2, pentamidine and ampicillin performed as expected, but DDI and Isoprinosine, which were inactive in rats, displayed activity here. Mefloquine showed no activity, but has not been tested in our animal model.

We were generally encouraged by these results, despite the discrepancies that were found with some drugs concerning their in vitro and in vivo anti-*P. carinii* activity. However, our later experiments were plagued by the same problems of consistency and reproducibility that occurred with our tissue culture studies. Technicians again displayed marked differences in their ability to make the axenic system work.

More recently, we have turned our attention to two systems that analyze *P. carinii* viability: fluorescent probes, Calcein AM and ethidium homodimer, which have proved superior over other vital stains in our hands (58); and ATP content, as determined by the luciferase reaction (59). It remains to be seen whether these systems will be more fruitful in testing anti-*P. carinii* drugs than our previous efforts.

IV. Conclusions

The immunosuppressed rat has long been the principal research tool for studying anti-*P. carinii* drugs. The choice of the type of rat is largely a matter of investigator preference. We continue to favor virus-positive animals with naturally acquired *P. carinii* infection over inoculated, virus-negative animals, because they are a highly reproducible experimental model, are easier to use, and more closely reflect the condition in humans. Although some investigators have found advan-

Table 7 Effects of Drugs on *Pneumocystis carinii* (Pc) In vitro

			Activity (% inhibition) (48 hr)[a]	
	Drug	Concentration (μg/mL)	Pc growth (%)	[^{3}H]hypoxanthine uptake (%)
Experiment 1[b]	Pentamidine	1	47	60
	Quinapyramine	0.1	24	49
	Quinapyramine	1	49	67
	DFMO	0.1	43	40
	DFMO	1	46	47
	MDL 27695	0.1	30	35
	MDL 27695	1	44	61
	9 DI	0.1	35	39
	9 DI	1	47	48
	Purine nucleoside 1	0.1	22	23
	Purine nucleoside 1	1	4	23
	Primaquine	0.1	1	7
	Primaquine	1	30	37
	Chloramphenicol	0.1	59	38
	Chloramphenicol	1	52	54
	Quinine	0.1	53	61
	Quinine	1	0	29
	Furazolidone	0.1	6	51
	Furazolidone	1	0	34
Experiment 2[c]	Pentamidine	1	40	
	Ampicillin	1	3	
	DDI	0.1	3	
	DDI	1	35	
	DDI	10	38	
	Isoprinosine	0.1	43	
	Isoprinosine	1	49	
	Isoprinosine	10	50	
	Mefloquine	0.1	0	
	Mefloquine	1	1	
	Mefloquine	10	0	

[a]Pc growth measured in organism nuclei per milliliter. [^{3}H]hypoxanthine uptake measured in cpm.
% Inhibition = $\frac{\text{Control} - \text{Rx}}{\text{Control}} \times 100$

[b]*Experiment 1*: Culture inoculated with 2×10^7 Pc/mL. At 48 hr, organism count in control culture was 7.9×10^7 mL. For [^{3}H]hypoxanthine uptake, 10^9 Pc were used in culture and [^{3}H]hypoxanthine was added at different time points. The [^{3}H]hypoxanthine uptake by Pc in control culture at 48 hr was 15,402 cpm.

[c]*Experiment 2*: Culture inoculated with 1×10^8 Pc/mL. At 48 hr, organism count in control culture was 7.2×10^8 Pc/mL.

tages of the inoculated rats, this has not been our experience. Other factors influencing the selection of rats include availability from commercial breeders and the regulations of the animal facility.

Regardless of the type of rat used, perhaps the major factors influencing their success in *P. carinii* studies are the housing and handling conditions. All immunosuppressed rats are at risk for infection with other opportunistic pathogens. The introduction of microisolater cages; laminar, HEPA-filtered air; and autoclaved food, water, and bedding at our institution resulted in improved survival of the rats and a reduction in the frequency of opportunistic infections.

The new classification system we have developed represents a simple quantitative, and reproducible method of comparing the anti-*P. carinii* activity of antimicrobial drugs. The system showed a hierarchy of antipneumocystis activity not only among classes of compounds, but also among individual members of a class. This classification system permits direct comparison of drugs studied at different times with each other and should be helpful in developing standard criteria for evaluating antipneumocystis agents that can be used by other investigators.

Despite the success of the rat model, it remains an expensive and inefficient system of screening drugs. Smaller animals, which require smaller quantities of these agents, would facilitate testing compounds that are in short supply. Corticosteroid-treated normal mice and congenitally immunodeficient (e.g., scid/scid) mice are promising alternatives.

The greatest impediment of *P. carinii* drug development is the lack of a reliable in vitro culture system. Although several approaches to drug testing have been proposed, none have yet gained widespread acceptance. Efforts to develop such a system remain a high priority in *P. carinii* research.

References

1. Frenkel JK, Good JT, Schultz JA. Latent pneumocystis infection of rats, relapse, and chemotherapy. Lab Invest 1966; 15:1559–1577.
2. Hughes WT, McNabb PC, Makres TD. Efficacy of trimethoprim and sulfamethoxazole in the prevention and treatment of *Pneumocystis carinii* pneumonitis. Antimicrob Agents Chemother 1974; 5:289–293.
3. Hughes WT. Limited effect of trimethoprim–sulfamethoxazole prophylaxis on *Pneumocystis carinii*. Antimicrob Agents Chemother 1979; 16:333–335.
4. Kluge RM, Spaulding DM, Spain JA. Combination of pentamidine and trimethoprim–sulfamethoxazole in the therapy of *Pneumocystis carinii* pneumonia in rats. Antimicrob Agents Chemother 1978; 13:975–978.
5. D'Antonio RG, Johnson DB, Winn RE, Van Dellen AF, Evans ME. Effect of folinic acid on the capacity of trimethoprim–sulfamethoxazole to prevent and treat *Pneumocystis carinii* pneumonia in rats. Antimicrob Agents Chemother 1986; 29:327–329.
6. Hughes WT, Smith BL. Intermittent chemoprophylaxis for *Pneumocystis carinii* pneumonia. Antimicrob Agents Chemother 1983; 24:300–301.

7. Hughes WT, Smith BL. Efficacy of diaminodiphenyl-sulfone and other drugs in murine *Pneumocystis carinii* pneumonitis. Antimicrob Agents Chemother 1984; 26: 436–440.
8. Hughes WT, Smith BL, Jacobus DP. Successful treatment and prevention of murine *Pneumocystis carinii* pneumonitis with 4,4'-sulfonylbisformanilide. Antimicrob Agents Chemother 1986; 29:509–510.
9. Hughes WT, Smith-McCain BL. Effects of sulfonylurea compounds on *Pneumocystis carinii*. J Infect Dis 1986; 153:944–947.
10. Hussain Z, Carlson ML, Craig ID, Lannigan R. Efficacy of tetroxoprim/sulfadiazone in the treatment of *Pneumocystis carinii* in rats. J Antimicrob Chemother 1985; 15: 575–578.
11. Kovacs JA, Allegra CJ, Kennedy S, Swan JC, Drake J, Parrillo JE, Chabner B, Masur H. Efficacy of trimetrexate, a potent lipid-soluble antifolate, in the treatment of rodent *Pneumocystis carinii* pneumonia. Am J Trop Med Hyg 1988; 39:491–496.
12. Queener SF, Bartlett MS, Jay MA, Durkin MM, Smith JW. Activity of lipid-soluble inhibitors of dihydrofolate reductase against *Pneumocystis carinii* in culture and in a rat model of infection. Antimicrob Agents Chemother 1987; 31:1323–1327.
13. Walzer PD, Kim CK, Foy J. Furazolidone and nitrofurantoin in the treatment of experimental *Pneumocystis carinii* pneumonia. Antimicrob Agents Chemother 1991; 35:158–163.
14. Walzer PD, Foy J, Steele PE, Kim CK, White M, Klein R, Otter B, Allegra A. Activities of antifolate, antiviral, and other drugs in an immunosuppressed rat model of *Pneumocystis carinii* pneumonia. Antimicrob Agents Chemother 1992; 36:1935–1942.
15. Yamada M, Takeuchi S, Shiota T, Matsumoto Y, Yoshikawa H, Okabayashi K, Tegoshi T, Yoshikawa T, Yoshida Y. Experimental studies on the chemoprophylaxis for *Pneumocystis carinii* pneumonia with intermittent administration of trimethoprim–sulfamethoxazole and pyrimethamine–sulfamonomethoxine. Jpn J Trop Med Hyg 1985; 13:287–294.
16. Yoshida Y, Takeuchi S, Ogino K, Ikai T, Yamada M. Studies on *Pneumocystis carinii* and *Pneumocystis carinii* pneumonia. III. Therapeutic experiment of the pneumonia with pyrimethamine + sulfamonomethoxine and trimethoprim + sulfamethoxazole. Jpn J Parasitol 1977; 26:367–375.
17. Hughes WT. Macrolide–antifol synergism in anti-*Pneumocystis carinii* therapeutics. J Protozool 1991; 38:160S.
18. Debs RJ, Blumenfeld W, Brunette EN, Straubinger RM, Montgomery AB, Lin E, Agabian N, Papahadjopoulos D. Successful treatment with aerosolized pentamidine of *Pneumocystis carinii* pneumonia in rats. Antimicrob Agents Chemother 1987; 31: 37–41.
19. Girard PM, Brun-Pascaud M, Farinotti R, Tamisier L, Kernbaum S. Pentamidine aerosol in prophylaxis and treatment of murine *Pneumocystis carinii* pneumonia. Antimicrob Agents Chemother 1987; 31:978–981.
20. Jones SK, Hall JE, Allen MA, Morrison SD, Ohemeng KA, Reddy VV, Geratz JD, Tidwell RR. Novel pentamidine analogs in the treatment of experiment *Pneumocystis carinii* pneumonia. Antimicrob Agents Chemother 1990; 34:1026–1030.

21. Tidwell RR, Jones SK, Geratz JD, Ohemeng KA, Cory M, Hall JE. Analogues of 1,5-bis(4-amidinophenoxy)pentane (pentamidine) in the treatment of experimental *Pneumocystis carinii* pneumonia. J Med Chem 1990; 33:1252–1257.
22. Walzer PD, Kim CK, Foy JM, Linke MJ, Cushion MT. Cationic antitrypanosomal and other antimicrobial agents in the treatment of experimental *Pneumocystis carinii* pneumonia. Antimicrob Agents Chemother 1988; 32:896–905.
23. Bartlett MS, Queener SF, Tidwell RR, Milhous WK, Berman JD, Ellis WY, Smith JW. 8-Aminoquinolines from Walter Reed Army Institute for Research for treatment and prophylaxis of *Pneumocystis carinii* in rat models. Antimicrob Agents Chemother 1991; 35:277–282.
24. Queener SF, Bartlett MS, Richardson JD, Durkin MM, Jay MA, Smith JW. Activity of clindamycin with primaquine against *Pneumocystis carinii* in vitro and in vivo. Antimicrob Agents Chemother 1988; 32:807–813.
25. Smith JW, Bartlett MS, Queener SF, Durkin MM, Jay MA, Hull MT, Klein RS, Marr JJ. *Pneumocystis carinii* pneumonia therapy with 9-deazainosine in rats. Diagn Microbiol Infect Dis 1987; 7:113–118.
26. Clarkson AB, Williams DE, Rosenberg C. Efficacy of DL-α-difluoromethylornithine in a rat model of *Pneumocystis carinii* pneumonia. Antimicrob Agents Chemother 1988; 32:1158–1163.
27. Clarkson AB Jr, Saric M, Grady RW. Deferoxamine and eflornithine (DL-α-difluoromethylornithine) in a rat model of *Pneumocystis carinii* pneumonia. Antimicrob Agents Chemother 1990; 34:1833–1835.
28. Walzer PD, Kim CK, Foy J. Furazolidone and nitrofurantoin in the treatment of experimental *Pneumocystis carinii* pneumonia. Antimicrob Agents Chemother 1991; 35:158–163.
29. Matsumoto Y, Yamada M, Amagai T. Yeast glucan of *Pneumocystis carinii* cyst wall: an excellent target for chemotherapy. J Protozool 1991; 38:6S–7S.
30. Schmatz DM, Romancheck MA, Pittarelli LA, Schwartz RE, Fromtling RA, Nollstadt KH, Van Middlesworth FL, Wilson KE, Turner MJ. Treatment of *Pneumocystis carinii* with 1,3-β-glucan synthesis inhibitors. Proc Natl Acad Sci USA 1990; 87:5950–5954.
31. Schmatz DM, Powles M, McFadden D, Pittarelli L. Treatment and prevention of *Pneumocystis carinii* pneumonia and further elucidation of the *Pneumocystis carinii* life cycle with 1,3-β-glucan synthesis inhibitor L-671-329. J Protozool 1991; 38: 151S–153S.
32. Hughes WT, Gray VL, Gutteridge WE, Latter VS, Pudney M. Efficacy of a hydroxynaphoquinone, 566C80, in experimental *Pneumocystis carinii* pneumonitis. Antimicrob Agents Chemother 1990; 34:225–228.
33. Brun-Pascaud M, Fay M, Zhong M, Bauchet J, Dux-Guyot A, Poeidalo JJ. Use of fluoroquinolones for prophylaxis of murine *Pneumocystis carinii* pneumonia. Antimicrob Agents Chemother 1992; 36:470–472.
34. Gigliotti F, Hughes WT. Passive immunoprophylaxis with specific monoclonal antibody confers partial protection against *Pneumocystis carinii* pneumonitis in animal models. J Clin Invest 1988; 81:1666–1668.
35. Shear HL, Valladares G, Narachi MA. Enhanced treatment of *Pneumocystis carinii*

pneumonia in rats with interferon-γ and reduced doses of trimethoprim/sulfmethoxazole. J AIDS 1990; 3:943–948.

36. Bartlett MS, Durkin MM, Jay MA, Queener SF, Smith JW. Sources of rats free of latent *Pneumocystis carinii*. J Clin Microbiol 1987; 9:1794–1795.
37. Bartlett MS, Fishman JA, Queener SF, Durkin MM, Jay MA, Smith JW. New rat model of *Pneumocystis carinii* infection. J Clin Microbiol 1988; 26:1100–1102.
38. Boylan CJ, Current WL. Improved rat models of *Pneumocystis carinii* pneumonia: induced laboratory infections in pneumocystis-free animals. Infect Immun 1992; 69:1589–1597.
39. Pifer LL, Pifer DD, Woods DR. Biological profile and response to anti-pneumocystis agents of *Pneumocystis carinii* in cell culture. Antimicrob Agents Chemother 1983; 24:674–678.
40. Cushion MT, Stanforth D, Linke MJ, Walzer PD. Method of testing the susceptibility of *Pneumocystis carinii* to antimicrobial agents in vitro. Antimicrob Agents Chemother 1985; 28:796–801.
41. Bartlett MS, Eichholtz R, Smith JW. Antimicrobial susceptibility of *Pneumocystis carinii* in culture. Diagn Microbiol Infect Dis 1985; 3:381–387.
42. Merali S, Meshnick SR. Susceptibility of *Pneumocystis carinii* to artemisinin in vitro. Antimicrob Agents Chemother 1991; 35:1225–1227.
43. Allegra CJ, Kovacs JA, Drake JC, Swan JC, Chabner BA, Masur H. Activity of antifolates against *Pneumocystis carinii* dihydrofolate reductase and identification of a potent new agent. J Exp Med 1987; 165:926–931.
44. Queener SF, Broughton MC. *Pneumocystis carinii* dihydrofolate reductase used to screen anti-pneumocystis drugs. Antimicrob Agents Chemother 1991; 35:1348.
45. Edman JC, Edman U, Cao M, Lundgren B, Kovacs JA, Santi DV. Isolation and expression of the *Pneumocystis carinii* dihydrofolate reductase gene. Proc Natl Acad Sci USA 1989; 86:8625–8629.
46. Volpe F, Dyer M, Scaife JG, Darby G. Stammers DK, Delves CJ. The multifunctional folic acid synthesis *fas* gene of *Pneumocystis carinii* appears to encode dihydropteroate synthase and hydroxymethyldihydropterin pyrophosphokinase. Gene 1992; 112:213–218.
47. Merali S, Zhang Y, Sloan D, Meshnick S. Inhibition of *Pneumocystis carinii* dihydropteroate synthetase by sulfa drugs. Antimicrob Agents Chemother 1990; 34:1075–1078.
48. Kovacs JA, Allegra CJ, Beaver J, Boarman D. Lewis M, Parrillo JE, Chabner B, Masur H. Characterization of de novo folate synthesis in *Pneumocystis carinii* and *Toxoplasma gondii*: potential for screening therapeutic agents. J Infect Dis 1989; 160:312–320.
49. Comley JCW, Mullin RJ, Wolfe LA, Hanlon MH, Ferone R. A microculture screen in assay for the primary in vitro evaluation of drugs against *Pneumocystis carinii*. Antimicrob Agents Chemother 1991; 35:1965–1974.
50. Walzer PD, Powell RD, Yoneda K, Rutledge ME, Milder JE. Growth characteristics and pathogenesis of experimental *Pneumocystis carinii* pneumonia. Infect Immun 1980; 27:929–937.
51. Kim CK, Foy JM, Cushion MT. Stanforth D, Linke MJ, Hendrix HL, Walzer PD. A

comparison of histologic and quantitative techniques in the evaluation of experimental *Pneumocystis carinii* pneumonia. Antimicrob Agents Chemother 1987; 31:197–201.
52. Walzer PD, Foy J, Steele P, White M. Treatment of experimental pneumocystosis: review of 7 years of experience and development of a new system for classifying antimicrobial drugs. Antimicrob Agents Chemother 1992; 36:1943–1950.
53. Walzer PD, Foy J, Steele P. Analysis of antifolate drug combinations in the treatment of experimental *Pneumocystis carinii* pneumonia. (submitted).
54. Walzer PD, Foy J, Sundberg R, Steele P. Guanylhydrazone derivatives in the treatment of experimental pneumocystosis. (in preparation).
55. Ulrich P, Cerami A. Trypanocidal 1,3-arylenediketonebis (quanylhydrazole)s. Structure–activity relationships among substituted and heterocyclic analogues. J Med Chem 1984; 27:35–40.
56. Sundberg RJ, Dahlausen DL, Manikumar G, Mavunkel B. Biswas A, Srinivasan V, Musallan HA, Reid WA Jr, Ager Al. Cationic antiprotozoal drugs. Trypanocidal activity of 2-(4'-formylphenyl)imidazo[1,2α]pyridinium guanylhydrazones and related derivatives of quarternary heteroatomic compounds. J Med Chem 1990; 33: 298–307.
57. Cushion MT, Ebbets D. Growth and metabolism of *Pneumocystis carinii* in axenic culture. J Clin Microbiol 1991; 28:1385–1394.
58. Kaneshiro ES, Wu YP, Cushion MT. Assays for testing *Pneumocystis carinii* viability. J Protozool 1991; 38:85S–87S.
59. Miyahira Y, Takeuchi T. Application of ATP measurement to evaluation of the growth of parasitic protozoa in vitro with a special reference to *Pneumocystis carinii*. Comp Biochem Physiol 1991; 100A:1031–1034.

26

Folate Antagonists in the Treatment of *Pneumocystis carinii* Pneumonia

DIANNE C. POLSEN
and JOSEPH A. KOVACS

Critical Care Medicine
National Institutes of Health
Bethesda, Maryland

GREGG Y. LIPSCHIK

Philadelphia Veterans Affairs Medical
  Center
and Medical College of Pennsylvania
Philadelphia, Pennsylvania

I. Introduction

The susceptibility of *Pneumocystis carinii* to inhibitors of folate metabolism is well documented by numerous in vivo and in vitro experiences. The combination of trimethoprim and sulfamethoxazole, two members of this class of drugs, is currently the recommended first-line therapy for the treatment of *P. carinii* pneumonia (1,2). Although this combination is clearly effective in treating *P. carinii* pneumonia, its use is somewhat limited by the high incidence of side effects, especially in patients with acquired immunodeficiency syndrome (AIDS), and by occasional treatment failures (3,4). Development of effective alternative therapies has, in the past, been hampered by the lack of rapid, high-processivity in vitro screening systems and the consequent need to rely on animal models that are more cumbersome, expensive, time-consuming, and that require large amounts of potential drugs.

Recognition that antifolates are effective in treating *P. carinii* pneumonia has focused research on folate metabolism in *P. carinii*, with a hope that greater understanding of these metabolic pathways will result in the identification of folate antagonists that are more potent or less toxic than conventional agents. These studies have resulted in the biochemical characterization of *P. carinii* dihydrofolate reductase (DHFR), thymidylate synthase (TS), and dihydropteroate synthase (DHPS); the cloning of these enzymes; the development of specific in vitro assays; and the identification of potential alternative therapeutic agents. This chapter will review our understanding of folate metabolism in *P. carinii* and the current status of folate antagonists in the treatment of *P. carinii* pneumonia.

II. Folate Metabolism: Overview

Folates are ubiquitous in nature and play an integral role in the synthesis of DNA, RNA, and proteins (reviewed in Ref. 5) (Fig. 1). Tetrahydrofolate, the reduced form of folic acid, or its derivatives, interact in multiple one-carbon transfers required in these metabolic pathways (6). Following these transfers, the folates remain as tetrahydrofolates, except when 5,10-methylenetetrahydrofolate serves as a methyl group donor in the synthesis of thymidylate by TS. In the latter reaction, the folate end-product is dihydrofolate, which cannot be reused until it is reduced to tetrahydrofolate by DHFR. Thus, DHFR is essential for repleting tetrahydrofolates, and inhibition of DHFR by methotrexate, trimethoprim, or similar drugs results in an accumulation of dihydrofolate and a depletion of the metabolically important tetrahydrofolates. The DHFRs are species-specific, and this characteristic has allowed the identification of inhibitors that differ markedly in their affinity for DHFRs from different species. The widely divergent minimum inhibitor concentrations (MICs) of the DHFR inhibitor trimethoprim in bacterial and mammalian enzymes illustrates the marked structural differences that exist in this enzyme. The average median inhibitory concentration (IC_{50}) of trimethoprim for four mammalian reductases is 235 μM, whereas typical bacterial DHFRs have IC_{50} values of about 0.008 μM (7). Several bacterial and mammalian DHFR genes have been sequenced and expressed, and these studies as well as three-dimensional structures deduced from crystallographic studies have confirmed structural differences in these enzymes (7).

Cells obtain their required folates by either active transport from their environment or by de novo synthesis. In almost all organisms these two pathways are mutually exclusive. Mammalian cells are unable to synthesize folates de novo, but have an active transport system for uptake of exogenous folates, which are highly charged molecules owing to the presence of terminal glutamic acid moieties, and thus cannot be taken up passively. This active transport system can also be used by hydrophilic folate analogues such as methotrexate.

Many microorganisms, including *P. carinii*, can synthesize folates de novo, but lack an active transport system and, hence, are unable to scavenge folates from the environment (8). A key enzyme in de novo folate synthesis is DHPS, which catalyzes the condensation of *para*-aminobenzoic acid (PABA) with 6-hydroxymethyldihydropteroate. Since mammalian cells do not possess this enzyme, it is a very attractive target for selective inhibition of an organism's metabolism. Sulfon-

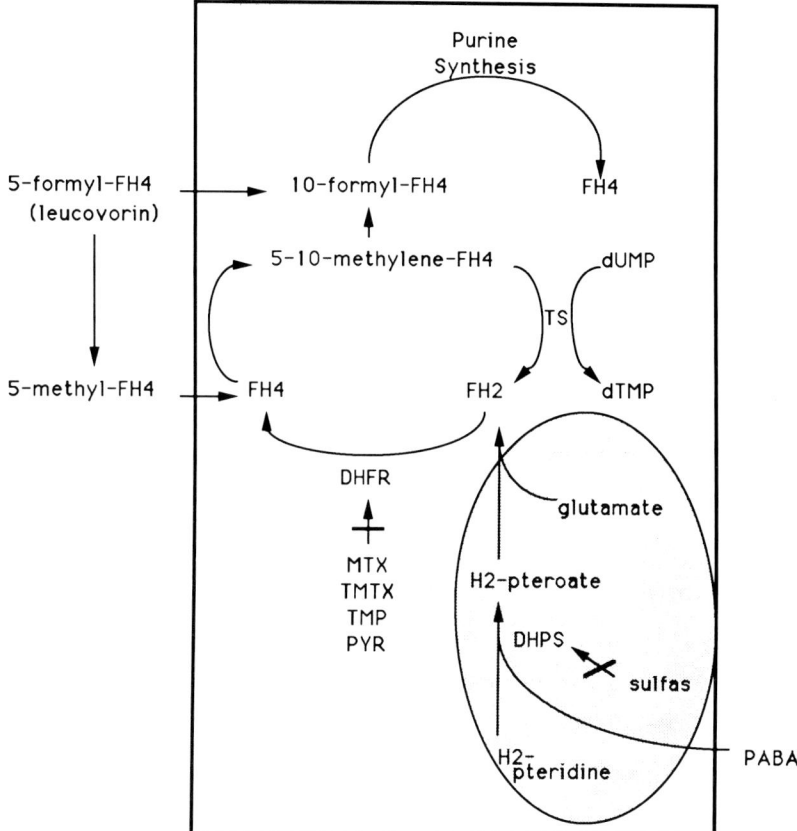

Figure 1 Schematic of folate metabolism in *P. carinii* and mammalian cells. The rectangle represents the cell membrane. The shaded area represents de novo folate synthesis and is present in *P. carinii*, but not host cells. Mammalian cell,s but not *P. carinii*, can take up reduced folates such as 5-formyl- or 5-methyltetrahydrofolate, by an active transport mechanism. Sulfonamides act by inhibiting DHPS; methotrexate, trimetrexate, trimethoprim, and pyrimethamine act by inhibiting DHFR. FH_2, dihydrofolate; FH_4, tetrahydrofolate. (From Lipschik GY, Kovacs JA. Chemotherapeutic targets in *Pneumocystis carinii*. In: Sutcliffe J, Georgopapadakou NH, eds. Emerging Targets in Antibacterial and Antifungal Therapy. New York: Chapman & Hull, 1992. Used with permission.)

amides and sulfones inhibit this enzyme, resulting in depletion of dihydrofolate and tetrahydrofolates.

Although inhibitors of DHFR and DHPS are potentially active as single agents against microorganisms, use of each agent alone will result in an accumulation of precursors, which may partially overcome the inhibition. The development of the classic agent trimethoprim–sulfamethoxazole, currently the standard antipneumocystis therapy, arose from the attempt to block the critical folate metabolic pathway in bacteria at two sequential points to produce a synergistic pharmacological effect. Synergy with the combination of trimethoprim and sulfamethoxazole has, in fact, been demonstrated in vitro for several microorganisms (9).

Because folate antagonists are known to be active against *P. carinii*, characterization of folate metabolism in *P. carinii* has been a major and very fruitful area of research, which may ultimately lead to the identification of improved therapeutic agents.

III. *Pneumocystis carinii* Dihydropteroate Synthase

Pneumocystis carinii has definitively been shown to possess the enzymes for de novo folate synthesis, including DHPS, in studies that employed rat-derived *P. carinii* maintained in short-term cultures (8). Organisms, pulsed overnight with [^{3}H]PABA in a PABA- and folate-free medium demonstrated the incorporation of [^{3}H]PABA into reduced folates, primarily 10-formyltetrahydrofolate and tetrahydrofolate. Incorporation of [^{3}H]PABA was inhibited by sulfamethoxazole at concentrations as low as 0.02 µg/mL, as well as by other agents active against *P. carinii*. Inclusion of two precursors of folate synthesis, dihydroneopterin and 6-hydroxymethyldihydropteridine, in the culture medium resulted in a 200–400% increase in [^{3}H]PABA incorporation, suggesting that precursors needed by *P. carinii* for folate metabolism are identical with other organisms.

The DHPS activity has recently been identified in crude *P. carinii* extracts using two assay systems. Characterization of the enzyme has been difficult in these studies because of low levels of enzymatic activity, but evaluation of the relative inhibitory activity of different sulfonamides as well as non–sulfa-containing analogues of PABA was possible (10,11).

The most important advance in the search for new, more potent inhibitors of *P. carinii* DHPS has been the recent cloning of this enzyme (12). By using oligonucleotides based on conserved regions in the DHPS of other organisms, Volpe and colleagues were able to identify a clone with an open-reading frame encoding a protein homologous to the DHPS of *Streptococcus pneumoniae* and *Bacillus subtilis*. The predicted protein contained 740 amino acids with a relative molecular mass (M_r) of 97,278. The protein appeared to be multifunctional, since it also contained regions homologous to bacterial 6-hydroxymethyldihydropterin pyrophosphokinase (DHPPK), the enzyme preceding DHPS in de novo folate synthesis. The authors have called this multifunctional gene the *fas* (folic acid synthesis) gene. An additional, as yet unidentified, function of the protein may be encoded by the first 160 amino acids, which do not have homology to any known protein.

The availability of large quantities of recombinant *P. carinii* DHPS should

Folate Antagonists 549

now allow large-scale screening of the extensive repositories of PABA analogues. In addition, agents specifically active against *P. carinii* DHPPK may also be identified and may prove useful in treating *P. carinii* pneumonia.

IV. *Pneumocystis carinii* Dihydrofolate Reductase

Since DHFR was a known target for anti-*P. carinii* therapy, it became an early focus of investigation and, thus, was one of the first enzymes of *P. carinii* to be characterized and cloned. Studies by Allegra et al. initially demonstrated DHFR activity in cytosolic preparations of partially purified rat *P. carinii* using a spectrophotometric assay that allowed the comparison of several DHFR inhibitors (13). The enzyme was subsequently partially purified and characterized by Kovacs et al., using high-performance liquid chromatography (14). Surprisingly, *P. carinii* DHFR was a small molecule of approximately 26,000 Da, similar to the M_r of the enzyme derived from bacteria, fungi, or mammalian cells. It was anticipated that enzyme characterization would identify a large molecule, with an M_r greater than 100,000 Da, similar to the enzyme size found in all protozoa. The protozoan DHFR is a component of a large, bifunctional molecule that also contains TS activity (15). The *P. carinii* DHFR and TS activity were readily separated by methotrexate affinity chromatography, indicating that they are not on the same molecule. The finding that *P. carinii* DHFR was a small, unifunctional, rather than large, bifunctional molecule was one of the first biochemical observations suggesting that *P. carinii* is accurately classified as a fungus, rather than a protozoan. The K_m of *P. carinii* DHFR for dihydrofolate was fourfold greater than the K_m of rat DHFR (17.6 vs 4.0 µM). These kinetic differences suggest a structural difference between the active site of the two enzymes that could allow identification of a DHFR inhibitor with greater affinity for the *P. carinii* DHFR than for the mammalian enzyme, resulting in an improved therapeutic index.

The gene encoding *P. carinii* DHFR has subsequently been cloned by Edman et al., using trimethoprim resistance as a selective marker, because trimethoprim had been shown to be a poor inhibitor of *P. carinii* DHPS (16). The predicted protein had an M_r of 23,868, similar to the size demonstrated by gel filtration. Trimethoprim was confirmed to be a poor inhibitor of *P. carinii* DHFR, with an IC_{50} of 20 µM, compared with 2 µM for human and 0.002 µM for *Escherichia coli* DHFR. The thymidylate synthase gene of *P. carinii* has also been cloned and was found to encode a protein of M_r 34,269 (17). Pulsed-field gel electrophoresis and Southern hybridization studies have documented that the genes encoding DHFR and TS of *P. carinii* reside on separate chromosomes, unambiguously demonstrating that in *P. carinii* these genes are not linked (16,17).

The availability of purified recombinant enzymes will allow the large-scale screening of DHFR and TS inhibitors, again with the hope that more effective, less toxic agents can be identified.

V. Methods of Identifying New Agents

Given the advances of the past few years, screening of potential new therapeutic agents is no longer dependent exclusively on studies in animal models. Enzyme assays using crude organism extracts or partially purified native DHFR and DHPS, as well as recombinant enzymes that can be produced in unlimited quantities, are available to use in an initial screening step to identify inhibitors of these targets with greater potency or selectivity than currently used agents. Promising agents can then be evaluated by short-term in vitro culture assays using intact organisms. Such assays are important because they demonstrate that the drug can cross into the organism and reach the target enzyme without being inactivated. In vitro culture assays can rely on nonspecific measurements on drug activity or on assays specific for folate metabolism, such as the [^{3}H]PABA incorporation assay (8,18,19). Assays that rely on enumeration of organisms are described elsewhere. The [^{3}H]PABA incorporation assay has been described earlier. This assay has recently been adapted to a 96-well microtiter plate in which membranes are assayed for radiolabeled folate products by scintillation counting (20). This technique greatly increases the number of studies that can be done at one time, and requires fewer *P. carinii* than had previously been needed in tissue culture studies.

As a last step, promising drugs can be evaluated in animal models, such as the corticosteroid-treated rat model (described elsewhere) in which *P. carinii* pneumonia spontaneously develops after 6–8 weeks (21). Preliminary identification of active compounds by the in vitro methods should facilitate screening by the animal model, and provide a target drug level to maximize efficacy. It is important to recognize, however, that drugs that show promise in vitro, but are inactive in the rat model, may in fact be active in humans. Limitations of the animal model include more rapid metabolism of most drugs compared with humans, as well as difficulties in administering the drugs with sufficient frequency to sustain high serum levels.

The cloning and expression of both DHPS and DHFR provides another mechanism for developing effective agents through rational drug design. Recombinant technology should provide enough protein to determine the crystal structure of both of these enzymes, which should allow development of agents that will optimally target the active site of the enzymes.

VI. Dihydropteroate Synthase Inhibitors

A. Preclinical Studies

Sulfonamides and Sulfones

The sulfonamides are class of chemotherapeutic agents that are derived from the compound *para*-aminobenzenesulfonamide (sulfanilamide). Their antimicrobial effect is achieved through antagonism of PABA and the inhibition of DHPS (Fig. 2). With the discovery, in the 1930s, of the antimicrobial Prontosil (sulfamidochrysoidine), sulfonamides heralded a new medical era. They were the first drugs used as effective therapy in the prevention and treatment of bacterial infections. The emergence of resistant bacteria and the development of penicillin and other antibiotics diminished their use in subsequent years. The p-aminobenzenesulfonyl unit is central to their effectiveness, and the N^1–substituted derivatives are the analogues with improved activity, in particular the N^1 heterocycle and N^1 acyl class (22). Sulfamethoxazole, the sulfa component of the currently recommended therapy for P. carinii pneumonia, has among the broadest antibacterial spectra and lowest MICs of the sulfonamides (22).

The sulfones, which are structurally related to sulfonamides, are chemically derived from 4,4′-diaminodiphenyl sulfone (dapsone); they were first used in the 1940s in the treatment of leprosy. Dapsone is the sulfone with the widest clinical application (see Fig. 2).

Sulfonamides were first shown to be effective in the rat model of P. carinii pneumonia by Frenkel et al., in 1966 (23). Sulfadiazine alone was shown to have partial efficacy; greater efficacy was seen in combination with pyrimethamine. This combination was subsequently used in humans, with some benefit (24). However, it was not until Hughes and colleagues demonstrated the efficacy of trimethoprim–sulfamethoxazole, both in animals and in humans, that this class of

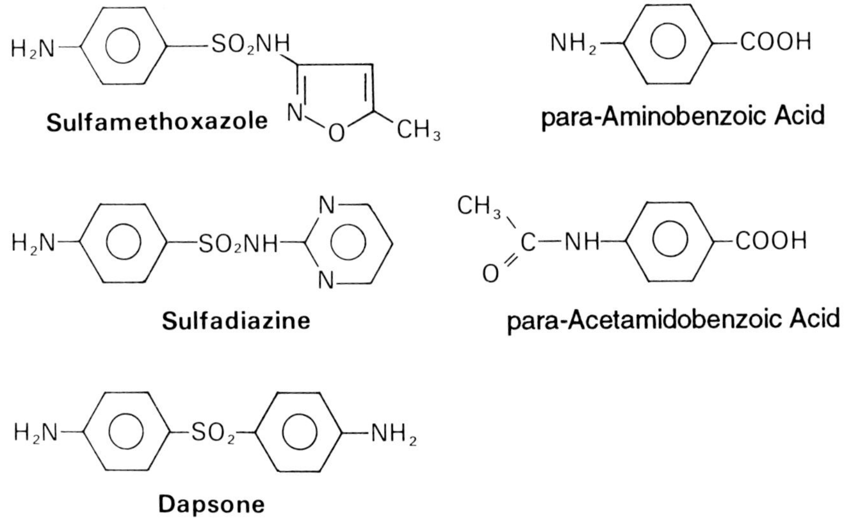

Figure 2 Structure of PABA and analogues that interfere with folate metabolism by inhibition of DHPS activity.

drugs became the treatment of choice for *P. carinii* pneumonia (21,25). These investigators also demonstrated the excellent prophylactic efficacy of trimethoprim–sulfamethoxazole in both rats and humans (21,26).

Because a wide variety of sulfonamides and related compounds have been developed, and because most of these have not been evaluated for treatment or prevention of *P. carinii* pneumonia, renewed attention has focused on alternative sulfa drugs as therapeutic agents. As noted earlier, enzyme assays with native *P. carinii* DHPS have been used to evaluate the relative potencies of a few sulfonamides. Merali et al. found that sulfaquinaxoline and sulfamethoxazole has IC_{50}s of 425 and 450 µM, respectively, with K_is of 92 and 59 µM; sulfadoxine and sulfadiazine had IC_{50}s greater than 500 µM, with K_i for sulfadoxine of 149 µM (11). In this assay dapsone was the most effective inhibitor, with an IC_{50} of 215 µM and a K_i of 9 µM. In contrast, Allegra and colleagues, using different assay conditions, found that most sulfonamides had an IC_{50} of between 0.5 and 10 µM; sulfamethoxazole and sulfadiazine were the most potent sulfonamides tested (IC_{50} = 0.7 and 0.4 µM, respectively) (10). Dapsone had an IC_{50} of 1.5 µM. Differences in assay conditions and methodology likely account for the disparate results seen in the two studies. The availability of recombinant enzyme should allow reassessment of the relative potency of these drugs, as well as rapid screening of the many previously synthesized sulfonamides and sulfones.

Sulfonamides have been evaluated to only a limited extent in short-term tissue culture assays. Sulfamethoxazole has been reported to inhibit [^{3}H]PABA incorporation, with an IC_{50} of approximately 0.1 µM; dapsone had similar activity (20). In addition, the combination trimethoprim–sulfamethoxazole has been inhibitory when cultures are evaluated by counting organisms, but not when evaluated by inhibition of [^{14}C]glucose utilization (18,19,27).

Evaluation of sulfa drugs in animal models has also been limited. Hughes and Smith demonstrated the effectiveness, in the immunosuppressed rat model, of dapsone as both a prophylactic and therapeutic agent, at doses of 25 mg/kg per day or greater; the addition of trimethoprim was marginally beneficial only at a low dose of dapsone (5 mg/kg per day) (28). Walzer et al. examined the effectiveness of several sulfa compounds for therapy in this model (29). Sulfamethoxazole, sulfadiazine, and sulfadoxine were similarly effective at a dose of 250 mg/kg per day, as was dapsone at a dose of 125 mg/kg per day. The effectiveness of the sulfa compounds was not improved in this model by the addition of a DHFR inhibitor. The diformyl derivative of dapsone, 4,4′-sulfonylbisformanilide also showed antipneumocystis activity in the immunosuppressed rat (30).

Other Compounds

Sulfonylureas are compounds structurally related to sulfonamides that have been used in humans as hypoglycemic agents. Two sulfonylurea agents, carbutamide

(N^1-sulfanilyl-N^2-butylcarbamide) and tolbutamide have been evaluated in the immunosuppressed rat model (31). Tolbutamide differs from carbutamide in that the functionally important amino group has been replaced with a methyl group; from studies in bacteria, such a substitution in a PABA analogue would be expected to dramatically reduce or eliminate antimicrobial activity (22). Carbutamide showed significant activity, similar to the improvement seen with trimethoprim–sulfamethoxazole, as both a prophylactic and therapeutic agent in the rat model. As predicted, tolbutamide showed no activity. The hypoglycemic effects of carbutamide have precluded further clinical evaluation.

Isoprinosine is a drug that was recently shown in a randomized placebo-controlled trial to slow the progression to AIDS amongst HIV-infected patients, primarily through diminishing the occurrence of *P. carinii* pneumonia (32). Although isoprinosine was evaluated because of potential immunostimulating properties, no changes in immune function correlating with benefit were noted. Isoprinosine is composed of three components, inosine and the salt of *para*-acetamidobenzoic acid (PAcBA) with dimethylaminopropanol. Because PAcBA is an analogue of PABA (see Fig. 2), Kovacs et al. investigated the possibility that isoprinosine exerted its benefit through a specific anti-*P. carinii* effect (33). In both an [^{3}H]PABA incorporation assay and a DHPS assay, isoprinosine as well as PAcBA alone were inhibitory (IC_{50} of 20–240 μM). No effect was seen in the immunosuppressed rat model; differences in metabolism of the drug by humans compared with rats may account for the lack of efficacy. The identification of nonsulfa-inhibitors of *P. carinii* DHPS is important, given the substantial number of adverse effects in HIV-infected patients attributed to the sulfa component of therapy. Large-scale screening, using recombinant enzyme, may result in the identification of a more potent nonsulfa DHPS inhibitor.

B. Clinical Trials

The only DHPS inhibitor other than sulfamethoxazole to be evaluated in clinical trials has been dapsone. In an open trial, dapsone as a single agent (100 mg/day) was associated with a success rate of 61% (11/18); this was felt to be lower than expected with standard therapy (34). In a smaller trial of seven patients, a higher dose of dapsone (200 mg/day) was poorly tolerated and appeared to be no more effective than the lower dose (35). Dapsone (100 mg/day) plus trimethoprim (20 mg/kg per day) was subsequently evaluated in 15 AIDS patients with mild to moderate *P. carinii* pneumonia (36). There was a 100% initial response rate and an overall efficacy of 87%, comparable to results seen with standard therapy. Results from a randomized trial comparing trimethoprim–dapsone with trimethoprim–sulfamethoxazole in patients with mild to moderate disease showed that both combinations were equally effective, but that trimethoprim–dapsone was associated with fewer side effects (37). Given these data, trimethoprim–dapsone is a currently accepted alternative to trimethoprim–sulfamethoxazole for the initial treatment of mild to moderate *P. carinii* pneumonia.

VII. Dihydrofolate Reductase Inhibitors

A. Preclinical Studies

Initial evaluation of inhibitors of *P. carinii* DHFR was prompted by the lack of information on the potency of available inhibitors and the development of new, potent lipid–soluble inhibitors of mammalian DHFR (Fig. 3). The 2,4-diaminopyrimidines, trimethoprim and pyrimethamine, which have been used in the treatment of *P. carinii* pneumonia, are active against *P. carinii* because they can enter organisms freely by passive diffusion. However, in initial enzyme inhibition studies by Allegra et al., these drugs were weak inhibitors of *P. carinii* DHFR, with an IC_{50} of 39.6 μM and 2.8 μM, respectively (30).

Cancer research has led to the development of more potent lipophilic DHFR

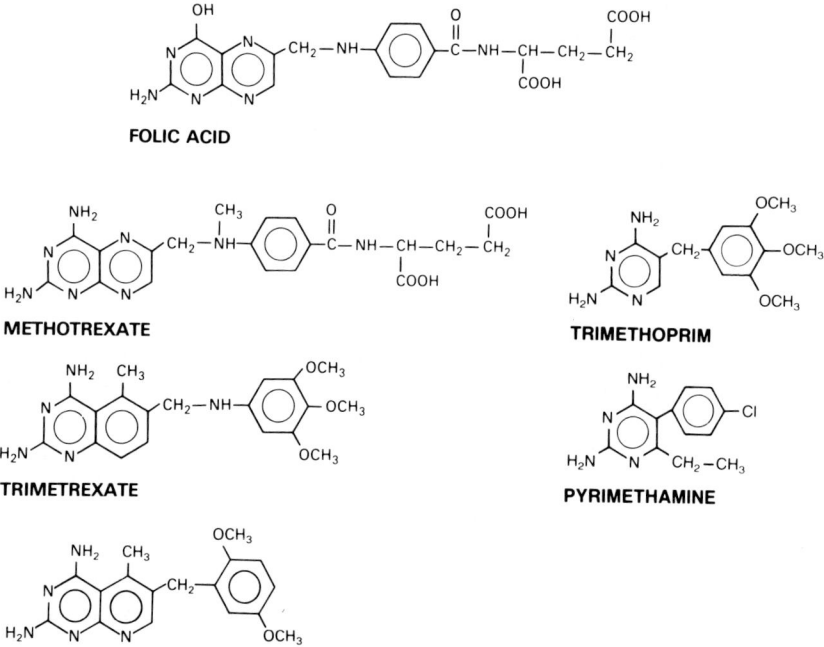

Figure 3 Structure of folic acid and analogues that interfere with folate metabolism by inhibition of DHFR activity.

inhibitors, such as trimetrexate and piritrexim, which are able to cross cell membranes without a transport mechanism (38–41). Such inhibitors would be expected to have activity against *P. carinii*, since they can enter the organism. Methotrexate, a potent inhibitor of mammalian DHFR, is 28,000-fold more potent than trimethoprim, with an IC_{50} of 0.0014 μM, but is inactive against *P. carinii* because it requires an active transport system for uptake (13).

Trimetrexate is a novel DHFR inhibitor that is a lipid-soluble quinazoline analogue of methotrexate. Initial studies with trimetrexate by Allegra et al. showed that it was 1500-fold more potent than trimethoprim in inhibiting *P. carinii* DHFR (IC_{50} = 0.026 μM) (13). Piritrexim, a similar compound, differs from trimetrexate in that it is a dimethoxy rather than trimethoxy analogue and has a shorter bridging link between its two ring structures. Piritrexim, unlike trimetrexate, is an orally bioavailable compound and has a shorter half-life in humans (4.5 hr vs 9–16 hr for trimetrexate (41–43). Piritrexim was as effective as trimetrexate in inhibiting *P. carinii* DHFR (IC_{50} = 0.019 μM) (44). The efficacy of both drugs was confirmed in tissue culture assays, in which concentrations as low as 14 μM trimetrexate and 1.6 μM piritrexim were inhibitory (45). Trimethoprim, at a concentration of 345 μM, had no inhibitory effects. Other DHFR inhibitors, some of which are more potent or more selective than currently available inhibitors, have been recently identified by screening with enzyme assays (46).

Both trimetrexate and piritrexim have also been evaluated in the immunosuppressed rat model. Since these drugs can enter host cells and *P. carinii* alike, host toxicity is a potential barrier to therapy. In preliminary dose escalation trials in humans, myelosuppression was the limiting adverse effect (43). Since host cells can use exogenous folates, the coadministration of leucovorin, which bypasses the blockade of DHFR, should minimize toxicity in host cells without affecting therapeutic efficacy when they are used in the treatment of *P. carinii* pneumonia. In the rat model, trimetrexate plus leucovorin was well tolerated and effective when administered parenterally alone or orally when combined with sulfamethoxazole, but was ineffective when administered orally without sulfamethoxazole (47). The half-life of trimetrexate in humans is 10 hr vs 1 hr in rats. Both trimetrexate and piritrexim were also effective in preventing or reducing the severity of *P. carinii* pneumonia when administered as prophylaxis from the start of immunosuppression (45). Of note, trimethoprim alone has been ineffective in treating or preventing *P. carinii* pneumonia in the rat model (29).

B. Clinical Trials

On the basis of the in vitro and animal data, a clinical trial evaluating trimetrexate plus leucovorin as therapy for documented *P. carinii* pneumonia was undertaken in 49 AIDS patients (42). Trimetrexate was evaluated in a nonrandom manner as a single agent for initial treatment and salvage therapy, and in combination with sulfadiazine for initial therapy. Response rates (no change in therapy) of 63–71% and survival rates of 69– 88% compared favorably with results published in studies using the standard regimens of trimethoprim–sulfamethoxazole and pentamidine. Trimetrexate plus leucovorin was well tolerated; 34% of patients had minor adverse reactions, but only one patient required discontinuation of trimetrexate because of adverse effects. However, the relapse rate within 3 months was unexpectedly high at 60% (six of ten patients) when trimetrexate was used as a single agent for primary therapy. Overall, this pilot study found trimetrexate to be safe and effective therapy.

Trimetrexate was subsequently compared with trimethoprim–sulfamethoxazole in a randomized, multicenter trial (ACTG protocol 029/031). This study was stopped prematurely because trimetrexate was found to be inferior, with 69% survival for trimetrexate, compared with 81% for trimethoprim–sulfamethoxazole (48). In an open-label trial of trimetrexate administered under a treatment IND mechanism to AIDS patients with *P. carinii* pneumonia who were intolerant of or had failed standard therapy, an overall response rate of 34% was seen; this compared favorably with historical controls (49).

Hypersensitivity reactions to trimetrexate have recently been reported in Phase II cancer trials, including hypotension and the systemic manifestations of flushing, pruritus, edema, and difficulty swallowing (50). These responses were reported in fewer than 2% of cancer patients treated with trimetrexate and have not been described in any patients with AIDS.

A recent pilot study evaluated the safety and efficacy of piritrexim for treatment of *P. carinii* pneumonia in humans (51). An open-label, dose-escalation trial was conducted, with simultaneous administration of leucovorin, in patients with mild to moderate *P. carinii* pneumonia. Oral piritrexim was effective, well tolerated, and capable of being used in the outpatient setting. It was effective in 60–77% of patients at a dose of 150–250 mg/m^2. Unfortunately, as with trimetrexate, the relapse rate was greater than anticipated, despite administration of prophylaxis after therapy. Given the experience with both trimetrexate and piritrexim, DHFR inhibitors appear not to be useful as single agents, except in patients unable to tolerate standard therapies. They may need to be administered with a sulfa agent for improved clearance of *P. carinii*.

VIII. Summary and Conclusions

The folic acid inhibitors trimethoprim, sulfamethoxazole, and dapsone constitute a vital part of currently available therapy for *P. carinii* pneumonia, but there are limitations to their use, primarily because of drug intolerance, but also because of occasional treatment failures. The goal of finding safer, more effective therapeutic regimens using folate antagonists should be enhanced by recent advances in understanding the metabolism of *P. carinii* coupled with new assays and the application of molecular biological techniques. Sulfonamides and sulfones, as single agents, are active against *P. carinii* in animal models, but dapsone as a single agent is ineffective in humans; sulfonamides as single agents have not been tested, but since most adverse reactions appear to be to the sulfonamide component, the advantages of such a regimen are probably small. The DHFR inhibitors alone are inadequate therapy; although potent inhibitors, such as trimetrexate, are clearly active in humans, when used as single agents they are associated with an unacceptably high relapse rate, despite prophylaxis. Accordingly, combination therapy seems to be necessary at present for maximum therapeutic benefit. An unresolved issue is the minimum dose of each drug necessary for efficacy as either therapy or prophylaxis. It is possible that much lower doses of sulfonamides, which may be associated with a lower incidence of toxicity, are effective as therapy; lower doses have already been shown to be effective for prophylaxis (52). Combining sulfa drugs with more potent DHFR inhibitors may also allow decreases in dose. The identification of non–sulfur containing PABA antagonists may overcome the toxic effects associated with sulfa drugs. Development of potent, selective DHFR inhibitors that can be used without leucovorin may offer advantages over available inhibitors. Folate inhibition is clearly an effective approach to the treatment and prevention of *P. carinii* pneumonia. The challenge for the future is to use our expanded knowledge base to identify more potent, less toxic regimens.

References

1. Hughes WT. *Pneumocystis carinii* pneumonitis [editorial]. N Engl J Med 1987; 317: 1021–1023.
2. Masur H, Lane HC, Kovacs JA, Allegra CJ, Edman JC. Pneumocystis pneumonia: from bench to clinic. Ann Intern Med 1989; 111:813–826.
3. Kovacs JA, Hiemenz JW, Macher AM, Stover D, Murray HW, Shelhamer J, Lane HC, Urmacher U, Honig C, Longo DL, Parker MM, Natanson C, Parrillo JE, Fauci AS, Pizzo PA, Masur H. *Pneumocystis carinii* pneumonia: a comparison between patients with the acquired immunodeficiency syndrome and patients with other immunodeficiencies. Ann Intern Med 1984; 100:663–671.
4. Gordin FM, Simon GL, Mills J, Wofsy CB. Adverse reactions to trimethoprim–sulfamethoxazole in patients with acquired immune deficiency syndrome. Ann Intern Med 1984; 100:495–499.
5. Siratonak FM, Burchall JJ, Ensminger WB, Montgomery JA, eds. Folate Antagonists as Therapeutic Agents. New York: Academic Press, 1984.
6. Hitchings GH. Functions of tetrahydrofolate and the role of dihydrofolate reductase in cellular metabolism. In: Hitchings GH, ed. Inhibition of Folate Metabolism in Chemotherapy. New York: Springer-Verlag, 1983:11–23.
7. Burchall JJ. Dihydrofolate reductase. In: Hitchings GH, ed. Inhibition of Folate Metabolism in Chemotherapy. New York: Springer-Verlag, 1983:55–74.

8. Kovacs JA, Allegra CJ, Beaver J, Boarman D, Lewis M, Parrillo JE, Chabner B, Masur H. Characterization of de novo folate synthesis in *Pneumocystis carinii* and *Toxoplasma gondii*: potential for screening therapeutic agents. J Infect Dis 1989; 160: 312–320.
9. Bushby SRM. Antibacterial activity. In: Hitchings GH, ed. Inhibition of Folate Metabolism in Chemotherapy. New York: Springer-Verlag, 1983:75–105.
10. Kovacs JA, Allegra CJ, Beaver J, Boarman D, Lewis M, Chabner B, Masur H. Evaluation of sulfonamides and sulfones as inhibitors of *Pneumocystis carinii* and *Toxoplasma gondii* dihydropteroate synthetase [abstract]. Abstr 28th Intersci Conf Antibiot Agents Chemother 1989:330, no. 1235.
11. Merali S, Zhang Y, Sloan D. Meshnick S. Inhibition of *Pneumocystis carinii* dihydropteroate synthetase by sulfa drugs. Antimicrob Agents Chemother 1990; 34: 1075–1078.
12. Volpe F, Dyer M, Scaife JG, Darby G, Stammers DK, Delves CJ. The multifunctional folic acid synthesis *fas* gene of *Pneumocystis carinii* appears to encode dihydropteroate synthase and hydroxymethyldihydropterin pyrophosphokinase. Gene 1992; 112: 213–218.
13. Allegra CJ, Kovacs JA, Drake JC, Swan JC, Chabner BA, Masur H. Activity of antifolates against *Pneumocystis carinii* dihydrofolate reductase and identification of a potent new agent. J Exp Med 1987; 165:926–931.
14. Kovacs JA, Allegra CJ, Masur H. Characterization of dihydrofolate reductase of *Pneumocystis carinii* and *Toxoplasma gondii*. Exp Parasitol 1990; 71:60–68.
15. Garrett CE, Coderre CE, Meek TD, Garvey EP, Claman DM, Beverley SM, Santi DV. A bifunctional thymidylate synthetase–dihydrofolate reductase in protozoa. Mol Biochem Parasitol 1984; 11:257–265.
16. Edman JC, Edman U, Cao M, Lundgren B, Kovacs JA, Santi DV. Isolation and expression of the *Pneumocystis carinii* dihydrofolate reductase gene. Proc Natl Acad Sci USA 1989; 86:8625–8629.
17. Edman U, Edman JC, Lundgren B, Santi DV. Isolation and expression of the *Pneumocystis carinii* thymidylate synthase gene. Proc Natl Acad Sci USA 1989; 86: 6503–6507.
18. Bartlett MS, Eichholtz R, Smith JW. Antimicrobial susceptibility of *Pneumocystis carinii* in culture. Diagn Microbiol Infect Dis 1985; 3:381–387.
19. Cushion MT, Stanforth D, Linke MJ, Walzer PD. Method of testing the susceptibility of *Pneumocystis carinii* to antimicrobial agents in vitro. Antimicrob Agents Chemother 1985; 28:796–801.
20. Comley JC, Mullin RJ, Wolfe LA, Hanlon MH, Ferone R. Microculture screening assay for primary in vitro evaluation of drugs against *Pneumocystis carinii*. Antimicrob Agents Chemother 1991; 35:1965–1974.
21. Hughes WT, McNabb PC, Makres TD. Efficacy of trimethoprim and sulfamethoxazole in the prevention and treatment of *Pneumocystis carinii* pneumonitis. Antimicrob Agents Chemother 1974; 5:289–293.
22. Anand N. Sulfonamides: structure–activity relationships and mechanism of action. In: Hitchings GH, ed. Inhibition of Folate Metabolism in Chemotherapy. New York: Springer-Verlag, 1983:25–54.

23. Frenkel JK, Good JT, Schultz JA. Latent *Pneumocystis* infection of rats, relapse and chemotherapy. Lab Invest 1966; 15:1559–1577.
24. Kirby HB, Kenamore B, Guckian JC. *Pneumocystis carinii* pneumonia treated with pyrimethamine and sulfadiazine. Ann Intern Med 1971; 75:505–509.
25. Hughes WT, Feldman S, Sanyal SK. Treatment of *Pneumocystis carinii* pneumonitis with trimethoprim–sulfamethoxazole. Can Med Assoc J 1975; 112:47–50.
26. Hughes WT, Kuhn S, Chaudhary S, Feldman S, Verzosa M, Aur RJ, Pratt C, George SL. Successful chemoprophylaxis for *Pneumocystis carinii* pneumonitis. N Engl J Med 1977; 297:1419–1426.
27. Pesanti EL. In vitro effects of antiprotozoan drugs and immune serum on *Pneumocystis carinii*. J Infect Dis 1980; 141:775–780.
28. Hughes WT, Smith BL. Efficacy of diaminodiphenylsulfone and other drugs in murine *Pneumocystis carinii* pneumonitis. Antimicrob Agents Chemother 1984; 26:436–440.
29. Walzer PD, Kim CK, Foy JM, Linke MJ, Cushion MT. Inhibitors of folic acid synthesis in the treatment of experimental *Pneumocystis carinii* pneumonia. Antimicrob Agents Chemother 1988; 32:96–103.
30. Hughes WT, Smith BL, Jacobus DP. Successful treatment and prevention of murine *Pneumocystis carinii* pneumonitis with 4,4′-sulfonylbisformanilide. Antimicrob Agents Chemother 1986; 29:509–510.
31. Hughes WT, Smith McCain BL. Effects of sulfonylurea compounds on *Pneumocystis carinii*. J Infect Dis 1986; 153:944–947.
32. Pedersen C, Sandstrom E, Petersen CS, Norkrans G, Gerstoft J, Karlsson A, Christensen KC, Hakansson C, Pehrson PO, Nielsen JO, Jurgensen HJ, The Scandinavian Isoprinosine Study Group. The efficacy of inosine pranobex in preventing the acquired immunodeficiency syndrome in patients with human immunodeficiency virus infection. N Engl J Med 1990; 322:1757–1763.
33. Kovacs JA, Gregory F, Boarman D, Allegra CJ. Inhibition of *Pneumocystis carinii* dihydropteroate synthase by *para*acetamidobenzoic acid may explain the activity of Isoprinosine in HIV infection [abstract]. Clin Res 1991; 39:143A.
34. Mills J, Leoung G, Medina I, Hopewell PC, Hughes WT, Wofsy C. Dapsone treatment of *Pneumocystis carinii* pneumonia in the acquired immunodeficiency syndrome. Antimicrob Agents Chemother 1988; 32:1057–1060.
35. Safrin S, Sattler FR, Lee BL, Young T, Bill R, Boylan CT, Mills J. Dapsone as a single agent is suboptimal therapy for *Pneumocystis carinii* pneumonia. J AIDS 1991; 4:244–249.
36. Leoung GS, Mills J, Hopewell PC, Hughes W, Wofsy C. Dapsone–trimethoprim for *Pneumocystis carinii* pneumonia in the acquired immunodeficiency syndrome. Ann Intern Med 1986; 105:45–48.
37. Medina I, Mills J, Leoung G, Hopewell PC, Lee B, Modin G, Benowitz N, Wofsy CB. Oral therapy for *Pneumocystis carinii* pneumonia in the acquired immunodeficiency syndrome. A controlled trial of trimethoprim–sulfamethoxazole versus trimethoprim–dapsone. N Engl J Med 1990; 323:776–782.
38. Bertino JR, Sawicki WL, Moroson BA, Cashmore AR, Elslager EF. 2,4-Diamino-5-methyl-6[3,4,5-trimethoxyanilino]quinazoline (TMQ). A potent non-classical folate antagonist inhibitor. Biochem Pharmacol 1979; 38:1983–1987.

39. Grivsky EM, Lee S, Sigal CW, Duch DS, Nichol CA. Synthesis and antitumor activity of 2,4-diamino-6-(2,5-dimethoxybenzyl)-5-methylpyridol[2,3-*d*]pyrimidine. J Med Chem 1980; 23:327–329.
40. Weir EC, Cashmore AR, Dreyer RN, Graham ML, Hsiao N, Moroson BA, Sawicki WL, Bertino JR. Pharmacology and toxicity of a potent "non-classical" 2,4-diaminoquinazoline folate antagonist, trimetrexate, in normal dogs. Cancer Res 1982; 42:1696–1702.
41. Iland H, Laszlo J, Brenckman W, Currie V, Young C, Williams T, Sigel C, Guaspari A, Blum R, Liao S. Preliminary Phase 1 clinical trials and pharmacokinetics of BW 301U, a new lipid-soluble folate antagonist [abstract]. Proc Am Soc Clin Oncol 1984; 3:29.
42. Allegra CJ, Chabner BA, Tuazon CU, Ogata-Arakaki D, Baird B, Drake JC, Simmons JT, Lack EE, Shelhamer JH, Balis F, Walker R, Kovacs JA, Lane HC, Masur H. Trimetrexate for the treatment of *Pneumocystis carinii* pneumonia in patients with the acquired immunodeficiency syndrome. N Engl J Med 1987; 317:978–985.
43. Lin JT, Cashmore AR, Baker M, Dreyer RN, Ernstoff M, Marsh JC, Bertino JR, Whitfield LR, Delap R, Grillo-Lopez A. Phase 1 studies with trimetrexate: clinical pharmacology, analytical methodology, and pharmacokinetics. Cancer Res 1987; 47:609–616.
44. Kovacs JA, Allegra CJ, Swan JC, Drake JC, Parrillo JE, Chabner BA, Masur H. Potent antipneumocystis and antitoxoplasma activities of piritrexim, a lipid-soluble antifolate. Antimicrob Agents Chemother 1988; 32:430–433.
45. Queener SF, Bartlett MS, Jay MA, Durkin MM, Smith JW. Activity of lipid-soluble inhibitors of dihydrofolate reductase against *Pneumocystis carinii* in culture and in a rat model of infection. Antimicrob Agents Chemother 1987; 31:1323–1327.
46. Broughton MC, Queener SF, *Pneumocystis carinii* dihydrofolate reductase used to screen potential antipneumocystis drugs. Antimicrob Agents Chemother 1991; 35:1348–1355.
47. Kovacs JA, Allegra CJ, Kennedy S, Swan JC, Drake JC, Parrillo JE, Chabner B, Masur H. Efficacy of trimetrexate, a potent lipid-soluble antifolate in the treatment of rodent *Pneumocystis carinii* pneumonia. Am J Trop Med Hyg 1988; 39:491–496.
48. Sattler FR, Feinberg J. New developments in the treatment of *Pneumocystis carinii* pneumonia. Chest 1992; 101:451–457.
49. Feinberg J, McDermott C, Nutter J. Trimetrexate salvage therapy for PCP in AIDS patients with limited therapeutic options. Abstr VIII Int Conf AIDS, 1992. Abstr PoB3297, p. B136.
50. Grem JL, King SA, Costanza ME, Brown TD. Hypersensitivity reactions to trimetrexate. Invest New Drugs 1990; 8:211–214.
51. Falloon JC, Allegra C, Kovacs J, O'Neill D, Ogata-Arakaki D, Feuerstein I. Piritrexim with leucovorin for the treatment of pneumocystis pneumonia in AIDS patients [abstract]. Clin Res 1990; 38:361A.
52. Hardy WD, Holzman RS, Feinberg J, et al. Trimethoprim–sulfamethoxazole vs aerosolized pentamidine for secondary prophylaxis of *Pneumocystis carinii* pneumonia in AIDS patients: a prospective, randomized controlled clinical trial (ACTG 021) [abstract]. Third European Conference on Clinical Aspects and Treatment of HIV Infection, 1992.

27

Pentamidine and Related Compounds in the Treatment of *Pneumocystis carinii* Infection

RICHARD R. TIDWELL
School of Medicine
University of North Carolina at Chapel Hill
Chapel Hill, North Carolina

CONSTANCE A. BELL
Walter Reed Army Institute of Research
Washington, D.C.

I. Introduction

The antiprotozoal activity of the diamidine class of compounds was first reported in the late 1930s by investigators searching for new agents with activity against African trypanosomiasis (1,2). Following the discovery of their antiprotozoal activity, many diamidine derivatives were synthesized (3) and subsequently tested for both in vivo and in vitro activity against several microorganisms. Aromatic diamidines have been demonstrated to have activity against several parasitic organisms including: *Acanthamoebla* (4); *Babesia canis* (5); *Crithidia fasciculata* (6); *Cryptosporidium parvum* (7); *Giardia lamblia* (8); *Leishmania* sp. (9,10); *Plasmodium* sp (10,11); *Pneumocystis carinii* (12–14); *Toxoplasma gondii* (15); and *Trypanosoma* sp. (1,2). Despite the broad range of activity exhibited by diamidines, the compounds have been used clinically only against African trypanosomiasis (16), antimony-resistant leishmaniasis (17), and *P. carinii* pneumonia (12,18).

The first use of diamidines to treat *P. carinii* pneumonia was in 1958, when it was reported that both pentamidine and a related compound, stilbamidine, were effective in treating *P. carinii* pneumonia in infants (12). Although both amidines were effective at doses of 4 mg/kg per day, pentamidine was better tolerated than stilbamidine. Therefore, most future studies were carried out with pentamidine. In

1963, Ivády et al. reported that prompt use of 4 mg/kg per day of pentamidine intramuscularly reduced the fatality rate of pneumocystosis in infants from 50 to 4% (19). In most later studies, the drug was given by intravenous injection because of the local toxicity associated with intramuscular injections (20). Before the advent of the acquired immune deficiency syndrome (AIDS) and after the discovery that the combination of trimethoprim and sulfamethoxazole (TMP–SMZ) was effective in the treatment of *P. carinii* pneumonia (18), pentamidine was rarely used for the treatment of this disease and was available only in the United States as an investigational drug from the Centers for Disease Control (CDC). However, with the sharp increase in pneumocystosis associated with AIDS patients, coupled with the reports that TMP–SMZ caused severe adverse reactions (21,22), the use of pentamidine as a therapy for *P. carinii* pneumonia dramatically

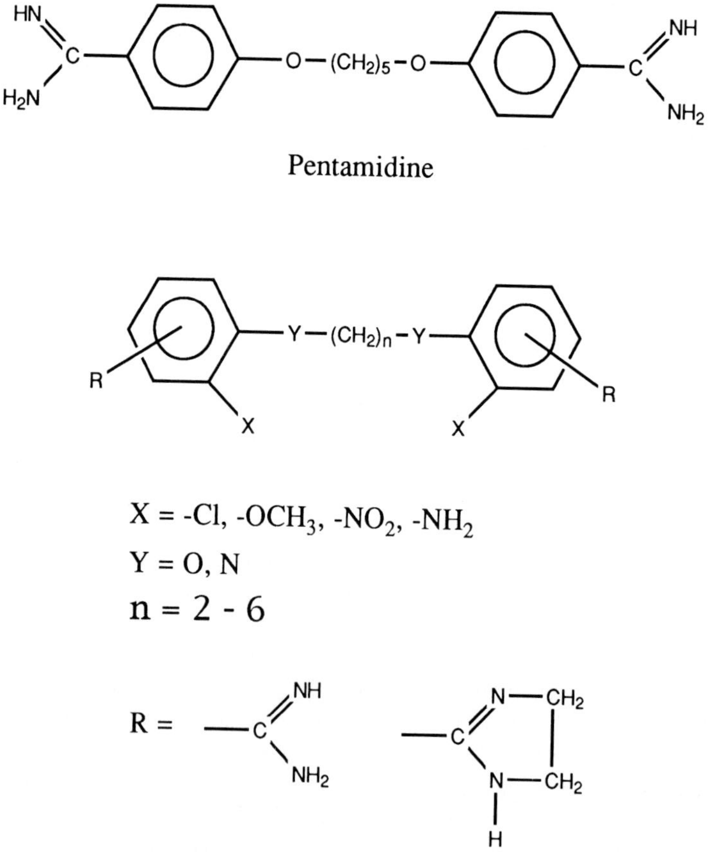

$X = -Cl, -OCH_3, -NO_2, -NH_2$
$Y = O, N$
$n = 2 - 6$

Figure 1 Structure of pentamidine and pentamidine analogues.

(21,22), the use of pentamidine as a therapy for *P. carinii* pneumonia dramatically increased. In 1985, pentamidine isethionate was licensed as an orphan drug in the United States for the treatment of *P. carinii* pneumonia (21) and, in 1987, the drug was found to be effective against *P. carinii* infection in an aerosolized form (23,24). Aerosolized pentamidine was associated with less adverse reactions than intravenous injections of the drug. Until recent studies demonstrated that TMP–SMZ or dapsone was as effective and much less costly than pentamidine, aerosolized administration of the drug was fast becoming the method of choice for primary prophylaxis for *P. carinii* pneumonia in AIDS patients (25–27).

The development of pentamidine-type molecules has been severely limited not only by the toxicity of several of the compounds, particularly pentamidine, but also by a lack of understanding of their mechanisms of toxicity and action, pharmacokinetics, and structure–activity relationships (see Refs. 20,21,28,29, for reviews on pentamidine). For the past 5 years, our laboratory has carried out research on the development of novel pentamidine analogues for the treatment of *P. carinii* pneumonia. This work has involved the synthesis of over 100 diamidine compounds and the testing of these compounds in the rat model of *P. carinii* pneumonia (13,14,30,31). In addition to the structure–activity studies, we have initiated investigation on the metabolism and the mechanism of action and toxicity of pentamidine (8,32–36). Data from these studies are summarized in the following, along with recent information on pentamidine from other laboratories.

II. Structure–Activity Studies

Before the studies carried out in our laboratory, only a handful of pentamidine-related drugs had been tested for activity against *P. carinii* infection. The initial clinical studies on pentamidine also showed that stilbamidine was effective in the treatment of *P. carinii* pneumonia in infants (12). In a later study, hydroxystilbamidine was demonstrated to have activity against *P. carinii* in a rat model of disease (37). In a more recent report, by Walzer et al., three compounds structurally related to pentamidine had efficacy greater than or equal to pentamidine in an immunosuppressed rat model of *P. carinii* pneumonia (38). In the past, the screening of large numbers of pentamidine-type drugs against *P. carinii* infection has been limited because of lack of a dependable in vitro assay system. Even though there are several in vitro screens that are now routinely used to test for drug activity against *P. carinii* (39–41), it is still not clear that these assays are dependable for quantitation of activity for agents such as pentamidine. Pentamidine appears to exert its primary effect against protozoan organisms by blocking DNA replication, rather than direct killing of the organism (unpublished data), and some of the current in vitro assays for *P. carinii* probably do not allow sufficient replication of the organism to measure static drug activity. In addition, it is still not clear to what extent the metabolism of these drugs plays on their activity and how this might affect quantitation differences seen between in vivo and in vitro systems. In a series of 20 pentamidine analogues tested for in vitro activity, according to the protocol of the Indiana group (39), all of the compounds showed activity at 1 µg/mL after seven days in the cell model system (unpublished data), and all of the drugs exhibited significant activity in our rat model of disease. However, the actual quantitative correlation between the two systems was poor.

The immunosuppressed rat model of *P. carinii* pneumonia was employed for all of the drug studies reported in this communication. Although several reports provide a detailed description of this model (13,14,37,38), the following outline of the method will allow an understanding of the data without referring to the previous publications.

Male Sprague–Dawley barrier-raised rats (150–200 g) were individually caged and begun on a regimen of low–protein (8%) diet and drinking water containing tetracycline (0.5 mg/mL) and dexamethasone (1.0 µg/mL) immediately upon arrival in the laboratory. This regimen was continued for the next 8 weeks, with fluid intake monitored daily and animals weighed weekly. At the beginning of week 6, animals were divided into groups of eight or more animals per group and the test compounds administered by iv injection at a daily dose of 10 mg/kg or the next highest soluble, nontoxic dose for 14 days, or by oral administration by gavage daily for 14 days. In each experiment, saline- and pentamidine-treated groups were included as negative and positive controls, respectively. The extent of disease and drug toxicity was quantitated according to the systems outlined in Table 1.

During the last 5 years we have tested more than 100 molecules related to pentamidine against a rat model of *P. carinii* pneumonia (13,14,30,31). Eighty of the compounds tested against *P. carinii* pneumonia can be represented by the general structure depicted in Figure 1. The compounds shown in Table 2 were selected from this group to illustrate the trends that were detected from the more extensive structure–activity analyses. In general, we found that changing the chain length between the two amidinophenoxy moieties had little effect on drug efficacy against *P. carinii* pneumonia (Table 2, compounds 1–4); however, the shorter-chain analogues clearly demonstrated lower toxicity. Moving the amidine group from a position *para* to the ether bond to the *meta* position (compound 5) resulted in a small drop in activity and somewhat reduced toxicity. Isosteric replacement of the ether oxygens with nitrogen (compound 6) resulted in reduced activity and increased toxicity. Whereas substitution on the aromatic ring with a nitro (compound 7) or methoxy (compound 9) group *meta* to the amidine group resulted in active compounds with increased toxicity, substitution with an amine group (compound 8) resulted in slightly increased activity and decreased toxicity. Substitution with chloro groups resulted in a compound (compound 10) with no detectable activity against *P. carinii* pneumonia at the highest soluble concentration. Replacement of the amidine groups with imidazoline moieties (compound 11) resulted in a highly active compound that showed no appreciable toxicity at the highest evaluated dose (10 mg/kg).

Table 1 Scoring of Histological Sections and Evaluation of Toxicity in Rats Treated with Pentamidine and Pentamidine Analogues

Histological scoring
- 0.5 = Fewer than 10 cysts counted per two fully examined sections.
- 1 = Scattered cysts with less than 10% of lung tissue involved.
- 2 = Scattered cysts with limited intense focal involvement and 10–25% of lung tissue involved.
- 3 = Scattered cysts with numerous intense areas of focal involvement and 26–50% of lung tissue involved.
- 4 = Cysts found throughout the tissue, with numerous very intense focal areas of involvement having greater than 50% of lung tissue involved.

Evaluation of toxicity
Toxicity of the test compounds was evaluated at 10mg/kg or the next highest soluble dose by the following criteria:
- 0 = No local, clinical, or histological toxicity.
- + = All animals survived the test dose without observable distress. Minimal or no signs of hypotension were observed. Some excess weight loss was noted or mild signs of local toxicity at the injection site. No histopathology was noted.
- ++ = All or most animals survived the test dose with marked signs of hypotension. All animals were observed to have other clinical side effects or some histopathology. Many animals had severe lesions at the injection site.
- +++ = An acute toxic effect was seen after a single dose, with symptoms compatible with severe hypotension or a sharp decrease in animals' health after multiple doses. Death occurred in fewer than 50% of the animals, resulting in a reduced screening dose.
- ++++ = Death occurred in more than 50% of the animals, with a resulting reduction in screening dose.

Source: Ref. 30.

An evaluation of the anti-*P. carinii* pneumonia screening data from the entire group of 80 pentamidine analogues identified several candidate compounds for more extensive evaluation (13,14,31). However, one compound [1,3-di(4-imidazolino-2-methoxyphenoxy)propane; DMP], appeared to be the most promising agent and was targeted for more extensive studies against rat *P. carinii* pneumonia (Fig. 2). This compound was originally screened in the *P. carinii* pneumonia rat model as the dihydrochloride salt (13). Although the dihydrochloride salt of DMP exhibited excellent activity at 2.5 mg/kg (iv) against *P. carinii* pneumonia, the low solubility of the drug limited its future development as a clinical agent (13). The compound was reformulated as the dilactate salt and evaluated in dose–response studies by both iv and oral administration and in studies for its prophylactic effect (42). The increased solubility of the dilactate salt allowed the evaluation of DMP toxicity. The compound showed no toxicity at the effective dose of 2.5 mg/kg (iv).

Table 2 Summary of Structure–Activity Relations of Pentamidine Analogues Against Rat PCP

Compound number	R[a]	Position R	n	X	Y	Dose (mg/kg per day)	Mean histological score (n)[b]	Toxicity[c]
Saline							3.3 (114)	0
1	Am	para	3	H	O	10.0	0.9 (8)	0
2	Am	para	4	H	O	10.0	0.6 (10)	0
3	Am	para	5	H	O	10.0	1.2 (87)	++
4	Am	para	6	H	O	10.0	1.1 (7)	+++
5	Am	meta	5	H	O	10.0	1.7 (16)	+
6	Am	para	5	H	N	10.0	1.6 (7)	+++
7	Am	para	5	NO_2	O	5.0[d]	2.0 (8)	++++
8	Am	para	5	NH_2	O	10.0	0.9 (15)	+
9	Am	para	5	OCH_3	O	5.0[d]	1.6 (14)	++++
10	Am	para	5	Cl	O	2.5[e]	3.5 (8)	0[f]
11	Im	para	5	H	O	10.0	0.7 (8)	0

[a]Am = −C(=NH)NH$_2$; Im = 2-imidazolinyl

[b]See Table 1 for explanation of histological scoring.
[c]See Table 1 for explanation of toxicity.
[d]Dose reduced because of toxicity.
[e]Dose reduced because of low solubility.
[f]Toxicity scored at 2.5 mg/kg.
n = number of animals per group.
Source: Revised from Ref. 30.

However, toxicity very similar to pentamidine (10 mg/kg, iv) was observed at 5 mg/kg (iv) (unpublished data).

From the dose–response data (Table 3), DMP appears approximately ten times more active against rat *P. carinii* pneumonia than pentamidine when administered by iv injection. Oral application of DMP (Table 4) also showed activity against *P. carinii* pneumonia in a dose-dependent manner (pentamidine shows no activity when given po). However, much higher drug doses were necessary when DMP was given orally, compared with iv dosing. For instance, 80 mg/kg per day of DMP lactate given orally achieved the same level of anti-*P. carinii* pneumonia activity (as measured by the mean histological score) as 1.0 mg/kg per day of the iv dose. More variability was noted within the groups

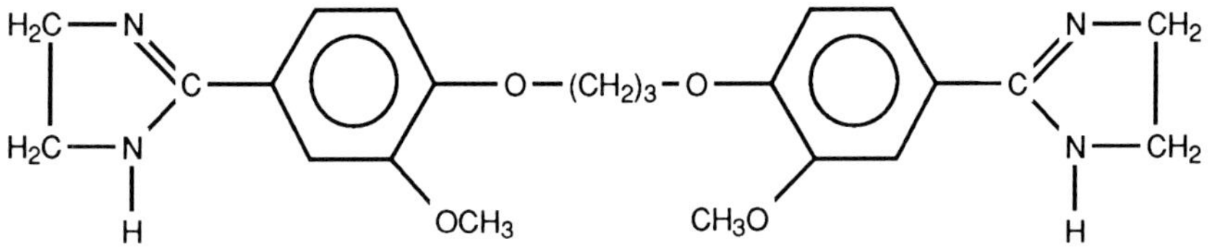

Figure 2 Structure of 1,3-di(4-imidazolino-2-methoxyphenoxy)propane (DMP). (From Ref. 13.)

receiving the oral doses, especially at the lower-dose levels. Experiments carried out at the University of Indiana confirmed the high potency of DMP against rat *P. carinii* pneumonia when the drug was administered by iv injection (Smith J, Bartlett M, personal communication). However, the studies conducted by the Indiana group failed to demonstrate oral activity of the drug. The differences seen in the oral-dosing experiments between the two laboratories may be the result of the variations in the rat model of *P. carinii* pneumonia used. A difference in the two animal models that may impinge on the oral availability of the drug is the diet. The Indiana protocol has the animals receiving normal rat chow (43), whereas our studies used animals on a low (8%)-protein diet (13,14,30,31). These data suggest that uptake of DMP may be retarded because of nonspecific binding of the strongly cationic drug with protein molecules. Since preliminary studies in our laboratory indicate that only 1–3% of the peak plasma levels are achieved when the drug is given orally, compared with the iv dose (unpublished data), small

Table 3 Dose–Response of DMP in the Treatment of Rat PCP by Daily Intravenous Injection

Compound	Dose (mg/kg)	Dose (mg/kg parent molecule)	Mean histological score (n)	Number of animals per histological score					Cysts/g lung[a] (% of control)
				0.5	1	2	3	4	
Saline			3.4 (38)	0	0	3	12	13	100.0
Pentamidine	10.0	7.5	1.4 (26)[b]	4	11	10	1	0	3.1
DMP lactate	2.5	1.75	0.7 (10)[b,c]	7	3	0	0	0	2.2
	1.0	0.7	1.1 (9)[b,d]	0	8	1	0	0	6.7
	0.5	0.35	1.4 (10)[b]	0	8	0	2	0	11.2

[a]Saline control = 2.2×10^7 cysts per gram of lung tissue.
[b]p vs saline controls >0.0001.
[c]p vs pentamidine controls >0.0001.
[d]p vs pentamidine >0.05.
n = number of animals.
Source: Revised from Ref. 41.

Table 4 Dose–Response of DMP in the Treatment of Rat PCP by Daily Oral Administration

Compound	Dose (mg/kg)	Dose (mg/kg parent molecule)	Mean histological score (n)	Number of animals per histological score					Cysts/g lung[a] (% of control)
				0.5	1	2	3	4	
Saline			3.2 (54)	1	0	11	18	24	100.0
Pentamidine[b]	10.0	7.5	1.6 (52)[c]	9	19	13	8	3	2.4
DMP lactate	80.0	56.0	1.1 (8)[c,d]	5	2	0	0	1	8.7
	40.0	28.0	1.8 (12)	1	4	3	1	3	11.9
	20.0	14.0	1.6 (11)	3	1	3	0	4	12.4
	10.0	7.0	2.7 (12)[e]	1	1	2	5	3	29.6

[a]Saline control = 3.78×10^7 cysts per gram of lung tissue.
[b]Pentamidine tested by daily iv injection.
[c]p vs saline controls >0.0001.
[d]p vs pentamidine controls >0.005.
[e]p vs pentamidine controls >0.01.
n = number of animals.
Source: Revised from Ref. 41.

decreases in oral bioavailability would greatly affect the activity of DMP. Studies are currently underway to establish the effect of diet on the oral bioavailability of DMP.

Table 5 records the effect of prophylactic treatment (twice weekly for 6 weeks beginning at the third week of immunosuppression) with DMP on rat *P. carinii* pneumonia. The iv dose of 2.5 mg/kg of DMP is highly effective in

Table 5 Prophylactic Study of DMP Lactate Against Rat PCP

Compound	Dose (mg/kg)	Toxicity	Mean histological score (n)	Number of animals per histological score					Cysts/g lung[a] (% of control)
				0.5	1	2	3	4	
Saline		0	3.8 (10)	0	0	0	2	8	100.0
Pentamidine	10.0	++	1.3 (10)[b]	3	4	2	1	0	7.3
DMP lactate	2.5	0	0.8 (11)[b]	8	1	2	0	0	1.1
	20.0[c]	0	2.5 (11)[b,d]	0	1	4	6	0	21.0

[a]Saline control = 3.7×10^7 cysts per gram of lung tissue.
[b]p vs saline controls >0.0001.
[c]Tested by oral adminstation, twice weekly for 6 weeks beginning at the third week of immunosuppression. All other drugs and doses tested by iv injection on the same dosing schedule.
[d]p vs pentamidine controls >0.0005.
n = number of animals.
Source: Revised from Ref. 41.

preventing pneumocystis pneumonia, whereas a dose of 20 mg/kg given orally significantly reduces both the mean histological score and cyst counts. Similar to the treatment studies, the oral prophylactic dose appears much less effective than the iv administration of the drug.

III. Pharmacology

Several studies (44–46) aimed at determining the distribution of pentamidine led to the following conclusions: (1) pentamidine is rapidly removed from plasma after administration; (2) the drug is associated with certain organs more than others; (3) the drug is excreted slowly over a relatively long period in the urine; and (4) only a small portion of the pentamidine administered can be accounted for by the total amount of drug found in tissue or excretory samples. The following account of distribution experiments carried out in our laboratory with rats receiving daily iv injections of pentamidine (10 mg/kg) for 14 days verifies the foregoing conclusions (32).

With use of high-performance liquid chromatography (HPLC) (47) the highest quantities of pentamidine per gram wet weight were found in kidneys (62.9 ± 53.2 µg/g), with moderate levels in lungs (66.8 ± 14.3 µg/g), spleen/pancreas (54.3 ± 25.5 µg/g), heart (45.7 ± 24.6 µg/g), muscle (32.0 ± 5.0 µg/g), and stomach (28.6 ± 4.4 µg/g). Low levels of drug were detectable in the liver (4.8 ± 2.6 µg/g), testes (8.9 ± 5.0 µg/g), and brain (2.9 ± 4.4 µg/g). No drug was detected in red blood cells, and only very small amounts were detected in plasma. Urine levels of pentamidine were low after the first dose (14.4 ± 8.8 µg/24 hr) and increased daily until a plateau value of 70.0 µg/24 hr was reached. The levels of pentamidine detected in the feces never exceeded 14.9 ± 1.3 µg/24 hr. The urine, plasma, fecal, and organ levels of pentamidine accounted for less than 20% of the total drug injected over the course of treatment. Although numerous reports suggested that pentamidine was not metabolized (48–50), it appeared that the best explanation for the low recovery of the drug was that pentamidine underwent metabolic transformation to products that were not detectable by our HPLC assay.

Since it had been reported that benzamidine is converted to N-hydroxybenzamidine by rat liver homogenates (51), the search for metabolites of pentamidine began with the development of an HPLC assay that would separate the N-hydroxy and N,N'-dihydroxy derivatives of pentamidine from the parent molecule. The use of an improved HPLC assay confirmed the presence, although in modest amounts, of both N-hydroxy (compound IV, Fig. 3) and the N,N'-dihydroxy (compound V) analogues of pentamidine in supernatants of rat liver homogenates (centrifuged at 9000 × g) (33). In addition to the N-hydroxy metabolites, four additional putative metabolites were observed and, subsequently, two of these were identified as the 2-pentanol (compound II) and 3-pentanol (compound I)

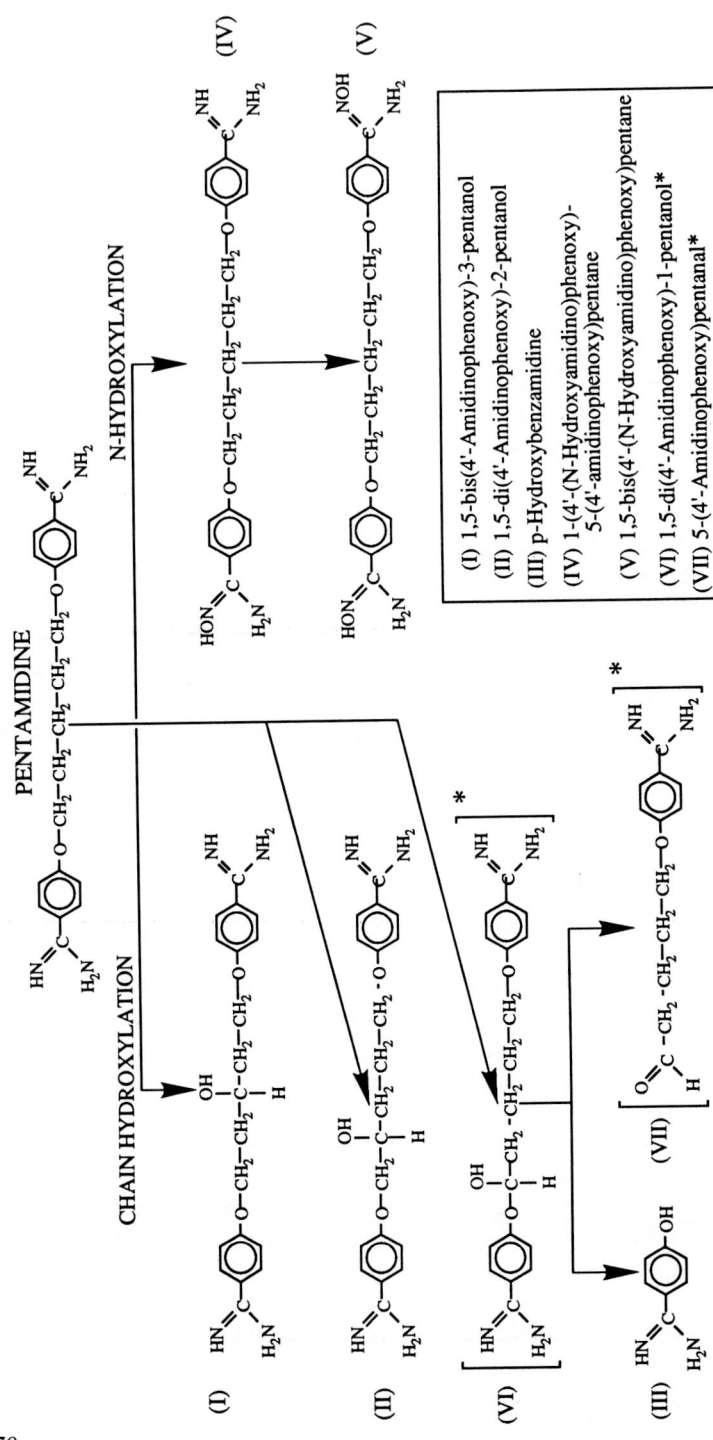

Figure 3 Primary metabolism of pentamidine. The presence of compounds marked by asterisk has not been confirmed. (From Ref. 33.)

analogues of pentamidine (34). These chain hydroxylated products accounted for most converted pentamidine in rat liver microsomes (34). An additional metabolic product was detected and identified as p-hydroxybenzamidine (compound III). The presence of p-hydroxybenzamidine was a strong indication that hydroxylation was occurring α to the ether bond, resulting in hemiacetal formation (compound VI), followed by cleavage of the hemiacetal into p-hydroxybenzamidine and the aldehyde (compound VII). The presence of the aldehyde has not been confirmed. However, it is likely that the aldehyde would be rapidly hydrolyzed into the corresponding acid. Attempts to confirm the presence of the acid product are now underway. In addition, the metabolic products of pentamidine are being evaluated for secondary metabolism and for their role in the antiprotozoal activity and toxicity of the parent molecule.

IV. Toxicity

The high rate of adverse reactions occurring in response to pentamidine therapy has been well documented clinically. Nearly 50% of all patients (AIDS and non-AIDS) treated with pentamidine have side effects (52–54), including abscesses at the site of intramuscular injection, severe hypotension following rapid injections, increased serum transaminase levels, leukopenia, thrombocytopenia, hypocalcemia, and rashes. Of the more serious side effects, hepatic, renal, and pancreatic complications occur fairly commonly. Nephrotoxicity occurs in approximately 25% of patients and can sometimes be quite severe, particularly in patients with preexisting renal conditions or diarrheal infections (52,55). Hyperglycemia or hypoglycemia occurs in up to 40% of patients in the United States (52,56). In vitro studies with insulinoma cell cultures have shown that pentamidine initially stimulates release of insulin, followed by inhibition of insulin release and cytolysis of cultured cells (57,58). Hepatic complications are also fairly common, although only rarely severe, with liver function adversely affected (54). Finally, little is currently known about the potential for pentamidine to target immune system components, even though numerous biochemical activities attributed to the drug (including inhibition of synthesis of DNA, RNA, phospholipids, and proteins; 20,48,59–61) would suggest that it is relatively potent here. The clinical studies demonstrating leukopenia in approximately 10% of treated patients add significantly to this hypothesis (20). Recent studies have demonstrated that interleukin-1 release was impaired in pentamidine-treated cells through an alteration in the posttranslational modification of precursor interleukin-1 (62). A similar effect was also observed for tumor necrosis factor (63). Any subtle immunotoxicological effects of a drug administered to an already profoundly immunosuppressed AIDS patient could exacerbate the susceptibility of the individual toward opportunistic disease and neoplasia, in addition to inadvertently decreasing the pharmacological value of the drug.

Although the clinical side effects have been well described, the mechanisms by which pentamidine causes these adverse reactions are unknown. Relatively few studies have been performed to examine the structural features of diamidines and related dicationic compounds that contribute to host cell toxicity. Two recent investigations were reported in which structure–toxicity relations relative to hepatotoxicity and cardiovascular effects were examined, but limited numbers of dicationic compounds were evaluated (64,65). The study on the hepatotoxic side effects of diamidines with trypanocidal activity clearly indicated that structural alterations resulting in decreased toxicity of the drugs could be achieved without compromising their trypanocidal effect (64). These studies, along with a handful of others, are the only demonstrated attempts to investigate specific mechanisms of toxicity of pentamidine analogues.

A thorough examination of the toxicity information available on pentamidine-type molecules reveals that this class of compounds possesses a wide range of toxic activity, both in the degree and nature of the toxicity exhibited by the numerous structural variations. For example, examination of the blood pressure-lowering properties of several dicationic molecules [propamidine, dibromopropamidine, pentamidine, and 2,7-di(*m*-amidinophenyldiazoamino)-10-ethyl-α-phenylphenanthridinium chloride] showed a great diversity in their hypotensive properties (66). The hypotensive activity of the compounds in dogs ranged from propamidine, which showed no significant blood pressure-lowering properties at 30 mg/kg, to dibromopropamidine, which produced a precipitous drop in blood pressure within 15 sec of an iv injection at a dose of 0.33 mg/kg (66; and unpublished data). The same diversity between structure modification and extent of toxic effect was

Table 6 Maximum Nontoxic Dose of Diamidines Against MA-104 and HEp-2 Cell Lines

Compound no.	n	R	MA-104 Cells (μM)	HEp-2 Cells (μM)
1	3	H	10	10
2	5	H	500	50
3	5	Br	0.1	ND[a]
4	5	NO_2	ND[a]	5
5	5	OCH_3	ND[a]	>1000
6	6	H	0.5	5

[a]ND = not done.
Source: Unpublished data.

observed when a sampling of the compounds were tested in vitro for their effect against HEp-2 (unpublished data) and M-104 (unpublished data) cell lines. The values from Table 6 show that a range of 3–4 logs in the concentration of selected compounds is required to produce a toxic effect against both cell lines. The values in Table 7 clearly show that there is also a large variation in the mutagenicity and toxicity to *Escherichia coli* of closely related structures (unpublished data). An analysis of the toxicity data available for pentamidine derivatives, including anecdotal toxicity information from our structure–activity studies against rat *P. carinii* pneumonia (13,14), clearly indicate that the toxic effect of these analogues is closely tied to specific molecular characteristics of the compounds and is not a general phenomenon credited solely to their strongly cationic properties. Additionally, their antiparasitic activity does not depend on structure alterations that contribute to host toxicity.

V. Mechanism of Action

The mechanism of antiparasitic activity by aromatic diamidines has not been determined. Although several suggested mechanisms of action remain viable, experimental evidence has virtually eliminated others as candidates. Many times, evidence suggesting a potential mode of action for diamidine compounds against one organism is contradicted by data from experiments with another organism. The inability to ascertain the specific interactions of these compounds related to their antiparasitic effect is compounded by the strongly cationic nature of the molecules, leading to nonspecific binding. Several mechanisms of antimicrobial action have been proposed for pentamidine and related compounds. These include interference with aerobic metabolism (2,60), inhibition of oxidative phosphorylation (67,68), inhibition of trypsin and related proteases (14), interference with amino acid transport (68,69), and inhibition of nucleic acid synthesis or metabolism. The specific interactions proposed for pentamidine that could interfere with nucleic acid synthesis or metabolism include the inhibition of phospholipid, polyamine, and protein synthesis (67,68,70,71); inhibition of polymerases (72); inhibition of ribosomal function (6,73,74); inhibition of dihydrofolate reductase–thymidylate synthetase (75); nucleic acid binding (8), and inhibition of topoisomerases (36,76,77).

Although most of the aforementioned mechanisms of action of pentamidine-type drugs remain to be proved or disproved, recent evidence makes several of the proposed mechanisms seem highly unlikely, and others become more attractive candidates. For instance, the inhibition of trypsin-like proteases can be eliminated as a potential mechanism of action because the substitution of imidazoline moieties for the amidine groups of pentamidine virtually eliminates the antiproteinase activity, while producing a molecule that is equally or more potent than the

Table 7 *Escherichia coli* Survival and Mutagenesis Frequency at *leuB* After Treatment with Dicationic Compounds[a]

Drug	Concentration (μg/mL)	% survival after 2 hr	[b]Leu+ reversion frequency × 10⁻³	Fold increase over wild-type	Bacteriostatic after 24 hr
Pentamidine	500	1.6	2.2	—	+
	5	100	1.3		—
DMP	500	20	5.8		+
	5	55	4.8		—
	500	32	5.3	—	+
	5	65	4.8		—
	500	2.9	11.0	5	+
	5	62	ND		—
	500	2	3.3	—	+
	5	44	ND		—
	500	0.069	1000	454	+
	5	2.0	3.3		+

[a]*E. coli* K12 strain AB1157 was used for this experiment.
[b]Cells were plated on leucine-omission medium in duplicate. The reversion frequency is listed as colonies per 10^3 survivors.
Source: Unpublished data.

parent drug against several parasitic organisms (8,10,13,14). Even though several pentamidine derivatives showed some activity against mammalian and bacterial thymidylate synthetase, the concentrations were much greater than would be necessary to produce a therapeutic effect (31). It has also been reported that pentamidine, although active against *C. fasciculata*, did not inhibit the activity of dihydrofolate reductase from the organism (68). A final point against folate antagonism as being a primary mode of action of pentamidine is the demonstrated activity of aromatic diamidines against *G. lamblia* (8), which is reported to lack both dihydrofolate reductase and thymidylate synthetase (78).

Meanwhile, the DNA-binding affinity of pentamidine analogues has become more attractive as a potential mode of action. Recent studies showed that the antigiardial effect of 39 pentamidine compounds had a strong correlation with the affinity of the compounds for calf thymus DNA ($r^2 = 0.81$) and poly(dA)·poly(dT) ($r^2 = 0.80$) (8). Also, a correlation was observed between DNA binding of a similar group of compounds and their activity against *L. mexicana amazonensis* and *P. falciparum* (10). However, the correlation coefficients were less than that observed for *G. lamblia*. A correlation was reported between trypanocidal activity of a series of bis-cationic drugs and petite mutagenesis in *Saccharomyces cerevisiae*. This activity was correlated with the degree of spatial separation of the cationic esters (79). The charge separation is a key factor in determining the DNA-binding strength of the dictation molecules (35). It is noteworthy that all of the over 100 dicationic molecules yet tested that have demonstrated activity against *P. carinii* pneumonia also bind to DNA (14,31; and unpublished data). Recent evidence has also indicated that DNA-binding agents, such as the pentamidine-type molecules, can inhibit enzymes that act directly on the DNA molecule (36,76,77). Two pentamidine-related antitrypanosomal drugs [diminazine (Berenil) and hydroxystilbamidine] were demonstrated to have inhibitory activity against the catenation–decatenation activity of topoisomerase II and relaxation activity of topoisomerase I isolated from trypanosomes (76). Pentamidine promoted the linearization of trypanosomal minicircle DNA at therapeutic concentrations (77). Finally, recent work in our laboratory demonstrated that pentamidine and several analogues of pentamidine exhibited inhibitory activity against an ATP-dependent topoisomerase from *P. carinii* (36). The data in Table 8 show that the diamidine compounds are more effective inhibitors of ATP-dependent topoisomerase than the ATP-independent enzyme activity. Also evidence from Table 8 shows that specificity for the *P. carinii* enzyme over the topoisomerase from *S. cerevisiae* was accomplished with DMP. It is noteworthy that the more effective agents against rat *P. carinii* pneumonia (13), DAMP and DMP, were the most potent inhibitors of ATP-dependent topoisomerase from rat *P. carinii* (36). Although the aforementioned data are too preliminary to provide a definitive conclusion on the mechanism of antimicrobial activity of pentamidine-related compounds, studies into the relations between DNA binding, topoisomerase

Table 8 Inhibition of Topoisomerase Activity by Pentamidine Analogues

Compound	50% inhibition (µM)		
	S. cerevisiae topoisomerase II	P. carinii ATP-independent topoisomerase	ATP-dependent topoisomerase
DAMP	1	>50	2.2
DMP	>500	>50	9.0
Pentamidine	ND	>50	>50

Source: Ref. 36.

inhibition, and antimicrobial action of these compounds should be a high priority of future investigations.

VI. Drug Resistance

The prophylactic use of aerosolized pentamidine, for the treatment of AIDS-associated *P. carinii* pneumonia, has led to growing concerns for the development of drug-resistant organisms (80,81). Unfortunately, the study of drug resistance by *P. carinii* is difficult in the laboratory setting owing to the limitation of the in vitro growth of the organism. The ability to develop pentamidine-resistant *P. carinii* strains could potentially aid in determining the mechanism of action of the drug. Resistance to pentamidine has been observed, in vitro, for several organisms including *S. cerevisiae* (82) and trypanosomes (69,83). The mode of resistance observed for *S. cerevisiae* is unclear, and the resistance seen with trypanosomes appears to result from altered pentamidine transport properties (69,83). The development of resistant strains resulting from reduced accumulation of the drug in the organism adds little information toward understanding the mechanism of action of the drug. In addition to the in vitro studies, resistance to pentamidine has been reported for patients with visceral leishmaniasis undergoing prolonged treatment with the drug (17). It is clear that additional studies should be undertaken to develop pentamidine-resistant organisms. These experiments could be carried out with any of the numerous organisms sensitive to the drug.

VII. Conclusions

Despite the absence of definitive information concerning the mechanism of activity of pentamidine-type compounds, the potency and broad spectrum of activity demonstrated by these molecules against AIDS-related opportunistic pathogens are more than sufficient to warrant further studies of these agents. Future development of pentamidine-type molecules is especially encouraging now that it appears that the mode of antimicrobial activity and toxicity are different and, more importantly, that toxicity and activity are linked to diverse structural components of the molecules. The recent work on pentamidine metabolism opens the door for studies designed to evaluate the role of metabolism on the activity and toxicity of the drug. Concerning the anti-*P. carinii* pneumonia effect of pentamidine-related compounds, it is important for future studies to focus on the mechanism of activity of the compounds. Once the specific molecular interactions of diamidines that result in their anti-*P. carinii* pneumonia effect are understood, a rational drug design approach can be undertaken. Only with this approach can the true potential of the pentamidine class of antimicrobial agents be attained.

Acknowledgments

The authors wish to thank Dr. James E. Hall, Dr. Christine C. Dykstra, Dr. Bradley J. Berger, and Susan K. Jones for their technical assistance in the preparation of this manuscript and Vicki J. Wingate for clerical assistance.

Studies reported in this paper and attributed to the research group at the University of North Carolina were supported by Public Health Service contract N01-AI-72648 and Public Health Service grant 1 R01-AI-32912-01 from the National Institute of Allergy and Infectious Diseases and funding from American Federation for AIDS Research and Fujisawa Pharmaceutical Corporation (Deerfield, Illinois).

References

1. King H, Lourie E, Yorke W. Studies in chemotherapy: XIX. Further report on new trypanocidal substances. Ann Trop Med Parasitol 1938; 32:177–192.
2. Lourie EM, Yorke W. Studies in chemotherapy: XXI. The trypanocidal action of certain aromatic diamidines. Ann Trop Med Parasitol 1939; 33:289–304.
3. Ashley J, Barber H, Ewings A, Newberry G, Self A. A chemotherapeutic comparison of the trypanocidal action of some aromatic diamidines. J Chem Soc Part I 1942; 20:103–116.
4. Kishore P, Shukla O. Antiamoebic action of diamidines of *Acanthamoeba culbertsoni*. Med Sci Res 1989; 17:601–602.
5. Lourie EM, Yorke W. Studies in chemotherapy. XXII. The action of certain aromatic diamidines on *Babesia canis* infections of puppies. Ann Trop Med Parasitol 1939; 33:305–312.
6. Wallis OC. The effect of pentamidine on ribosomes of the parasitic flagellate *Crithidia (Strigomonas) oncopelti*. J Protozool 1966; 13:234–239.
7. Blagburn BL, Sundermann CA, Lindsay DS, Hall JE, Tidwell RR. Inhibition of *Cryptosporidium parvum* in neonatal Hsd: (ICR)BR Swiss mice by polyether ionophores and aromatic amidines. Antimicrob Agents Chemother 1991; 35:1520–1523.
8. Bell CA, Cory M, Fairley TA, Hall JE, Tidwell RR. Structure–activity relationships of pentamidine analogs against *Giardia lamblia* and correlation of antigiardial activity with DNA-binding affinity. Antimicrob Agents Chemother 1991; 35:1099–1107.
9. Kirk R, Sati MH. The use of certain aromatic diamidines in the treatment of kala-azar. Ann Trop Med Parasitol 1940; 34:181–197.
10. Bell CA, Hall JE, Kyle DE, Grogl M, Ohemeng KA, Allen MA, Tidwell RR. Structure–activity relationships of analogs of pentamidine against *Plasmodium falciparum* and *Leishmania mexicana amazonensis*. Antimicrob Agents Chemother 1990; 34:1381–1386.
11. Fulton JD. The course of *Plasmodium relictum* infection in canaries and the treatment of bird and monkey malaria with synthetic bases. Ann Trop Med Parasitol 1940; 34: 53–66.

12. Ivády VG, Páldy L. Ein neues behandlungsverfahren der interstitiellen plasmazelligen pneumonie frühgeborener mit fünfwertigem stibium und aromatischen diamidinen. Monatsschr Kinderheilkd 1958; 106:10–14.
13. Jones SK, Hall JE, Allen MA, Morrison SD, Ohemeng KA, Reddy VV, Geratz JD, Tidwell RR. Novel pentamidine analogs in the treatment of experimental *Pneumocystis carinii* pneumonia. Antimicrob Agents Chemother 1990; 34:1026–1030.
14. Tidwell RR, Jones SK, Geratz JD, Ohemeng KA, Cory M, Hall JE. Analogues of 1,5-bis(4-amidinophenoxy)pentane (pentamidine) in the treatment of experimental *Pneumocystis carinii* pneumonia. J Med Chem 1990; 33:1252–1257.
15. Lindsay DS, Blagburn BL, Hall JE, Tidwell RR. Activity of pentamidine and pentamidine analogs against *Toxoplasma gondii* in cell cultures. Antimicrob Agents Chemother 1991; 35:1914–1916.
16. Apted FIC. Present status of chemotherapy and chemoprophylaxis of human trypanosomiasis in the Eastern Hemisphere. Pharmacol Ther 1980; 11:391–413.
17. Bryceson ADM, Chulay JD, Mugambi M, Were JB, Gachihi G, Chunge CN, Muigai R, Bhatt SM, Ho M, Spencer HC, Meme J, Anabwani G. Visceral leishmaniasis unresponsive to antimonial drugs. II. Response to high dosage sodium stibogluconate or prolonged treatment with pentamidine. Trans R Soc Trop Med Hyg 1985; 79: 705–714.
18. Hughes WT, McNabb PC, Makres TD, Feldman S. Efficacy of trimethoprim and sulfamethoxazole in the prevention and treatment of *Pneumocystis carinii* pneumonitis. Antimicrob Agents Chemother 1974; 5:289–293.
19. Ivády G, Páldy L, Unger G. Weitere erfahrungen bei der behandlung der interstitiellen plasmacellulären pneumonie mit pentamidin. Monatsschr Kinderheilkd 1963; 111:297–299.
20. Kapusnick JE, Mills J. Pentamidine. In: Antimicrobial Agents Annual 3. New York: Elsevier, 1988:299–311.
21. Pearson RD, Hewlett EL. Pentamidine for the treatment of *Pneumocystis carinii* pneumonia and other protozoal diseases. Ann Intern Med 1985; 103:782–786.
22. Gordin FM, Simon GL, Wofsy CB, Mills J. Adverse reactions to trimethoprim-sulfamethoxazole in patients with the acquired immunodeficiency syndrome. Ann Intern Med 1984; 100:495–499.
23. Montgomery AB, Luce JM, Turner J, Lin ET, Debs RJ, Corkery KJ, Brunette EN, Hopewell PC. Aerosolised pentamidine as sole therapy for *Pneumocystis carinii* pneumonia in patients with acquired immunodeficiency syndrome. Lancet 1987; 2: 480–483.
24. Debs RJ, Blumenfeld W, Brunette EN, Straubinger RM, Montgomery AB, Lin E, Agabian N, Papahadjopoulos D. Successful treatment with aerosolized pentamidine of *Pneumocystis carinii* pneumonia in rats. Antimicrob Agents Chemother 1987; 31: 37–41.
25. Freedberg KA, Tosteson ANA, Cohen CJ, Cotton DJ. Primary prophylaxis for *Pneumocystis carinii* pneumonia in HIV-infected people with CD4 counts below 200/ mm^3: a cost effectiveness analysis. J AIDS 1991; 4:521–531.
26. Golden JA, Chernoff D, Hollander H, Feigal D. Conte JE. Prevention of *Pneumocystis carinii* pneumonia by inhaled pentamidine. Lancet 1989; 1:654–657.

27. Lawson L, Montaner JSG, Falutz J, Hyland R, Rachlis A, Gervais A, Rennzi P, McFadden D, Fong IW, Garber GE, Martel A, Schlech W, Louie T. Placebo controlled Canadian cooperative trial of aerosolized pentamidine for the secondary prophylaxis of AIDS-related PCP. Clin Invest Med 1989; 12:B93.
28. Drake S, Lampasona V, Nicks HL, Schwarzmann SW. Drug reviews. Pentamidine isethionate in the treatment of *Pneumocystis carinii* pneumonia. Clin Pharm 1985; 4: 507–516.
29. Goa KL, Campoli-Richards DM. Pentamidine isethionate: a review of its antiprotozoal activity, pharmacokinetic properties and therapeutic use in *Pneumocystis carinii* pneumonia. Drugs 1987; 33:242–258.
30. Tidwell RR, Kilgore SG, Ohemeng KA, Geratz JD, Hall JE. Treatment of experimental *Pneumocystis carinii* pneumonia with analogs of pentamidine. J Protozool 1989; 36:74S–76S.
31. Tidwell RR, Jones SK, Geratz JD, Ohemeng KA, Bell CA, Berger BJ, Hall JE. Development of pentamidine analogues as new agents for the treatment of *Pneumocystis carinii* pneumonia. Ann NY Acad Sci 1990; 616:421–441.
32. Berger BJ, Hall JE, Tidwell RR. The distribution of multiple doses of pentamidine in rats. Pharmacol Toxicol 1990; 66:234–236.
33. Berger BJ, Lombardy RJ, Marbury GD, Bell CA, Dykstra CC, Hall JE, Tidwell RR. Metabolic *N*-hydroxylation of pentamidine in vitro. Antimicrob Agents Chemother 1990; 34:1678–1684.
34. Berger BJ, Reddy VV, Le ST, Lombardy RJ, Hall JE, Tidwell RR. Hydroxylation of pentamidine by rat liver microsomes. J Pharmacol Exp Therap 1991; 256:883–889.
35. Cory M, Tidwell RR, Fairley TA. Structure and DNA binding activity of analogs of 1,5-di(4-amidinophenoxy)pentane (pentamidine). J Med Chem 1992; 35:431–438.
36. Dykstra CC, Tidwell RR. Inhibition of topoisomerases from *Pneumocystis carinii* by aromatic dicationic molecules. J Protozool 1991; 6:78S–81S.
37. Frenkel JK, Good JT, Shultz JA. Latent pneumocystis infection of rats, relapse and chemotherapy. Lab Invest 1966; 15:1559–1577.
38. Walzer PD, Kim CK, Foy J, Linke MJ, Cushion MT. Cationic antitrypanosomal and other antimicrobial agents in the therapy of experimental *Pneumocystis carinii* pneumonia. Antimicrob Agents Chemother 1988; 32:896–905.
39. Bartlett MS, Eichholtz R, Smith JW. Antimicrobial susceptibility of *Pneumocystis carinii* in culture. Diagn Microbiol Infect Dis 1985; 3:381–387.
40. Cushion MT, Walzer PD. Growth and serial passage of *Pneumocystis carinii* in the A549 cell line. Infect Immun 1984; 44:245–251.
41. Comley JC, Mullin RJ, Wolfe LA, Hanlon MH, Ferone R. Microculture screening assay for primary in vitro evaluation of drugs against *Pneumocystis carinii*. Antimicrob Agents Chemother 1991; 35:1965–1974.
42. Tidwell RR, Jones SK, Dykstra CC, Gorton L, Hall JE. Treatment of experimental *Pneumocystis carinii* pneumonia with 1,3-di(4-imidazolino-2-methoxyphenoxy)-propane lactate. J Protozool 1991; 6:148S–150S.
43. Bartlett MS, Queener SF, Tidwell RR, Milhous WK, Berman JD, Ellis WY, Smith JW. 8-Aminoquinolones from Walter Reed Army Institute for Research for treatment

and prophylaxis of pneumocystis pneumonia in rat models. Antimicrob Agents Chemother 1991; 35:277–282.
44. Waalkes TP, Denham C, DeVita VT. Pentamidine: clinical pharmacologic correlations in man and mice. Clin Pharmacol Ther 1970; 11:505–512.
45. Waldman RH, Pearce DE, Martin RA. Pentamidine isothionate levels in lungs, livers, and kidneys of rats after aerosol or intramuscular administration. Am Rev Respir Dis 1973; 108:1004–1006.
46. Conte JE, Upton RA, Phelps RT, Wofsy CB, Zurlinden E, Lin ET. Use of a specific and sensitive assay to determine pentamidine pharmacokinetics in patients with AIDS. J Infect Dis 1986; 154:923–929.
47. Berger BJ, Hall JE, Tidwell RR. High-performance liquid chromatographic method for the quantification of several diamidine compounds with potential chemotherapeutic value. J Chromatogr Biomed Appl 1989; 494:191–200.
48. Sands M, Kron MA, Brown RB. Pentamidine: a review. Rev Infect Dis 1985; 7:625–634.
49. Bernard EM, Donnelly HJ, Maher MP, Armstrong D. Use of a new bioassay to study pentamidine pharmacokinetics. J Infect Dis 1985; 152:750–754.
50. Hughes WT. Treatment and prophylaxis for *Pneumocystis carinii* pneumonia. Parasitol Today 1987; 3:332–335.
51. Clement B. The *N*-oxidation of benzamidine in vitro. Xenobiotica 1983; 13:467–473.
52. Kovacs JA, Hiemenz JW, Macher AM, Stover D, Murray HW, Shelhamer J, Lane HC, Urmacher C, Honig C, Longo DL, Parker MM, Natanson C, Parrillo JE, Fauci AS, Pizzo PA, Masur H. *Pneumocystis carinii* pneumonia: a comparison between patients with the acquired immunodeficiency syndrome and patients with other immunodeficiencies. Ann Intern Med 1984; 100:663–671.
53. Navin TR, Fontaine RE. Intravenous versus intramuscular administration of pentamidine. N Engl J Med 1984; 311:1701–1702.
54. Walzer PD, Perl DP, Krogstad DJ, Rawson PG, Schultz MG. *Pneumocystis carinii* pneumonia in the United States. Epidemiologic, diagnostic, and clinical features. Ann Intern Med 1974; 80:83–93.
55. Stehr-Green JK, Helmick CG. Pentamidine and renal toxicity. N Engl J Med 1985; 313:694–695.
56. Murdoch JK, Keystone JS. Pentamidine and hypoglycemia. Ann Intern Med 1983; 99:879.
57. Bouchard P, Sai P, Reach G, Chaubarrere I, Ganeval D, Assan R. Diabetes mellitus following pentamidine-induced hypoglycemia in humans. Diabetes 1982; 31:40–45.
58. Osei K, Falko JM, Nelson KP, Stephens R. Diabetogenic effect of pentamidine. In vitro and in vivo studies in a patient with malignant insulinoma. Am J Med 1984; 77:41–46.
59. Sansom CE, Laughton CA, Neidle S, Schwalbe CH, Stevens MFG. Structural studies on bioactive compounds. Part XIV. Molecular modelling of the interactions between pentamidine and DNA. Anti-Cancer Drug Design 1990; 5:243–248.
60. Schoenbach EB, Greenspan EM. The pharmacology, mode of action and therapeutic

potentialities of stilbamidine, pentamidine, propamidine and other aromatic diamidines. Medicine 1948; 27:327–377.
61. Waalkes TP, Makulu DR. Pharmacologic aspects of pentamidine. J Nat Canc Inst 1976; 43:171.
62. Rosenthal GJ, Corsini E, Craig WA, Comment CE, Luster MI. Pentamidine: an inhibitor of interleukin-1 that acts via a post-translational event. Toxicol Appl Pharmacol 1991; 107:555–561.
63. Corsini E, Craig W, Rosenthal GJ. Modulation of tumor necrosis factor release from alveolar macrophages treated with pentamidine isethionate. Int J Immunopharmacol 1992; 14:121–130.
64. Sippel H, Estler C-J. Comparative evaluation of hepatotoxic side effects of various new trypanocidal diamidines in rat hepatocytes and mice. Arzneimittel-Forschung 1990; 40:290–293.
65. Steinmann U, Estler CJ, Dann O. Hemodynamic effects of a series of new trypanocidal indoleamidino compounds. Drug Dev Res 1986; 7:153–163.
66. Geratz JD, Webster WP. Inhibition of the amidase and kininogenase activities of pancreatic kallikrein by aromatic diamidines and an evaluation of diamidines for their in vivo use. Arch Int Pharmacodyn 1971; 194:359–370.
67. Bornstein RS, Yarbro JW. An evaluation of the mechanism of action of pentamidine isethionate. J Surg Oncol 1970; 2:393–398.
68. Gutteridge WE. Some effects of the pentamidine di-isethionate on *Crithidia fasciculata*. J Protozool 1969; 16:306–311.
69. Damper D, Patton CL. Pentamidine transport in *Trypanosoma brucei*—kinetics and specificity. Biochem Pharmacol 1976; 25:271–276.
70. Bachrach U, Brem S, Wertman SB, Schnur LF, Greenblatt CC. Effect of inhibitors on growth and on polyamine and macromolecular syntheses. Exp Parasitol 1979; 48: 464–470.
71. Bitonti AJ, Dumont JA, McCann PP. Characterization of *Trypanosoma brucei* S-adenosyl-L-methionine decarboxylase and its inhibition by Berenil, pentamidine, and methylglyoxal bis(guanylhydrazone). Biochem J 1986; 237:685–689.
72. Waring MJ. The effects of antimicrobial agents on ribonucleic acid polymerase. Mol Pharmacol 1965; 1:1–13.
73. MacAdam RF, Williamson J. Drug effects on the fine structure of *Trypanosoma rhodesiense*: diamidines. Trans R Soc Trop Med Hyg 1972; 66:897–904.
74. Hentzer B, Kobayasi T. The ultrastructural changes of *Leishmania tropica* after treatment with pentamidine. Ann Trop Med Parasitol 1977; 71:157–166.
75. Kaplan HG, Myers CE. Complex inhibition of thymidylate synthetase by aromatic diamidines: evidence for both rapid, freely reversible and slowly progressive, nonequilibrium inhibition. J Pharmacol Exp Ther 1977; 201:554–563.
76. Douc-Rasy S, Kayser A, Riou J-F, Riou G. ATP-independent type II topoisomerase from trypanosomes. Proc Natl Acad Sci USA 1986; 83:7152–7156.
77. Shapiro TA, England PT. Selective cleavage of kinetoplast DNA minicircles promoted by antitrypanosomal drugs. Proc Natl Acad Sci USA 1990; 87:950–954.
78. Wang CC. Purine and pyrimidine metabolism in *Trichomonadidae* and *Giardia*. In: Molecular Parasitology. Orlando: Academic Press, 1983:13.

79. Ferguson LR, Sundberg RJ. Petite mutagenesis in *Saccharomyces cerevisiae* by a series of bis-cationic trypanocidal drugs. Antimicrob Agents Chemother 1991; 35: 2318–2321.
80. Smaldone G, Dickinson G, Marcial E, Young E, Seymour J. Deposition of aerosolized pentamidine and failure of pneumocystis prophylaxis. Chest 1992; 101: 82–87.
81. Walzer PD. *Pneumocystis carinii*—new clinical spectrum? N Engl J Med 1991; 324: 263–265.
82. Hatfield C, Kasarskis A, Staben C. Pentamidine sensitivity and resistance in *Saccharomyces cerevisiae* as a model for pentamidine effects on *Pneumocystis carinii*. J Protozool 1991; 38:70S–71S.
83. Frommel TO, Balber AE. Flow cytofluorimetric analysis of drug accumulation by multidrug-resistant *Trypanosoma brucei brucei* and *T. b. rhodesiense*. Mol Biochem Parasitol 1987; 26:183–192.

28

Primaquine, Other 8-Aminoquinolines, and Clindamycin

SHERRY F. QUEENER, JOHN R. BLACK, MARILYN S. BARTLETT, and JAMES W. SMITH

Indiana University School of Medicine
Indianapolis, Indiana

I. Introduction

In vivo and in vitro models for *Pneumocystis carinii* were developed at Indiana University in the mid-1970s to foster research on the organism, which at that time was causing infections in pediatric patients receiving a new chemotherapeutic regimen for control of leukemia (1). With the advent of the acquired immunodeficiency syndrome (AIDS) epidemic, interest in these models grew, and our work was expanded to include drug discovery, as it became obvious that existing drugs had exceptional toxicity in AIDS patients, and therapy commonly failed. Our initial drug discovery effort using both in vivo and in vitro models began in 1983 and was designed to search rapidly and systematically for anti-*P. carinii* activity among as many different classes of drugs as could reasonably be procured (2–6). To speed the movement of effective agents into clinical use, the search emphasized drugs that were currently in use in humans for other purposes or had been tested in humans.

Among the first groups of drugs tested were antimalarial agents. Chloroquine, a 4-aminoquinoline, had originally been tested against *P. carinii* by Frenkel (7), who concluded the compound was not effective in his latently infected rats. The 8-aminoquinoline primaquine had been tested only in combination with chloroquine in a fixed dosage combination supplied by Winthrop (8). This combination was also judged ineffective.

We chose to test primaquine and chloroquine alone in both our in vitro and our in vivo models to evaluate these classes of compounds more systematically. We were also aware of studies in malaria for which primaquine had been combined with mirincamycin, a chemical relative of clindamycin and synergy of the combination had been observed (9). No mechanism specific for malaria was proposed to explain the synergy. In fact, clindamycin alone has a broad antimicrobial spectrum that includes not only bacteria, but also plasmodia (10) and *Toxoplasma gondii* (11). The appeal of these drugs was that they were already widely used in humans; consequently, they could be more rapidly applied to clinical use against *P. carinii* pneumonia. In this chapter we will review the research findings that support use of primaquine plus clindamycin and use of other 8-aminoquinolines for *P. carinii* pneumonia, as well as summarize the current clinical trials that document effectiveness of these agents for *P. carinii* pneumonia in AIDS patients.

II. In Vitro Data

Compounds to be evaluated were first tested for activity in an in vitro culture system that has been extensively used for screening (2–6,12,13). Human embryonic lung (HEL) cells or WI-38 human embryonic lung fibroblasts served as the feeder layer for *P. carinii*. The WI-38 cells were grown to confluency in minimum essential medium with Earle's salts (Sigma) supplemented with 2 mM L-glutamine, 26 mM sodium bicarbonate, and 10% fetal bovine serum. The HEL cells required, in addition, 0.1 mM nonessential amino acids (Sigma), 1 mM sodium pyruvate, and 0.1% w/v lactalbumin hydrolysate. All cultures received 100 units/mL of penicillin G and 0.1 mg/mL of streptomycin. Cell monolayers grown in 12- or 24-well plates were inoculated with a suspension of *P. carinii* obtained from infected rat lung so that the final concentration of organisms was between 3×10^5 and 7×10^5/mL. Drugs were added at the time of inoculation; replicates were prepared so that four wells could be harvested at each time point for each condition. Each experiment contained control wells to which no drug was added to confirm adequate growth of organisms and to serve as the basis of comparison for drug effects; an increase in counts greater than 2.5-fold from day 1 to day 7 was required before the study was considered valid. Trimethoprim–sulfamethoxazole at 50/250 μg/mL was included as a positive control in each experiment. Plates were incubated at 35°C with 5% O_2, 10% CO_2, 85% N_2. Plates were harvested over 7 days, and the medium was evaluated for numbers of organisms. Counts of organisms, which are based upon 10-μL samples, are performed on Giemsa-stained preparations; multiplying counts per field by 4×10^5 yields numbers of *P. carinii* per milliliter of culture medium. Enzyme-linked immunosorbent assay (ELISA) evaluations were performed on 300-μL aliquots of culture medium from each well and employed pooled convalescent rat sera as the primary antibody. The second antibody was goal antirat IgG, conjugated with alkaline phosphatase. After development of color with substrate, the samples were quantitated using a Thermomax plate reader (14).

When tested alone in this standard in vitro culture system, primaquine, chloroquine, and hydroxychloroquine (Plaquenil) effectively inhibited growth of *P. carinii* at 1 μg/mL, 10 μg/mL, and 10 μg/mL, respectively (Fig. 1). Neither chloroquine at 0.1 μg/mL (190 nM) nor hydroxychloroquine at 0.1 μg/mL (230

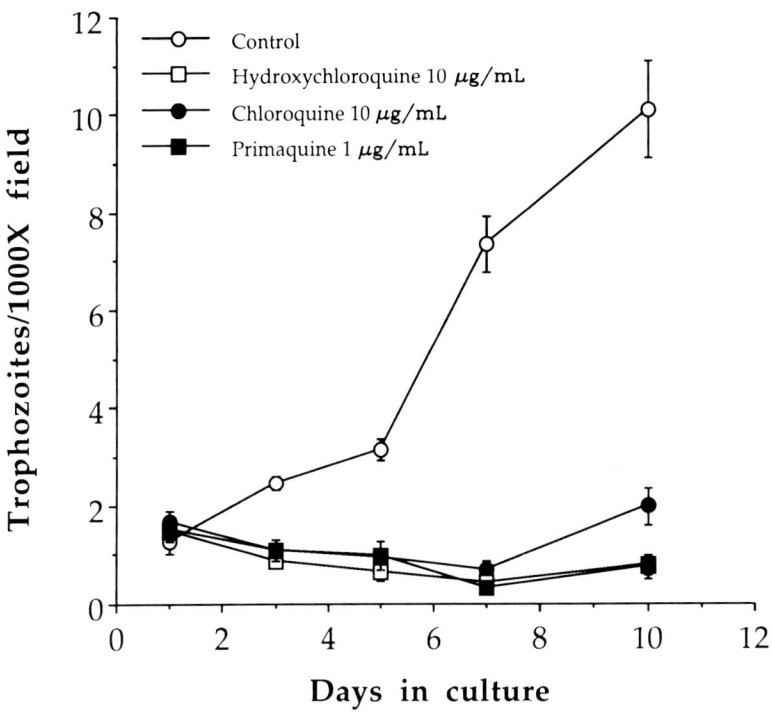

Figure 1 Effect of primaquine, chloroquine, and hydroxychloroquine on growth of cultured *P. carinii*. Cultures were grown in standard medium alone (control) or supplemented with test drugs at the concentrations shown (see text). Growth was assessed by counting the numbers of trophozoites in the culture supernatant. No toxicity toward the host cell monolayer was observed.

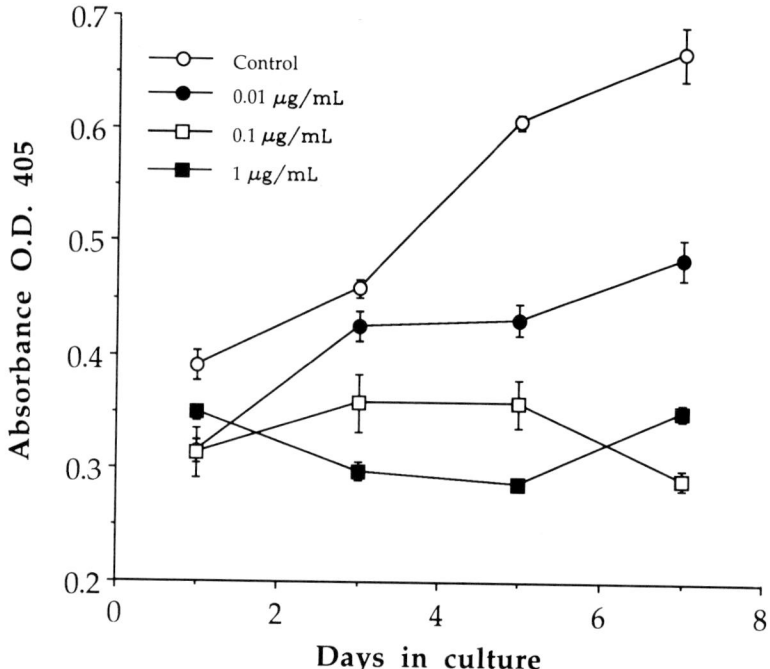

Figure 2 Dose response of primaquine inhibition of cultured *P. carinii*. Cultures were established as previously reported (5). Growth was assessed in this study by ELISA detection of *P. carinii* antigen in the culture (14).

nM) was an effective inhibitor of growth in culture (data not shown), but primaquine was effective, even at concentrations as low as 0.01 μg/mL, or 22 nM (Fig. 2). Clindamycin alone did not show an effect until concentrations exceeded 50 μg/mL (0.1 mM) in the culture fluid (Fig. 3).

Various combinations of clindamycin with primaquine were also assessed in the culture system. For the combinations tested, all activity observed could be attributed to the primaquine content of the culture medium. We have not yet been able to demonstrate unequivocal synergy of these compounds in culture.

The activity of chloroquine and primaquine in culture against *P. carinii* led us to evaluate related compounds (Table 1). Of these compounds, the bisaminoquinoline (4,7-quinolinediamine-$N^4N^{4'}$-1,6-hexanediylbis[N^7N^7-dimethyl]) was the most potent. A variety of 8-aminoquinolines have also been tested in culture (Table 2). Compounds WR242511 and 80/53 show activity at least equivalent to that of primaquine in vitro.

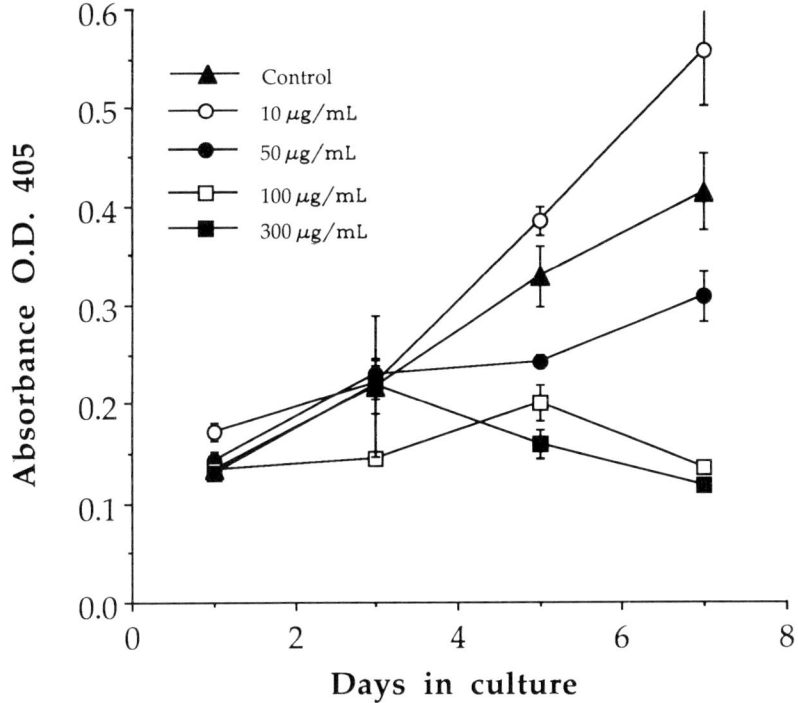

Figure 3 Dose response of clindamycin inhibition of cultured *P. carinii*. Conditions were as reported in the legend for Figure 2.

III. Studies in Animal Models

A. Therapy Protocols

As a result of in vitro studies, several drugs were selected for testing in vivo. Chloroquine was not effective in an early pilot study and was not included in subsequent tests. Likewise, the bisaminoquinolines were not effective in animal tests because of difficulties with solubility and toxicity. The 8-aminoquinolines were better tolerated and studied in more detail.

Primaquine alone given in daily doses of up to 2 mg/kg was ineffective for therapy of *P. carinii* pneumonia in a standard model using latently infected rats (5). Likewise, clindamycin alone at 225 mg/kg per day (in three divided doses) was without effect, which was expected, based on the results of Hughes et al. with doses of 400 mg/kg daily (15). Combinations of clindamycin with primaquine reduced the numbers of *P. carinii* detected in treated rat lungs to fewer than 10% of the untreated control (Fig. 4).

Table 1 Efects of 4-Aminoquinolines and Related Compounds on Growth of *P. carinii* in Culture

Compound	Structure	Lowest effective dose in culture (μg/mL)
Chloroquine		10
Hydroxychloroquine		10
Mefloquine		10
4,7-Quinoline-diamine, $N^4N^{4'}$-1,6-hexanediylbis [N^7N^7-dimethyl-		0.1

Other 8-aminoquinolines, originally developed as antimalarials by Walter Reed Army Institute for Research (WRAIR), were also tested in therapy protocols (12). The drugs selected for testing were WR 6026, WR 238605, and WR 242511. All three of these agents were much more effective alone at a dose of 2 mg/kg per day than was primaquine (Table 3). The efficacy of these three WRAIR compounds, demonstrated at Indiana University with rats infected by transtracheal inoculation, was confirmed by studies at the University of North Carolina in studies using rats with latent infections (12).

Table 2 Effects of 8-Aminoquinolines on Growth of *P. carinii* in Culture

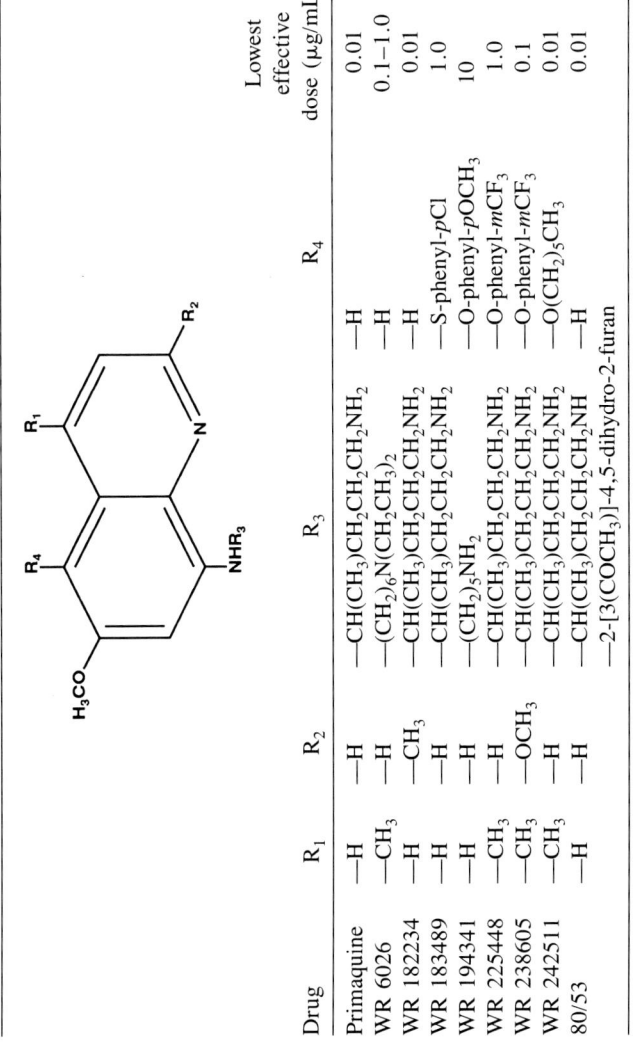

Drug	R_1	R_2	R_3	R_4	Lowest effective dose (µg/mL)
Primaquine	—H	—H	—CH(CH$_3$)CH$_2$CH$_2$CH$_2$NH$_2$	—H	0.01
WR 6026	—CH$_3$	—H	—(CH$_2$)$_6$N(CH$_3$)$_2$	—H	0.1–1.0
WR 182234	—H	—CH$_3$	—CH(CH$_3$)CH$_2$CH$_2$CH$_2$NH$_2$	—H	0.01
WR 183489	—H	—H	—CH(CH$_3$)CH$_2$CH$_2$CH$_2$NH$_2$	—S-phenyl-*p*Cl	1.0
WR 194341	—H	—H	—(CH$_2$)$_5$NH$_2$	—O-phenyl-*p*OCH$_3$	10
WR 225448	—CH$_3$	—H	—CH(CH$_3$)CH$_2$CH$_2$CH$_2$NH$_2$	—O-phenyl-*m*CF$_3$	1.0
WR 238605	—CH$_3$	—OCH$_3$	—CH(CH$_3$)CH$_2$CH$_2$CH$_2$NH$_2$	—O-phenyl-*m*CF$_3$	0.1
WR 242511	—CH$_3$	—H	—CH(CH$_3$)CH$_2$CH$_2$CH$_2$NH$_2$	—O(CH$_2$)$_5$CH$_3$	0.01
80/53	—H	—H	—CH(CH$_3$)CH$_2$CH$_2$CH$_2$NH —2-[3(COCH$_3$)]-4,5-dihydro-2-furan	—H	0.01

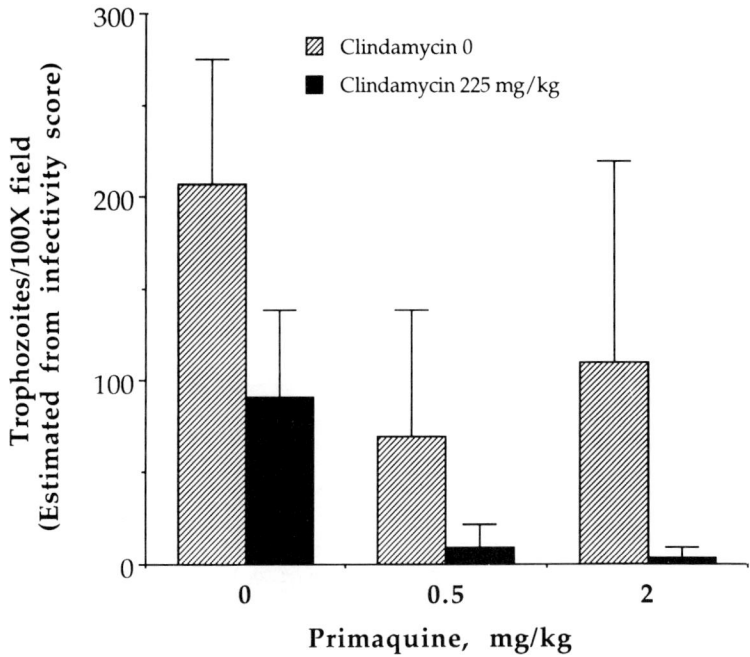

Figure 4 Therapy of *P. carinii* pneumonia in rats with primaquine and clindamycin. Female Sprague–Dawley rats developed spontaneous *P. carinii* infections over 8 weeks of immunosuppression, according to standard protocols (5). Primaquine was given in drinking water, but clindamycin was injected subcutaneously three times daily to achieve the daily dose of 225 mg/kg. Therapy was for 15 days; there were ten rats in each group. For this illustration, infectivity scores were used to estimate numbers of organisms per 1000× field in samples from two separate experiments. Infectivity scores are assigned, based on estimation of numbers of organisms in sampled 1000× fields: 0, no organisms per 50 fields; 1, fewer than 1 organism per 10 fields; 2, 2–9 organisms per 10 fields; 3, 1–10 organisms per field; 4, 11–100 organisms per field; 5, more than 100 organisms per field (5,12). Control infectivity scores were 4.4 and 4.7; the lowest score in the chart (clindamycin 225 mg/kg with 2 mg/kg primaquine) was 2.8. This conversion of infectivity score to estimated numbers of organisms illustrates logarithmic nature of the scoring system previously published. The only values statistically significantly different from control are the combination of 225 mg/kg clindamycin with 0.5 or 2 mg/kg primaquine.

Because potency was so great with the three WRAIR compounds, the drugs were tested in a dose-ranging study to determine the lowest effective doses for therapy (see Table 3). The lowest effective dose for WR 6026 and WR 238605 was 0.5 mg/kg per day, but no lower doses were tested for WR 238605. WR 242511 was effective at 0.25 mg/kg per day, but not at 0.1 mg/kg per day.

Table 3 Effect of 8-Aminoquinolines for Therapy of *P. carinii* Pneumonia in Rats

Compound	Dose (mg/kg per day)	Giemsa stain infectivity score	Silver stain infectivity score
Untreated		4.2 ± 0.2	3.6 ± 0.2
Primaquine	2.0	4.3 ± 0.3	3.4 ± 0.3
	0.5	4.1 ± 0.3	3.2 ± 0.3
WR 6026	2.0	0.3 ± 0.1	0.4 ± 0.2
	1.0	1.1 ± 0.2	0.9 ± 0.4
	0.5	1.8 ± 0.6	2.1 ± 0.4
	0.25	4.7 ± 0.2	3.9 ± 0.1
WR 238605	4.0	0.03 ± 0.1	0.3 ± 0.2
	2.0	0.9 ± 0.4	1.0 ± 0.4
	1.0	2.3 ± 0.9	2.4 ± 0.6
	0.5	2.6 ± 0.2	2.7 ± 0.1
WR 242511	2.0	0.16 ± 0.2	0.5 ± 0.2
	1.0	0.5 ± 0.2	0.8 ± 0.3
	0.5	2.4 ± 0.8	2.2 ± 0.6
	0.25	1.8 ± 0.6	1.8 ± 0.5
	0.1	4.0 ± 0.3	3.6 ± 0.2
Trimethoprim–sulfamethoxazole	50/250	0.9 + 0.6	0.4 ± 0.1

Data from three experiments with similar values for untreated controls are included in this table. All drugs were administered in drinking water.

B. Prophylaxis Protocols

Primaquine, used alone for prophylaxis against *P. carinii* in latently infected rats, was effective at 0.5 mg/kg per day when administered in drinking water, but was not effective with doses at or below 0.2 mg/kg per day (Table 4). Clindamycin seemed synergistic when used at 5 mg/kg per day along with primaquine at 0.5 mg/kg per day, but when combined with lower doses of primaquine, was less effective. When tested using transtracheally inoculated rats in a prophylaxis protocol, primaquine alone at 0.57 mg/kg per day lowered the level of infection by 1 unit on our scoring scale, which corresponds to about a 90% reduction relative to controls. Primaquine at that same dose was strongly effective when combined with 225 mg/kg daily of clindamycin; the infectivity score for this treatment fell to 1.4, which corresponds to an average of less than one organism per 1000× field, compared with the control score of 4.4, which represents about 100 organisms per 1000× field.

WR 6026, WR 238605, and WR 242511, which were effective in therapy

Table 4 Effect of Primaquine on Prophylaxis of *P. carinii* Pneumonia in Rats

Treatment	Dose (mg/kg per day)	Giemsa stain infectivity score	Silver stain infectivity score
Latent infection model			
Control		3.2 ± 0.2	3.2 ± 0.2
Primaquine	0.5	0.9 ± 0.2	1.4 ± 0.2
	0.2	3.3 ± 0.3	3.0 ± 0.2
	0.1	3.2 ± 0.2	2.9 ± 0.2
Clindamycin	5.0	3.7 ± 0.1	3.7 ± 0.2
Primaquine + clindamycin	0.5 5.0	0.1 ± 0.1	0.2 ± 0.1
Primaquine + clindamycin	0.2 5.0	2.5 ± 0.3	3.0 ± 0.3
Primaquine + clindamycin	0.1 5.0	2.2 ± 0.2	2.5 ± 0.3
Transtracheally infected model			
Control		4.4 ± 0.3	3.9 ± 0.1
Primaquine	0.57	3.3 ± 0.3	3.2 ± 0.2
Primaquine + clindamycin	0.57 225	1.4 ± 0.4	1.8 ± 0.3

Immunosuppression was with cortisone acetate (250 mg/kg given subcutaneously twice weekly). Drugs were administered in drinking water.

protocols against *P. carinii* pneumonia, were also tested in prophylaxis protocols using transtracheally inoculated rats (Table 5). The dose selected was 0.57 mg/kg per day, which corresponded to 1.4, 0.98, and 1 μmol/kg per day for WR 6026, WR 238605, and WR 242511, respectively. A 0.57 mg/kg per day dose of primaquine corresponds to 1.25 μmol/kg per day. The three WRAIR compounds were much more potent alone for prophylaxis than was primaquine. Not only were scores significantly lower than those for primaquine, but significant numbers of animals receiving the WRAIR compounds were free of detectable infection at the end of the study (12).

C. Intermittent Dosing Protocols

The half-life of primaquine in humans is about 4 hr, but for WR 6026 it is 8–24 hr, and for WR 238605 it is 52 hr (16). On the basis of these longer half-lives, we reasoned that certain 8-aminoquinolines given on an intermittent-dosing schedule might be effective against *P. carinii* pneumonia, if the potency of the compounds were sufficiently high and the tissue distribution favorable. The studies using

Table 5 Prophylaxis of Rats with *P. carinii* Pneumonia with 8-Aminoquinolines from WRAIR

Drug	Dose (mg/kg per day)	Giemsa stain infectivity score	Silver stain infectivity score
WR 6026	0.57	0.09 ± 0.1	0.4 ± 0.1
WR 238605	0.57	0.4 ± 0.2	0.4 ± 0.2
WR 242511	0.57	0	0.1 ± 0.1
Trimethoprim–sulfamethoxazole	50/250	0.07 ± 0.1	0.1 ± 0.1
Control		4.0 ± 0.3	3.3 ± 0.2

Animals were immunosuppressed with dexamethasone and received test drugs in drinking water.

intermittent-dosing included primaquine and the two other 8-aminoquinolines most studied in humans: WR 6026 and WR 238605 (17).

Primaquine, given at a total dose of about 24 mg/kg, was equally effective for prophylaxis of *P. carinii* pneumonia in transtracheally inoculated rats when given as a single weekly dose, as two divided doses, or as daily doses (Table 6),

Table 6 Prophylaxis of *P. carinii* Pneumonia in Rats with Primaquine Administered Intermittently

Drug (mg/kg per dose)	Dosing schedule	Total dose (mg/kg)	Giemsa stain infectivity score	Silver stain infectivity score
Untreated			4.4 ± 0.3	3.9 ± 0.1
Primaquine (0.57)	Daily	23.4	3.3 ± 0.3	3.2 ± 0.2
+ clindamycin (225)	Daily	9200	1.4 ± 0.4	1.9 ± 0.3
+ clindamycin (50)	Daily	2100	3.8 ± 0.2	3.4 ± 0.1
Primaquine (2)	Twice weekly	24	2.8 ± 0.5	2.7 ± 0.3
+ clindamycin (225)	Daily	9200	1.9 ± 0.3	2.2 ± 0.3
+ clindamycin (50)	Daily	2100	2.7 ± 0.5	2.6 ± 0.4
Primaquine (4)	Once a week	24	3.0 ± 0.5	3.1 ± 0.3
+ clindamycin (225)	Daily	9200	2.9 ± 0.3	2.7 ± 0.2
+ clindamycin (50)	Daily	2100	3.1 ± 0.4	3.0 ± 0.3

Immunosuppresion of transtracheally inoculated rats was with cortisone acetate. Doses of drugs administered daily were given in drinking water; those given once or twice weekly were given by gavage.

although the effect reduced the scores by only about 1 unit (about a 90% reduction in organisms). Clindamycin at 225 mg/kg per day greatly improved effectiveness for the divided doses of primaquine, but not when primaquine was given as a single weekly dose.

Primaquine, WR 6026, and WR 238605 were directly compared in a dose-ranging prophylaxis study in which the doses were given every fourth day (Table 7). Primaquine was effective at 4 mg/kg per dose on this schedule, but not at 1 mg/kg per dose. In contrast, WR 6026 retained a degree of effectiveness at 1 mg/kg per dose, reducing the numbers of organisms about 2 logs relative to untreated controls. WR 238605 at 1 mg/kg per dose reduced the numbers of organisms about 3 logs relative to untreated controls when given on this same schedule.

The schedule of dosing every fourth day was also applied in a therapy protocol using transtracheally inoculated rats (Fig. 5). Primaquine was significantly effective only at doses of 16 mg/kg per dose, or a total dose of 64 mg/kg for the study. The highest dose of WR 6026 that was tested was 8 mg/kg per dose, or 32 mg/kg for the study; no statistically significant effect was noted in Giemsa scores, but numbers of cysts were significantly reduced. In contrast, WR 238605 was effective in this intermittent therapy protocol, even in doses as low as 2 mg/kg per dose, corresponding to a total study dose of 8 mg/kg.

Table 7 Dose-ranging Studies of 8-Aminoquinolines Used Intermittently for Prophylaxis of *P. carinii* in Rats

Drug (mg/kg per dose)	Dosing schedule	Total dose (mg/kg)	Giemsa stain infectivity score	Silver stain infectivity score
Untreated			4.4 ± 0.1	3.5 ± 0.1
Primaquine				
4	Every 4th day	40	0.2 ± 0.2	0.9 ± 0.2
1	Every 4th day	10	4.2 ± 0.3	3.6 ± 0.2
0.25	Daily	10	4.5 ± 0.2	3.7 ± 0.1
WR 6026				
4	Every 4th day	40	0.1 ± 0.1	0.1 ± 0.1
1	Every 4th day	10	2.6 ± 0.3	2.4 ± 0.2
0.25	Daily	10	2.9 ± 0.4	2.7 ± 0.2
WR 238605				
4	Every 4th day	40	0.1 ± 0.1	0.1 ± 0.1
1	Every 4th day	10	1.5 ± 0.3	2.0 ± 0.2
0.25	Daily	10	3.6 ± 0.2	3.1 ± 0.1

Immunosuppression of transtracheally inoculated animals was with dexamethasone in drinking water. Doses of drugs given daily were in drinking water; those administered every fourth day were by gavage.

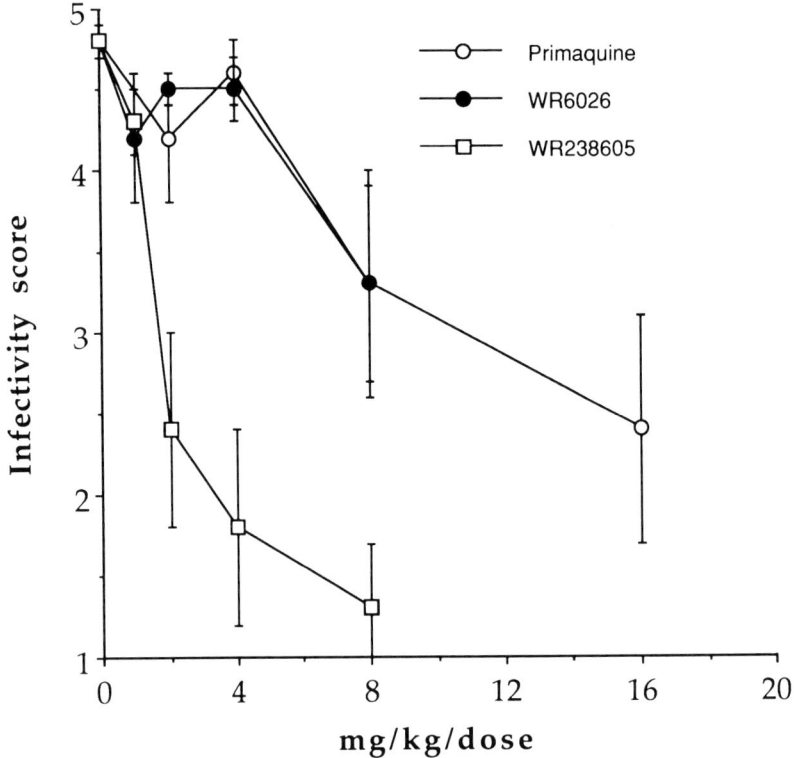

Figure 5 Therapy of *P. carinii* pneumonia in rats, using 8-aminoquinolines administered every 4 days. Female Sprague–Dawley rats were transtracheally inoculated with *P. carinii*, according to published procedures (17). Infectivity scores were assigned as described in legend to Figure 4. Immune suppression was with dexamethasone in drinking water (1.2 mg/liter). Therapy with ten animals per group began 5 weeks after inoculation and continued for 16 days.

IV. Treatment Studies of Clindamycin and Primaquine for *Pneumocystis carinii* Pneumonia in Humans

Our enthusiasm for initiating treatment studies for patients with AIDS and *P. carinii* pneumonia was based primarily on the activity of the combination of clindamycin and primaquine in vitro and in the rat treatment and prophylaxis models discussed previously. The combination had additional potential appeal because both drugs could be given orally and inexpensively. Moreover, both drugs appeared to be concentrated at the site of infection. Clindamycin is concentrated more than 50-fold in pulmonary alveolar macrophages (18), and primaquine is concentrated in mammalian lung tissue (19). Both drugs had been used safely and extensively to treat a variety of bacterial and protozoal infections in non-AIDS patients.

Our first study was a prospective, noncomparative, multicenter pilot study designed to assess the safety and efficacy of clindamycin and primaquine in the treatment of AIDS patients with acute *P. carinii* pneumonia of mild to moderate severity (20). Histologically confirmed *P. carinii* pneumonia and an alveolar minus arterial oxygen gradient $[(A-a)DO_2]$ less than 40 mmHg were required for entry. Patients were excluded if they had received any prior treatment for the current episode of *P. carinii* pneumonia, or if they had significant pancytopenia or renal or liver disease. Patients with known glucose-6-phosphate dehydrogenase (G6PD) deficiency, significant diarrhea, nausea, vomiting, or ileus, precluding oral treatment, were excluded. Treatment with corticosteroids was not permitted.

Twenty-two patients were treated with intravenous clindamycin at 900 mg every 8 hr for the first 10 days and then switched to oral clindamycin at 450 mg every 6 hr after satisfying specific criteria for clinical improvement. Primaquine, 30 mg base per day, was administered orally as two 26.3 mg primaquine phosphate tablets (26.3 mg primaquine phosphate = 15 mg primaquine base) daily throughout the 21-day course of treatment. The particular doses of both drugs were chosen because they were likely to represent the highest doses that would be well tolerated. Twenty of the 22 patients (91%) treated with the intravenous–oral regimen showed marked clinical improvement by the day 7 evaluation. Of the two therapeutic failures, one was declared as such inappropriately because a venous blood gas sample was mistakenly thought to be arterial. The other patient, who was considered a *P. carinii* pneumonia therapeutic failure, actually died of concomitant *Haemophilus influenzae* pneumonia. Four patients (18%) were withdrawn owing to adverse effects of clindamycin and primaquine therapy.

The study protocol was then modified to assess the safety and efficacy of an entirely oral treatment regimen (21). The oral dosing regimen used was clindamycin, 600 mg every 8 hr and primaquine, 30 mg (base) per day. Thirty-five of 38 patients (92%) treated with the oral regimen experienced clinical improvement by day 7. Five were withdrawn for adverse effects.

Overall, 55 of 60 patients (92%) in this study had a favorable therapeutic response, and 46 patients (77%) completed a full course of clindamycin and primaquine treatment. All but 1 patient survived. One patient relapsed 6 weeks following completion of treatment, and 9 were withdrawn for adverse effects.

Other investigators have also reported successful treatment of *P. carinii* pneumonia in AIDS patients with the combination of clindamycin and primaquine. All 19 of a series of consecutively hospitalized patients with first episode *P. carinii* pneumonia of mild to moderate severity [median baseline room air arterial oxygen tension (PaO_2) was 60.1 mmHg] treated with clindamycin and primaquine responded favorably (22). There were no differences in time to defervescence and resolution of radiographic infiltrates in this series of patients when compared with a matched group of patients treated with trimethoprim–

sulfamethoxazole. No patient in the clindamycin and primaquine treatment group required dosage modification or treatment termination because of side effects.

The combination of clindamycin and primaquine has also been used as "salvage" therapy. Twenty-six patients, including 4 requiring mechanical ventilation, who either showed intolerance to or were failing standard therapies were treated with clindamycin and primaquine (23). Twenty-four of the 28 episodes of *P. carinii* pneumonia in these patients (86%) were treated successfully. All patients survived at least 30 days following treatment. In another series of 109 patients, most of whom had failed or were intolerant to standard therapies, treatment consisted of only 15 mg of primaquine base daily along with intravenous clindamycin (24). Twenty-eight patients were characterized as having mild *P. carinii* pneumonia ($Pao_2 > 75$ mmHg), 59 as having moderately severe *P. carinii* pneumonia (Pao_2 50–75 mmHg), and 22 as having severe *P. carinii* pneumonia ($Pao_2 < 50$ mmHg). Twenty-two patients required mechanical ventilation. Sixty-four of the 70 proved cases of *P. carinii* pneumonia were rescued with clindamycin and primaquine therapy. As with all salvage therapies, the contribution of prior therapies and spontaneous healing of alveolar damage to the ultimate outcome is impossible to assess.

TMP/SMX and pentamidine produce serious side effects in a majority of AIDS patients. The reported toxicity of clindamycin and primaquine in AIDS patients with *P. carinii* pneumonia has been generally mild and easily managed. The most commonly encountered minor toxicity has been an erythematous macular or macular–papular rash, which developed on or about day 10 of treatment in 105 of 197 (53%) patients in the foregoing studies. Development of this rash was the most common reason for termination of clindamycin and primaquine therapy in these studies. However, as these studies progressed and the generally benign and self-limited nature of the rash became apparent, primary care providers and investigators became more comfortable with continuing clindamycin and primaquine treatment, despite development of rash. Clindamycin may have been the culpable agent in most cases, since a similar eruption has been described in 50% of AIDS patients receiving clindamycin and pyrimethamine for toxoplasmosis (25). Clindamycin may cause clinically significant diarrhea and pseudomembranous colitis (26). Diarrhea occurred in 9% of the foregoing patients, but no cases of pseudomembranous colitis were seen. Primaquine, like dapsone, is an oxidant drug that causes methemoglobinemia (27). Nearly half of the patients in our study developed methemoglobinemia above 10% at some time during therapy, but this did not result in clinical deterioration in any patient.

V. Summary

The high potency of primaquine in culture tests against *P. carinii* suggested that the 8-aminoquinolines should be explored as anti-*P. carinii* agents. Animal studies demonstrated that, when combined with clindamycin, primaquine was effective for therapy and prophylaxis of *P. carinii* pneumonia, and that primaquine alone could be effective for prophylaxis when given on an intermittent-dosing schedule. Related compounds from Walter Reed Army Institute for Research were even more potent than primaquine. These animal studies, along with the in vitro data, formed the rationale for clinical trials.

Clinical trials to date show that the combination of clindamycin and primaquine is an effective and well-tolerated treatment for *P. carinii* pneumonia of mild to moderate severity. It is inexpensive, can be given orally, and is ideally suited to outpatient therapy. The combination may be especially useful for patients who are failing or intolerant to TMP–SMX pentamidine.

Clinical trials directly comparing clindamycin and primaquine to TMP–SMX and dapsone–trimethoprim are currently underway in the United States and Canada. In addition, Phase I trials of WR 6026 have begun for developing the drug for *P. carinii* pneumonia in AIDS patients. The drug is already in Phase II trials for treatment of leishmaniasis. It is hoped that Phase I trials of WR 238605 will begin soon.

Acknowledgments

The studies reported in this chapter were supported in part by funds from the following sources: National Institutes of Health projects HO1-AI-42543, NO1-AI-72647, UO1-AI-25859; The Upjohn Company; Indiana University School of Medicine. Thanks also to our colleagues at the AIDS Division of the National Institutes of Health for their scientific advice and assistance in procuring compounds: Dr. Barbara Laughon and Dr. M. Nasr. We wish to thank the scientists at Walter Reed Army Institute for Research for their contributions to the development of these compounds.

References

1. Ruebush TK, Weinstein RA, Baehner RL, Wolff D, Bartlett MS, Gonzales-Cressi F, Sulzer AJ, Schultz MG. An outbreak of *Pneumocystis carinii* pneumonia in children with acute lymphocytic leukemia. Am J Dis Child 1978; 132:143–148.
2. Bartlett MS, Eichholtz R, Smith JW. Antimicrobial susceptibility of *Pneumocystis carinii* in culture. Diagn Microbiol Infect Dis 1985; 3:381–387.
3. Bartlett MS, Marr JJ, Queener SF, Klein RS, Smith JW. Activity of inosine analogs against *Pneumocystis carinii* in culture. Antimicrob Agents Chemother 1986; 30:181–183.
4. Queener SF, Bartlett MS, Jay MA, Durkin MM, Smith JW. Activity of lipid-soluble inhibitors of dihydrofolate reductase against *Pneumocystis carinii* in culture and in a rat model of infection. Antimicrob Agents Chemother 1987; 31:1323–1327.

5. Queener SF, Bartlett MS, Richardson JD, Durkin MM, Jay MA, Smith JW. Activity of clindamycin with primaquine against *Pneumocystis carinii* in vitro and in vivo. Antimicrob Agents Chemother 1988; 32:807–813.
6. Rosowsky A, Freisheim JH, Hynes JB, Queener SF, Bartlett MS, Smith JW. Tricyclic 2,4-diaminopyrimidines with broad antifolate activity and the ability to inhibit *Pneumocystis carinii* growth in cultured human lung fibroblasts in the presence of leucovorin. Biochem Pharmacol 1989; 38:2677–2684.
7. Frenkel JK, Good JT, Shultz JA. Latent pneumocystis infection of rats, relapse, and chemotherapy. Lab Invest 1966; 15:1559–1577.
8. Hughes WT, Smith BL. Efficacy of diaminodiphenylsulfone and other drugs in murine *Pneumocystis carinii* pneumonitis. Antimicrob Agents Chemother 1984; 26: 436–440.
9. Schmidt LH. Enhancement of the curative activity of primaquine by concomitant administration of mirincamycin. Antimicrob Agents Chemother 1985; 27:151–157.
10. Kremsner PG. Clindamycin in malaria treatment. J Antimicrob Chemother 1990; 25: 9–14.
11. Hofflin JM, Remington JS. Clindamycin in a murine model of toxoplasmic encephalitis. Antimicrob Agents Chemother 1987; 31:492–496.
12. Bartlett MS, Queener SF, Tidwell RR, Milhous WK, Berman JD, Ellis WY, Smith JW. 8-Aminoquinolines from Walter Reed Army Institute for Research for treatment and prophylaxis of pneumocystis pneumonia in rat models. Antimicrob Agents Chemother 1991; 35:277–282.
13. Queener SF, Fujioka H, Nishiyama Y, Furukawa H, Bartlett MS, Smith JW. In vitro activities of acridone alkaloids against *Pneumocystis carinii*. Antimicrob Agents Chemother 1991; 35:377–379.
14. Durkin MM, Bartlett MS, Queener SF, Shaw MM, Lee CH, Smith JW. An ELISA method for quantitation of *Pneumocystis carinii* in culture and lung. J Protozool 1991; 38:208S–210S.
15. Hughes WT, McNabb PC, Makres TD, Feldman S. Efficacy of trimethoprim and sulfamethoxazole in the prevention and treatment of *Pneumocystis carinii* pneumonitis. Antimicrob Agents Chemother 1974; 5:289–293.
16. Coleman RE. Sporontocidal activity of the antimalarial WE-238605 against *Plasmodium berghei anka* in *Anopheles stephensi*. Am J Trop Med Hyg 1990; 42: 196–205.
17. Queener SF, Dean RA, Bartlett MS, Milhous WK, Berman JD, Ellis WY, Smith JW. Efficacy of intermittent dosage of 8-aminoquinolines for therapy of prophylaxis of pneumocystis pneumonia in rats. J Infect Dis 1992; 165:764–768.
18. Hand WL, Boozer RM, King-Thompson NL. Antibiotic uptake by alveolar macrophages of smokers. Antimicrob Agents Chemother 1991; 27:42–45.
19. Clark AM, Baker JK, McChesney JD. Excretion, distribution, and metabolism of primaquine in rats. J Pharm Sci 1984; 73:502–506.
20. Black JR, Feinberg J, Murphy RL, Fass RJ, Carey J, Sattler FR. Clindamycin and primaquine as primary treatment for mild and moderately severe *Pneumocystis carinii* pneumonia. Eur J Clin Microbiol Infect Dis 1991; 10:204–207.
21. Black JR, Akil B, Murphy RL, Fass RJ, Feinberg J, Mills J, Sattler FR. Oral

clindamycin plus primaquine therapy for *Pneumocystis carinii* pneumonia in AIDS patients. Seventh Int Conf on AIDS, Florence, Italy, June 1991: abstr Th.B.42.
22. Ruf B, Rohde I, Pohle HD. Efficacy of clindamycin/primaquine versus trimethoprim/ sulfamethoxazole in primary treatment of *Pneumocystis carinii* pneumonia. Eur J Clin Microbiol Infect Dis 1991; 10:207–210.
23. Noskin GA, Murphy RL, Black JR, Phair JP. Salvage therapy with clindamycin/ primaquine for *Pneumocystis carinii* pneumonia. Clin Infect Dis 1992; 14:183–188.
24. Toma E. Clindamycin/primaquine for treatment of *Pneumocystis carinii* pneumonia in AIDS. Eur J Clin Microbiol Infect Dis 1991; 10:210–213.
25. Danneman B, McCutchan A, Israelski D, et al. Treatment of toxoplasmic encephalitis in patients with AIDS. A randomized trial comparing pyrimethamine plus clindamycin to pyrimethamine plus sulfadiazine. Ann Intern Med 1992; 116:33–43.
26. Hermans PE. Lincosamides. Antimicrob Agents Annu 1986; 1:103–114.
27. Grewal RS. Pharmacology of 8-aminoquinolines. Bull WHO 1981; 59:397–406.

29
Hydroxynaphthoquinones

WALTER T. HUGHES

St. Jude Children's Research Hospital
Memphis, Tennessee

I. Introduction

In 1946, Wendel reported certain 2-hydroxy-3-alkyl-naphthoquinones inhibited the respiratory processes of *Plasmodium* species (1). Later these observations were confirmed by Fieser and colleagues (2). However, no drug suitable for human use was found. The antiprotozoal activity of several naphthoquinones was also demonstrated for trypanosomes (3–6), *Toxoplasma* species (7), *Theileria parva* (7,8), and *Eimeria* species (7). The mechanism and site of action have been elucidated for a few protozoa. Some hydroxynaphthoquinones have been shown to inhibit the mitochondrial electron chain of the cytochrome bc1 complex (complex III). The enzyme dihydroorotate dehydrogenase plays a key role in the pyrimidine synthesis pathway and is linked to the mitochondrial electron transport chain by ubiquinone. Thus, the inhibition of electron transport by hydroxynaphthoquinones will result in inhibition of pyrimidine synthesis (9).

Because certain drugs with antiprotozoal activity also have anti-*Pneumocystis carinii* activity, a hydroxynaphthoquinone compound known to have potent efficacy in experimental malaria was studied.

II. Initial Studies to Determine Anti-*Pneumocystis carinii* Activity of a 1,4-Hydroxynaphthoquinone

A drug designated 566C80 and with the generic name of atovaquone, 2-[trans-4-(chlorophenyl)cyclohexyl]-3-hydroxy-1,4-naphthoquinone, was investigated in the murine animal model, wherein *P. carinii* pneumonia is provoked in Sprague–Dawley rats by continuous corticosteroid immunosuppression (11). In all experiments, 566C80 was administered orally. Assessment of efficacy was based on the extent of *P. carinii* pneumonia (PCP) in the lungs of rats after courses of 566C80. Lung specimens obtained at necropsy were studied under code and rated 0–3+ for the extent of *P. carinii* infection.

When 566C80 was given prophylactically in doses of 100 mg/kg per day or more, the drug was highly effective and equal to the drug combination trimethoprim–sulfamethoxazole in current use for prophylaxis (Table 1).

Once pneumonitis was established, the therapeutic administration of 566C80 resulted in cure of all animals receiving 100 mg/kg per day (Table 2).

After 3 weeks of treatment with 566C80, animals were continued on immunosuppression, but without 566C80. No *P. carinii* developed in any of the ten rats given 566C80, but in the comparative group treated with TMP–SMX and pentamidine, the recurrent infection was found in more than 40% of animals. This finding suggested 566C80 may have a "cidal," or killing effect, whereas the other drugs have a "static" effect against *P. carinii*. To achieve this total response, plasma concentrations of more than 60 µg/mL were required (11).

In preparation for clinical trials, an experiment was done to determine the effect of ingestion with food on absorption of 566C80. The drug was administered at four dose levels, ranging from 10 to 100 mg/kg per day, either by gavage or mixed in food pellets. The results, demonstrated in plasma concentrations and extent of PCP, are summarized in Table 3. The data show that 566C80 was more effective and plasma concentrations were higher in the animals receiving 566C80 with food than in those given the drug without food (10).

III. Pharmacokinetics and Safety

In Phase I studies of human immunodeficiency virus (HIV)-infected adults, 566C80 was found to be safe, and an oral dosage range was established (9). The HIV-seropositive men were studied at dose levels of 100, 250, 750, 1500, and 3000 mg of 566C80, given orally once daily for periods of 12 or 21 days. An additional group was given 750 mg three times daily for 5 days, then twice daily at 12-hr intervals for an additional 16 days. The drug was administered in 250-mg yellow tablets.

Twenty-four cases were studied. All of the men tolerated 566C80 well. Some abnormalities that occurred while the drug was administered included a

Table 1 Extent of *P. carinii* After Prophylaxis: Histopathology of Lung Sections[a]

Site and drug group	Dose (mg/kg per day)[b]	No. of rats tested	No. of rats evaluated[c]	Extent of disease				Total (% of evaluated rats)
				None	1+	2+	3+	
Control	No drug	10	9	0	1	0	8	9 (100)
566C80	200 (r)	10	9	9	0	0	0	0 (0)
566C80	100 (r)	10	10	10	0	0	0	0 (0)
566C80[d]	100 (g)	10	8	8	0	0	0	0 (0)
566C80	100 (g)	10	9	8	1	0	0	1 (11)
566C80	50 (g)	10	9	7	0	1	1	2 (22)
566C80	25 (g)	10	8	1	2	1	4	7 (88)
566C80	10 (g)	10	10	1	1	0	8	9 (90)
TMP-SMZ	50/250 (r)	10	10	10	0	0	0	0 (0)

[a]Lung sections stained with Grocott–Gomori stain.
[b]Mode of administration in parentheses. r, rations; g, gavage.
[c]Excludes accidental deaths from gavage and loss from cannibalism.
[d]Initial screening study.
Source: Ref. 11.

Table 2 Extent of *P. carinii* After Treatment: Histopathology of Lung Sections[a]

Site and drug group[d]	Dose (mg/kg per day)[b]	No. of rats tested	No. of rats evaluated	No. of rats with *P. carinii* pneumonitis				
				Extent of disease				Total (% of evaluated rats)
				None	1+	2+	3+	
Control	No drug[c]	10	10	0	1	3	6	10 (100)
Control	No drug	10	9	0	1	0	8	9 (100)
566C80	100 (g)	10	8	8	0	0	0	0 (0)
566C80	50 (g)	10	9	2	0	3	4	7 (78)
566C80	25 (g)	10	8	1	0	1	6	7 (88)
TMP-SMZ	50/250 (r)	10	10	8	1	1	0	2 (20)

[a]Lung sections stained with Grocott–Gomori stain.
[b]Mode of administration in parentheses. g, gavage; r, rations.
[c]Five of ten rats scrificed at 4 weeks of immunosuppression when therapeutic drugs were started.
[d]Started on 566C80 treatment after 6 weeks of dexamethasone administration.
Source: Ref. 10.

Table 3 Enhancement of 566C80 Absorption and Efficacy by Administration with Food in Experimental Rats

Dose of 566C80 (mg/kg per day)	Plasma concentration of 566C80 (μg/mL) median (range)		% Rats with *Pneumocystis carinii* pneumonia after 6 weeks of 566C80	
	No food[a]	With food[b]	No food[a]	With food[b]
None (control)	0	0	100	67
10	24 (17–31)	72 (11–115)	90	0
25	52 (7–75)	120 (115–124)	88	0
50	71 (63–94)	143 (81–191)	22	0
100	74 (61–88)	NA	0	0

Note: NA, plasma not available. There were eight to ten rats per dose level.
[a]Drug administered by gavage.
[b]566C80 given orally as a component of food pellets.
Source: Ref. 10.

transient maculopapular rash that resolved before the drug was discontinued. Three patients had increased appetite, and one had a transient sinus arrhythmia. No hematological, hepatic, gastrointestinal, or renal abnormalities could be attributed to 566C80.

The essentials of pharmacokinetics of 566C80 in adult men with HIV infection are summarized in Table 4. The steady-state maximum concentration (C_{max}) increased in a linear manner with doses from 4.5 μg/mL at the 100 mg/day to 37.9 μg/mL at 750 mg/day. The area under plasma concentration–time curve at steady state (AUC_{ss}) also increased linearly with dose from 79 hr·μg/mL at 100 mg to 781 hr·μg/mL at 750 mg. However, little increase occurred at the next dose level of 1500 mg. At the 3000 mg dose and on the regimen of 750 mg three times daily for 5 days and twice daily for 16 days, increases in the C_{max} and AUC occurred, but not linearly, as recorded for doses of 750 mg or less. These data indicated the rate of absorption of 566C80 decreases at doses greater than 705 mg. Figure 1 shows the mean peak plasma concentration of 566C80 (4 hr postdose) and the trough (24 hr postdose) concentrations when single doses were given daily. The mean concentration at steady state from day 12 and for the subsequent 336 hr (2 weeks) after the last dose are shown in Figure 2. The highest plasma concentration achieved in this study was 87 μg/mL. The absence of toxicity at these spurious concentrations suggests larger doses could be tolerated, but with the current formulation the limited bioavailability precludes a significant increase in plasma concentrations, even if higher doses are given.

Table 4 Plasma Pharmacokinetic Parameters of 566C80 at Steady State After 12 days (Cohorts 1–5) of Single Daily Doses and 21 Days (Cohort 6) of Multiple Daily Doses

Cohort ($n = 4$)	Dosage (mg/day)	C_{max} (μg/mL)	T_{max} (hr)	AUC^{ss} (hr·μg/mL)	AUC.N (hr·μg/mL)	$t\frac{1}{2}$ (hr)	CL/F (L/hr)
1	100	4.5 ± 1.0	4.0 ± 0.0	79 ± 10	94 ± 17	45 ± 11	1.28 ± 0.15
2	250	14.3 ± 5.7	6.5 ± 1.9	273 ± 129	308 ± 104	56 ± 12	1.10 ± 0.6
3	750	37.9 ± 1.1	7.0 ± 1.4	781 ± 36	738 ± 93	57 ± 2	0.96 ± 0.04
4	1500	33.4 ± 7.9	6.5 ± 3.8	654 ± 160	688 ± 68	55 ± 21	2.38 ± 0.47
5[a]	3000	39.0 ± 5.5	8.0 ± 2.0	1088 ± 501	1057 ± 305	51 ± 8	4.09 ± 0.86
6	750 three times daily for 5 days, then twice daily for 16 days	51.0 ± 24.6	6.0 ± 2.8	843 ± 142	870 ± 159	77 ± 43	1.56 ± 0.55

Note: C_{max}, maximum plasma concentration; T_{max}, time to maximum plasma concentration; AUC_{ss}, area under plasma concentration–time curve at steady state (day 12); AUC.N, AUC normalized by body weight and elimination rate of a 70-kg man; $t\frac{1}{2}$, plasma half-life; CL/F, total plasma clearance/extent of oral bioavailability of drug.
[a]$n = 3$.

Hydroxynaphthoquinones

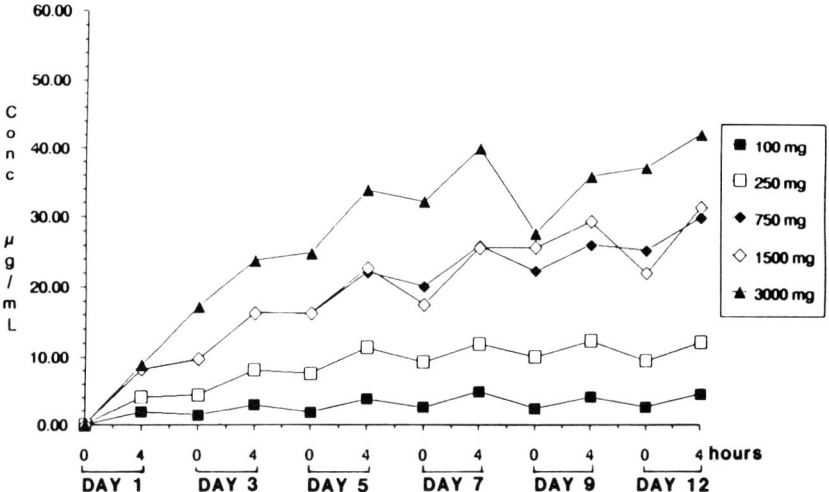

Figure 1 Mean plasma peak-and-trough concentrations (Conc) of 566C80 in patients over 12-day period at escalating daily oral doses. Plasma concentrations were measured at 4 hr after this single daily dose (0) and again at 24 hr after each daily dose (immediately before daily dose). (From Ref. 10.)

IV. Therapeutic Efficacy

In a pilot open-label trial of 566C80, AIDS patients with mild to moderately severe PCP (Pao$_2$ >60 mmHg while breathing room air) were enrolled in a study to determine the efficacy of the drug. Three cohorts of patients were studied at different dose levels: 750 mg three times daily for 5 days, then twice daily for 16 days; 750 mg three times daily for 21 days; and 750 mg four times daily for 21 days. The drug was given orally.

Thirty-four patients were enrolled in the study, and all survived the episode of PCP. Whereas 29 of the 34 cases (85%) improved while receiving 566C80, 27 (79%) of the patients were considered therapeutic successes (Table 5).

A possible toxic effect led to the discontinuation of 566C80 in four patients (12%), two because of rash and two because of fever. A rash was noted in seven patients. Table 6 summarizes the possible adverse effects.

The mean steady-state plasma concentrations of 566C80 were similar for the three groups: 16 ± 2.1 (b.i.d.); 20.4 ± 2.5 (t.i.d.); and 18.9 ± 3.1 (q.i.d.). These values are considerably lower than expected, but can be accepted as satisfactory for reasonable rates of therapeutic efficacy. This study shows 566C80 has therapeutic efficacy because cases such as those studied here would end fatally if not treated with a specific anti-*P. carinii* drug.

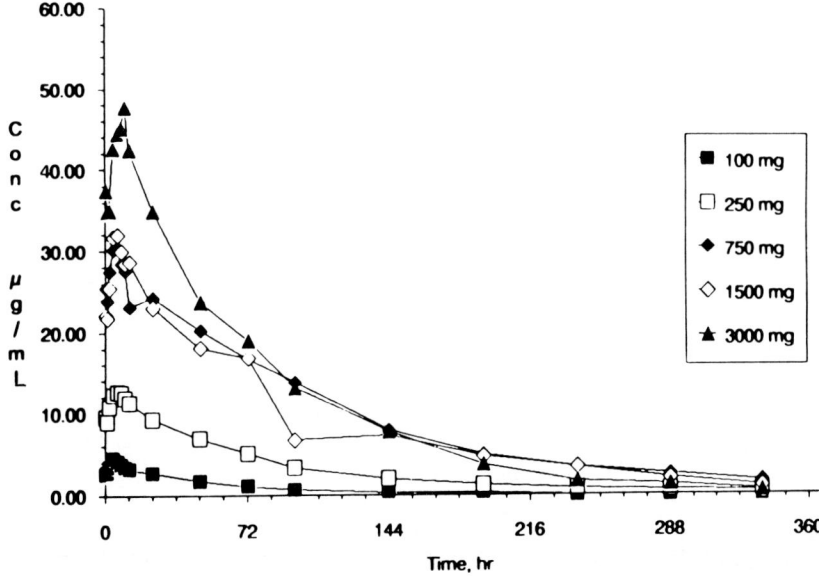

Figure 2 Mean plasma 566C80 concentrations (Conc) in patients at day 12 steady state at escalating oral doses. Time is in hours after last dose on day 23 of drug administration. (From Ref. 10.)

Table 5 Response to Therapy of Patients Treated with 566C80 for Pneumocystis Pneumonia

Response	750 mg b.i.d.	750 mg t.i.d.[a]	750 mg q.i.d.	Total no. (%)
Therapeutic success	9/10	13/15	5/9	27/34 (79)
Therapeutic failure	1/10	2/15	4/9	7/34 (21)
Failure for lack of response	1/10	2/15	2/9	5/34 (15)
Failure for toxicity	0/10	0/10	2/9	2/29 (3)
Duration of 566C80 therapy before failure for lack of response (days)	2	5, 21	10, 11	
Survived episode of pneumocystis pneumonia	10/10	15/15	9/9	34/34 (100)

[a]One patient received concomitant corticosteroids.
Source: Ref. 12.

Table 6 Adverse Reactions in Patients Treated with 566C80 for Pneumocystis Pneumonia

Adverse reaction	Number of patients			
	750 mg b.i.d. $n = 10$	750 mg t.i.d. $n = 15$	750 mg q.i.d. $n = 9$	Total no. (%)
Not requiring discontinuation of 566C80				
Rash	1	2	4	7/34 (21%)
Alanine aminotransferase >100 U/L	2	4	3	9/34 (26%)
Neutropenia[a]	1	1	1	3/34 (9%)
Anemia[b]	2	1	3	6/34 (18%)
Requiring discontinuation of 566C80				
Rash	0	0	2	2/34 (6%)
Drug fever	0	0	2[c]	2/34 (6%)

[a]Total neutrophil count <1000/mm³.
[b]Decrease in hemoglobin of 2 g or transfusion.
[c]Received >14 days of therapy and were therapeutic successes.
Source: Ref. 12.

A multicenter study comparing 566C80 and TMP–SMZ for the treatment of mild to moderate *P. carinii* pneumonia in patients with AIDS has recently been completed (13). A randomized, double-blind study enrolled 322 patients; 160 received 750 mg 566C80 and 162 received 320 mg TMP–1600 mg SMZ orally three times a day for 21 days. In the group with mild *P. carinii* pneumonitis (A−a (Do_2) <35 mmHg), 63% of the 111 treated with 566C80 and also 63% of those treated with TMP–SMZ met the criteria for therapeutic success. Therapeutic failures because of adverse effects to the drug occurred in 6 and 19% ($p = 0.005$) and because of inadequate therapeutic response in 18 and 7% ($p = 0.015$) of the 566C80 and TMP–SMZ-treated groups, respectively. Similar responses were found in moderately severe cases of *P. carinii* pneumonitis (A−a (Do_2), 35–45 mmHg) with overall therapeutic successful responses in 59 and 66% of the 566C80- and TMP–SMZ-treated cases, respectively ($p = 0.532$). Like the mild cases, the moderately ill patients had more therapeutic failures because of toxicity (23 vs 8%) in the TMP–SMZ group and because of lack of therapeutic efficacy (16 vs 4%) in the 566C80 group.

The treatment-limiting adverse effects included leukopenia (0 vs 3%), rash (3 vs 7%), fever (0.5 vs 5%), liver dysfunction (0.5 vs 7.5%), and vomiting (1 vs 6.5%) in the 566C80 and TP–SMX groups, respectively.

There was a definite relation to steady-state plasma concentrations of 566C80 and therapeutic success.

V. Conclusion

566C80 (Atovaquone) is a safe, well-tolerated, and effective drug for the treatment of mild to moderately severe PCP. Its effect in the initial treatment of severe PCP has not been determined.

Several hydroxynaphthoquinone compounds have been synthesized and deserve investigation for anti-*P. carinii* activity. At present only 566C80 has been studied in detail.

Note Added in Proof

Since the preparation of this chapter, atovaquone (formerly BW 566C80) has been licensed by the U.S. Food and Drug Administration for the treatment of mild to moderate episodes of *P. carinii* pneumonia in patients who are intolerant to TMP-SMX.

References

1. Wendell WB. Influence of naphthoquinones upon respiratory and carbohydrate metabolism of malarial parasites. Fed Proc 1946; 5:406–407.
2. Fieser LF, Schirmer JP, Archer S, Lorenz RR, Pfaffenbach PI. Naphthoquinone antimalarials. XXIX. 2-Hydroxy-3-(omega-cyclohexylalkyl)-1, 4-naphthoquinones. J Med Chem 1967; 10:513–518.
3. Boveris A, Stoppani AOM, Docampo R, Cruz FS. Superoxide anion production and trypanocidal action of naphthoquinones on *Trypanosoma cruzi*. Comp Biochem Physiol 1978; 61:327–329.
4. Docampo R, Cruz FS, Boveris A, Muniz RP, Esquivel DM. Lipid peroxidation and the generation of free radicals, superoxide anion, and hydrogen peroxide in beta-lapachone-treated *Trypanosoma cruzi* epimastigotes. Arch Biochem Biophys 1978; 186:292–297.
5. Lopes JN, Cruz FS, Docampo R, Vasconcellos ME, Sampalo MC, Pinto AV, Gilbert B. In vitro and in vivo evaluation of the toxicity of 1,4-naphthoquinone and 1,2-naphthoquinone derivatives against *Trypanosoma cruzi*. Ann Trop Med Parasitol 1978; 72:523–531.
6. Meshnick SR, Blobstein SH, Grady RW, Cerami A. An approach to the development of new drugs for African trypanosomiasis. J Exp Med 1978; 148:569–579.
7. Hudson AT, Randall AW, Ginger CD, Hill B, Latter V, McHardy N, Williams RB. Novel anti-malarial hydroxynaphthoquinones with potent broad spectrum anti-protozoal activity. Parasitology 1985; 90:45–55.
8. McHardy N, Haigh AJB, Dolan TT. Chemotherapy of *Theileria parva* infection. Nature 1976; 261:698–699.
9. Hammond DJ, Burchell JR, Pudney M. Inhibition of pyrimidine biosynthesis de novo in *Plasmodium falciparum* by 2-(4-*t*-butylcyclohexyl)-3-hydroxy-1,4-naphthoquinone in vitro. Mol Biochem Parasitol 1985; 14:97–109.

10. Hughes WT, Kennedy W, Shenep JL, Flynn PM, Hetherington SV, Fullen G, Lancaster DJ, Stein DS, Palte S, Rosenbaum D, Liao SHT, Blum MR, Rogers DM. Safety and pharmacokinetics of 566C80, a hydroxynaphthoquinone with anti-*Pneumocystis carinii* activity: a Phase I study in human immunodeficiency virus-infected men. J Infect Dis 1991; 163:843–848.
11. Hughes WT, Gray VL, Gutteridge WE, Latter VS, Pudney M. Efficacy of a hydroxynaphthoquinone, 566C80, in experimental *Pneumocystis carinii* pneumonitis. Antimicrob Agents Chemother 1990; 34:225–228.
12. Falloon J, Kovacs J, Hughes W, O'Neill D, Polis M, Parvey R, Rogers M, LaFon S, Feuerstein I, Lancaster D, Land M, Tuazon C, Dohn M, Greenberg S, Lane HC, Masur H. 566C80, a hydroxynaphthoquinone for the treatment of *Pneumocystis* pneumonia in patients with the acquired immunodeficiency syndrome. N Engl J Med 1991; 325:1534–1538.
13. Hughes W, Leoung G, Kramer F, Bozzette S, Frame P. Clumeck H, Masur H, Lancaster D, Hyland R, Lavelle J, Safrin S, Sampson J, Weinberg W, Falloon J, Feinberg J, LaFon S, Rogers M, Sattler S, and others. Comparison of 566C80 and trimethoprim–sulfamethoxazole for the treatment of *P. carinii* pneumonitis. N Engl J Med, 1993 (in press).

30

The Use of β-1,3-Glucan Synthesis Inhibitors for the Treatment and Prevention of *Pneumocystis carinii* Pneumonia

DENNIS M. SCHMATZ

Merck Research Laboratories
Rahway, New Jersey

I. History of β-1,3-Glucan Synthesis Inhibitors

There are two structurally distinct classes of β-1,3-glucan synthesis inhibitors: the echinocandins (Fig. 1) and the papulacandins (Fig. 2). Both classes are natural products and were initially identified as antifungal agents (1–13). Of these two classes, the echinocandins have been more extensively explored because of their superior in vivo activity against *Candida albicans* in rodent models (13–18). The discovery of the first echinocandin, echinocandin B, was initially reported by Benz et al., in 1974 (1), occurring as a natural product produced by the fermentation of a strain of *Aspergillus nidulans* var. *echinulatus*. Subsequently, other laboratories identified this product in fermentation broths of *A. rugulosis* (2,19). The basic echinocandin structure (see Fig. 1) features a cyclic hexapeptide nucleus containing all L-amino acids, several of which are modified, and a fatty acid side chain. A variety of naturally occurring echinocandins have been identified with different side chains or different amino acids in their nucleus, several of which are shown in Figure 1. Most of these compounds are specifically active against *Candida* species (1,17,20–22), but are thought to have little therapeutic value against other important fungal pathogens such as *Aspergillus* and *Cryptococcus*. The narrow antifungal spectrum and the limited need for systemic

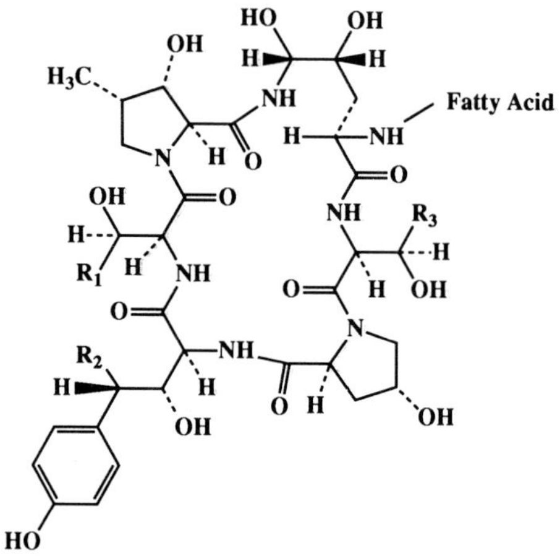

Figure 1 Naturally occurring echinocandins.

Compound	R_1	R_2	R_3	Fatty acid	Refs.
Echinocandin B	CH_3	OH	CH_3	Linoleic acid	1,2,19
Aculeacin A	CH_3	OH	CH_3	Palmitic acid	12,20
L-671,329	CH_2CONH_2	OH	CH_3	Dimethylmyristate	8,9
S31794	CH_2CONH_2	OH	CH_3	Myristic acid	10
Sporiofungin A	CH_2CONH_2	H	H	Dimethylmyristate	11
Mulundocandin	H	OH	CH_3	Methylmyristate	6,7

antifungal agents in the 1970s made the echinocandins unattractive for further development.

A rise in systemic fungal infections in the 1980s, owing to the acquired immunodeficiency syndrome (AIDS) epidemic and the use of immunosuppressive agents for cancer chemotherapy and organ transplants, initiated a renewed interest in the echinocandins. The "cidal" nature of these compounds against *Candida* (13–17,23) is a possible advantage over azole antifungals, which are "static" and have had limited success against deep mycoses in the immunocompromised patient (24,25). The compound currently used for treating fungal infections, amphotericin B, is cidal and effective against *Candida* and *Aspergillus*; however, this drug has a narrow therapeutic index and, as a consequence, is rarely used prophylactically (26,27).

II. Mechanism of Action

The observed effects of echinocandins and papulacandins on growing yeast suggested that these compounds altered cell wall biosynthesis (28–32). Mizoguchi

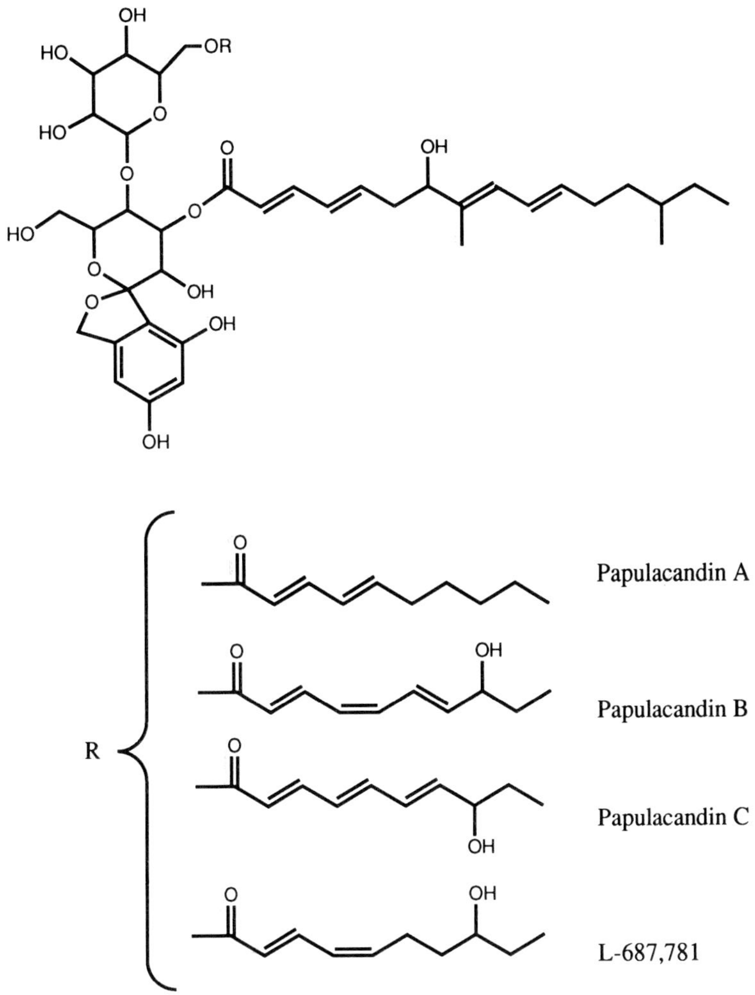

Figure 2 Naturally occurring papulacandins.

et al. (1977) found that aculeacin A (see Fig. 1) lysed the buds of actively growing *Saccharomyces cerevisae* and that high levels of sorbitol (0.8–1.0 M) effectively prevented this lysis by acting as an osmotic stabilizer. They also noted a reduction of radiolabeled glucose incorporation into the cell wall of these organisms, suggesting an alteration of cell wall biosynthesis (32). Similar experiments conducted by Baguley et al. (1979) with papulacandin B (see Fig. 2) and echinocandin B, using both *S. cerevisiae* and *C. albicans* suggested specific inhibition of β-glucan synthesis, based on inhibition of the alkali-insoluble fraction of glucan products known to contain predominantly β-glucans and the lack of inhibition of mannan synthesis (33). More specifically, Perez et al. (1981) claimed that β-1,3-glucan synthesis was inhibited, based on the lack of inhibition of the synthesis of other cell wall components and the sensitivity of the inhibitable product to β-1,3 glucanase (34). These results have subsequently been confirmed by several other laboratories (31,35–39). Although some laboratories claim direct inhibition of β-1,3-glucan synthase, the enzyme has not been purified, and the compounds appear to be noncompetitive inhibitors (34,36). In fact, it has been suggested that papulacandin B inhibits β-1,6-linkage formation between linear β-1,3-glucans. This is based on the fact that the β-1,3-glucan synthesis assay measures the synthesis of alkali-insoluble product; the linear β-1,3-glucan is alkali-soluble, whereas the branched form is alkali-insoluble (40). A more detailed review of glucan synthesis in fungi and its inhibition has recently been published by Tkacz (41).

III. Antipneumocystis Activity of β-1,3-Glucan Synthesis Inhibitors

In an effort to determine its taxonomic position, several laboratories have been looking at biochemical and molecular aspects of *Pneumocystis carinii* to identify characteristics that show similarity to fungi or protozoa (42–44). One indication that *P. carinii* might be related to fungi was the observation that the cyst wall, when stained with Aniline Blue, resembled the appearance of fungal cell walls known to contain β-1,3,-glucan (45). Additional evidence of this polymer was the sensitivity of *P. carinii* cysts to zymolyase, an enzymatic preparation that contains predominantly β-1,3-glucanase (46–48). To explore the potential of β-1,3-glucan synthesis as a chemotherapeutic target, rats with acute *P. carinii* pneumonia were treated with L-671,329 (49,50), a naturally occurring echinocandin analogue (see Fig. 1), previously shown to have anticandida activity (17). The compound effectively eliminated *P. carinii* cysts in the lungs of rats after only 4 days of therapy and had an effective dose for eliminating 90% of the cysts (ED_{90}) of 0.15 mg/kg when administered twice daily subcutaneously (50). Subsequently, aculeacin A (see Fig. 1) was also found to be efficacious against *P. carinii* when administered intraperitoneally for 2 weeks at 10 mg/kg per day to rats with moderate disease (51).

The efficacy of papulacandin analogue L-687,781 (see Fig. 2) provides additional evidence of the potential antipneumocystis activity of β-1,3-glucan inhibitors (50,52). Although this compound is not as potent as L-671,329, it significantly eliminated cysts after 4 days of therapy at a dose of 10 mg/kg. The rapid elimination of cysts by both structural classes of β-1,3-glucan synthesis inhibitors is unique relative to other known antipneumocystis agents, such as intravenous pentamidine isethionate and oral trimethoprim–sulfamethoxazole, which require several weeks of continued therapy to show a similar degree of cyst clearance in the rat model (50,53). However, when a *P. carinii*-specific DNA probe was used to quantitate trophozoite forms (54), this stage appeared to persist even after several weeks of therapy with L-671,329. This was in contrast with conventional therapies for *P. carinii* pneumonia during which both stages are gradually eliminated over the 2–3 weeks of treatment (53).

Although trophozoites persist with L-671,329 therapy, the total number of organisms does not increase during treatment, suggesting that the compound prevents the expansion of the trophozoite population, and that the cyst stage may be required for proliferation (53). In one study, echinocandin B was reported to reduce trophozoites in the lung with therapy (55). However, treatment was initiated early during the infection (3–4 weeks of immunosuppression) and the reduction in trophozoites relative to untreated controls at the completion of therapy may reflect more of a prophylactic effect. Despite trophozoite persistence, these compounds may restore respiratory function in patients with acute *P. carinii* pneumonia soon after initiating therapy, as is suggested in one rat study in which lung involvement improved rapidly with aculeacin A treatment (51,56).

Although short-term therapy with β-1,3-glucan synthesis inhibitors appears to selectively affect the development of cyst forms, prophylactic administration of L-671,329 (53) prevents the proliferation of both forms. A daily subcutaneous dose of 1 mg/kg of L-671,329 administered to rats with latent *P. carinii* during 6 weeks of continuous immunosuppression prevented the development of both cyst and trophozoite forms, demonstrating the potential use of this compound for preventing *P. carinii* pneumonia in immunocompromised patients (53) and suggesting the presence of an obligatory trophozoite–cyst life cycle. If trophozoites were capable of expanding independently of cysts, one would have expected to see trophozoite forms in rats receiving L-671,329 prophylaxis.

IV. Structure–Activity Relations and Chemically Modified Echinocandins

Several other lipopeptide analogues present in the L-671,329 fermentation broth were also isolated and evaluated in vivo against *P. carinii* and *C. albicans*. All of the compounds contained a dimethylmyristoyl side chain, but differed in the total number of hydroxyl groups or by the deletion of the methyl group on the 3-hydroxy-4 methylproline residue (Fig. 3). Because of their activity against *P. carinii*, these compounds are now identified as pneumocandins (57) with L-671,329 being identified as pneumocandin A_0. In addition to naturally occurring pneumocandins, analogues with similar changes were synthesized to explore the structure–activity relation (SAR) between the lipopeptide structure and

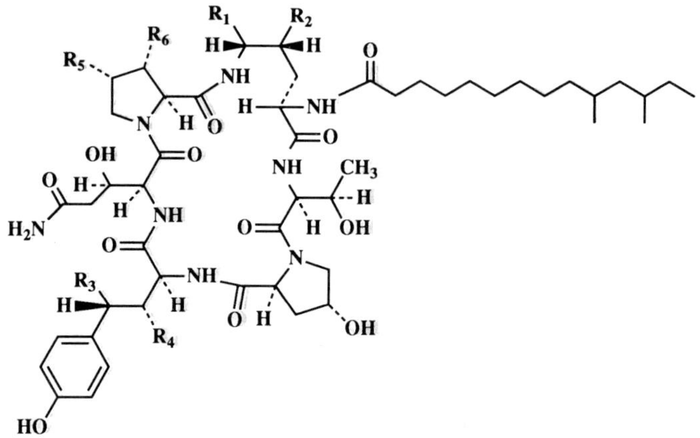

Compound	R_1	R_2	R_3	R_4	R_5	R_6	PCP[a] ED_{90} (mg/kg)	TOKA[b] ED_{90} (mg/kg)
Pneumocandin A_0	OH	OH	OH	OH	CH_3	OH	0.25	1.15
Pneumocandin A_2	H	H	OH	OH	CH_3	OH	<1.25	>6.00
Pneumocandin A_4	H	H	H	H	CH_3	OH	>2.50	>6.00
L-691,936	H	OH	H	OH	CH_3	OH	>1.00	2.00
Pneumocandin B_0	OH	OH	OH	OH	H	OH	0.15	0.35
Pneumocandin B_2	H	H	OH	OH	H	OH	0.60	>6.00
L-733,686	H	OH	OH	OH	H	OH	0.15	>6.00
L-706,577	OH	OH	H	OH	H	OH	>1.25	1.46
L-692,289	H	OH	H	OH	H	OH	1.25	1.66
Pneumocandin C_0	OH	OH	OH	OH	OH	H	0.30	>6.00

[a]PCP, 90% reduction in acute rat PCP model (50,58).
[b]TOKA, 90% reduction of *C. albicans* colony-forming units in mouse target kidney organ (TOKA) assay (23).

Figure 3 The pneumocandins.

antipnuemocystis–anticandidal activities. These compounds are represented by L-numbers in Figure 3 (58,59,60).

Evaluation of these analogues demonstrates divergence in the SAR for in vivo anticandidal and antipneumocystis activity (see Fig. 3). Anticandidal activity is sensitive to the absence of a hydroxyl group at the R_1 and the R_2 positions on the ornithine residue of the hexapeptide ring (see Fig. 3) and is also diminished when R_6 on the 3-hydroxy-4-methylproline is hydrogen and a new hydroxyl is present at the R_5 position. The antipneumocystis activity is minimally altered by any of these changes and is affected in this series only by reduction at the R_3

benzylic hydroxyl on the dihydroxyhomotyrosine residue. There are insufficient data to determine the role of the R_4 position for either of the biological activities. It is important to mention that the anticandidal activity was measured as the reduction in *C. albicans* in the kidney of DBA/2 mice, whereas the antipneumocystis activity was determined as the reduction of cysts in the lungs of immunocompromised rats with acute *P. carinii* pneumonia. Therefore, the divergent activity of the pneumocandins seen between *C. albicans* and *P. carinii* could be attributed to differences in biological distribution to specific organs or pharmacological differences between rats and mice (58). The lack of an in vitro efficacy model for *P. carinii* further complicates the effort to determine the intrinsic activity of these compounds.

Another aspect of the echinocandins that has been explored is the SAR of the lipophilic side chain. It is required for antifungal activity and β-1,3-glucan synthesis inhibition, as proved by evaluating the deacylated nucleus (61). Enzymatic deacylation of echinocandin B, followed by synthetic reacylation (16,62,63) has also permitted comparison of various side chain substitutions. The length of the side chain on echinocandin B alters the anticandidal activity with C_{14}–C_{16} being optimal for in vitro activity and C_{18} for in vivo activity (62,64). One negative characteristic of echinocandin B is the potential for red blood cell hemolysis at therapeutic levels. By focusing on this aspect, it was found that some side chain substitutions reduced this hemolytic potential while retaining the in vivo antifungal activity (16). These studies led to the development of cilofungin (Fig. 4), a semisynthetic echinocandin with an octyloxybenzoyl side chain, that was efficacious against systemic candidiasis in human clinical trials (65–67). Unfortunately, anion gap acidosis and acute renal failure were reported in some patients receiving cilofungin; however, these adverse effects may have been attributable to the polyethylene glycol vehicle that was used to solubilize the compound (67). These studies were the first human trials with an echinocandin against candidiasis. At present, none of the β-1,3-glucan synthesis inhibitors have been tested against *P. carinii* pneumonia in humans.

Information concerning the effects of side chain substitutions on in vivo antipneumocystis activity in rodent models is quite limited. One distinct SAR difference that has been observed is that cilofungin is much less active than tetrahydroechinocandin B (68) (see Fig. 4) and echinocandin B (see Fig. 1) (55) against *P. carinii* in the rat. In contrast, cilofungin is similar in potency to tetrahydroechinocandin B (see Fig. 4) (23,69) and superior to echinocandin B (16) against candidiasis in the mouse, again suggesting an SAR difference for anticandidal and antipneumocystis activity.

All of the pneumocandins have a dimethylmyristoyl side chain and appear to be much less hemolytic than echinocandin B and aculeacin A (17,58). Therefore, chemical modification of these compounds to reduce hemolytic activity is not required. Reacylation experiments designed to directly compare the effect of the

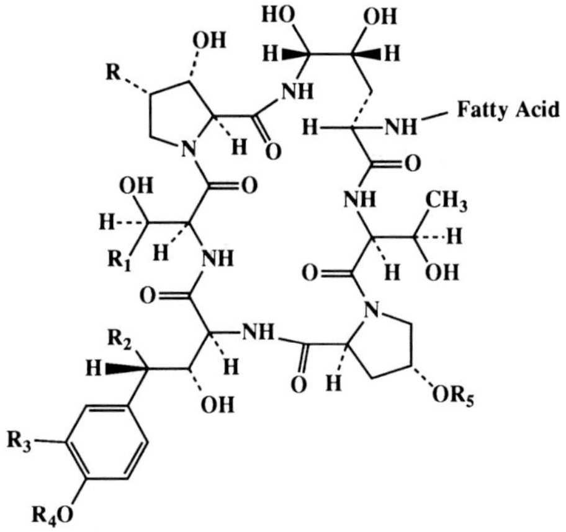

Compound	R	R_1	R_2	R_3	R_4	R_5	Fatty acid	Ref.
Cilofungin	CH_3	CH_3	OH	H	H	H	Octyloxybenzoate	62
Tetrahydroechino-candin B	CH_3	CH_3	OH	H	H	H	Stearic acid	62
Aculeacin Dα	CH_3	CH_3	H	H	H	H	Myristic acid	73
Aculeacin Dγ	CH_3	CH_3	H	H	H	H	Palmitic acid	73
FR131535	CH_3	CH_2CONH_2	OH	OSO_3Na	H	H	Myristic acid	72
FR 901379	CH_3	CH_2CONH_2	OH	OSO_3Na	H	H	Palmitic acid	72
Compound IIIA	H	CH_2CONH_2	OH	H	H	PO_3Na	Dimethylmyristate	74
L-693,989	H	CH_2CONH_2	OH	H	PO_3Na	H	Dimethylmyristate	75

Figure 4 Semisynthetic and novel echinocandins.

side chain versus that of the nucleus on hemolysis indicate that the dimethylmyristoyl side chain of the pneumocandins is less hemolytic than the tetrahydroechinocandin B C_{18} side chain. However, the single amino acid difference between the echinocandin B nucleus and the pneumocandin B nucleus (threonine versus 3-hydroxyglutamine) also accounts for some of the enhanced hemolytic activity of tetrahydroechinocandin B (70).

In vitro evaluation of cilofungin analogues that were produced by total synthesis (71) has also provided some interesting SAR data. These studies demonstrate that the homotyrosine residue is critical for the potent in vitro anticandidal activity of cilofungin and that the hydroxyl group on the 3-hydroxy-4-methylproline residue is also important, but to a lesser degree. A more complete review of the SAR for the echinocandin lipopeptides has recently been compiled by Hammond (70).

Additional echinocandin analogues with activity against *P. carinii* have recently appeared in the patent literature (see Fig. 4), including two naturally occurring water-soluble echinocandins FR 131535 and FR 901379 (72), several new aculeacin D analogues that lack the benzylic hydroxyl (R_2 position in Fig. 4) (73), and a biophosphorylated form of pneumocandin B_0 (compound IIIA), which is phosphorylated at the proline residue (see Fig. 4) using the microorganism *Rhizopus oryzae* (74).

V. Development and Evaluation of Water-Soluble Prodrug L-693,989

Similar to all of the previously discovered naturally occurring echinocandins, the pneumocandins have very poor water solubility, which limits their therapeutic use. As an alternative to cosolvent systems for solubilizing the compound, a series of prodrugs of pneumocandin B_0 were synthesized and evaluated in vivo (75). These studies led to the identification of L-693,989, a phosphate ester prodrug of pneumocandin B_0 (see Figs. 3 and 4) that is freely soluble in water (50–100 mg/mL) and that retains all of the in vivo biological activity of pneumocandin B_0 (68,75,65). It also appears to have improved pharmacokinetics over the parent compound, apparently owing to a slower clearance rate (77). Conversion of the prodrug to pneumocandin B_0 is presumed to occur as a result of cleavage of the phosphate ester by endogenous phosphatases.

Extensive studies have been conducted to evaluate the antipneumocystis (68) and antifungal activity of L-693,989 (76). As with L-671,329, L-693,989 also selectively eliminated cyst forms when used therapeutically and prevented the development of cysts and trophozoites when used prophylactically (68). The compound was also orally efficacious in rats when given at higher doses with an oral therapeutic ED_{90} of 30 mg/kg (b.i.d.) and an oral prophylactic ED_{90} of 5 mg/kg (once daily). From the parenteral therapeutic ED_{90} of 0.15 mg/kg (b.i.d.) and oral bioavailability studies, L-693,989 appears to be approximately 0.5–1.0% orally bioavailable in the rat. The relevance of these results to humans are unclear because oral bioavailability studies have not yet been conducted in other species.

The lack of significant oral bioavailability of the echinocandins may limit these compounds to parenteral or aerosol use. Methods for enhancing the bioavailability of a cyclic peptide with a molecular weight of approximately 1000–1100 are not apparent; however, the immunosuppressive agent cyclosporine, which is a cyclic undecapeptide with a molecular weight of 1203, is used as an oral therapeutic agent, and enhanced absorbance is achieved with an olive oil-glyceride formulation (78). Attempts to use similar vehicles with the pneumocandins have met with little success (Schwartz RE, et al., unpublished), and there have been no indications of any progress toward achieving an orally bioavailable echinocandin.

VI. Antipneumocystis Activity of Aerosolized Echinocandins

Oral absorption is also minimal for pentamidine isethionate, which is currently used to treat *P. carinii*, and parenteral use has resulted in toxicity problems (79,80). As an alternative, an aerosol formulation of pentamidine was developed for use in the prevention of *P. carinii* pneumonia (81–83). Patients with AIDS, who present a reduced CD4 count of fewer than 200/mm^3 or have had an episode of *P. carinii* pneumonia, are treated once or twice a month with nebulized pentamidine for the duration of their illness. This approach has had some success in the clinic and has provided an alternative for patients intolerant to oral prophylactic agents such as TMP–SMZ or dapsone. To explore the potential use of L-693,989 by this route, an aerosol prophylaxis study was conducted on rats with latent *P. carinii* infections using nebulized compound (84). Before the start of this experiment, a biodeposition study with radiolabeled pneumocandin B_0, injected parenterally, demonstrated that only a small percentage of compound ($\leq 0.5\%$) was deposited in the lungs; the required dose for aerosol prophylaxis was estimated to be between 1 and 100 μg delivered to the lungs (approximately 6–600 μg/kg body weight). Bioconversion of L-693,989 to active pneumocandin B_0 in the lungs occurred rapidly, with almost complete conversion in 15 min (84). Rats with latent *P. carinii* infections were placed on L-693,989 aerosol prophylaxis during a 6-week period of continuous immunosuppression. Three doses were used: 1, 10, and 100 μg, delivered to the lungs by inhalation, and two treatment regimens were chosen: daily or weekly. The lowest daily dose of 1 μg was fully effective in preventing the onset of *P. carinii* infection, whereas a weekly dose of 100 μg was required to achieve the same degree of control. Further evidence of the effectiveness of L-693,989 prophylaxis was seen histologically and upon review of the mean lung weights of treated animals, which were significantly lower than control rats with acute *P. carinii*. These reduced lung weights were most likely due to the lack of edema seen in the treated animals. The amount of L-693,989 required to prevent the onset of *P. carinii* pneumonia is quite low relative to the dose of aerosolized pentamidine required (4.8–8.6 mg/kg thrice weekly) to achieve a comparable degree of cyst clearance in a similar rat model (85).

Aerosolized cilofungin and echinocandin B have also been evaluated for the treatment and prevention of *P. carinii* pneumonia in the rat (55). Echinocandin B was very effective as an aerosol prophylactic agent at the lowest level tested of 12.5 mg/kg per day. Without further titration, it is not possible to determine the potency of echinocandin B relative to L-693,989, which was fully effective at ≤ 6 μg/kg per day. Cilofungin was tested in parallel with echinocandin B and was much less efficacious, with both cysts and trophozoites still present at the highest dose tested of 50 mg/kg per day (55). These results again indicate a difference in antipneumo-

β-1,3-Glucan Synthesis Inhibitors

cystis activity as a result of a side-chain substitution. Since the compounds were delivered directly to the lungs, it suggests that the change is in the intrinsic activity of the compounds and not a pharmacokinetic difference.

One concern with aerosol prophylaxis is the potential for disseminated disease. Although disseminated *P. carinii* infections are still rare, there appears to be some correlation between occurrence and the use of aerosolized pentamidine (86–88). This may result from the lack of drug in other tissues, since the compound remains in the lung (89–92). Blood levels in rats treated with aerosolized echinocandins have not been measured, and it is important that this determination be made before developing these compounds for aerosol use.

VII. Conclusion and Future Prospects

The echinocandins have a narrow antifungal spectrum, with significant activity against a variety of *Candida* species. The lack of activity of these compounds against other clinically important fungi such as *Aspergillus* and *Cryptococcus* has been a concern in introduction of these agents for clinical use, since most systemic fungal infections cannot be diagnosed by blood culture (93,94); consequently, clinicians commonly treat fungal infections empirically (95). Although most fungal infections are candidiasis, aspergillosis, a rapidly progressing fungal infection, may be present and is fatal if untreated. The currently used agent for treating fungemia is amphotericin B, since this compound is a broad-spectrum antifungal agent. However, because of side effects it is rarely used prophylactically following transplant surgery or cancer chemotherapy. Patients would be at reduced risk if a safe antifungal agent were available for the treatment and prevention of a variety of systemic fungal infections. The need for such an agent is becoming more urgent with the continuously increasing number of systemic fungal infections appearing in the hospital setting (96–98), and a broad-spectrum echinocandin would be an exciting new entry into clinical medicine.

Although the echinocandins are not fungicidal against *Aspergillus* species in vitro, alterations in the growth of this organism and the inhibition of *Aspergillus* β-1,3-glucan synthesis has been observed (99). Also, cilofungin, at high doses, has a therapeutic effect against experimental *Aspergillus* infections in mice (100). Thus, the antifungal spectrum of the echinocandins may be broadened through the discovery of new analogues.

Now that the echinocandins have been shown to be active in vivo against *Candida* and *P. carinii* and possibly *Aspergillus*, the viability of β-1,3-glucan synthesis as a broad-spectrum antifungal target is becoming more evident. A clearer understanding of the mechanism by which these compounds inhibit β-1,3-glucan synthesis and the search for inhibitors of this target may lead to future agents for the treatment and prevention of a variety of infectious diseases.

References

1. Benz F, Knüsel F, Nüesch J, Treichler H, Voser W, Nyfeler R, Keller-Schierlein W. Stoffwechselprodukte von mikroorganismen. Echinocandin B, ein neuartiges polypeptid–antibioticum aus *Aspergillus nidulans* var. *echinulatus*: isolierung und bausteine. Helv Chim Acta 1974; 57:2459–2477.
2. Keller-Juslén C, Kuhn M, Loosli HR, Petcher TJ, Weber HP, von Wartburg A. Struktur des cyclopeptid–antibioticums SL7810 (=echinocandin B). Tetrahedron Lett 1976; 4147–4150.
3. Traxler P, Fritz H, Richter WJ. Zur struktur von papulacandin B, einem neuen antifungischen antibiotikum. Helv Chim Acta 1977; 60:578–584.
4. Traxler P, Gruner J, Auden JAL. Papulacandins, a new family of antibiotics with antifungal activity. I. Fermentation, isolation, chemical and biological characterization of papulacandins A, B, C, D and E. J Antibiot 1977; 30:289–296.
5. Traxler P, Fritz H, Fuhrer H, Richter WJ. Papulacandins, a new family of antibiotics with antifungal activity. Structures of papulacandins A, B, C and D. J Antibiot 1980; 33:967–978.
6. Roy K, Mukhopadhyay T, Reddy GCS, Desikan KR, Ganguli BN. Mulundocandin, a new lipopeptide antibiotic I. Taxonomy, fermentation, isolation, and characterization. J Antibiot 1987; 40:275–280.
7. Mukhopadhyay T, Ganguli BN. Mulundocandin, a new lipopeptide antibiotic II. Structure elucidation. J Antibiot 1987; 40:281–289.
8. Schwartz RE, Giacobbe RA, Bland JA, Monaghan RL. L-671,329, a new antifungal agent I. Fermentation and isolation. J Antibiot 1989; 42:163–167.
9. Wichmann CF, Liesch JM, Schwartz RE. L-671,329, A new antifungal agent II. Structure determination. J Antibiot 1989; 42:168–173.
10. Dreyfuss MM, Tscherter H. Antibiotic S 31794/F-1. US Patent 4,173,629, 1979.
11. Pache W, Dreyfuss M, Traber R, Tscherter H. Sporiofungins, new antifungal antibiotics of the cyclopeptide group. Proc 13th Int Congr Chemother, Vienna, Austria, 1983: PS 4.8/3, Part 115 abstr. 10.
12. Mizuno K, Yagi A, Satoi S, Takada M, Hayashi M, Asano K, Matsuda T. Studies on aculeacin I. Isolation and characterization of aculeacin A. J Antibiot 1977; 30:297–302.
13. Traxler P, Tosch W, Zak O. Papulacandins—synthesis and biological activity of papulacandin B derivatives. J Antibiot 1987; 40:1146–1164.
14. Gordee RS, Zeckner DJ, Ellis LF, Thakkar AL, Howard LC. In vitro and in vivo anti-*Candida* activity and toxicology of LY 121019. J Antibiot 1984; 37:1054–1065.
15. Gordee RS, Zeckner DJ, Howard LC, Alborn WE, Debono M. Anti-*Candida* activity and toxicology of LY 121019, a novel semisynthetic polypeptide antifungal antibiotic. Ann NY Acad Sci 1988; 544:294–309.
16. Debono M, Abbott BJ, Turner JR, Howard LC, Gordee RS, Hunt AS, Barnhart M, Mollloy RM, Willard KE, Fukuda D, Butler TF, Zeckner DJ. Synthesis and evaluation of LY 121019, a member of a series of semisynthetic analogues of the antifungal lipopeptide echinocandin B. Ann NY Acad Sci 1988; 544:152–167.

17. Fromtling RA, Abruzzo G. L-671,329, a new antifungal agent. III. In vitro activity, toxicity and efficacy in comparison to aculeacin. J Antibiot 1989; 42:174–178.
18. Hanson LH, Perlman AM, Clemons KV, Stevens DA. Synergy between cilofungin and amphotericin B in a murine model of candidiasis. Antimicrob Agents Chemother 1991; 35:1334–1337.
19. Traber R, Keller-Juslën C, Loosli H-R, Kuhn M, von Wartburg A. Cyclopeptid-antibiotika aus *Aspergillus* arten. Struktur der echinocandine C und D. Helv Chim Acta 1979; 62:1252–1267.
20. Iwata K, Yamamoto Y, Yamaguchi H, Hiratani T. In vitro studies of aculeacin A, a new antifungal antibiotic. J Antibiot 1982; 35:203–209.
21. Satoi S, Yagi A, Asano K, Mizuno K, Watanabe T. Studies on aculeacin. II. Isolation and characterization of aculeacins B, C, D, E, F, and G. J Antibiot 1977; 30:303–307.
22. Sakaitani M, Ohfune Y. Stereoselective hydroxylation of a peptide side chain. The synthesis of the echinocandin right-half equivalent. Tetrahedron Lett 1989; 30:2251–2254.
23. Bartizal K, Abruzzo G, Trainor C, Krupa D, Nollstadt K, Schmatz D, Schwartz R, Hammond M, Balkovec J, Van Middlesworth F. In vitro antifungal activities and in vivo efficacies of 1,3-β-D-glucan synthesis inhibitors L-671,329, L-646,991, tetrahydroechinocandin B, and L-687,781, a papulacandin. Antimicrob Agents Chemother 1992; 36:1648–1657.
24. de Almeida OP, Scully C. Oral lesions in the systemic mycoses. Curr Opin Dent 1991; 1:423–428.
25. Just-Nubling G, Stille W. Therapie von systemmykosen bei abwehrschwache. Immun Infekt 1991; 19:116–120.
26. Gallis HA, Drew RH, Pickard WW. Amphotericin B: 30 years of clinical experience. Rev Infect Dis 1990; 12:308–329.
27. Thomas AH. Suggested mechanism for the antimycotic activity of the polyene antibiotics and the *N*-substituted imidazoles. J Antimicrob Chemother 1986; 17:269–279.
28. Traxler P, Fritz H, Richter WJ. Zur struktur von papulacandin B, einem neuen antifungischen antibiotikum. Helv Chim Acta 1977; 60:578–584.
29. Cassone A, Mason RE, Kerridge D. Lysis of growing yeast-form cells of *Candida albicans* by echinocandin: a cytological study. Sabouraudia 1981; 19:97–110.
30. Bozzola JJ, Mehta RJ, Nisbet LJ, Valenta JR. The effect of aculeacin A and papulacandin B on morphology and cell wall ultrastructure in *Candida albicans*. Can J Microbiol 1984; 30:857–863.
31. Yamaguchi H, Hiratani T, Baba M, Osumi M. Effect of aculeacin A, a wall-active antibiotic, on synthesis of the yeast cell wall. Microbiol Immunol 1981; 29:609–623.
32. Mizoguchi J, Saito T, Mizuno K, Hayano K. On the mode of action of a new antifungal antibiotic, aculeacin A: inhibition of cell wall synthesis in *Saccharomyces cerevisiae*. J Antibiot 1977; 30:308–313.
33. Baguley BC, Römmele G, Gruner J, Wehrli W. Papulacandin B: an inhibitor of glucan synthesis in yeast spheroplasts. Eur J Biochem 1979; 97:345–351.

34. Perez P, Varona R, Garcia-Acha I, Duran A. Effect of papulacandin B and aculeacin A on β-(1,3)-glucan synthase from *Geotrichum lactis*. FEBS Lett 1981; 129: 249–252.
35. Kang MS, Szaniszlo PJ, Notario V, Cabib E. The effect of papulacandin B on (1→3)-β-D-glucan synthetases. A possible relationship between inhibition and enzyme conformation. Carbohydr Res 1986; 149:13–21.
36. Quigley DR, Selitrennikoff CP. β(1,3)Glucan synthase activity of *Neurospora crassa*: kinetic analysis of negative effectors. Exp Mycol 1984; 8:320–333.
37. Taft C, Stark T, Selitrennikoff CP. Cilofungin LY-121019 inhibits *Candida albicans* 1,3-β-D-glucan synthase activity. Antimicrob Agents Chemother 1988; 32:1901–1903.
38. Varona R, Perez P, Duran A. Effect of papulacandin B on β-glucan synthesis in *Schizosaccharomyces pombe*. FEMS Microbiol Lett 1983; 20:243–247.
39. Yamaguchi H, Hiratani T, Iwata K, Yamamoto Y. Studies on the mechanism of antifungal action of aculeacin A. J Antibiot 1982; 35:210–219.
40. Kopecka M. Papulacandin B: inhibitor of biogenesis of (1→3-β-D-glucan fibrillar component of the cell wall of *Saccharomyces cerevisiae* protoplasts. Folia Microbiol (Praha) 1984; 29:441–449.
41. Tkacz J. Glucan biosynthesis in fungi and its inhibition. In: Sutcliffe J, Georgopapadakou NH, eds. Emerging Targets in Antibacterial and Antifungal Chemotherapy. New York: Chapman & Hall, 1992:495–523.
42. Edman JC, Kovacs JA, Masur H, Santi DV, Elwood HJ, Sogin ML. Ribosomal RNA sequence shows *Pneumocystis carinii* to be a member of the fungi. Nature 1988; 334:519–522.
43. Stringer S, Stringer J, Blase M, Walzer P, Cushion M. *Pneumocystis carinii* sequence from ribosomal RNA implies a close relationship with fungi. Exp Parasitol 1989; 68: 450–461.
44. Edman U, Edman JC, Lundgren B, Santi DV. Isolation and expression of the *Pneumocystis carinii* thymidylate synthase gene. Proc Natl Acad Sci USA 1989; 86: 6503–6507.
45. Matsumoto Y, Matsuda S, Tegoshi T. Yeast glucan in the cyst wall of *Pneumocystis carinii*. J Protozool 1989; 36:21S–22S.
46. DeStefano JA, Cushion MT, Puvanesarajah V, Walzer PD. Analysis of *Pneumocystis carinii* cyst wall. II. Sugar composition. J Protozool 1990; 37:436–441.
47. Matsumoto Y, Yoshida Y. Advances in *Pneumocystis* biology. Parasitol Today 1986; 2:137–142.
48. Kitamura K, Kaneko T, Yamamoto Y. Lysis of viable yeast cells by enzymes of *Arthrobacter luteus*. II. Purification and properties of an enzyme, zymolyase, which lyses viable yeast cells. J Gen Appl Microbiol 1974; 20:323–344.
49. Schmatz DM. Method for the control of *Pneumocystis carinii*. U.S. Patent #5,166,135, 1992.
50. Schmatz DM, Romancheck MA, Pittarelli LA, Schwartz RE, Fromtling RA, Nollstadt KH, Van Middlesworth FL, Wilson KE, Turner MJ. Treatment of *Pneumocystis carinii* pneumonia with 1,3-β-glucan synthesis inhibitors. Proc Natl Acad Sci USA 1990; 87:5950–5954.

51. Matsumoto Y, Yamada M, Amagai T. Yeast glucan of *Pneumocystis carinii* cyst wall: an excellent target for chemotherapy. J Protozool 1991; 38:6S–7S.
52. Van Middlesworth F, Omstead MN, Schmatz D, Bartizal K, Fromtling R, Bills G, Nollstadt K, Honeycutt S, Zweerink M, Garrity G, Wilson K. L-687,781, A new member of the papulacandin family of β-1,3-D-glucan synthesis inhibitors I. Fermentation, isolation, and biological activity. J Antibiot 1991; 44:45–51.
53. Schmatz DM, Powles MA, McFadden DC, Pittarelli LA, Liberator PA, Anderson JW. Treatment and prevention of *Pneumocystis carinii* pneumonia and further elucidation of the *P. carinii* life cycle with 1,3-β-glucan synthesis inhibitor L-671,329. J Protozool 1991; 38:151S–153S.
54. Liberator PA, Anderson JW, Powles M, Pittarelli LA, Graves DC, Schmatz DM. A comparative study of antipneumocystis agents in the rat using a *Pneumocystis carinii* specific DNA probe to quantitate infection. J Clin Microbiol 1992; 30:2968–2974.
55. Current WL. Method for treating *Pneumocystis* pneumonia. Australia Patent Application 72041/91, 1991.
56. Yamada M, Matsumoto Y, Amagai T. Activity of aculeacin A, an inhibitor of β-1,3-glucan synthesis, against *Pneumocystis carinii* pneumonia [abstract]. Int Congr Parasitol, Paris, Aug 1990: S9.A98.
57. Schwartz RE, Sesin DF, Joshua H, Wilson KE, Kempf AJ, Goklen KE, Kuehner D, Gailliot P, Gleason C, White R, Inamine E, Bills G, Salmon P, Zitano L. Pneumocandins from *Zalerion arboricola* I. Discovery and isolation of pneumocandins from *Zalerion arboricola*. J Antibiot 1992; (in press).
58. Schmatz DM, Abruzzo G, Powles MA, McFadden DC, Balkovec J, Black R, Nollstadt K. Bartizal K. Pneumocandins from *Zalerion arboricola* III. Biological evaluation of the pneumocandins and semisynthetic lipopeptides for activity against *Pneumocystis carinii* and *Candida* species. J Antibiot 1992; 45:1886–1891.
59. Black RM, Balkovec JM, Hammond ML, Abruzzo G, Bartizal K, Marrinan J, Trainor C, McFadden DC, Nollstadt K, Pittarelli L, Powles MA, Schmatz DM. Selective reductions of the echinocandin ring-system—investigation of the antifungal and antipneumocystis activity of L-688,786 and related analogs [abstract]. In: Abstr Pap Am Chem Soc 1992; 203:63.
60. Balkovec JM, Black RM. Reduction studies of antifungal echinocandin lipopeptides. One step conversion of echinocandin B to echinocandin C. Tetrahedron Lett 1992; 33:4529–4532.
61. Boeck LD, Fukuda DS, Abbott BJ, Debona M. Deacylation of echinocandin B by *Actinoplanes-Utahensis*. J Antibiot 1989; 42:382–388.
62. DeBono M, Abbott BJ, Fukuda DS, Barnhart M, Willard KE, Molloy RM, Michel KH, Turner JR, Butler TF, Hunt AH. Synthesis of new analogs of echinocandin B by enzymatic deacylation and chemical reacylation of the echinocandin B peptide: synthesis of the antifungal agent cilofungin (LY121019). J Antibiot 1989; 42: 389–397.
63. Pache W, Keller C, Kuhn M. Cleavage of echinocandin B with polymyxin acylase liberating the fatty acid and reacylation of the peptide moiety. Experientia 1978; 34: 1670–1671.

64. DeBono M, Abbott BJ, Molloy RM, Fukuda DS, Hunt AH, Daupert VM, Counter FT, Ott JL, Carrell CB, Howard LC, Boeck LD, Hamill RL. Enzymatic and chemical modifications of lipopeptide antibiotic A21978C: the synthesis and evaluation of daptomycin (LY 146032). J Antibiot 1988; 41:1093–1105.
65. Copley-Merriman CR, Gallis H, Graybill JR, Doebbling BN, Hyslop DL. Cilofungin treatment of disseminated candidiasis. Preliminary phase II results [abstract]. Abstr 30th Intersci Conf Antimicrob Agents Chemother, Atlanta, October 21–24, 1990:582.
66. Copley-Merriman CR, Ransburg NJ, Crane LR, Kerkering TM, Pappas PG, Pottage JC, Hyslop DL. Cilofungin treatment of *Candida* esophagitis. Preliminary phase II results [abstract]. Abstr 30th Intersci Conf Antimicrob Agents Chemother, Atlanta, October 21–24, 1990:581.
67. Doebbling BN, Fine BD, Pfaller MA, Sheetz CT, Stokes JB, Wenzel RP. Acute tubular necrosis and anionic gap acidosis during therapy with cilofungin (LY121019) in polyethylene glycol [abstract]. Abstr 30th Intersci Conf Antimicrob Agents Chemother, Atlanta, October 21–24, 1990:583.
68. Schmatz DM, Powles MA, McFadden DC, Pittarelli L, Balkovec J, Hammond M, Zambias R, Liberator P, Anderson J. Evaluation of the antipneumocystis activity of water soluble lipopeptide L-693,989 in the rat. Antimicrob Agents Chemother 1992; 36:1964–1970.
69. Bartizal K, Abruzzo G, Trainor C, Krupa D, Nollstadt K, Schmatz D, Schwartz R, Hammond M, Balkovec J, Vanmiddlesworth F. β-1,3 glucan synthesis inhibitors L-671,329, L-646,991, tetrahydroechinocandin B and papulacandin in a new target organ kidney assay (TOKA) of systemic candidiasis [abstract]. Abstr 30th Intersci Conf Antimicrob Agents Chemother, Atlanta, October 21–24, 1990:584.
70. Hammond ML. Chemical and structure activity studies of the echinocandin lipopeptides. In: Rippon JW, Fromtling RA, eds. Cutaneous Antifungal Agents. New York: Marcel Dekker, 1992, (in press).
71. Zambias RA, Hammond ML, Heck JV, Bartizal K, Trainor C, Abruzzo G, Schmatz DM, Nollstadt KM. Preparation and structure activity relationships of simplified analogues of the antifungal agent cilofungin: a total synthesis approach. J Med Chem 1992; 35:2843–2855.
72. Fujisawa Pharmaceutical Co. Pharmaceutical composition against *Pneumocystis carinii*. European Patent Application No. 91119421.5, 1991.
73. Toyo Jozo. Agents acting on *Pneumocystis carinii*. International Patent Application No. 034470/90, 1990.
74. Chen SS, Petuch BR, Hsu AT, Arison BH, Dumont F, White RF, Mathre DJ, Wu JT, So LT, Reamer RA. New process for biophosphorylating organic compounds. International Patent Application No. PCT/US91/06816, 1991.
75. Balkovec JM, Black RM, Hammond ML, Heck JV, Zambias RA, Abruzzo G, Bartizal K, Kropp H, Trainor C, Schwartz RE, McFadden DC, Nollstadt KH, Pittarelli LA, Powles MA, Schmatz DM. Synthesis, stability and biological evaluation of water soluble prodrugs of a new echinocandin lipopeptide. Discovery of a potential clinical agent for the treatment of systemic candidiasis and *Pneumocystis carinii* pneumonia (PCP). J Med Chem 1992; 35;194–198.

76. Bartizal K, Abruzzo G, Trainor C, Puckett J, Ponticas S, Krupa D, Schmatz D, Nollstadt K, Schwartz R, Hammond M, Balkovec J, Zambias R, Kropp H. Antifungal activity of L-693,989 a new water soluble prodrug derivative of an echinocandin analog L-688,786 [abstract]. Abstr 31st Intersci Conf Antimicrob Agents Chemother, Chicago, September 29–October 2, 1991:206.
77. Hajdu R, Sundelof JG, Bartizal K, Abruzzo G, Trainor C, Thompson R, Kropp H. Comparative pharmacokinetics in four animal species of L-688,786 and its water soluble prodrug, L-693,989 [abstract]. Abstr 31st Intersci Conf Antimicrob Agents Chemother, Chicago, September 29–October 2, 1991:209.
78. Smith PL, Wall DA, Gochoco CH, Wilson G. Routes of delivery: case studies (5) oral absorption of peptides and proteins. Adv Drug Deliv Rev 1992; 8: 253–290.
79. Herchline TE, Plouffe JF, Para MF. Diabetes mellitus presenting with ketoacidosis following pentamidine therapy in patients with acquired immunodeficiency syndrome. J Infect 1991; 22:41–44.
80. Monk JP, Benfield P. Inhaled pentamidine. An overview of its pharmacological properties and a review of its therapeutic use in *Pneumocystis carinii* pneumonia. Drugs 1990; 39:741–756.
81. Montgomery AB, Luce JM, Turner J, Lin ET, Debs RJ, Corkery KJ, Brunette EN, Hopewell PC. Aerosolized pentamidine as sole therapy for *Pneumocystis carinii* pneumonia in patients with acquired immunodeficiency syndrome. Lancet 1987; 2: 480–483.
82. Montgomery AB, Debs RJ, Luce JM, Corkery KJ, Turner J, Hopewell PC. Aerosolized pentamidine as second line therapy in patients with AIDS and *Pneumocystis carinii* pneumonia. Chest 1989; 95:747–750.
83. Centers for Disease Control. Guidelines for prophylaxis against *Pneumocystis carinii* pneumonia for persons infected with human immunodeficiency virus. MMWR 1989; 38:1–9.
84. Schmatz DM, Powles M, McFadden DC, Vadas E, Meisner D, Hajdu R. Treatment and prevention of *P. carinii* pneumonia in the rat using aerosolized water soluble lipopeptide L-693,989 [abstract]. Abstr 31st Intersci Conf Antimicrob Agents Chemother, Chicago, September 29–October 2, 1991; 208.
85. Girard PM, Brun-Pascaud M, Farinotti R, Tamisier L, Kernbaum S. Pentamidine aerosol in prophylaxis and treatment of murine *Pneumocystis carinii* pneumonia. Antimicrob Agents Chemother 1987; 31:978–981.
86. Witt K, Nielsen TN, Junge J. Dissemination of *Pneumocystis carinii* in patients with AIDS. Scand J Infect Dis 1991; 23:691–695.
87. Noskin GA, Murphy RL. Extrapulmonary infection with *Pneumocystis carinii* in patients receiving aerosolized pentamidine. Rev Infect Dis 1991; 13:525.
88. Northfelt DW. Extrapulmonary pneumocystosis in patients taking aerosolised pentamidine. Lancet 1989; 2:1454.
89. Debs RJ, Blumenfield W, Brunette EN, Straubinger RM, Montgomery AB, Lin E, Agabain N, Papahadjopoulos D. Successful treatment with aerosolized pentamidine of *Pneumocystis carinii* pneumonia in rats. Antimicrob Agents Chemother 1987; 31: 37–41.

90. Dickenson G, Smaldone GC. Particle deposition and failure of prophylaxis using aerosolized pentamidine. Am Rev Respir Dis 1990; 141:A150.
91. Amin MB, Abrash MP, Mezger E, Sekerak GF. Systemic dissemination of *Pneumocystis carinii* in a patient with acquired immunodeficiency syndrome. Henry Ford Hosp Med J 1990; 38:68–71.
92. Deroux SJ, Volkan Adsay N, Ioachim HL. Disseminated pneumocystosis without pulmonary involvement during prophylactic aerosolized pentamidine therapy in a patient with the acquired immunodeficiency syndrome. Arch Pathol Lab Med 1991; 115:1137–1140.
93. Young RC, Bennett JE, Vogel CL, Carbone PP, De Vita VT. Aspergillosis: the spectrum of the disease in 98 patients. Medicine 1970; 49:147–173.
94. Meyer RD, Young LS, Armstrong D, Yu B. Aspergillosis complicating neoplastic disease. Am J Med 1973; 54:6–15.
95. Holleran WM, Wilbur JR, DeGregorio MW. Empiric amphotericin B therapy in patients with acute leukemia. Rev Infect Dis 1985; 7:619–624.
96. Walsh TJ, Jarosinski PF, Fromtling RA. Increasing usage of systemic antifungal agents. Diagn Microbiol Infect Dis 1990; 13:37–40.
97. Walsh TJ, Pizzo PA, Nosocomial fungal infections: a classification of hospital acquired fungal infections and mycoses arising from endogenous flora or reactivation. Annu Rev Microbiol 1988; 42:517–545.
98. Mills J, Masur H. AIDS-related infections. Sci Am 1990; Aug:50–57.
99. Douglas C, Marrinan J, Curotto J, Onishi J, Kurtz M. Activity of a new echinocandin, L-688,786, against filamentous fungi [abstract]. Abstr Annu Meet Soc Microbiol, New Orleans, Louisiana, May 26–30, 1992:1845.
100. Denning DW, Stevens DA. Efficacy of cilofungin alone and in combination with amphotericin B in a murine model of disseminated aspergillosis. Antimicrob Agents Chemother 1991; 35:1329–1333.

31

Corticosteroids and Other Adjunctive Agents

SAMUEL A. BOZZETTE

University of California, San Diego
and RAND
Santa Monica, California

I. Introduction

Severe moribidity and mortality continue to occur in patients receiving effective therapy for *Pneumocystis carinii* pneumonia, and crossover from one effective therapy to another does not seem to improve prognosis in deteriorating patients (1–4). Rather than being a direct result of the failure of antimicrobial therapy, severe morbidity and mortality often appear to occur because of early severe lung injury, which actually may be exacerbated by the institution of therapy. Substantial evidence now exists to indicate that adjunctive corticosteroids can mitigate lung damage and improve clinical outcomes in *P. carinii* pneumonia (5–7). An expert panel convened under the joint sponsorship of the University of California and the National Institutes of Health (NIH) has recommended the early use of adjunctive corticosteroids in moderate and severe *P. carinii* pneumonia, and the Working Group on Steroid Use of the Infectious Diseases Society of America has

---

This chapter was adapted in part from Bozzette SA: The use of corticosteroids in *Pneumocystis carinii* pneumonia. J Infect Dis 1990; 162:1365–1369.

endorsed this recommendation (8,9). Specifically, the University of California–National Institutes of Health panel recommendations are that patients older than 13 years with moderate or severe *P. carinii* pneumonia, as denoted by an arterial oxygen pressure of less than 70 mmHg on room air (or an alveolar–arterial oxygen gradient of greater than 35 mmHg), should receive adjunctive corticosteroids initiated when specific therapy for *P. carinii* pneumonia is begun. The currently recommended schedule was that used in a trial conducted by the California Collaborative Treatment Group: 40 mg of prednisone twice daily for 5 days, followed by 40 mg a day for 5 days, followed by 20 mg daily until the conclusion of therapy (5).

II. Rationale

The rationale for adjunctive corticosteroid use is that death in *P. carinii* pneumonia is secondary to respiratory failure caused by severe lung injury that, in part, may be due to the immune response to the infection. The lungs of persons dying of acute *P. carinii* pneumonia show histological evidence of severe lung injury, including interstitial inflammation, edema, hyperplasia of type II pneumocytes, microatelectasis, alveolar filling, often fibrosis, and occasionally hyaline membranes or pulmonary cyst formation with or without pneumothorax (10–17). Additionally, the major poor prognostic factors in acute *P. carinii* pneumonia also appear to be markers of lung injury; these include poor oxygenation, high lactate dehydrogenase (LDH) levels, severe abnormalities on chest radiograph, and the presence of interstitial edema or fibrosis on biopsy (18–20).

The host response to *P. carinii* has not been fully characterized (21). However, it appears that lymphocytes, alveolar macrophages, neutrophils and their products, and the direct effects of the organism on pneumocytes are all involved in the pathogenesis of lung injury, which is not prevented by depletion of CD4-positive lymphocytes (22–25). These facts, coupled with the knowledge that corticosteroids interfere with function of inflammatory cells as well as the release and action of many mediators of inflammation, constitute the preclinical basis for use of adjunctive corticosteroid therapy (26–29). However, no direct experimental data addressing the specific nature of the corticosteroid effect in this infection now exists. Further exploration of the pulmonary response to *P. carinii* as modulated by corticosteroids will require the use of models that do not rely on corticosteroid suppression of immunity to induce disease (30,31).

The specific rationale for initiating adjunctive corticosteroids early, rather than later, in the course of antimicrobial treatment is that deterioration in oxygenation shortly after initiation of standard treatment is usual and is often associated with an adverse clinical outcome. In fact, several series have documented that even the typical successfully treated patient suffers early deterioration in oxygenation and does not recover to admission oxygen levels until approximately day 5 of treatment (2,5,7). In both a prospective cohort of 251 patients and a retrospective cohort of 327 patients with *P. carinii* pneumonia, the magnitude of early deterioration in oxygenation was the most powerful predictor of eventual mortality (5,32; unpublished data). Finally, in these same series, over 75% of cases of respiratory failure occurred within 3 days of instituting therapy, despite the fact that the median patient developing respiratory failure had been symptomatic for nearly 4 weeks before admission (5,32; unpublished data).

III. Clinical Trials

Some clinicians have suspected a role for corticosteroids in the treatment of *P. carinii* pneumonia for some time; it has long been noted that symptoms of *P. carinii* pneumonia often appeared only after corticosteroids were tapered in transplant or cancer patients (33–35). In the acquired immunodeficiency syndrome (AIDS) era, several case reports and small series have appeared suggesting clinical or radiographic improvement related to the inadvertent use of corticosteroids alone or the intentional use of corticosteroids as an adjunct to antimicrobial therapy (36–43). However, convincing data did not appear until the completion of randomized clinical trials.

The largest of these studies was a large, broad, open-label, multicenter randomized trial conducted by the California Collaborative Treatment Group (5). Participants had received less than 72 hr of antipneumocystis therapy at entry and were not in respiratory failure. The operational definition of respiratory failure was not receiving mechanical ventilation and having a hypoxemia ratio greater than 75. A hypoxemia ratio (partial alveolar pressure/fraction of inspired oxygen or Pao_2/Fio_2 ratio) of 75 indicates profound hypoxemia and is equivalent to a Pao_2 of 60 or an a-A gradient of greater than 450 while receiving 80% oxygen. In this study, there was convincing evidence for a physiological and clinical benefit from adjunctive corticosteroids, whether evaluating all 333 patients enrolled, the 251 with confirmed or presumed disease, or only the 225 with confirmed disease.

Early deterioration in oxygenation was significantly blunted by adjunctive corticosteroids, with the average change in hypoxemia (Pao_2/Fio_2) ratio at 3 days of treatment being -41 in the standard therapy group and $+4$ in the adjunctive corticosteroid group (Fig. 1). The risk of unfavorable clinical outcomes was significantly higher in the standard treatment group. For example, the relative hazards for respiratory failure and death within 31 days in the standard therapy group versus adjunctive corticosteroids were both 2.3 (30 vs 14% and 23 vs 11%, respectively), whereas the relative hazard for death at 84 days was 1.8 (26 vs 16%). Finally, a nonsignificant trend toward a reduced incidence of dose-limiting toxicity to *P. carinii* treatment was observed in the adjunctive corticosteroid group (22 vs 31% of standard therapy patients), along with a statistically significant reduction in some symptoms including fever, cough, and dyspnea at rest.

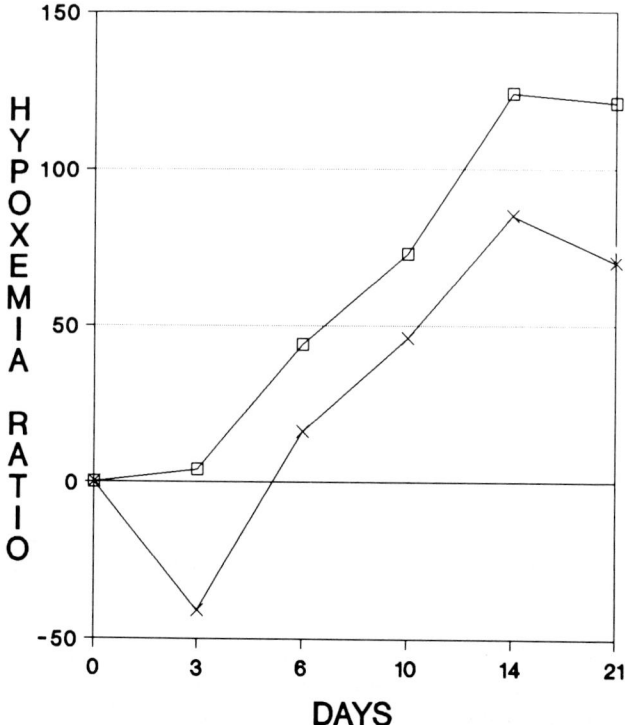

Figure 1 Change in hypoxemia ratio over time in patients receiving standard therapy alone (X) or standard therapy plus adjunctive corticosteroids. The average hypoxemia ratio was significantly greater in the group receiving adjunctive corticosteroids after 3 days of treatment and over the entire 21-day treatment period. A 50-point change in the hypoxemia or Pao_2/Fio_2 ratio is equal to a 10-torr change in Pao_2 while receiving room air. (From Ref. 5.)

Although the estimate of the effect size for clinical benefit was similar at a relative risk of 1.9–2.5 for all categories of patients, statistical significance could be demonstrated only for patients with moderate or severe disease (Table 1 and Fig. 2). However, since the mildly ill group included only 62 patients who experienced only four episodes of respiratory failure, and no deaths attributable to *P. carinii* pneumonia, the study had low power to detect clinical benefit in this group. The study also did not detect significant complications of corticosteroid therapy or a significant increase in the incidence of cancers or infections other than localized herpetic outbreaks. Of note, there was a strikingly high rate of incident Kaposi's sarcoma in both groups in the 12 weeks after enrollment, affecting approximately 10% of participants. This suggests that factors other than corticosteroid use per se

Table 1 Crude Risk of Unfavorable Outcome at 31 days of Follow-up in 251 Patients with Mild (I), Moderate (II), or Severe (III) *P. carinii* Pneumonia

Stratum	I	II	III	All
Total patients	62	121	68	251
Standard therapy	34 (55%)	61 (50%)	33 (49%)	128 (51%)
Corticosteroid	28 (45%)	60 (50%)	35 (51%)	123 (49%)
Respiratory failure				
Standard therapy	3 (9%)	19 (31%)	16 (49%)	38 (30%)
Corticosteroid	1 (4%)	7 (12%)	9 (26%)	17 (14%)
Relative risk (95% CI)	2.5 (0.2,69)	2.7 (1.3,5.6)	1.9 (1,3.6)	2.3 (1.4,3.6)
p	0.38	0.01	0.05	0.001
Death				
Standard therapy	1[a] (3%)	13 (21%)	14 (43%)	28 (22%)
Corticosteroid	0 (0%)	6 (10%)	7 (19%)	13 (11%)
Relative risk (95% CI)		2.1 (0.9,5.1)	2.1 (1,4.5)	2.2 (1.2,3.9)
p	0.55	0.09	0.05	0.01

[a]Death was attributed to *Staphylococcus aureus* sepsis; all other deaths were attributed dirctly or indirectly to pneumocystis pneumonia.
Source: Ref. 5.

may account for the reports of explosive Kaposi's sarcoma after corticosteroid-treated *P. carinii* pneumonia (44).

Two small single-institution, placebo-controlled, double-blind studies are crucial in confirming key findings of the California Collaborative Treatment Group trial. A group at St. Paul's Hospital demonstrated that, even in mildly ill patients, adjunctive corticosteroids prevent early deterioration in oxygenation and improve other manifestations of lung injury (7). Thirty-seven patients with an oxygen saturation of 85–90% at rest or a 5% drop in oxygen saturation with exercise were studied. Corticosteroids were administered as 60 mg of prednisone once daily for 7 days, followed by every-other-day dose reductions in a 14-day taper. A sequential design was used in which the data were examined for extreme differences between treatment groups after each patient's outcome was known. A difference extreme enough to require discontinuation of the study under the previously established stopping rule was observed when 8 of 19 (42%) patients receiving placebo, but only 1 of 18 (6%) receiving corticosteroids had a 10% decline in oxygen saturation at rest by the third day of the study. However, this study was not designed to address "hard" clinical endpoints, and only one true clinical failure occurred.

Mitigating concern about the "soft" nature of the oxygen saturation endpoint were the findings that several other clinical and laboratory markers of disease severity were improved by corticosteroid administration. These included serum LDH, respiratory rate, and exercise tolerance. Moreover, the difference in exercise

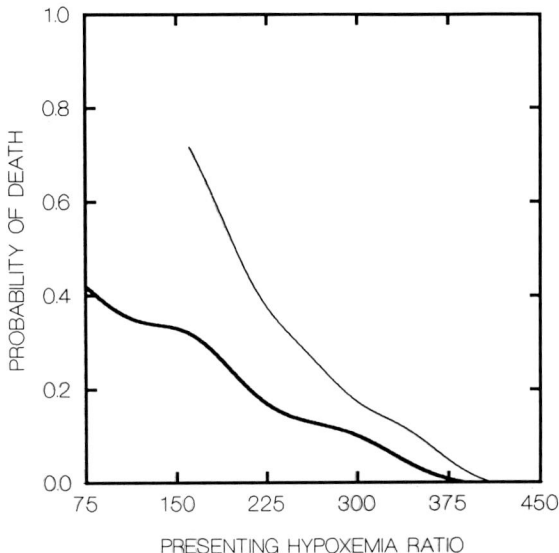

Figure 2 Probability of death versus presenting hypoxemia (Pao_2/Fio_2) ratio. The approximately 50% reduction in the risk of death appears to be present across the entire range of observed presenting hypoxemia ratios. Note that a hypoxemia ratio of 300 is equal to a Pao_2 of 63 while breathing room air and a ratio of 75 is equal to a Pao_2 of 60 with 80% inspired oxygen. (From Ref. 5.)

tolerance was persistent at 30 days, even though many of the placebo patients crossed over to corticosteroid at 3 days. This suggests that early corticosteroid use may interrupt mechanisms leading to long-term impairment of pulmonary reserve, such as the development of pulmonary fibrosis (18,45).

A group at the University of Miami confirmed the clinical benefit of adjunctive corticosteroids in severely ill patients (6). Twenty-three patients with a respiratory rate of more than 30 breaths per minute and an arterial oxygen tension of less than 75 torr while breathing at least 35% oxygen were studied. Corticosteroid were administered as 40 mg of methylprednisolone every 6 hr for 7 days. The study was stopped before its scheduled close at the recommendation of an independent data safety and monitoring board because an unexpectedly high number [9 of 11 (82%)] of patients suffered respiratory failure and died in the placebo group, whereas only 3 of 12 (25%) in the adjunctive corticosteroid group experienced these endpoints. Additionally, oxygenation, fever, and dyspnea score were all improved in the corticosteroid group. Of note, 4 of the 9 surviving corticosteroid patients had clinical deterioration, which responded to reinstitution and tapering of corticosteroids. Other comparisons were limited by the few survivors in the placebo group.

Three unpublished randomized studies have been presented only orally or in abstract form. An unblinded trial conducted in Copenhagen and Amsterdam had similar findings to those observed in the moderate and severe group in the California Collaborative Treatment Group study (8). Fifty-three patients with an arterial oxygen pressure of less than 67.5 mmHg while breathing room air were studied. The experimental regimen was methylprednisolone given parenterally at a dose of 0.5 mg/kg every 6 hr for 10 days. In a report of interim data, current as of May 1990, a significant benefit in the reduction of respiratory failure (7 vs 32%) and death (11 vs 44%) was evident.

A multicenter, placebo-controlled blinded trial conducted by a group at the University of Toronto did not find a statistically significant benefit for adjunctive corticosteroids (46). One hundred twenty patients characterized as having moderate to severe *P. carinii* pneumonia were studied, but entry criteria and arterial oxygen at admission to the study were not reported. The authors excluded 20 patients in whom pneumocystis infection was not confirmed and 22 other in whom unspecified protocol violations occurred. Death occurred in 4 of 40 (10%) patients receiving corticosteroids and in 6 of 38 (16%) patients receiving standard therapy, and mechanical ventilation was administered to 1 patient in each group. Additionally, 10 patients in the placebo group and 6 in the corticosteroid group received off-protocol high-dose corticosteroids because of clinical deterioration. The interpretation of these partially reported result is complicated both by the low case fatality rate, which resulted in a low statistical power and, given the frequent off-protocol use of corticosteroids and the infrequent use of mechanical ventilation, by the lack of a physiological definition of early respiratory failure.

The third unpublished study was a double-blind, placebo-controlled trial conducted at San Francisco General Hospital that evaluated adjunctive corticosteroids begun anytime during the course of therapy when the arterial oxygen pressure dropped below 51 mmHg (47). Of the 41 patients enrolled within 48 hr of starting therapy, 19 received the study regimen of 60 mg of methylprednisolone given every 6 hr. There was no difference in oxygenation or in the risk of death (31 vs 37%) between treatment groups. However, 3 patients suffered complications that may have been related to corticosteroid use (1 with gastrointestinal bleeding and 2 with acute psychosis), and infectious complications were observed only in the corticosteroid group (47).

Taken as a group, these five clinical studies provide compelling evidence for clinical benefit from early adjunctive corticosteroids in moderate to severe pneumocystosis. Table 2 summarizes the data from the randomized trials of corticosteroids in moderate to severe disease. Mortality data are presented because death is the only endpoint for which comparable data is available from all the studies. The odds ratio for death favored corticosteroids in all five studies. A test for

Table 2 Summary of Mortality Data from Six Clinical Trials of Early Adjunctive Corticosteroids[a]

Study	N	Corticosteroids: (dead/alive)	Standard therapy: (dead/alive)	Odds ratio
1. California Collaborative Treat Group[b]	189	13/82	27/67	2.5 (1.2–5.0)
2. Toronto	78	4/36	6/32	1.7 (0.4–6.3)
3. European	53	2/26	8/17	5.1 (1.2–20.1)
4. University of Miami	23	3/9	9/2	9.7 (1.9–50.1)
5. San Francisco General[c]	11	1/4	2/4	1.7 (0.1–28.1)
All studies				2.9 (1.7–5.0)[d]
Only blinded studies (2–4)				3.1 (1.2–8.2)[d]
Only studies brought to scheduled completion (1,2,4)				2.2 (1.2–4.1)[d]

[a]The simple arithmetic mean of the odd ratios is 4.2.
[b]Includes only the 189 patients with moderate to severe disease.
[c]Includes only the 11 patients treated within 48 hr of admission.
[d]"Typical" odds ratio computed using a Mantel–Haenszel procedure to stratify by study.

homogeneity did not reject the null hypothesis that the studies have an underlying common odds ratio (48). Therefore, the apparently common effect is estimated by the typical odds ratio. The typical odds ratio combines the studies' individual odds ratios, using weights proportional to the variance (and thus the sample size) in a manner that avoids the direct comparisons of patients in different trials, which would result from simple pooling (49).

The typical odds ratio for the five studies is 2.9, with a 95% confidence interval of 1.7–5.0 for all studies ($p < 0.001$; see Table 1). Because a lack of blinding can introduce bias even when objective endpoints are employed, the typical odds ratio for the three double-blind, placebo-controlled trials was calculated and is 3.1 with a 95% confidence interval of 1.2–8.2 ($p < 0.02$; see Table 1). Because early termination of a trial is often associated with an overestimate of effect size, the typical odds ratio for the three studies that were completed according to an a priori schedule was calculated, and is 2.2 with a 95% confidence interval of 1.2–4.0 ($p < 0.01$; see Table 1). Thus, a statistically significant benefit is indicated, even when employing the conservative technique of entirely excluding studies that do not meet specified quality criteria.

IV. Controversies

Controversies do exist concerning the use of corticosteroids in *P. carinii* pneumonia. First is the appropriateness of generalizing the findings in patients with AIDS to other populations. Although data are lacking, there is little reason to believe that the pathophysiology of *P. carinii* pneumonia is fundamentally different in immunocompromised patients without human immunodeficiency virus (HIV) infection. Given the potential for a lifesaving benefit and the absence of convincing clinical evidence to the contrary, I routinely recommend the immediate use of adjunctive corticosteroids when such persons present with moderate to severe disease, because of the high mortality and often fulminant course of disease in this setting (50). Pregnancy may lead me to withhold corticosteroids in women with marginal indications because of the possibility of fetal damage, but I again routinely recommend immediate use in severe disease because of the high risk of maternal mortality and the potentially devastating effect of profound maternal hypoxemia on the fetus. Corticosteroids may not be indicated in infants who are generally immunologically naive before the onset of clinical pneumonia, but they are often used by neonatologists, because of the dismal prognosis of severe disease in this population (51). Extra caution must be employed when using methylprednisolone in infants because of the possibility of toxicity from the benzyl alcohol preservative in the parenteral preparation.

The optimal adjunctive corticosteroid regimen is unknown. Given the variations encountered in clinical practice and that the studies indicating a benefit for adjunctive corticosteroids all used different regimens, it is reasonable to use the generally recommended California Collaborative Treatment Group regimen. However, one must recognize that it merely represents the most rigorously validated regimen, rather than the optimal one for all patients. Some clinicians prefer higher-dose corticosteroids or, particularly in patients who are doing well after the initial phases of therapy, shorter courses (6,39,47,52). One should note that the media duration of adjunctive corticosteroid therapy actually received by survivors in the California study was only 16 days (53). However, true dose-finding studies do not exist, and there are reports of "rebound" deterioration after very short courses or with rapid taper of corticosteroids that has not been seen with longer courses or slower tapers (5,6,54).

The role of pulses of corticosteroids in high doses (500 mg to several grams of methylprednisolone per day) for patients who deteriorate while receiving therapy has not been completely established (39,47,50,51). The results of the San Francisco study and the fact that corticosteroids for respiratory distress syndrome seem to be effective only when given before the inciting insult suggest no dramatic benefit from the practice (55–57). However, the former study was small, and the latter analogy is imperfect. Most experts would seem to agree that there is little harm in initiating corticosteroids in the usually recommended doses to the regimen of an individual with an established diagnosis who steadily deteriorates from mild to severe disease on standard therapy alone (8).

There has been concern over the potential for harm from corticosteroids (44,50). However, the contribution of corticosteroids to the variety of observed adverse outcomes seen in various small series is unclear, because patients with *P. carinii* pneumonia are already at risk for complications such as gastrointestinal bleeding, Kaposi's sarcoma, or reactivation of granulomatous disease. Furthermore, larger-cohort studies and randomized trials have not uncovered a pattern of adverse outcomes that would warrant foregoing adjunctive corticosteroids, and further studies are unlikely to do so (5,8,58). For example, it is unlikely that even a substantial increase in the reactivation rate for tuberculosis, estimated to be 2.1 cases per 100 high-risk HIV-infected patient-years of observation, could outweigh a 50% reduction in the 20–30% acute case fatality rate in *P. carinii* pneumonia (5,6,8,53,59,60). However, importantly, the overall benefit demonstrated from early corticosteroid use in randomized trials may not have been seen in these studies without a policy of rapidly pursuing a morphological diagnosis of *P. carinii* pneumonia and of ruling out other potential pathogens in all participants (5,7,8). Extrapolation of these results to situations of empiric therapy is unwarranted and represents poor clinical practice (8).

Finally, some controversy remains over how severe an illness should be before one considers the use of adjunctive corticosteroids. Although expert panel guidelines are necessarily specific and conservative, the risk for unfavorable outcome appears to increase continuously over the range of presenting arterial oxygen pressures, and the relative physiological effect of corticosteroids appears to be relatively constant (see Fig. 2) (5,7). That clinical benefit has not been demonstrated in the mildly ill may be because no net benefit exists or because the few patients studied and their generally good prognosis has led to a low power to detect a benefit.

Therefore, judgment is required to determine whether the likely clinical effect of corticosteroids is worthwhile in individual patients at the margin of the current guidelines. I sometimes choose to use adjunctive corticosteroids in patients with Pao_2 greater than 75 while breathing room air if the patient appears distressed, is hyperventilating, has a severely abnormal chest radiograph, or possibly a very high LDH level. On the other hand, I may choose to withhold adjunctive corticosteroids in patient's with a room air Pao_2 of 70 torr who is comfortable, communicative, and has no other severe abnormalities.

V. Other Agents

There are no clinical data available on the use of other adjunctive agents in the treatment of *P. carinii* pneumonia. However, a variety of other agents thought to mitigate lung damage, particularly damage related to oxidant injury, are being considered for clinical trial in patients with *P. carinii* pneumonia. These agents include nonsteroidal anti-inflammatory drugs, pentoxifylline, *N*-acetylcysteine, and inhaled corticosteroids (61–66). Also, because steroid-induced pneumocystosis in the rat is associated with a decrease in the level of surfactant phospholipids, consideration is being given to human trials of both artificial and natural surfactant replacement therapy (67).

Finally, an immune stimulant is in clinical trial. Inhaled interferon gamma stimulates both rat and human pulmonary macrophages and is active in both the prophylaxis and treatment of steroid-induced *P. carinii* pneumonia in the rat (68–70). Because altered pulmonary macrophage function and altered cytokine production appear to be features both of rats with steroid-induced pneumocystosis and of patients with AIDS, a pilot clinical trial is underway to assess the safety of inhaled interferon gamma in patients with HIV-associated *P. carinii* pneumonia (71–73). The emphasis in this trial will be both on determining if enhancement of the immune response has occurred and if such an enhancement is likely to lead to clinical benefit or harm.

Acknowledgment

The author wishes to think Dr. Sally Morton, for her assistance in the performance of the meta-analysis contained in this chapter.

References

1. Hughes WT, Feldman S, Chaudhary SC, et al. Comparison of pentamidine isethionate and trimethoprim sulfamethoxazole in the treatment of *Pneumocystis carinii* pneumonia. J Pediatr 1978; 92:285–291.
2. Haverkos HW, the PCP Therapy Project Group. Assessment of therapy for *Pneumocystis carinii* pneumonia. Am J Med 1984; 76:501–508.
3. Wharton JM, Coleman DL, Wofsy CB, et al. Trimethoprim–sulfamethoxazole or pentamidine for *Pneumocystis carinii* pneumonia in the acquired immunodeficiency syndrome. A prospective randomized trial. Ann Intern Med 1986; 105:37–44.
4. Sattler FR, Cowan R, Nielsen DM, Ruskin J. Trimethoprim–sulfamethoxazole compared with pentamidine for treatment of *Pneumocystis carinii* pneumonia in the acquired immunodeficiency syndrome. A prospective non-crossover study. Ann Intern Med 1988; 109:280–287.
5. Bozzette SA, Sattler FR, Chiu J, et al. A controlled trial of early adjunctive treatment with corticosteroids for *Pneumocystis carinii* pneumonia in the acquired immunodeficiency syndrome. N Engl J Med 1990; 323:1451–1457.
6. Gagnon S, Boota AM, Fischl MA, Baier N, Kiersey OW, LaVoie L. Corticosteroids as adjunctive therapy for severe *Pneumocystis carinii* pneumonia in the acquired immunodeficiency syndrome. N Engl J Med 1990; 323:1444–1450.
7. Montaner JSG, Lawson LM, Levitt N, Belsberg A, Schechter MT, Ruedy J. Corticosteroids prevent early deterioration in patients with moderately severe *Pneumocystis carinii* pneumonia and the acquired immunodeficiency syndrome. Ann Intern Med 1990; 113:14–20.
8. The National Institutes of Health–University of California Expert Panel for Corticosteroids as Adjunctive Therapy for *Pneumocystis carinii* Pneumonia. Consensus statement on the use of corticosteroids as adjunctive therapy for *Pneumocystis* pneumonia in the acquired immunodeficiency syndrome. N Engl J Med 1990; 323: 1500–1504.
9. McGowan JE, Chestney PJ, Crossley KB, LaForce FM. Guidelines for the use of systemic glucocorticosteroids in the management of selected infections. J Infect Dis 1992; 165:1–13.
10. Maxfield RA, Surkin BI, Fazzini EP, Rapaport DM, Stenson WM, Goldring RA. Respiratory failure in patients with acquired immunodeficiency syndrome and *Pneumocystis carinii* pneumonia. Crit Care Med 1986; 14:443–449.
11. Marchevsky A, Rosen MJ, Chrystal G, et al. Pulmonary complications of the acquired immunodeficiency syndrome: a clinicopathologic study of 70 cases. Hum Pathol 1985; 16:659–670.
12. Nash G, Fligiel S. Pathologic features of the lung in the acquired immune deficiency syndrome: an autopsy study of homosexual males. Am J Clin Pathol 1984; 81:6–12.
13. Askin FB, Katqenstein ALA. Pneumocystis infection masquerading as diffuse alveolar damage: a potential source of diagnostic error. Chest 1981; 79:420–422.
14. Sandhu JS, Goodman PC. Pulmonary cysts associated with *Pneumocystis carinii* pneumonia in patients with AIDS. Radiology 1989; 173:33–35.
15. Liu YC, Tomashefski JF, Tomfors JW, Green H. Necrotizing *Pneumocystis carinii*

vasculitis associated with lung necrosis and cavitation in a patient with acquired immunodeficiency syndrome. Arch Pathol Lab Med 1989; 113:494–497.
16. Beers MF, Sohn M, Swartz M. Recurrent pneumothorax in AIDS with pneumocystis pneumonia: a clinicopathologic report of three cases and review of the literature. Chest 1990; 98:266–270.
17. Eng RH, Bishberg E, Smith SM. Evidence for destruction of lung tissues during *Pneumocystis carinii* pneumonia. Arch Intern Med 1987; 149:746–749.
18. Brenner M, Ognibene FP, Lack EE, et al. Prognostic factors and life expectancy of patients with acquired immunodeficiency syndrome and *Pneumocystis carinii* pneumonia. Am Rev Respir Dis 1987; 136:1199–1206.
19. Zaman MK, White DA. Serum lactate dehydrogenase levels and *Pneumocystis carinii* pneumonia. Diagnostic and prognostic significance. Am Rev Respir Dis 1988; 137:796–800.
20. Garay SM, Greene J. Prognostic indicators in the initial presentation of *Pneumocystis carinii* pneumonia. Chest 1989; 95:769–772.
21. Walzer PD. Immunopathogenesis of *Pneumocystis carinii* infection. J Lab Clin Med 1991; 118:206–216.
22. Beck JM, Warnock ML, Curtis JL, et al. Inflammatory responses to *Pneumocystis carinii* in mice selectively depleted of helper T lymphocytes. Am J Respir Cell Mol Biol 1991; 5:186–187.
23. Smith RL, El-Sadr WM, Lewis ML. Correlation of bronchoalveolar cell populations with clinical severity of *Pneumocystis carinii* pneumonia. Chest 1988; 92:60–64.
24. Mason GR, Hashimoto CH, Dickman PS, Foutty LF, Cobb CJ. Prognostic implications of bronchoalveolar lavage neutrophilia in patients with *Pneumocystis carinii* pneumonia and AIDS. Am Rev Respir Dis 1989; 139:1336–1342.
25. Spragg RG, Smith RM, Harrell JH. Evidence of lung inflammation in patients with AIDS and *P. carinii* pneumonia [abstract]. Am Rev Respir Dis 1987; 135:A169.
26. Fauci AS, Dale DC, Balow JE. Glucocorticosteroid therapy: mechanisms of action and clinical considerations. Ann Intern Med 1976; 84:304–315.
27. Blackwood L, Pennington JE. Dose-dependent effect of glucocorticoids in pulmonary defenses in a steroid-resistant host. Am Rev Respir Dis 1982; 126:1045–1049.
28. Peters-Golden M, Thebert P. Inhibition by methylprednisolone of zymosan-induced leukotriene synthesis in alveolar macrophages. Am Rev Respir Dis 1987; 135:1020–1026.
29. Morris HG. Mechanisms of glucocorticoid action in pulmonary disease. Chest 1985; 88(suppl):133S–141S.
30. Shellito J, Suzara VV, Blumenfeld W, Beck JM, Steger HJ, Ermak THE. A new model of *Pneumocystis carinii* infection in mice selectively depleted of helper T lymphocytes. J Clin Invest 1990; 85:1686–1693.
31. Roths JM, Marshall JD, Allen RD, Carlson GA, Sidman CL. Spontaneous *Pneumocystis carinii* pneumonia in immunodeficient mutant scid mice. Am J Pathol 1990; 136:1173–1186.
32. Bozzette SA, Arcia J, McGlynn L, et al. The impact of *Pneumocystis carinii* and cytomegalovirus on the course and outcome of atypical pneumonia in patients with advanced HIV disease. J Infect Dis 1992; 165:93–98.

33. Rifkind D, Starzl TE, Marchioro TL, et al. Transplantation pneumonia. JAMA 1964; 189:808–812.
34. Burke BA, Good RA. Pneumocystis carinii infection. Medicine 1973; 52:23–51.
35. Singer C, Armstrong D, Rosen PP, et al. Pneumocystis carinii pneumonia: a cluster of eleven cases. Ann Intern Med 1975; 82:772–777.
36. MacFadden DK, Edelson JD, Rebuck AJ. Pneumocystis carinii pneumonia in the acquired immunodeficiency syndrome: response to inadvertent steroid therapy. Can Med Assoc J 1985; 132:1161–1163.
37. Foltzer MA, Hannan SE, Kozak AJ. Pneumocystis pneumonia. Response to corticosteroids [letter]. JAMA 1985; 253:979.
38. Rankin JA, Pella JA. Radiographic resolution of Pneumocystis carinii pneumonia in response to corticosteroid therapy. Am Rev Respir Dis 1987; 136:182–183.
39. El-Sadr W, Sidhu G, et al. High dose corticosteroids as adjunct therapy in severe Pneumocystis carinii pneumonia. AIDS Res 1986; 4:349–355.
40. MacFadden DK, Edelson JD, Hyland RH, et al. Corticosteroids as adjunctive therapy of Pneumocystis carinii pneumonia in patients with acquired immunodeficiency syndrome. Lancet 1987; 2:1477–1479.
41. Montaner JS, Russell JA, Lawson L, Ruedy J. Acute respiratory failure secondary to Pneumocystis carinii pneumonia in the acquired immunodeficiency syndrome. A potential role for systemic corticosteroids. Chest 1989; 95:881–884.
42. Mottin D, Denis M, Dombret H, Rossert J, Mayard CH, Akoun G. Role for steroids in treatment of Pneumocystis carinii pneumonia in AIDS [letter]. Lancet 1987; 2:519.
43. Walmsley S, Salit IE, Brunton J. The possible role of corticosteroid therapy for pneumocystis pneumonia in the acquired immunodeficiency syndrome (AIDS). J AIDS 1988; 1:354–360.
44. Gill PS, Loureiro C, Bernstein-Singer M, Dorick MU, Sattler F, Levine AM. Clinical effect of glucocorticoids on Kaposi's sarcoma related to the acquired immunodeficiency syndrome. Ann Intern Med 1989; 110:937–940.
45. Zapol WM, Trelstad RI, Coffey JW, Tsai I, Salvador RA. Pulmonary fibrosis in severe acute respiratory failure. Am Rev Respir Dis 1979; 119:547–554.
46. Walmsley S, Spence D, Bast M, O'Rorke K, Bruton J, Salit IE. Double-blind randomized controlled trial of the role of corticosteroids in Pneumocystis carinii pneumonia in AIDS. Abstr VII Int Conf AIDS, Florence, 1991; 2:241, WB 2237.
47. Clement M, Edison R, Turner J, et al. Corticosteroids as adjunctive therapy in severe Pneumocystis carinii pneumonia: a prospective placebo-controlled trial [abstract]. Am Rev Respir Dis 1989; 139:A250.
48. Laird N, Mosteller F. Some statistical methods for combining experimental results. Int J Tech Assess Health Care 1990; 6:5–30.
49. Yusuf S, Peto R, Lewis J, Collins R, Sleight P. beta Blockade during and after myocardial infarction: an overview of the randomized trails. Prog Cardiovasc Dis 1985; 27:335–371.
50. Kovacs JA, Hiemenz JW, Macher AM, et al. Pneumocystis carinii pneumonia: a comparison between patients with the acquired immunodeficiency syndrome and patients with other immunodeficiencies. Ann Intern Med 1984; 100:663–666.
51. Peglow SL, Smulian AG, Linke MJ, Pogue CL, Nurrie S, Crisler J, Phair J, Gold JW,

Armstrong D, Walzer PD. Serologic responses to *Pneumocystis carinii* antigens in health and disease. J Infect Dis 1990; 161:296–306.
52. Rahal JJ. Corticosteroids as adjunctive therapy for pneumocystis pneumonia in patients with AIDS [letter]. N Engl J Med 1991; 324:1666.
53. American Thoracic Society and the Centers for Disease Control. Treatment of tuberculosis and tuberculosis infection in adults and children. Am Rev Respir Dis 1986; 134:355–363.
54. LaRocco A, Oldfield EC. Corticosteroids as adjunctive therapy for pneumocystis pneumonia in patients with AIDS [letter]. N Engl J Med 1991; 324:1668.
55. Bernard GR, Luce JM, Sprung CL, et al. High-dose corticosteroids in patients with the adult respiratory distress syndrome. N Engl J Med 1987; 317:1565–1570.
56. Luce JM, Montgomery AB, Marks JD, Turner J, Metz CA, Murray JF. Ineffectiveness of high-dose methylprednisolone in preventing parenchymal lung injury and improving mortality in patients with septic shock. Am Rev Respir Dis 1988; 138: 62–68.
57. Brigham KL, Bowers RE, McKeen CR. Methylprednisolone prevention of increased lung vascular permeability following endotoxemia in sheep. J Clin Invest 1981; 67: 1103–1110.
58. Lambertus MW, Goltz MB, Murthy AR, Mathisen GE. Complications of corticosteroid therapy in patients with AIDS and *Pneumocystis carinii* pneumonia. Chest 1990; 98:38–43.
59. Selwyn PA, Hartel D, Lewis VA, et al. A prospective study of the risk of tuberculosis among intravenous drug users with human immunodeficiency virus infection. N Engl J Med 1989; 320:545–550.
60. Bozzette SA. Corticosteroids in adjunctive therapy for pneumocystis pneumonia in patients with AIDS. N Engl J Med 1991; 324:1669.
61. Vane RJ. Inhibition of prostaglandin synthesis as a mechanism of action for aspirin-like drugs. Nature 1971; 231:232–235.
62. Kennedy TP, Rao NV, Noah W, et al. Ibuprofen prevents oxidant lung injury and in vitro lipid peroxidation by chelating iron. J Clin Invest 1990; 86:1565–1573.
63. Sullivan GW, Carper HT, Novick WJ, Mandell GL. Inhibition of the inflammatory action of interleukin-1 and tumor necrosis factor (alpha) on neutrophil function by pentoxifylline. Infect Immun 1988; 56:1722–1729.
64. McDonald RJ. Pentoxifylline reduces injury to isolated lungs perfused with human neutrophils. Am Rev Respir Dis 1991; 144:1347–1350.
65. Hammerschmidt D, Kotasek D, McCarthy T, et al. Pentoxifylline inhibits granulocyte and platelet function including granulocyte priming by platelet activating factor. J Lab Clin Med 1988; 112:254–263.
66. Pacht ER, Timerman AP, Lykens MG, Merola AJ. Deficiency of alveolar fluid glutathione in patients with sepsis and the adult respiratory distress syndrome. Chest 1991; 100:1397–1403.
67. Sheehan PM, Stokes DC, Yeh Y, Hughes WT. Surfactant phospholipids and lavage phospholipase A^2 in experimental *Pneumocystis carinii* pneumonia. Am Rev Respir Dis 1986; 134:526–531.
68. Debs RJ, Fuchs HJ, Philip R, et al. Lung-specific delivery of cytokines induces

sustained pulmonary and systemic immunomodulation in rats. J Immunol 1988; 140: 3482–3448.
69. Jaffe HA, Buhl R, Mastrangeli A, et al. Organ-specific cytokine therapy: local activation of mononuclear phagocytes by delivery of an aerosol of recombinate interferon-gamma to the human lung. J Clin Invest 1991; 88:297–302.
70. Shear HL, Valladares G, Narachi MA. Enhanced treatment of *Pneumocystis carinii* pneumonia in rats with interferon-gamma and reduced doses of trimethoprim/sulfamethoxazole. J AIDS 1990; 3:943–948.
71. Shear HL, El-Sadar W, Rubinstein BE, Ferreira M. Effects of steroid-induced *Pneumocystis carinii* on alveolar macrophages in the rat. J Protozool 1989; 36: 49S–50S.
72. Pesanti EL. Interaction of cytokines and alveolar cells with *Pneumocystis carinii in vitro*. J Infect Dis 1991; 163:611–616.
73. Murray HW, Gellene RA, Libby DM, et al. Activation of tissue macrophages from AIDS in patients: in vitro response of AIDS alveolar macrophages to lymphokines and interferon-gamma. J Immunol 1985; 135:2374–2377.

AUTHOR INDEX

Italic numbers give the page on which the complete reference is listed.

A

Aarnaes, S.L., 390, 391, *398*
Abbadini, M., 238, *247*
Abbott, B.J., 615, 616, 621, *626*, *629*, *630*
Abd, A.G., 419, *433*
Abouya, Y.L., 336, *353*
Abramowitz, J.A., 337, *354*
Abrams, D.I., 423, *434*, 468, *483*
Abramson, I., 302, *313*, 339, 342, 347, *355*
Abrash, M.P., 173, *179*, 625, *632*
Abruzzo, G., 615, 616, 618, 620, 621, 622, 623, *627*, *629*, *630*, *631*
Ackerson, J.E., 290, *307*
Adams, D.O., 240, *249*
Adams, J.A., 326, *329*, 387, *398*
Adams, S.R., 477, *484*
Adamson, I.Y.R., 301, *312*
Adinoff, A.D., 280, *286*
Adler, J.H., 102, *105*
Afchain, D., 238–39, *248*
Afessa, B., 161, 173, *177*, 363, *377*
Agabian, N., 495, *508*, 563, *579*, 625, *631*
Ager, A.L., 529, *543*
Agostini, C., 299, *312*
Aguirre, T., 94, *103*

Ahers, P.V., 135, *140*
Ahmad, M., 430, *435*
Aikawa, M., 26, 27, *41*, 255, *263*
Akerman, M., 416, 418, 423, 425, *432*
Akil, B., 302, *313*, 339, 342, 347, *355*, 468, *483*, 598, *601–2*
Akiva, L., 349, *359*
Akoun, G., 428, *435*, 635, *646*
Alampur, S.K., 343, 349, *356–57*
Albelda, S.M., 238, *247*
Albertson, T.E., 385, *397*
Alborn, W.E., 615, 616, *626*
Albrecht, H., 135, *140*, 336, *353*
Albright, J.T., 241, *249*
Alcindor, L.G., 58, *70*, 258, 259, *264*, 302, 304, *312–13*
Alderson, P.O., 258, *264*, 428, *435*
Aliouat, E.M., 26, *40*, 203, *220*
Allaudeen, H.S., 3, 4, *22*, 215, *222*
Allegra, A., 512, 527, 530, 531, *540*
Allegra, C.J., 20, 21, *24*, 51, 53, *68*, 192, *218*, 292, 305, *308*, 332, 334, 338, *350*, 352, 381, *395*, 446, *462–63*, 468, *483*, 488, 495, 499, *506*, *508*, *509*, 512, 514, 515, *540*, *542*, 545, 546, 548, 549, 550, 552, 553, 555, 556, *557*, *558*, *559*, *560*

649

Allen, A.G., 129, *139*
Allen, M.A., 512, *540*, 561, 563, 565, 567, 573, 575, *578*, *579*
Allen, R.D., 195, 196, 197, *218*, 223, 224, 225, 231, *233*, 253, 255, 261, *263*, 634, *645*
Allet, B., 299, *311*
Alroy, J., 63, *71*
Altman, L.C., 184, *217*
Alvares, O.F., 184, *217*
Alvira, R., 173, *180*
Aly, A.G., 290, *307*
Aly, R., 237, *247*
Amagai, T., 59, 62, *71*, 129, *139*, 512, *541*, 618, 619, *629*
Amendolea, M.A., 115, *119*, 341, *356*
Ament, M.E., 333, *351*
Amin, M.B., 173, *179*, 625, *632*
Ammann, A.J., 468, *483*
Amundson, D.E., 302, *313*
Anand, N., 551, 553, *558*
Ancarani, F., 349, *359*
Andersen, H.K., 143, 146, *150*, 269, 272, 274, 279, *283*
Anderson, C.D., 334, *352*, 361, 363, *375*
Anderson, F.J., 143, 147, *150*
Anderson, J.W., 62, 63, *71*, 255, *263*, 619, 621, 623, *629*, *630*
Anderson, R., 131, *140*
Ando, M., 292, *308*
Andrada, R., 479, *484*
Andrawis, V.A., 125, *138*
Angritt, P., 163, *178*
Angulo, O., 290, 301, *307*
Ankobiah, W., 382, *396*
Ansfield, M.J., 303, *314*
Anthony, L.B., 290, 301, *307*
Antinori, A., 299, *312*
Appel, D., 162, *178*, 385, *398*, 419, *433*
Aprung, C.L., 347, *358*
Apted, F.I.C., 561, *579*
Arai, T., 294, *308-9*
Aranda, C.P., 381, 385, *395*
Araujo, F. G., 447, *463*

Archer, A., *177*, 373, *378*
Archer, S., 603, *612*
Archibald, R.W.R., 363, *376*
Arcia, J., 338, 345, *354*, 635, *645*
Arena, C., 4, 5, 7, 9, 14, 16, 18, 20, *22*
Arheart, K., 143, 147, *150*
Arich, C., 361, 363, *376*
Arison, B.H., 623, *630*
Arizono, N., 210, *222*
Arlen, Z., 332, *350*
Armstrong, D.A., 115, *119*, 124, 134, *137*, *140*, 144, 147, 149, *151*, 155, *174*, 187, 191, 194, *217*, *218*, 229, *234*, 252, 256, *261*, *263*, 268, 269, 273, 274, 275, 276, 278, *283*, *286*, 290, 291, *306*, 332, 336, 341, 347, *350*, *353*, 362, 363, 373, 374, *376*, *378*, 381, 384, 392, *395*, 411, *413*, 569, *581*, 625, *632*, 635, 641, 642, *646–47*
Armstrong, M.Y.K., 4, 5, 6, 7, 9, 10, 14, 16, 18, 19, 20, 21, *22*, *23*, *24*, 29, *43*, 49, 50, 52, 53, 54, 55, 59, 63, 64, *66*, *69*, *71*, 73, 74, 78, *89*, 108, 111, 114, *118*, *119*, 182, 185, 186, 201, *216*, 243, 245, *249*, *250*, 252, 259, *262*, *265*, 280, *286*, 294, 296, 304, *309*, *310*, 488, *506*
Arraj-Peffer, S.M., 200, *219*, 261, *265*
Asano, K., 615, *626*, 627
Asch, A., 238, *247*
Ashihara, T., 363, *377*
Ashley, J., 561, *578*
Askanazi, J., 349, *359*
Askin, F.B., 156, 157, 158, 159, 163, 165, 169, *176*, 634, *644*
Aspock, H., 115, *119*
Assan, R., 571, *581*
Athos, L., 155, *175*
Auden, J.A.L., 615, *626*
Aur, R.J.A., 349, *359*, 552, *559*
Autran, B., 428, *435*
Avery, M.E., 301, *312*
Avron, B., 63, *71*
Awen, C.F., 361, 363, *375*

Author Index

B

Baba, M., 616, 618, *627*
Babcock, G.F., 56, *70*
Bacellar, H., 131, *140*
Bachmann, K.D., 416, *432*
Bachrach, U., 573, *582*
Baehner, R.L., 135, *140*, 149, *151*, 440, 441, 442, *461*, 488, *507*, 585, *600*
Bagarazzi, M., 459, *466*
Baggott, B.B., 347, *358*
Baggott, L.A., 347, *358*
Bagheri, K., 347, *357*
Baguley, B.C., 618, *627*
Baier, H., 155, *175*, *176*, 302, *313*, 342, 347, *356*, 381, 382, *395*, 633, 638, 642, *644*
Baier, N., 633, 638, 642, *644*
Bailey, C.L., 229, *234*
Bailey, D., 173, *179*
Bains, M.S., 416, 428, *432*
Baird, B., 334, 335, 338, *352*, 499, *509*, 555, *560*
Baker, E.L., 363, 371, *378*
Baker, J.K., 598, *601*
Baker, M., 555, *560*
Baker, P., 304, *314*
Balaan, M., 27, 29, 31, 34, *42*
Balachandran, I., 25, 26, 27, *39*, 161, 163, 169, *177*
Balber, A.E., 577, *583*
Baldwin, J.C., 268, *282*, 333, *351*
Balis, F., 334, 338, *352*, 555, *560*
Balkovec, J., 616, 620, 621, 623, *627*, *629*, *630*, *631*
Ballardie, F.W., 268, *282*, 333, *351*
Ballou, L.R., 49, 52, 53, 59, *67*, 108, *118*, 130, *139*, 210, *221*, 274, *285*, 296, *309*
Balow, J.E., 634, *645*
Balthazar, E.J., 363, 371, *378*, 425, 426, *434*
Baltzan, M.A., 361, 363, *375*
Bandarizadch, B., 422, 423, *434*
Banerjee, D.K., 299, *311*

Banerji, S., 47, 49, 50, 53, *65-66*, 83, 90, 101, *104*, 116, 117, *119*, 126, 127, 129, 130, 137, *138*, *139*, 405, 406, 408, 411, *413*, *414*
Bankhurst, A.D., 303, *314*
Banks, K.L., 208, *221*
Banner, H., 428, *435*
Bar, M.H., 363, *376*
Barber, H., 561, *578*
Barbers, R., 385, *397*
Bardenstein, D.S., 363, *376*
Barham, S.S., 169, *179*
Barlow, J.L.R., 448, *463-64*
Barnard, C.N., 422, *434*
Barnett, R.N., 361, 363, *375*
Barnhart, M., 615, 616, 621, *626*, *629*
Baron, R.B., 340, *355*, 393, 394, *399*
Barrie, H.J., 334, *352*, 361, 363, *375*
Barrio, J.L., 160, *177*, 393, *400*, 416, 419, 425, *432*
Barron, T.F., 428, *435*
Barta, K., 142, 145, 149, *149*
Barthold, S.W., 26, *42*, 184, 185, 193, 194, 197, *217*, *218*, *219*, 232, *235*
Bartizal, K., 616, 618, 620, 621, 622, 623, *627*, *629*, *630*, *631*
Bartlett, J.G., 427, *434*
Bartlett, M.S., 4, 5, 7, 8, 9, 13, 19, 20, 22, *24*, 26, 27, 30, 34, 36, *40*, *41*, 48, 49, 51, 52, 53, 55, 56, 59, 63, *66*, *67*, *68*, *69*, *70*, 71, 80, 83, *89*, *90*, 135, *140*, 149, *151*, 191, 193, 212, 215, *218*, 222, 252, *261*, 273, 274, *285*, 305, *315*, 448, *463*, 481, 482, *485*, 488, 489, 492, 494, 495, 496, 499, 501, *506*, *507*, *508*, *509*, 512, 514, *540*, *541*, *542*, 550, 552, 555, *558*, *560*, 563, 564, 567, *580-81*, 585, 586, 587, 588, 589, 590, 592, 594, 595, 597, *600*, *601*
Bartley, D.L., 124, *138*
Bartok, A., 302, *313*, 338, 339, 342, 345, 347, *354*, *355*
Barton, E.G., Jr., 26, 37, *40*, 46, 47, 48, 53, 55, 59, 63, *65*, 92, *103*, 123, *137*, 210, *221*

Barton, S.E., 338, *354*
Baseler, M., 334, 335, *352*
Baselski, V.S., 391, *399*
Basgoz, N., 163, *178*
Baskerville, A., 290, 291, 296, *306*
Baskin, M.I., 419, *433*
Bassan, H., 334, *352*
Bassis, M., 363, *377*
Bast, M., 639, *646*
Bastin, R., 25, 26, 30, 31, 37, *39*
Bate, C.A.W., 299, *311*
Bates, F.T., 160, *176*, 419, 425, 428, *433*
Batra, P., 173, *179*
Bauchet, J., 512, *541*
Baud, L., 428, *435*
Bauer, M., 336, 341, 342, *353*
Bauer, N.L., 49, *67*, 273, 274, *285*
Baughman, R.P., 47, 52, *65*, 129, 130, 137, *139*, 192, 212, *218*, 260, *265*, 338, 339, 340, 341, 343, 344, 345, 346, *354*, *356*, *357*, 381, 384, 385, 389, 390, 391, 392, 393, 394, *396*, *397*, *398*, *399*, *400–401*
Baumann, W., 155, *175*
Bazaz, G.R., 130, *139*
Beach, D.H., 94, 102, *103*
Beach, R.S., 322, *328*
Beachey, E.H., 237, 238, *247*
Beall, G.N., 343, 349, *357*
Beals, T.F., 27, 29, *43*
Beamer, W.G., 229, *234*
Bean, G.A., 102, *104*
Beard, L.J., 272, 281, *284*
Beaumel, A., 336, *353*
Beaver, J., 20, 21, *24*, 51, *68*, 292, 305, *308*, 488, *506*, 514, 515, *542*, 546, 548, 550, 552, *558*
Beck, J.M., 199, 200, *219*, 253, 261, *262*, *265*, 268, 278, *283*, 300, *312*, 503, *509*, 634, *645*
Beck, K., 343, 349, *357*
Becker, J.M., 3, 4, *22*, 215, *222*
Becker, R.P., 27, 29, 31, 34, *42*
Becker-Hapak, M., 410, *413*
Beckers, P.J.A., 25, 26, 27, 30, 34, 35,

[Beckers, P.J.A.]
37, *39*, *40*, *42*, 123, 125, *137*, *138*, 142, 146, *150*, 252, *262*, 269, 274, 279, *283*, 291, *308*, 320, *328*, 345, *357*
Beckwith, A.L., 155, *175*
Bedos, J.P., 342, *356*
Bedrossian, C.W.M., 25, 26, 27, 30, 31, 33, 34, 35, 38, *39*, *176*
Beers, M.F., 161, *177*, 347, *357*, 634, *645*
Bekerman, C., 418, 423, 427, 428, 430, *433*, *435*
Bell, C.A., 561, 563, 565, 567, 569, 570, 573, 575, *578*, *580*
Bellanti, J.A., 302, 303, *312*
Belsberg, A., 633, 634, 637, 642, 643, *644*
Belshem, J., 184, *217*
Benfield, P., 624, *631*
Bengler, C., 361, 363, *376*, *378*
Beniz, J., 363, *377*
Bennett, C., 427, 428, *435*
Bennett, C.L., 338, 342, 347, *354*
Bennett, J.E., 625, *632*
Benowitz, N., 553, *559*
Benowitz, N.L., 479, *484*
Benson, B.J., 259, *264–65*, 303, *314*
Benson, C.A., 336, 338, 340, 341, *353*
Bensousan, T., 336, *353*
Benua, R.S., 416, 428, *432*
Benz, F., 615, *626*
Berens, R.L., 94, 102, *103*
Bereziat, G., 410, *413*
Berger, B.B., 363, *377*
Berger, B.J., 563, 565, 567, 569, 570, 571, 575, *580*, *581*
Bergers, A.M.G., 26, 35, *42*
Berges, A., 341, *356*
Berman, J.D., 19, *24*, 482, *485*, 492, 494, 496, 499, *507*, *508*, 512, *541*, 567, *580–81*, 586, 590, 592, 594, 595, 597, *601*
Berman, S.M., 173, *179*
Bernard, E., 339, *355*, 373, *378*, 411, *413*

Author Index 653

Bernard, E.M., 336, 341, 347, *353*, 373, 374, *378*, 381, 385, 392, 394, *395*, 569, *581*
Bernard, G.R., 642, *646–47*
Bernaudin, J.F., 169, 170, *178*
Bernstein, L.J., 327, *328*
Bernstein-Singer, M., 637, 642, *646*
Berstein, M.T., 267, *282*
Bertino, J.R., 555, *559*, *560*
Bertram, J.F., 301, *312*
Bevelaqua, F.A., 381, 385, *395*
Beverley, S.M., 98, *104*, 549, *558*
Beyer, D., 339, *355*
Bezahler, G., 385, *398*
Bhat, S., 339, *355*
Bhatt, O.N., 427, *435*
Bienz, K.A., 298, *310*
Bier, S., 161, *177*, 416, *432*
Bigby, T.D., 155, *176*, 381, 382, *395*
Bill, R., *559*
Bille-Hansen, V., 204, 205, *220*
Bills, G., 618, 619, *629*
Birk, M.G., 26, 27, 29, 30, 34, 37, 38, *42*
Birnbaum, B.A., 363, 371, *378*, 425, 426, *434*
Birnbaum, N.S.A., 428, *435*
Birriel, J.A., 326, *329*, 387, *398*
Bisetti, I., 6, *23*
Bishberg, E., 162, *178*, 347, *357*, 425, *434*, 634, *645*
Biswas, A., 529, *543*
Biswas, J., 363, *377*
Bitonti, A.J., 573, *582*
Bitran, J., 418, 423, 426, 427, 428, 430, *433*, *434*, *435*
Bjorneby, J.M., 208, *221*
Black, J.R., 448, *463*, 481, *485*, 598, 599, *601–2*
Black, R.M., 620, 621, 623, *629*, *630*
Blackie, S.P., 163, *178*
Blackwelder, W., 334, *352*
Blackwood, L., 634, *645*
Blagburn, B.L., 561, *578*, *579*
Blanc, P., 373, *378*, 393, 394, *400*
Bland, J.A., 615, *626*

Blankenship, C., *328–29*
Blase, J.P., 470, *483*
Blase, M., 25, *39*, 618, *628*
Blase, M.A., 49, 50, *67*, *69*, 78, 84, 89, *90*, 91, 95, *103*
Blase, M.H., 408, *413*
Blaser, M.J., 298, *310*
Blecka, L.J., 389, *398*
Bleiweiss, I.J., 163, *178*
Blendis, L.M., 419, 427, *433*
Bleyer, W.A., 468, *483*
Blezberg, A., 302, *313*
Blobstein, S.H., 603, *612*
Bloch, D.A., 302, *313*, 348, *358*
Bloch, K., 102, *104*
Blodi, C.F., 363, *377*
Bloom, B.R., 303, *314*
Bloom, F.L., *328*
Blum, M.R., 604, 606, 607, 609, 610, *612*
Blum, R., 555, *560*
Blum, R.N., 349, *359*
Blum, S., 336, 341, 347, *353*, 374, *378*
Blumenfeld, L.V., 381, 383, 384, 392, *395*
Blumenfeld, W., 4, 7, 8, 20, *22*, *23*, 163, *178*, 200, *219*, 243, *249–50*, 253, *262*, 268, 272, 278, 280, *283*, *284*, *286*, 468, *483*, 488, 495, 503, 506, *508*, *509*, 512, *540*, 563, *579*, 625, *631*, 634, *645*
Blumershine, R., 26, 27, *40*, 489, *507*
Boarman, D., 20, 21, *24*, 51, *68*, 292, 305, *308*, 488, *506*, 514, 515, *542*, 546, 548, 550, 552, 553, *558*, *559*
Bobby, J., 338, *354*
Bodey, G.P., 336, *353*
Boeck, L.D., 621, *629*
Boland, M., 324, 325, *329*
Bolender, R.P., 301, *312*
Bonagura, V.R., 290, 295, 302, *306*
Bonfils-Roberts, E.A., 385, *398*
Bonk, S., 298, *310*
Bonnafoux, J., 363, *378*
Bonney, R.J., 299, *311*
Boota, A.M., 302, *313*, 342, 347, *356*, 633, 638, 642, *644*

Boozer, R.M., 597, *601*
Borkowsky, W., 298, *310*, 323, *328*
Bornstein, R.S., 573, *582*
Borst, P., 78, *89*
Bosken, C.H., 394, *400–401*
Bosma, G.C., 195, *218*, 223, 225, *233*
Bosma, M.J., 195, *218*, 223, 225, *233*
Bosniak, M.A., 363, 371, *378*, 425, 426, *434*
Botha, W.S., 205, 206, *220*
Bouchard, P., 571, *581*
Boudes, P., 340, *355*
Bourbigot, B., 336, *353*
Bouton, C., 25, 26, 30, 31, 37, *39*, 58, 70, 258, 259, *264*, 302, 304, *312–13*
Boveris, A., 603, *612*
Bovlen, C.T., 381, 384, *395*
Bowden, D.H., 301, *312*
Bower, M., 338, *354*
Bowers, R.E., 642, *646–47*
Boyer, D., 160, 173, *176*, 363, *377*
Boylan, C.J., 182, 191, 192, 193, 215, *216*, 224, 231, 233, *234*, *235*, 497, *509*, 512, *542*
Boylen, T., 155, *175*
Boylen, C.T., 302, *313*, 339, 342, 347, *355*, 385, *397*, 468, *483*, *559*
Bozzette, S.A., 302, *313*, 338, 339, 342, 345, 347, *354*, *355*, 482, *485*, 611, *613*, 633, 634, 635, 636, 637, 638, 642, 643, *644*, *645*, *646–47*
Bozzola, J.J., 616, *627*
Bradburne, R.M., 416, 419, *432*
Bradshaw, M., 332, *350*
Brandstein, L., 191, *217–18*
Brasfield, D.M., 293, *308*
Bray, M.V., 197, *219*, 232, *235*
Braza, F., 290, 301, *307*
Brazinsky, J.H., 135, *140*
Breda, S.D., 363, *376*, *377*
Breidbart, D., 347, *358*, 384, 394, *397*, 420, *433*
Breitschwerdt, E.B., 93, *103*
Brem, S., 573, *582*
Brenckman, W., 555, *560*
Brenner, M., 258, *264*, 338, 339, 341,

[Brenner, M.]
344, *354*, 449, *464*, 469, *483*, 634, 638, *645*
Breslow, A., 290, 295, *306*
Brettle, R.P., 143, 146, *150*, 275, *285*
Brettman, L., 268, *282*, 332, 336, *350*
Brevig, J.K., 347, *357*
Bridge, P.D., 129, *139*
Brigham, K.L., 642, *646–47*
Broaddus, C., 381, 383, 384, 392, *395*
Broaddus, V.C., 338, *354*
Brodine, S., 302, *313*
Brody, J.S., 301, *312*
Broughton, M.C., 488, 494, *506*, 514, *542*, 555, *560*
Brown, A.E., 362, *376*
Brown, J.F., 277, *286*
Brown, L.K., 155, *175*
Brown, R.B., 569, 571, *581*
Brown, T.D., 556, *560*
Browne, M.J., 135, *140*, 381, 385, *395*
Browne, M.T., 268, *282*
Brownstein, D.G., 26, *42*, 193, 194, *218*
Brozna, J.P., 299, *311*
Brug, S.L., 319, *327*, 332, *350*
Brunette, E.N., 199, *219*, 300, *312*, 495, *508*, 512, *540*, 563, *579*, 624, 625, *631*
Brun-Pascaud, M., 258, *264*, 512, *540*, *541*, 624, *631*
Bruns, G., 114, *119*
Brunton, J., 635, *646*
Brunvand, M.W., 333, *351*
Bruton, J., 639, *646*
Bryant, C.G., 348, *359*
Bryceson, A.D.M., 561, 577, *579*
Brzosko, W.J., 6, *23*, *67*, 142, 145, *149*, 272, *284*
Bucala, A., 373, *378*
Bucala, R., 411, *413*
Buck, B.E., *328*
Buck, C.A., 238, *247*
Buck, G.A., 49, 50, *66*, 73, 74, 84, *89*, 210, *222*
Buckley, D., 259, *264–65*
Buergelt, C.D., 207, *221*

Author Index 655

Buescher, E.S., 293, *308*
Buhl, R., 643, *648*
Bujak, J.S., 230, *234*
Bujes, D., 268, *282*
Bukholm, G., 298, *310*
Bulian, P., 299, *312*
Burchall, J.J., 546, *557*
Burchell, J.R., 447, *463*, 603, 604, *612*
Burdge, D.R., 363, *377*
Burke, B.A., 267, 272, *281*, 290, 291, 294, 295, 301, *306*, 332, 333, *350*, 362, *376*, 635, *646*
Burns, J., 405, *413*
Burns, S.M., 143, 146, *150*, 275, *285*
Burnstein, T., 13, *23*, 27, 38, *42*
Burroughs, M., *328–29*
Bursztein, S., 349, *359*
Burt, M.E., 427, *435*
Busch, D.F., 163, *178*
Bushby, S.R.M., 548, *558*
Busuttil, R.W., 333, *351*
Butler, T.F., 615, 616, 621, *626*, *629*
Bye, M.R., 327, *328*
Byrd, R.B., 425, *434*
Byrd, T.F., 305, *315*
Byrne, G.I., 305, *315*
Byrnes, T.A., 347, *357*

C

Cabib, E., 618, *628*
Cahdwani, S., 323, *328*
Caillaux, M., 203, *220*, 293, *308*
Caldwell, P., 47, 52, *65*
Callahan, R.J., 430, *435*
Campbell, A., 155, *175*
Campbell, B.N., Jr., 48, *66*
Campbell, S.W., 256, *263*, 362, 363, *376*
Campbell, W.G., Jr., 26, 27, 30, 31, 33, 34, 35, 37, *40*, 46, 47, 48, 53, 55, 59, 63, *65*, 92, *103*, 123, *137*, 182, 183, 208, 209, 210, *216*, *221*
Campoli-Richards, D.M., 563, *580*
Camus, F., 290, *307*
Camus, D., 26, 27, 30, 31, 34, 37, *40*,

[Camus, D.]
41, 46, 47, 53, 59, 60, 62, 63, *65*, 70, 124, *138*, 203, *220*, 293, *308*
Candy, D.A., 239, *248*
Cane, R.D., 348, *358*
Cantanzaro, A., 382, *397*
Cao, M., 49, 51, *67*, 73, 74, 81, 83, 89, 99, *104*, 514, *542*, 549, *558*
Capron, A., 124, *138*, 238–39, *247*, *248*
Car, N.G., 20, *24*, 290, *306*
Carbone, P.P., 625, *632*
Carbonera, D., 98, *104*
Carette, M.F., 428, *435*
Carey, J., 481, *485*, 598, *601*
Carlson, G.A., 195, 196, 197, *218*, 223, 224, 225, 231, *233*, 253, 255, 261, *263*, 634, *645*
Carlson, M.L., 495, *508*, 512, *540*
Carnevale, G., 26, 27, 35, *40*
Carosi, G., 26, 27, 35, *40*
Carpenter, H.A., 169, *179*
Carper, H.T., 643, *646–47*
Carr, D.H., 333, *351*
Carrasquillo, J.A., 428, *435*
Carrow, M., 336, 341, 347, *353*, 374, *378*
Carson, J.L., 26, 27, 30, 38, *41*, 240, 249, 252, *262*
Carter, T.R., 363, *377*
Cartun, R.W., 173, *179*, 363, 371, *377–78*
Casalino, E., 342, *356*
Cashmore, A.R., 555, *559*, 560
Cassens, B., 302, *313*, 339, 342, 347, *355*
Cassone, A., 616, *627*
Castelli, F., 26, 27, 35, *40*
Caughey, G., 155, *175*, 385, *397–98*
Causey, D., 363, *377*
Cella, R., 98, *104*
Celo, J.S., 363, *376*
Cerami, A., 373, *378*, 411, *413*, 529, *543*, 603, *612*
Cesbron, J.-Y., 124, *138*
Chabner, B.A., 20, 21, *24*, 51, *68*, 292, 305, *308*, 334, 338, *352*, 446, *462*, 488, 495, 499, *506*, *508*, *509*, 512, 514, 515, *540*, *542*, 546, 548, 549, 550, 552, 555, *558*, 560

Chadwick, E., 323, *328*
Chaffey, M.H., 373, *378*, 393, 394, *400*
Chagas, C., 91, *103*, 129, *139*, 332, *349*
Chaisson, R.E., 363, *377*, 381, 391, *396*
Champion, L.A.A., 160, *176*, 416, 420, *432*
Chandler, F.W., 26, 27, 34, *42*, 155, 158, *174*, *176*, 182, 183, 208, 209, *216*, *221*
Chandra, P., 155, *176*, 390, *398*
Chandra, R.K., 267, *282*, 332, 333, 336, *350*
Chandrasekar, P.H., 333, *351*
Chanez, P., 334, *352*
Chapel, H.M., 297, *310*
Charet, P., 203, *220*, 293, *308*
Charles, M.A., 425, 431, *434*
Chastang, C., 492, *507*
Chatterton, J.M.W., 52, *69*, 143, 146, *150*, 275, *285*
Chaubarrere, I., 571, *581*
Chaudhary, S.C., 51, *68*, 349, *359*, 427, 428, *435*, 440, 441, 442, 451, *461*, *464*, 552, *559*, 633, *644*
Chave, J.-P., 136, *140*, 336, 348, 349, *353*, *359*, 470, *483*
Cheatham, A.B., 49, 59, *67*, 108, 110, *118*
Chechani, V., 416, 419, 425, 431, *432*
Chen, L.B., 238, *247*
Chen, S.S., 623, *630*
Chen, W., 198, *219*, 300, 302, *312*
Chen, Y., 237, *246*
Chen, Y.S., 102, *104*
Cheng, S.-C., 323, *328*
Chernoff, D., 446, *462*, 475, 476, *484*, 563, *579*
Chesnut, R.W., 229, *234*
Chestney, P.J., 633, *644*
Chevrolet, J.C., 160, *176*
Child, C., 457, *466*
Chinchilla, M., 298, *310*
Chinchinian, H., 134, *140*, 334, *352*
Chiu, J., 302, *313*, 339, 342, 347, *355*, 633, 634, 635, 636, 637, 638, 642, 643, *644*

Cho, Y.J., 298, *310*
Chopard, P., 349, *359*, 455, *465*
Chrisp, C.E., 193, 194, 195, 210, *218*, *221*, 226, 233, *234*, 273, 274, 276, *285*, *286*, 291, *307*
Christensen, K.C., 553, *559*
Christol, D., 25, 26, 30, 31, 37, *39*, 58, *70*, 258, 259, *264*, 302, 304, *312–13*
Chrystal, G., 155, *174*, 634, *644*
Chuang, M.T., 155, *175*
Chulay, J.D., 561, 577, *579*
Church, J., *329*, 459, *466*
Chusid, M.J., 135, *140*
Claman, D.M., 98, *104*, 549, *558*
Claman, H.N., 184, 189, *217*
Claps, A.A., 130, *139*
Clark, A.M., 598, *601*
Clark, B.F.C., 100, *104*
Clarkson, A.B., Jr., 49, *66*, 512, *541*
Claypool, W., 27, 29, 31, 34, *42*
Cledes, J., 336, *353*
Clement, B., 569, *581*
Clement, M., 343, *356*, 639, 642, *646*
Clement, M.J., 362, 371, *376*, 456, *465*
Clements, J.A., 259, *264*
Clemons, K.V., 615, *627*
Clinton, B.A., 381, 390, 391, 392, *396*
Clotet, B., 457, *466*
Clumeck, H., 611, *613*
Clumeck, N., 482, *485*
Cobb, C.J., 260, *265*, 281, *287*, 341, *356*, *399*, 634, *645*
Coburn, T., 423, 427, 428, *434*, *435*
Cochran, J.E., 290, *307*
Coderre, C.E., 549, *558*
Coderre, J.A., 98, *104*, 549, *558*
Coffey, J.W., 638, *646*
Coffman, J., 302, *313*, 339, 342, 347, *355*
Cohen, B.A., 416, *432*
Cohen, C.J., 563, *579*
Cohen, J., 333, *351*
Cohen, K.L., 363, *376*
Cohen, O.J., 173, *179*, 326, *329*, 362, *376*

Author Index

Cohn, D.L., 341, 347, 349, *356*, *357*, *359*
Colangelo, G., 341, 344, 345, 346, *356*, *357*, 389, 391, 392, *398*
Cole, P., 383, *397*
Colella, S., 238, *247*
Coleman, D.L., 260, *265*, 339, *355*, 394, *400*, 428, *435*, 440, 441, 442, 444, *461*, 468, *483*, 633, *644*
Coleman, R.E., 594, *601*
Coll, J., 341, *356*
Collier, A.M., 26, 27, 30, 38, *41*, 240, *249*, 252, *262*
Collins, C., 333, *351*, 393, *399*
Collins, J., 383, *397*
Collins, J.V., 125, 127, 128, 130, 131, 136, 137, *138*, 411, *413*
Collins, R., 641, *646*
Colthurst, D., 100, *104*
Coman, D.R., 229, *234*
Comley, J.C.W., 10, 21, *23*, 52, *68*–*69*, 488, *506*, 514, 515, *542*, 550, 552, *558*, 563, 567, 568, *580*
Comment, C.E., 571, *582*
Conforti, C., 238, *247*
Conley, M.E., 422, 423, *434*
Connolly, M., 341, *356*
Connor, E., 323, 324, 325, *328*, *329*, 459, *466*
Connors, T.A., 201, *219*
Conri, C., 347, *358*
Constans, J., 347, *358*
Conte, J.E., Jr., 440, 441, 446, *461*, *462*, 475, 476, 477, *484*, 563, 569, *579*, *581*
Contini, C., 55, 56, 58, *70*, 115, *119*, 341, *356*
Cook, R.T., 25, 26, 27, 30, 31, 35, 37, *39*, 92, *103*
Cook, W.W., 303, *314*
Cooley, A.J., 277, *286*
Coonrod, J.D., 302, 303, *312*, *314*
Cooper, D.K.C., 422, *434*
Cooper, P.H., 363, *377*
Copland, J.W., 205, 206, *220*
Copley-Merriman, C.R., 621, 623, *630*

Corkery, K.J., 563, *579*, 624, *631*
Cornelius, M.J., 383, *397*
Cornette, J., 238, 239, *247*, *248*
Cornhauser, D.M., 482, *485*
Corsini, E., 571, *582*
Cory, M., 512, *541*, 561, 563, 565, 567, 573, 575, 576, *578*, *579*, *580*
Costanza, M.E., 556, *560*
Costello, A.H., 239, *248*
Cote, R.J., 173, *179*, 256, *263*, 362, 363, 371, *376*, *377*–*78*
Cott, G.R., 290, *307*
Cotton, D., 381, 385, *395*
Cotton, D.J., 563, *579*
Cotton, R., 7, *23*, 49, 50, 51, 52, 53, 66, 73, 74, 75, 84, *89*, 210, *222*
Coulaud, J., 290, *307*
Coulibaly, G., 336, *353*
Coulman, C.U., 363, *376*
Courtney, H.S., 237, 238, *247*
Cowan, R., 338, *354*, 440, 441, 442, 443, *461*, 468, 469, 470, 473, 474, *483*, 633, *644*
Cox, C., 20, *24*, 46, 47, 48, 49, 51, 55, *65*, 292, 305, *308*
Cox, F., 427, 428, *435*
Cox, H., 51, *68*
Cox, P.H., 343, 349, *357*
Craft, A.W., 143, 146, *150*, 274, *285*
Craig, I.D., 512, *540*
Craig, W.A., 571, *582*
Crain, J.D., 495, *508*
Cranage, M.P., 290, 291, 296, *306*
Crane, L.R., 621, *630*
Crawczynski, K., 6, *23*, 272, *284*
Crawford, T.B., 208, *221*
Crawley, J.C.W., 394, *401*
Crayton, H.E., 333, *351*
Credle, X.V.F., 383, *397*
Cregan, P., 390, 391, *398*
Crisalli, M.P., 457, *465*
Crisler, J., 115, *119*, 144, 147, *151*, 268, 269, 273, 274, 275, 278, *283*, 641, 642, *646*–*47*
Crocco, J.A., 336, 338, 340, 341, *353*
Croft, S.L., 94, *104*

Cross, A.S., 373, *378*, 416, 418, *432*
Crossley, K.B., 633, *644*
Crowle, A.J., 291, *307*
Cruciani, M., 457, *465*
Cruz, F.S., 603, *612*
Crystal, R.G., 299, *311*, 383, *397*
Csillag, A., 191, *217–18*
Cucco, R.A., 347, *358*
Cunningham, C., 173, *180*
Cunningham-Rundles, S., 268, *282*, 290, 295, 302, *306*, 332, 336, *350*
Cupples, J.B., 163, *178*
Curotto, J., 625, *632*
Curran, J.W., 361, *375*
Current, W.L., 3, 4, *22*, 182, 191, 192, 193, 215, *216*, *222*, 224, 231, 233, *234*, *235*, 497, *509*, 512, *542*, 619, 621, 624, *629*
Currie, D.L., 348, *358*
Currie, V., 555, *560*
Curry, A., 26, 30, 35, 37, *41*
Curtis, J.L., 155, *176*, 200, *219*, 261, *265*, 381, 382, *395*, 634, *645*
Cushion, M.T., 4, 5, 7, 8, 9, 10, 13, 14, 15, 16, 19, 20, *22*, *23*, *24*, 25, 26, 27, 29, 30, 31, 34, 35, 36, 37, 38, *39*, *40*, 49, 50, 51, 52, 53, 55, 56, 57, 58, 59, 60, 62, 63, *66*, *67*, *68*, *69*, *70*, *71*, 75, 77, 78, 84, *89*, *90*, 91, 95, *103*, 108, 113, 114, 115, *118*, *119*, 123, 125, 127, 129, 130, 131, 136, 137, *137*, *138*, *139*, *140*, 182–86, 192, 193, 210, 212, 213, *216*, *217*, *218*, *222*, 231, *235*, 245, *250*, 253, 255, 256, 260, *262*, *263*, 268, 269, 270, 273, 274, 276, *282*, *284*, *285–86*, 290, 293, 296, 304, 305, *307*, *308*, *309*, *310*, *315*, 391, *399*, 408, *413*, 488, 495, *506*, *508*, 512, 514, 516, 517, 518, 529, 530, 534, 536, 537, *541*, *542–43*, 550, 552, 555, *558*, *559*, 563, 565, *580*, 618, *628*
Custer, R.P., 195, *218*, 223, 225, *233*
Czuprynski, C.J., 277, *286*

D

Dacosta-Iyer, M., 173, *179*
Daggett, P.-M., 21, *24*
Dago-Akribi, A., 336, *353*
Dahlausen, D.L., 529, *543*
Dahnert, W.F., 427, *434*
Dahr, W., 239, *248*
Dake, M.D., 381, 383, 384, 392, *395*
Dale, D.C., 634, *645*
Daley, C., 347, *357*, 416, *432*
Dal Nogare, A.R., 239, *248*
Damm, D., 259, *264*
Damper, D., 573, 577, *582*
Dandurand, R., 290, 301, *307*
Dann, O., 572, *582*
Danneman, B., 599, *602*
Danovitch, G.M., 333, *351*
D'Antonio, R.G., 495, *508–9*, 512, *539*
Danzi, M.C., 457, *465*
Darby, G., 514, *542*, 548, *558*
D'Argenio, D., 471, *483–84*
Dauber, J.H., 125, 127, 128, 130, 136, 137, *138*, 333, *351*, 381, 391, *396*, 420, 421, *433*
Daupert, V.M., 621, *630*
Davalos, A.M., 205, *220*
Davey, R.T., Jr., 161, 169, 173, *177*, 334, 335, *352*, 363, *377*, 381, *395*
David, S., 136, *140*, 336, *353*
Davidian, M.M., 172, *179*, 431, *435*
Davidson, M.M., 52, *69*
Davies, P., 299, *311*
Davies, S., 448, *463*, *464*
Davis, C.B., 48, *66*
Davis, D.E., 268, *282*
Davis, D.S., 49, 59, *67*, 108, 110, *118*
Davis, R., 468, *483*
Day, L., 114, *119*
Dayan, D., 238, *248*
de Almeida, O.P., 616, *627*
Dean, R.A., 492, 499, *508*, 595, 597, *601*
DeBaetselier, P., 229, *234*
DeBona, M., 615, 616, 621, *626*, *629*, *630*

Debre, P., 428, *435*
Debs, R.F., 495, *508*, 625, *631*
Debs, R.J., 199, *219*, 300, *312*, 446, 462, 512, *540*, 563, *579*, 624, 625, *631*, 643, *647–48*
de Cock, K.M., 336, *353*
Dee, P., 416, *431*
Deepe, G.S., 278, 279, *286*
de Faucal, H., 334, *352*
Define, L.A., 384, 389, *397*
Degre, M., 298, *310*
DeGregorio, M.W., 625, *632*
Dehner, L.P., 156, 157, 163, 165, 169, *176*
Dei-Cas, E., 26, 27, 30, 31, 34, 37, *40*, *41*, 46, 47, 53, 59, 60, 62, 63, *65*, *70*, 124, *138*, 203, *220*, 293, *308*
Deigan, E., 114, *119*
Dejana, E., 238, *247*
de Jonge, P., 73, 74, 78, *89*
de Jongh, F.C.M., 73, 74, 78, *89*
Dekker, A., 363, *378*, 381, 391, *396*
Dekmezian, R., 336, *353*
Delage, A., 361, 363, *376*, *378*
Delaney, M.D., 155, *176*, 390, 394, *398*, *400*, 428, *435*
Delanoe, M., 91, *103*
Delanoe, P., 91, *103*
Delap, R., 555, *560*
del Arco Galan, C., 347, *358*
Delcamp, T.J., 98, *104*
de le Maza, L., 390, 391, *398*
Dell, A., 16, 20, 21, *24*, 29, *43*, 59, 63, *71*
Dellers, R.W., 26, *41*, 207, 210, *221*, *222*
DeLorenzo, L.J., 172, *179*, 341, *355*, 373, *378*, 393, *400*, 416, 419, 425, 431, *432*, *435*
Del Rio, C., 382, *396–97*
DeLuca, A., 299, *312*
Delves, C.J., 514, *542*, 548, *558*
Dembinski, A.S., 173, *179*
Denham, C., 569, *581*
Denis, M., 428, *435*, 635, *646*
Denning, D.W., 625, *632*
Dennis, M.J., 290, 291, 296, *306*
Denny, T., 323, 324, 325, *328*, *329*

Derouin, F., 492, *507*
Deroux, S.J., 625, *632*
DeRubertis, F.R., 363, *378*
Desikan, K.R., 615, *626*
DeStefano, J.A., 26, 27, 34, *40*, 53, 54, 56, 58, 59, 60, 61, 62, *70*, *71*, 182, *216*, 245, *250*, 296, 304, *309*, *310*, 618, *628*
Detecs, R., 393, *399*
Detels, R., 268, *282*, 323, *328*, 334, 335, *352*, 450, *464*
DeTruchis, P., 290, *307*, 457, *466*
Deutsch, R.M., 63, *71*
DeVita, V.T., 160, *176*, 361, 373, *375*, 416, 418, 423, *431*, 569, *581*, 625, *632*
Deyton, L., 161, 169, 173, *177*, 334, 335, *352*, 363, *377*, 381, *395*
Dialynas, D.P., 503, *509*
DiCelle, P.F., 299, *312*
Dickenson, G., 452, *464*, 577, *583*, 625, *632*
Dickinson, C.M., 477, *484*
Dickman, P.S., 260, *265*, 281, *287*, 341, *356*, *399*, 634, *645*
Dickmeiss, E., 143, 146, *150*, 269, 272, 274, 279, *283*
Dickmeyer, M., 336, 341, 347, *353*, 374, *378*
Dietrich, R.A., 419, 423, *433*
Diffley, P., 303, *314*
Dillard, T.A., 347, *358*
Dines, D.E., 169, *179*
Di Perri, G., 457, *465*
DiPrima, M.A., 55, 56, 58, *70*, 115, *119*, 341, *356*
Dixit, V.M., 237–38, *247*
Dobbs, G.L., 259, *264*
Dobbs, L., 259, *264*
Dobrzanski, D., 163, *178*
Dobson, K., 303, *314*
Docampo, R., 603, *612*
Dockrell, H.M., 299, *311*
Dodek, P.M., 260, *265*, 339, *355*, 394, *400*, 428, *435*
Dodge, W., 471, *483*
Doebbling, B.N., 621, 623, *630*

Dohn, M.N., 47, 52, *65*, 338, 339, 340, 341, 343, 344, 345, 346, *354, 356, 357*, 385, 389, 391, 392, *397, 398, 399*, 610, 611, *613*
Dolan, S.A., 155, 171, *174*
Dolan, T.T., 603, *612*
Dolen, S., 280, *286*
Dombret, H., 635, *646*
Domer, J., 304, *314*
Domingo, J., 381, *396*
Donelson, J.E., 303, *314*
Dong, S.R., 363, *377*
Donnelly, H.J., 569, *581*
Donnelly, W.H., 418, *432*
Donta, S.T., 297, 304, *310*
Dooley, D.P., 442, *462*
Doppman, J.L., 160, *176*, 361, 373, *375*, 416, 418, 423, *431*
Dorick, M.U., 637, 642, *646*
Doshi, S., 363, *378*
Douc-Rasy, S., 573, 575, *582*
Douglas, C., 625, *632*
Dow, F.T., 348, *359*
Downs, J.D., 210, *221*
Downs, T.D., 108, 112, 114, *118*, 273, 274, *284–85*, 296, *309*
Dowsett, A.B., 290, 291, 296, *306*
Drake, J.C., 51, *68*, 334, 338, *352*, 446, *462*, 495, 499, *508, 509*, 512, 514, *540, 542*, 549, 555, *558, 560*
Drake, S., 563, *580*
Drake, T.A., 363, *377*
Draper, D., 338, 342, 347, *354*
Drew, R.H., 616, *627*
Drew, W.L., 383, *397*
Dreyer, R.N., 555, *560*
Dreyfuss, M.M., 615, *626*
Drickamer, K., 259, *264–65*
Drucker, D.J., 173, *179*
Duane, G.B., 259, *265*, 394, *400*
Dubois, A., 361, 363, *376*
DuBois, R.E., 457, *466*
Duch, D.S., 555, *560*
Dudley, J., 334, *352*
Dugdale, M., 457, *465*
Duggan, M.A., 155, *175*

Dummer, J.S., 333, *351*, 420, 421, *433*, 451, *464*
Dumont, F., 623, *630*
Dumont, J.A., 573, *582*
Duncan, J., 239, *248*
Duncanson, F.P., 343, 349, *356–57*, 452, *465*
Duquesnoy, R.J., 333, *351*, 421, *433*
Duran, A., 618, *628*
Durkin, M.M., 4, 5, 7, 8, 9, 19, *22, 24*, 26, 34, 36, *40*, 51, 52, *68, 69*, 191, 193, 215, *218*, 252, *261*, 481, 485, 488, 489, 492, 494, 495, 496, 501, *507, 508, 509*, 512, *540, 541*, 542, 555, *560*, 585, 586, 587, 588, 589, 592, *600, 601*
Dutz, W., 130, *139*, 155, 164, *174, 178*, 272, *284*, 332, *350*, 422, 423, *434*
Dux-Guyot, A., 512, *541*
Dwork, A., 363, *376*
Dwyer, D.M., 48, *66*
Dyer, M., 514, *542*, 548, *558*
Dykstra, C.C., 49, *68*, 563, 565, 569, 570, 573, 575, *580*
Dyner, T.S., 163, *178*

E

Easmon, C.S.F., 47, 53, *65*
Easterly, J.A., 126, *138*
Ebbets, D., 10, 20, *23*, 51, 55, 63, *68*, 293, *308*, 536, *543*
Echevarria, R.A., 165, *178*
Echols, R.M., 363, *376*
Eckel, M., 298, *310*
Eddy, T., 458, *466*
Edelson, J.D., 302, *313*, 635, *646*
Edelson, P.J., *328–29*, 444, 446, *462*
Eden, O.B., 143, 146, *150*, 274, *285*
Edison, R., 475, *484*, 639, 642, *646*
Edlind, T.D., 52, 53, *69*, 83, *90*, 488, *507*
Edman, J.C., 7, *23*, 25, *39*, 49, 50, 51, 52, 53, *66, 67, 68*, 73, 74, 75, 78, 81, 83, 84, *89, 90*, 91, 95, 98, 99, *103, 104*, 129, *138*, 155, *175*, 210,

Author Index

[Edman, J.C.]
  222, 332, *350*, 381, *395*, 408, *413*, 514, *542*, 545, 549, *557*, *558*, 618, *628*
Edman, U., 49, 51, *67*, 73, 74, 81, 83, 89, 98, 99, *104*, 514, *542*, 549, *558*, 618, *628*
Ed-Sadr, W., 338, 348, *354*
Edwards, B.L., 290, 295, 302, *306*
Edwards, C.C., 50, 59, 63, *69*, 78, *89*, 130, *139*, 143, 147, *150*
Efferen, L.S., 348, *359*
Effros, R.M., 259, *265*, 394, *400*
Egawa, K., 55, 59, 63, 64, *69*, 108, 111, *118*, 411, *413*
Ehahi, N., 9, 11, *23*, 488, *507*
Ehlers, S., 277, *286*
Eicher, E.M., 229, *234*
Eichholtz, R., 19, *24*, 488, 489, *506*, 514, *542*, 550, 552, *558*, 563, 564, *580*, 585, 586, *600*
Eijking, E.P., 258, 259, 261, *264*, 348, *358*
Eisen, S., 495, *508*
Eledjam, J.J., 363, *378*
El-Helaly, S.M., 290, *307*
Elkins, K., 304, *314*
Eller, A., *329*
Elliott, R.C., 383, *397*
Ellis, D.H., 93, *103*
Ellis, L.F., 615, 616, *626*
Ellis, W.Y., 19, *24*, 482, *485*, 492, 494, 496, 499, *507*, *508*, 512, *541*, 567, *580-81*, 586, 590, 592, 594, 595, 597, *601*
Elmendorf, S.L., 363, *376*
El-Sadr, W.M., 172, *179*, 281, *287*, 341, *356*, 391, *399*, 441, 449, *461*, *464*, 634, 635, 642, 643, *645*, *646*, 648
El-Sebai, M.M., 290, *307*
Elslager, E.F., 555, *559*
Elting, L., 336, *353*
Elwood, H.J., 25, *39*, 49, 50, *67*, 78, 83, 84, *89*, *90*, 91, 95, 96, *103*, *105*, 129, *138*, 155, *175*, 408, *413*, 618, *628*

Elwood, L.J., 163, *178*
Emak, T.H.E., 200, *219*, 253, *262*, 268, 278, *283*, 503, *509*, 634, *645*
Eng, R.H.K., 162, *178*, 347, *357*, 425, *434*, 634, *645*
England, P.T., 573, 575, *582*
Ennist, D., 304, *314*
Enriquez, R.E., 363, *376*
Ensminger, W.B., 546, *557*
Erb, P., 298, *310*
Erdegem, T.D., 446, *462-63*
Erlandsen, S.L., 14, *24*
Ernst, J.A., 332, *350*
Ernstoff, M., 555, *560*
Eron, L.J., 363, *376*
Errasfa, M., 299, *311*
Ersurum, S.C., 290, *307*
Escudier, E., 169, 170, *178*
Eshdat, Y., 239, *248*
Esquivel, D.M., 603, *612*
Essig, L.J., 50, *69*
Estler, C.-J., 572, *582*
Ettensohn, D.B., 416, 419, *432*
Evans, D.A., 155, *176*, 381, 382, *395*
Evans, M.E., 495, *508-9*, 512, *539*
Eveland, W.C., 111, *118*
Ewig, S., 363, 372, *378*
Ewings, A., 561, *578*
Ezekowitz, R.A.B., 114, *119*, 245, *250*, 252, *262*, 280, *286*, 294, *309*

F

Fairley, T.A., 561, 563, 573, 575, 576, *578*, *580*
Fajardo, L.F., 299, *311*
Falenback, K.H., 416, *432*
Falko, J.M., 571, *581*
Falloon, J., 334, 335, *352*, 373, *378*, 447, 457, 458, *463*, *465*, *466*, 556, *560*, 610, 611, *613*
Falutz, J., 563, *580*
Fan, P.T., 92, *103*, 268, 282, 332, *350*
Farber, B.F., 302, *313*
Farber, C., 238, *247*

Farinotti, R., 290, *307*, 512, *540*, 624, *631*
Faris, L., 290, *307*
Farrow, B.R.H., 205, 206, *220*
Fass, R.J., 481, *485*, 598, *601–2*
Fast, D.J., 299, *311*
Fauci, A.S., 21, *24*, 165, *178*, 258, *264*, 334, 335, 338, 339, 341, 343, 344, *352*, *354*, *357*, 468, 469, *483*, 545, 557, 571, *581*, 634, *645*
Fay, M., 512, *541*
Fayer, R., 298, *310*
Fazzini, E.P., 348, *358*, 634, *644*
Federic, M.P., 423, *434*
Feigal, D.W., Jr., 338, 343, *354*, *356*, 446, 455, *462*, *465*, 475, 476, *484*, 563, *579*
Feinberg, J., 3, 4, *22*, 215, *222*, 443, 447, 448, 452, 457, *462*, *463*, 468, 481, *483*, *485*, 556, 557, *560*, 598, *601–2*, 611, *613*
Feld, M.K., 383, *397*
Feldman, A.H., 418, *432*
Feldman, M., 229, *234*
Feldman, S., 51, *68*, 111, *118*, 349, *359*, 423, 427, 428, *434*, *435*, 440, 441, 442, *461*, 487, 495, *506*, 552, *559*, 561, 562, *579*, 589, *601*, 633, *644*
Fels, A.O.S., 333, *351*
Fenwick, J.C., 348, *358*
Ferguson, L.R., 575, *582–83*
Fernandez, M., 394, *400–401*
Fernandez-Ulloa, M., 394, *401*
Ferone, R., 10, 21, *23*, 52, *68–69*, 488, *506*, 514, 515, *542*, 550, 552, *558*, 563, 567, 568, *580*
Ferrante, A., 272, 281, *284*
Ferreira, M., 643, *648*
Ferri, G., 98, *104*
Festing, M.F.W., 201, *219*
Feuerstein, I.M., 163, 168, 173, *177*, *178*, 373, *378*, 556, *560*, 610, 611, *613*
Fieser, L.F., 603, *612*
Filice, G., 26, 27, 35, *40*

Finch, P.J.P., 382, *396*, 416, 419, 425, 431, *432*
Fine, B.D., 621, *630*
Fine, J.M., 419, 423, *433*
Finikiotis, M.W., 363, *378*
Finley, T.N., 383, *397*
Finne, J., 239, *248*
Fischl, M.A., 302, *313*, 342, 347, *356*, *358*, 451, *464*, 633, 638, 642, *644*
Fischman, A.J., 429, 430, *435*
Fisher, A.G., 384, *397*
Fisher, D.J., 113, *118*, 274, 278, *285*, 296, 297, *309*
Fisher, R., 135, *140*, 268, 282
Fishl, M.A., 452, *464*
Fishman, A.P., 26, 30, 34, 38, *41*, 252, *262*, 291, 296, 303, *308*
Fishman, E.K., 373, *378*, 418, 419, 423, 424, 425, 426, *433*, *434*
Fishman, J.A., 49, 50, *66*, 73, 74, 78, *89*, 191, 193, 215, *218*, 252, 258, 259, *261*, *264*, 265, 430, *435*, 496, 509, 512, *542*
Fitch, F.W., 503, *509*
Fitzgerald, W., 381, 385, *395*
Fleisher, A.G., 347, *358*
Flesch, I.E.A., 299, *311*
Fleury-Feith, J., 169, 170, *178*
Fligiel, S., 155, *174*, 634, *644*
Flint, A., 155, *175*
Flower, C.D.R., 420, 421, *433*
Flye, M.W., 427, *435*
Flynn, P.M., 604, 606, 607, 609, 610, *612*
Foa, R., 299, *312*
Foley, N.M., 133, *140*, 299, *311*
Folk, J.C., 363, *377*
Foltzer, M.A., 635, *646*
Fong, I.W., 563, *580*
Fontaine, R.E., 571, *581*
Forbes, I.J., 361, 363, *375–76*
Forder, A.A., 422, *434*
Forrest, J.V., 373, *378*, 416, *432*
Forseter, G., 343, 349, *356–57*
Forster, S.M., 155, *175*
Foust, R.T., 363, *377*

Author Index

Foutty, L.F., 260, 265, 281, 287, 341, 356, 399, 634, 645
Fox, C., 165, 178
Foy, J.M., 192, 218, 253, 255, 263, 495, 508, 512, 516, 517, 518, 519, 523, 526, 527, 528, 529, 530, 531, 532, 533, 540, 541, 542–43, 552, 555, 559, 563, 565, 580
Frame, D.L., 338, 339, 340, 343, 344, 354
Frame, P.T., 47, 52, 65, 341, 344, 345, 346, 356, 357, 381, 385, 389, 390, 391, 392, 393, 394, 396, 397, 398, 399, 482, 485, 611, 613
Francioli, P., 136, 140, 336, 353
Francis, N.D., 155, 175
Francis, P.S., 168, 173, 178, 373, 378
Franklin, C., 302, 313, 348, 349, 358, 359
Fraser, R.S., 162, 178
Frazier, W.A., 237–38, 247
Frederick, T., 329, 459, 466
Frederick, W.R., 363, 377
Freedberg, K.A., 563, 579
Freels, S., 302, 313, 349, 359
Freeman, W.R., 173, 180
Freisheim, J.H., 98, 104, 585, 586, 601
French, M.A., 160, 176
Frenkel, J.K., 3, 4, 22, 26, 27, 41, 51, 68, 181, 182, 183, 191, 202, 203, 210, 215, 216, 222, 224, 234, 252, 253, 255, 262, 263, 276, 285, 290, 298, 306, 310, 487, 495, 501, 506, 512, 539, 551, 559, 563, 565, 580, 585, 601
Fried, E.D., 136, 140, 212, 222, 334, 352
Fried, J.C., 336, 341, 342, 353
Friedman, A.H., 173, 180
Friedman, H.B., 334, 352
Friedman, Y., 302, 313, 348, 349, 358, 359
Friedman-Kien, A., 444, 446, 462
Fritz, H., 615, 616, 626, 627
Froman, G., 238, 247
Frommel, T.O., 577, 583

Fromtling, R.A., 59, 62, 71, 304, 314, 495, 508, 512, 534, 541, 615, 616, 618, 619, 620, 621, 625, 627, 628, 629, 632
Fuchs, H.J., 199, 219, 300, 312, 643, 647–48
Fuhrer, H., 615, 626
Fuhrman, C., 340, 355
Fujioka, H., 586, 601
Fujita, S., 49, 66–67, 82, 90
Fujiwara, K., 26, 27, 30, 31, 41, 193, 194, 201, 218, 219, 229, 234, 270, 272, 276, 278, 284, 286
Fukuda, D.S., 615, 616, 621, 626, 629, 630
Fulkerson, W.J., 290, 301, 307
Fullen, G., 604, 606, 607, 609, 610, 612
Fulton, J.D., 561, 578
Furata, T., 229, 234
Furrer, H.-J., 349, 359
Furukawa, H., 586, 601
Furuta, T., 26, 27, 30, 31, 41, 143, 151, 194, 201, 218, 219, 270, 272, 276, 278, 284

G

Gabriel, O., 239, 248
Gabriel, V., 349, 359
Gachihi, G., 561, 577, 579
Gaggini, L.C., 349, 359
Gagliardi, A.J., 161, 177, 259, 265, 339, 340, 355, 394, 400
Gagnon, S., 302, 313, 342, 347, 356, 633, 638, 642, 644
Gail, D.B., 301, 312
Gailit, J., 238, 247
Gailliot, P., 619, 629
Gaither, T., 293, 308
Gajdusek, D.C., 267, 281, 320, 328, 362, 376
Gal, A.A., 163, 178, 381, 384, 395
Galan, F., 410, 413
Gale, R.P., 442, 461
Gallant, J.E., 363, 376

Gallimore, P.H., 238, *247*
Gallin, J.I., 230, *234*, 293, *308*
Gallis, H.A., 616, 621, 623, *627*, *630*
Gamsu, G., 155, 161, 162, 163, *175*, *177*, 373, *378*, 384, 385, 393, 394, *397–98*, *400*, 416, 423, *432*, *434*
Ganeval, D., 571, *581*
Ganguli, B.N., 615, *626*
Ganjei, P., 155, *176*, 381, 382, *395*
Garaazzi, M., 324, 325, *329*
Garay, S.M., 338, 340, 345, *354*, *357*, 381, 385, *395*, 416, 428, *432*, *435*, 634, *645*
Garber, G.E., 563, *580*
Garbisa, S., 299, *312*
Garces, J.M., 341, *356*
Garcia, E.R., 322, *328*
Garcia, R.L., 155, 173, *176*, *179*
Garcia-Acha, I., 618, *628*
Garfinkel, D.J., 258, *264*, 428, *435*
Garfinkle, J.B., 338, 342, 347, *354*
Garner, G.R., 363, *377*
Garner, R.E., 26, 27, 29, 34, *40*, *43*, 59, 63, *71*
Garo, B., 336, *353*
Garre, M., 336, *353*
Garrett, C.E., 98, *104*, 549, *558*
Garrity, G., 618, *629*
Garvey, E.P., 98, *104*, 549, *558*
Gatti, R.A., 267, *282*
Gaudebout, C., 456, *465*
Gautier, V., 334, *352*
Gazzard, B.G., 338, *354*
Gedroyc, W.M., 416, 417, *432*
Geelhoed, G.W., 160, *176*, 361, 373, *375*, 416, 418, 423, *431*
Geisinger, K.R., 161, 163, *177*, 418, *433*
Gelfand, D.H., 404, *413*
Gelfand, E.W., 267, *282*, 290, *306*
Gelfman, N., 290, 301, *307*
Gellei, B., 334, *352*
Gellene, R.A., 155, *176*, 339, 340, *355*, 643, *648*
Gelman, R., 323, *328*
Gelmont, D.M., 136, *140*, 212, *222*, 334, *352*

Genner, J., 126, 127, 137, *138*, 155, *174*, 183, 210, *216*, *222*
George, S.L., 349, *359*, 552, *559*
Geratz, J.D., 512, *540*, *541*, 561, 563, 564, 565, 566, 567, 572, 573, 575, *579*, *580*, *582*
Gerber, M., 155, *175*
Gerein, A.N., 347, *358*
German, V.F., 292, *308*
Gerrard, M.P., 143, 146, *150*, 274, *285*
Gerstoft, J., 143, 146, *150*, 269, 272, 274, 279, *283*, *284*, 553, *559*
Gertler, P., 338, 342, *354*
Gervais, A., 456, *465*, 563, *580*
Gervais, C., 361, 363, *376*
Gherman, C.R., 363, *377*
Giacobbe, R.A., 615, *626*
Giancotti, F., 238, *247*
Gibson, B.B., 384, 389, *397*
Gibson, W.C., 78, *89*
Gigliotti, F., 49, 52, 53, 59, *67*, *68*, *70*, *90*, 108, 110, 111, 112, 113, 115, *118*, *119*, 130, *139*, 202, 210, *220*, *221*, 253, *263*, 268, 272, 273, 274, 278, *283*, *285*, 290, 296, 297, *306*, *309*, *310*, 363, *377*, 512, *541*
Gilbert, B., 603, *612*
Gill, P.S., 637, 642, *646*
Gill, V.J., 49, *68*, 115, *119*, 125, *138*, 334, 335, *352*, 381, 391, *396*, *399*, 456, *465*
Gilman, T.M., 448, *464*
Gilmore, M., 50, 53, *69*, 78, *89*
Gilroy, S.A., 343, 349, *356–57*
Ginger, C.D., 603, *612*
Ginsburg, V., 237–38, 239, *247*, *248*
Giorgi, J.V., 323, *328*
Giovanni, P., 457, *465*
Girard, P.-M., 290, *307*, 456, 457, *465*, 466, 512, *540*, 624, *631*
Giron, J.A., 137, *140*, 149, *151*, 272, *284*, 332, 336, 345, *350*, *353*
Giuntoli, D., 49, 53, *67*, *70*, 75, 77, 78, 80, 84, *89*
Glancy, T.P., 56, *70*
Gleason, C., 619, *629*

Hayes, G.V., 107, *118*, 142, 143, 147, *150*, 269, 274, 279, *283*, 345, *357*, 382, *396*
Haynes, R.H., 99, *104*
Heald, A., 349, *359*
Heck, J.V., 622, 623, *630*
Hedrich, H.J., 201, *219*
Heeb, M.J., 239, *248*
Hegedis, C., 363, *377*
Heidelberger, K.P., 163, 173, *178*, 361, 363, *376*, 425, *434*
Heimann, A., 341, *356*
Helmick, C.G., 473, *484*, 571, *581*
Helmke, R.J., 292, *308*
Helprin, G.A., 160, *176*
Hemler, M.E., 238, *247*
Henderson, D.K., 348, *359*
Henderson, D.W., 361, 363, *375–76*
Hendley, J.O., 93, *103*, 124, *137*, 495, *508*
Hendrix, H.L., 253, *263*, 516, 517, 518, *542–43*
Henningar, G.R., 334, *352*
Henriksen, S.A., 204, 205, *220*
Henshaw, N.G., 26, 27, 30, 38, *41*, 240, *249*, 252, *262*
Henson, J.W., 333, *351*
Hentzer, B., 573, *582*
Hepburn, B., 268, *282*
Herchline, T.E., 624, *631*
Herman, G.A., 114, *119*
Hermans, P.E., 599, *602*
Hernandez-Avila, M.A., 144, 148, *151*
Herriott, M.J., 299, *311*
Herrod, H.G., 279, *286*
Heryet, A.R., 411, *414*
Herzenberg, L.A., 229, *234*
Heseltine, P.N.R., 448, *464*
Hesketh, P.J., 290, *307*
Hess, C.B., 298, *310*
Hetherington, S.V., 604, 606, 607, 609, 610, *612*
Heurich, A.E., 155, *175*, 384, *397*
Hewlett, E.L., 563, *579*
Heyman, M.R., 173, *179*, 363, *376*
Heyrman, K.A., 135, *140*

Hidalgo, H., 292, *308*
Hiemenz, J.W., 336, 337, 338, 345, *353*, 416, *432*, 441, 442, 444, *461*, 468, *483*, 545, *557*, 571, *581*, 641, 642, *646*
Higenbottam, T.W., 420, 421, *433*
Hignette, C., 342, *356*
Hill, B., 603, *612*
Hinds, G., *328–29*
Hines, D., 336, 338, 340, 341, *353*
Hipkiss, J.A., 405, *413*
Hiratani, T., 615, 616, 618, *627*, *628*
Hirsch, C.S., 419, 425, *433*
Hirschel, B., 133, *140*, 349, *359*, 455, *465*
Hirschfield, L.S., 363, *377*
Hisano, S., 26, 27, *41*, 240, *249*
Hitchings, G.H., 546, *557*
Hnatiuk, O.W., 347, *358*
Ho, M., 268, *282*, 333, *351*
Hoag, W.G., 226, *234*
Hoan, M., 299, *311*
Hofflin, J.M., 268, *282*, 333, *351*, 586, *601*
Hoffman, A.G.D., 260, *265*
Hofmann, B., 143, 146, *150*, 269, 272, 274, 279, *283*, *284*
Hokanson, J., 471, *483*
Ho-Kyun, K., 272, *284*, 411, *414*
Holland, B., 324, 325, *329*
Holland, E., 451, *464*
Hollander, H., 384, *397*, 440, 441, 446, *461*, 475, *484*, 563, *579*
Holleran, W.M., 625, *632*
Holten-Andersen, W., 143, 146, *150*, 269, 272, 274, 279, *283*, *284*
Holz, G.J., 94, 102, *103*
Holzman, B., 326, *329*
Holzman, R.S.W., 268, *282*, 298, *310*, 332, 336, *350*, 443, 452, 457, *462*, 557, *560*
Honeycutt, S., 618, *629*
Hong, S.M., 305, *315*
Hong, S.-T., 7, *23*, 49, 50, 53, *66*, *67*, *70*, 75, 77, 78, 80, 84, *89*, 144, 148, *151*, 210, 212, 222, 231, *235*

Author Index

Haidaris, C.G., 53, *70*, 115, *119*
Haidaris, P.J., 53, *70*, 115, *119*
Haigh, A.J.B., 603, *612*
Hajdu, R., 623, 624, *631*
Hajdu, S.I., 381, 384, 392, *395*
Hakala, T.R., 268, *282*, 333, *351*
Hakansson, C., 553, *559*
Hale, T.L., 298, *310*
Hall, E., 193, 194, 195, 210, *218*, *221*, 226, 233, *234*, 273, 274, 276, *285*, *286*
Hall, G.S., 129, *139*
Hall, J.E., 512, *540*, *541*, 561, 563, 564, 565, 566, 567, 569, 570, 571, 573, 575, *578*, *579*, *580*, *581*
Halpern, J.L., 49, *67*, 108, 114, *118*, 130, *139*, 144, 147, *151*, 273, 274, *285*, 320, *328*
Halsey, N.H., 144, 148, *151*
Halton, K., 161, *177*, 416, *432*
Ham, E.K., 240, *249*
Hamada, S., 49, *66–67*, 82, *90*
Hammers, L.W., 363, *376*
Hammerschlag, P.E., 363, *376*, *377*
Hammerschmidt, D., 643, *646–47*
Hammes, G.G., 48, *66*
Hammond, D.J., 447, *463*, 603, 604, *612*
Hammond, M., 616, 620, 621, 622, 623, *627*, *629*, *630*, *631*
Hamper, U.M., 427, *434*
Hancock, D.E., 50, *69*
Hancock, V., 9, 11, *23*, 26, *40*, 100, *104*, 203, *220*, 488, *507*
Hand, W.L., 597, *601*
Hanlon, M.H., 10, 21, *23*, 52, *68–69*, 488, *506*, 514, 515, *542*, 550, 552, *558*, 563, 567, 568, *580*
Hanly, P.J., 303, *314*
Hannan, S.E., 635, *646*
Hannappel, E., 258, 259, 261, *264*, 348, *358*
Hansen, B.D., 14, *24*, 489, *507*
Hansen, S., 173, *180*
Hanson, L.H., 615, *627*
Hanssen, H.A., 237, *246*
Harcup, C., 155, *175*

Hardesty, R.L., 333, *351*, 421, *433*
Hardt, C., 268, *282*
Hardy, A.M., 268, *282*, 333, *351*
Hardy, R.R., 229, *234*
Hardy, W.D., 363, *377*, 443, 452, 457, *462*, 557, *560*
Harmsen, A.G., 113, *118*, 198, *219*, 253, *263*, 268, 270, 272, 274, 278, *283*, *285*, 296, 297, 300, 302, *309*, *312*, *313*
Haron, E., 336, *353*
Harrell, J.H., 634, *645*
Harrington, T.M., 268, *282*
Hart, M.N., 25, 26, 27, 30, 31, 35, 37, *39*, 92, *103*
Hartel, D., 642, *646–47*
Hartley, W.J., 205, 206, *220*
Hartman, B.J., 136, *140*, 155, *175*, 212, 222, 334, *352*
Hartz, J.W., 161, 163, *177*, 418, *433*
Hashimoto, C.H., 260, *265*, 281, *287*, 341, *356*, 399, 634, *645*
Haskins, R.H., 102, *104*
Hasleton, P.S., 26, 30, 35, 37, *41*
Hasselager, E., 205, *220*
Hassl, A., 115, *119*
Hasty, D.L., 238, *247*
Hatfield, C., 577, *583*
Hattner, R.S., 428, *435*
Hausman, R.E., 241, *249*
Havell, E.A., 198, *219*, 300, 302, *312*
Havenhill, M.A., 181, 182, 191, *216*
Haverkos, H.W., 143, 147, *150*, 337, 338, 345, *353*, 392, 393, *399*, 633, 634, *644*
Havran, W., 503, *509*
Havron, W.S., 182, *216*, 267, 276, *281*, 290, *307*, 332, 333, 336, *350*
Hawgood, S., 259, *264–65*
Hawksworth, D.L., 129, *139*
Hay, R.J., 8, *23*
Hayakawa, K., 229, *234*
Hayano, K., 616–17, *627*
Hayashi, M., 615, *626*
Hayashi, Y., 391, *399*
Hayes, D.J., 53, 55, *69*, 495, *508*

Grant, D., 347, *358*
Grasmasse, H., 239, *248*
Grau, G.E., 299, *311*
Graves, D.C., 49, 50, *66*, *67*, 80, 81, 84, *89*, 108, 112, 114, *118*, 130, *139*, 210, *221*, 268, 269, 273, 274, 276, 277, *283*, *284–85*, *286*, 296, *309*, 410, *413*, 619, *629*
Gray, V.L., 47, *65*, 447, *463*, 482, *485*, 495, *508*, 512, *541*, 604, 605, *612–13*
Graybill, H.R., 299, *311*
Graybill, J.R., 621, 623, *630*
Greaves, T.S., 155, *175*, 381, 391, *396*
Grebe, S.F., 428, *435*
Greco, F.A., 290, 301, *307*
Greco, M.J., 341, *356*
Green, H., 160, 161, 162, 169, *177*, 634, *644–45*
Green, W.R., 161, 173, *177*, 363, *377*
Greenaway, P.J., 290, 291, 296, *306*
Greenberg, S.D., 240, *249*, 610, 611, *613*
Greenblatt, C.C., 573, *582*
Greenblatt, C.L., 303, 304, *314*
Greene, I., 363, *376*
Greene, J., 338, 340, *354*, 634, *645*
Greene, J.B., 268, *282*, 332, 336, *350*, 428, *435*
Greenfield, S., 338, 342, 347, *354*
Greeno, R.A., 259, *265*, 339, 340, *355*, 385, 394, *397*, *400*
Greenspan, E.M., 571, 573, *581–82*
Gregory, F., 553, *559*
Grem, J.L., 556, *560*
Gress, J., 381, 385, *395*
Grewal, R.S., 599, *602*
Grey, H.M., 229, *234*
Griffel, B., 334, *352*
Griffis, J.M., 8, *23*, 243, *249–50*, 272, 280, *284*, *286*
Griffith, B.P., 333, *351*, 421, *433*
Griffiths, M.H., 155, *175*
Grigsby, D., 423, *434*
Grillo-Lopez, A., 555, *560*
Grimaud, J.A., 238–39, *248*
Grimes, M.M., 363, *376*

Grivsky, E.M., 555, *560*
Grocott, R.G., 389, *398*
Grogl, M., 561, 575, *578*
Gronbeck, C., 160, *177*
Gross, J.G., 173, *180*
Grundy, J.E., 338, *354*
Gruner, J., 615, 618, *626*, *627*
Gryzan, S., 333, *351*, 421, *433*, 451, *464*
Guadebout, C., 290, *307*
Guarda, L.A., 155, *174*
Guarner, J., 155, *175*, 382, *396–97*
Guaspari, A., 555, *560*
Guckian, J.C., 551, *559*
Guerrant, R.L., 239, *248*, 363, *377*
Guerry, D., 290, 295, *306*
Guida, B., 457, *465*
Guillon, J.M., 428, *435*
Guiver, L.A., 129, *139*, 391, *399*, 408, 409, 411, *413*
Gumbs, R.V., 363, *377*
Gupta, P.K., 155, *175*
Gurney, J.W., 160, *176*, 419, 425, 428, *433*
Gutierrez, Y., 25, 26, 27, 31, 37, 38, *39*
Gutman, L., 25, 26, 30, 31, 37, *39*
Gutteridge, W.E., 47, *65*, 94, *104*, 447, *463*, 482, *485*, 495, *508*, 512, *541*, 573, 575, *582*, 604, 605, *612–13*
Guyre, P.M., 298, *310*
Guze, P.A., 338, 342, *354*
Guzzo, F.P., 165, *178*
Gyorkey, F., 155, *174*

H

Haagsman, H.P., 259, *264–65*
Hackney, R.L., 363, *377*
Hadley, W.K., 338, *354*, 381, 382, 383, 384, 392, *395*, 468, *483*
Hafner, R., 3, 4, 22, 215, *222*
Haggerty, M.F., 347, *358*
Haggie, M.H.K., 183, *216*
Hagler, D.N., 205, *220*, 278, 279, *286*
Hagler, N.G., 363, *377*
Hagopian, W.A., 363, *377*
Hahn, H., 277, *286*

Gleason, W.A., Jr., 267, *281*, 332, 333, 334, 336, *350*
Glencross, D., 20, *24*, 290, *306*
Glode, L.M., 230, *235*
Gluckstein, D., 302, *313*, 339, 342, 347, *355*
Gnarpe, H., 184, *217*
Goa, K.L., 563, *580*
Goad, L.J., 94, 102, *103*
Gochoco, C.H., 623, *631*
Godard, P., 334, *352*
Godbold, H.J., Jr., 208, *221*
Godfrey-Faussett, P., 155, *175*
Goedbloed, E., 205–6, *220*
Goesch, T.R., 135, *140*, 336, *353*
Goetz, A., 334, *352*
Goheen, M.P., 26, 27, *40*, 59, 63, *71*, 489, *507*
Goklen, K.E., 619, *629*
Gold, J.W.M., 115, *119*, 144, 147, *151*, 256, 260, *263*, *265*, 268, 269, 273, 274, 275, 278, *283*, 332, 336, 339, 341, 347, *350*, *353*, *355*, 362, 363, 374, *376*, *378*, 381, 384, 392, 394, *395*, *397*, 641, 642, *646–47*
Goldblum, L.E., 427, *434*
Golden, E., 260, *265*, 339, *355*
Golden, J.A., 155, *175*, 260, *265*, 305, *315*, 339, *355*, 373, *378*, 381, 383, 384, 385, 392, 393, 394, *395*, *397–98*, *400*, 416, 423, 428, *432*, *434*, *435*, 440, 441, 446, 448, *461*, *462*, *463*, 468, 475, 476, *483*, *484*, 563, *579*
Goldenberg, A.S., 363, 371, *378*, 425, 426, *434*
Goldfinger, S., 326, *329*
Goldin, R.D., 155, *175*
Goldring, R.M., 348, *358*, 634, *644*
Goldsmith, J.C., 173, *179*, *180*
Goldsmith, S.J., 428, *435*
Goldstein, D.S., 162, *178*, 419, *433*
Goldstein, L.I., 333, *351*
Goltz, M.B., 642, *646–47*
Gomis, P., 471, *483*
Gonzales-Crussi, F., 135, *140*, 149, *151*, 488, *507*, 585, *600*

Gonzalez, J., 173, *180*
Gonzalez, R., 259, *264*
Good, J.T., 51, *68*, 182, 183, 202, 203, 210, *216*, 224, *234*, 252, 253, *262*, 276, *285*, 290, *306*, 487, 495, 501, *506*, 512, *539*, 551, *559*, 563, 565, *580*, 585, *601*
Good, R.A., 267, 272, *281*, *282*, 290, 291, 294, 295, 301, *306*, 322, *328*, 332, 333, *350*, 362, *376*, 635, *646*
Goodman, J.L., 419, 420, *433*
Goodman, P.C., 347, *357*, 373, *378*, 416, *432*, 634, *644*
Goodwin, J.S., 303, *314*
Goodwin, S.D., 442, *462*
Goold, S.D., 363, *378*
Gootz, T.D., 404, *413*
Gopinath, N., 419, 427, *433*
Gordee, R.S., 615, 616, 621, *626*
Gordin, F.M., 226, *234*, 420, *433*, 442, *461–62*, 468, *483*, 545, *557*, 563, *579*
Gordon, C.J., 333, *351*
Gordon, J., 229, *234*
Gordon, K.P., 404, *413*
Gordon, P.R., 163, *178*
Gorton, L., 565, *580*
Gosey, L.L., 381, 391, *396*
Goto, Y., 26, 27, 30, 31, *41*, 193, 194, *218*, 276, *286*
Gotoh, S., 209, *221*
Gottlieb, J.E., 393, *400*
Gottlieb, M.S., 92, *103*, 268, *282*, 332, *350*
Gottlieb, S., 362, *376*
Gottschall, J.I., 184, *217*, 257, *263*
Gotz, G., 135, *140*, 336, *353*
Gould, I.A., 163, *178*, 393, *400*
Gradus, M.S., 50, 53, *69*, 78, *89*
Grady, D., 340, *355*, 393, 394, *399*
Grady, R.W., 49, *66*, 512, *541*, 603, *612*
Graham, B.S., 290, 301, *307*, 333, *351*
Graham, M.L., 555, *560*
Graham, N.M.H., 131, *140*
Grant, A.D., 133, *140*

Honig, C., 468, *483*, 545, *557*, 571, *581*
Honig, E.G., 382, *396–97*
Hook, M., 238, *247*
Hoover, D.R., 131, *140*
Hopewell, P.C., 302, *313*, 332, 337, 338, 339, 340, 347, 348, 349, *350*, *354*, *355*, *358*, *359*, 381, 382, 383, 384, 392, *395*, 444, *462*, 468, 475, 479, 481, *483*, *484*, 553, *559*, 563, 579, 624, *631*
Hopkin, J.N., 143, 147, *150*
Hopkin, J.M., 47, 49, 50, 53, *65–66*, 83, *90*, 101, *104*, 116, 117, *119*, 125–31, 136, 137, *138*, *139*, 240, *249*, 391, *399*, 403, 405, 406, 408, 409, 411, *412*, *413*, *414*
Hori, H., 49, 50, *67*, 84, *90*, 100, *104*
Horio, S., 292, *308*
Horn, B.R., 425, *434*
Horne, N.W., 303, *313*
Horowitz, H.W., 343, 349, *356–57*, 452, *465*
Horst, M.N., 26, 27, 29, 34, *40*, *43*, 59, 63, *71*
Horwitz, M.A., 305, *315*
Hossfeld, D.K., 135, *140*, 336, *353*
Howard, L.C., 615, 616, 621, *626*
Howard, R.G., 130, *139*
Howard, R.J., 237–38, *247*
Howard, R.M., 381, 391, *396*
Howes, E.L., 258, *264*
Hoxie, J.A., 422, 423, *434*
Ho-Yen, D.O., 52, *69*, 143, 146, *150*, 275, *285*
Hruban, R.H., 418, 419, 423, 424, 425, *433*
Hryniewicki, J., 390, 391, *398*
Hsiao, N., 555, *560*
Hsu, A.T., 623, *630*
Hsu, F.S., 207, *221*
Hsu, L.C., 302, *312*
Hu, L., 471, *483–84*
Huang, C.T., 238, *247*, 341, *355*, 373, *378*, 393, *400*, 416, 419, 425, 431, *432*
Huang, S.-N., 26, *41*, *42*

Hubbard, S.M., 135, *140*, 268, *282*
Huberman, R., 431, *435*
Hudson, A.T., 603, *612*
Hudson, D., 25, *39*
Hudson, K., 49, *67*
Huerkamp, M.J., 193, 194, 195, 210, *218*, *221*, 226, 233, *234*, 273, 274, 276, *285*, *286*, 291, *307*
Hug, E., 276, *286*
Hughes, J., 394, *401*
Hughes, W.T., 3, 4, 5, 7, 8, 20, *22*, 26, 27, 37, *41*, *42*, *43*, 47, 49, 51, 52, 53, 59, *65*, *67*, *68*, *90*, 92, 93, *103*, 108, 110, 111, 113, 114, *118*, *119*, 124, 126, 130, *138*, *139*, 142, 146, *150*, 182, 183, 202, 210, 215, *216*, *219*, 220, *221*, 222, 226, *234*, 252, 253, 258, 259, *261*, *262*, *263*, *264*, 267, 268, 269, 272, 273, 274, 276, 278, 279, *281*, *283*, *284*, *285*, 290, 293, 296, 297, 302, 304, 305, *306*, *307*, *308*, *309*, *310*, *313*, *315*, 320, 321, 327, *328*, 332, 333, 336, 345, 349, *350*, *357*, *359*, 382, *396*, 411, *414*, 422, 423, 427, 428, *434*, *435*, 440, 441, 442, 447, 451, 457, *461*, *463*, *464*, *465*, 479, 481, 482, *484*, *485*, 487, 488, 495, 499, *506*, *508*, *509*, 512, 527, *539*, *540*, *541*, 545, 550, 552, 553, 554, *557*, *558*, *559*, 561, 562, 569, *579*, *581*, 586, 589, *601*, 604, 605, 606, 607, 609, 610, 611, *612–13*, 633, 643, *644*, *646–47*
Hughlett, C., 302, *313*, 339, 342, 347, *355*, 468, *483*
Hui, A.N., 155, *174*, *175*
Hull, J.G., 361, 363, *375*
Hull, M.T., 26, 27, *40*, 489, 492, 494, 495, *507*, *508*, 512, *541*
Hull, S., 239, *248*
Hull, W., 260, *265*
Hultgren, S., 239, *248*
Humason, G.L., 208, *221*
Humeniuk, V., 361, 363, *375–76*
Humphrey, D.M., 25, 26, 27, *39*, 161, 163, 169, *177*

Hunninghake, G.W., 394, *400*
Hunt, A.H., 621, *629*, *630*
Hunt, A.S., 615, 616, 621, *626*
Hurtubise, P., 394, *400–401*
Huseby, J.S., 363, *377*
Huskinson, J., 447, *463*
Hussain, Z., 495, *508*, 512, *540*
Hutchins, G.M., 427, *434*
Hutchinson, S.A., 102, *104*
Huxtable, C.R.R., 205, 206, *220*
Hyland, R.H., 302, *313*, 563, *580*, 611, *613*, 635, *646*
Hynes, J.B., 98, *104*, 585, 586, *601*
Hynes, R.O., 238, 243, *248*
Hyslop, D.L., 621, 623, *630*

I

Iadarola, P., 98, *104*
Iannini, P., 290, 301, *307*
Ihde, D.C., 135, *140*
Ihde, D.H., 268, *282*
Ikai, T., 205, *220*, 512, *540*
Ikeda, H., 49, 50, *67*, 81, *90*, 391, *399*
Ikegami, M., 301, *312*
Iland, H., 555, *560*
Ilowite, J.S., 419, *433*
Ilowite, N.T., 290, 295, 302, *306*
Inamine, E., 619, *629*
Inber, M.S., 240, *249*
Ingram-Drake, L., 468, *483*
Inouye, T., 302, *313*
Ioachim, H.L., 625, *632*
Isaacson, C., 160, *177*
Islam, S., 336, *353*
Israel, H.I., 393, *400*
Israelski, D., 599, *602*
Itatani, C.A., 26, 27, 31, 34, 37, 38, *41*, 46, 47, 48, 52, 53, *65*, 240, *249*
Ivády, G., 422, *434*, 440, *460*, 561, 562, 563, *579*
Ivey, M.E., 49, 50, *66*, 80, 81, 84, *89*, 107, 108, 112, 114, *118*, 130, *139*, 142, 143, 147, *150*, 210, *221*, 269, 273, 274, 279, *283*, *284–85*, 296, *309*, 345, *357*, 382, *396*

Iwamoto, G.K., 443, *462*
Iwata, K., 615, 618, *627*, *628*

J

Jackson, H.C., 9, 11, *23*, 26, *40*, 100, *104*, 203, *220*, 488, *507*
Jackson, P.R., 14, *24*, 489, *507*
Jacob, P., 479, *484*
Jacobs, J.L., 136, *140*, 212, *222*, 334, *352*
Jacobs, M.P., 394, *401*
Jacobs, T., 201, *219*
Jacobson, M.A., 338, *354*, 457, *466*
Jacobus, D.P., 479, *484*, 512, *540*, 552, 554, *559*
Jaffe, H.A., 643, *648*
Jaffe, H.S., 468, *483*
Jagirdar, J.S., 163, *178*
Jakobsen, P.H., 299, *311*
Jalaj, J.K., 333, *351*
James, M.A., 299, *311*
Jameson, B., 142, 143, 146, *150*, 274, 285, 333, *351*
Janbon, C., 361, 363, *376*
Jarnum, S., 361, 363, *375*
Jarosinski, P.F., 625, *632*
Jarrells, Mc., 303, *314*
Jarvis, G.A., 243, *249–50*, 272, *284*
Javaly, K., 343, 349, *356–57*
Jay, M.A., 19, *24*, 51, *68*, 191, 193, 215, *218*, 252, *261*, 481, *485*, 492, 494, 495, 496, *508*, *509*, 512, *540*, *541*, *542*, 555, *560*, 585, 586, 588, 589, 592, *600*, *601*
Jayasimhulu, K., 55, 56, 57, 58, *70*
Jeffrey, R.B., 423, 427, *434*, *435*
Jeliffe, R., 471, *483–84*
Jenne, J.W., 303, *313–14*
Jimenez-Lucho, V., 239, *248*
Jirovec, O., 4, *22*, 319, *327*, 332, *350*, 487, *506*
Jobe, A., 301, *312*
Joe, L., 420, *433*
Johansen, K.S., 280, *286–87*, 293, *308*
Johnson, D.B., 495, *508–9*, 512, *539*
Johnson, D.L., 385, *397*

Johnson, H.D., 135, *140*, 252, *262*, 422, 423, *434*
Johnson, J.E., 291, *307*
Johnson, J.R., 303, *313–14*
Johnson, M.P., 442, *462*
Johnson, N.McI., 299, *311*
Johnson, W., 451, *464*
Johnson, W.S., 240, *249*
Johnson, W.W., 135, *140*, 422, 423, *434*
Johnston, R.B., 280, *286*
Joiner, K.A., 294, *309*
Joly, P., 428, *435*
Jones, D.B., 25, 26, 27, *39*, 161, 163, 169, *177*
Jones, J.G., 394, *401*
Jones, S.K., 512, *540*, *541*, 561, 563, 565, 567, 573, 575, *579*, *580*
Jones, T.C., 189, *217*, 243, *249*, 252, 253, *262*, 273, 280, *284*, 291, 292, 294, 298, *308*, *310*
Joos, B., 470, *483*
Jorsal, S.E., 204, 205, *220*
Jose, D.G., 267, *282*
Joseph, P., 475, 476, *484*
Joshua, H., 619, *629*
Joss, A.W.L., 52, *69*, 143, 146, *150*, 275, *285*
Joyner, R.E., 50, 59, 63, *69*, 78, *89*, 143, 147, *150*
Judson, M.A., 160, *176*
Juers, J.A., 303, *314*
Jules-Elysee, K.M., 373, *378*, 381, 385, 392, 394, *395*, 456, *465*
Junge, J., 625, *631*
Juranek, D.D., 143, 147, *150*, 477, *484*
Jurgensen, H.J., 553, *559*
Just-Nubling, G., 616, *627*

K

Kabat, L., 422, 423, *434*
Kabbash, L., 238, *247*
Kabelac, L.P., 207, *221*
Kaelis, M., 210, 213, *222*
Kafatos, A.G., 182, *216*, 267, 276, *281*, 290, *307*, 332, 333, 336, *350*

Kaftori, J.K., 334, *352*
Kagan, I.A., 111, *119*, 142, 145, *150*
Kagawa, F.T., 340, 341, *355*, 394, *400*
Kales, C.P., 336, 338, 340, 341, *353*
Kalica, A., 4, 7, 20, *22*, 488, *506*
Kallenbach, J.M., 20, *24*, 160, *177*, 290, *306*
Kalo, A., 238, *248*
Kaltreider, H.B., 200, *219*, 261, *265*, 303, *314*
Kamani, N., 422, 423, *434*
Kamholz, S.L., 382, *396*
Kaneko, T., 62, *71*, 618, *628*
Kaneshima, H., 195, *219*
Kaneshiro, E.S., 14, 15, 16, *24*, 55, 56, 57, 58, *70*, 537, *543*
Kang, M.S., 618, *628*
Kanouse, D.E., 338, 342, 347, *354*
Kaplan, H.G., 573, *582*
Kaplan, M.H., 302, *313*
Kappler, F., 503, *509*
Kapusnick, J.E., 562, 563, 571, *579*
Karlsson, A., 553, *559*
Karlsson, K.A., 239, *248*
Karnovsky, M.J., 296, *309*
Karpel, J.P., 162, *178*, 385, *398*, 419, *433*
Kasarskis, A., 577, *583*
Kaselis, M.T., 7, *23*, 137, *140*, 192, 193, 212, 213, *218*
Kaslow, R.A., 131, *140*, 323, *328*, 334, 335, *352*
Kassel, S.H., 165, *178*
Katlama, C., 441, *461*
Katz, D.R., 338, *354*
Katz, K., 173, *180*
Katz, M.H., 340, *355*, 393, 394, *399*
Katz, P., 293, *308*
Katz, S.M., 26, 27, 30, 34, *40*
Katzenstein, A.L., 158, 159, *176*, 334, *352*, 634, *644*
Kaufmann, S.H.E., 276, *286*, 299, *311*
Kavuru, M., 373, *378*
Kay, H.E.M., 333, *351*
Kay, R., 457, *466*
Kayser, A., 573, 575, *582*

Keech, F., 430, *435*
Keely, S., 231, 233, *235*
Kefatos, A.G., 267, 276, *281*
Keller, C., 621, *629*
Keller-Juslën, C., 615, *626*, 627
Keller-Schierlein, W., 615, *626*
Kelly, J.W., 442, *462*
Kemper, C., 302, *313*, 339, 342, 347, *355*, 457, *465*
Kempf, A.J., 619, *629*
Kenamore, B., 551, *559*
Kennedy, M.J., 299, *311*
Kennedy, S., 51, *68*, 495, *508*, 512, *540*, 555, *560*
Kennedy, T.P., 643, *646–47*
Kennedy, W., 457, *465*, 482, *485*, 604, 606, 607, 609, 610, *612*
Keogh, B.A., 383, 394, *397*, *400*
Kerkering, T.M., 621, *630*
Kernbaum, S., 25, 26, 30, 31, 37, *39*, 58, *70*, 258, 259, *264*, 302, 304, *312–13*, 512, *540*, 624, *631*
Kerridge, D., 616, *627*
Kessler, H.A., 336, 338, 340, 341, *353*
Keusch, G.T., 63, *71*, 237, *246*
Keystone, J.S., 571, *581*
Khaw, B.A., 430, *435*
Khodadad, E.J., 164, *178*
Khoo, K.-H., 16, 20, 21, *24*, 29, *43*, 59, 63, *71*
Kidd, P., 393, *399*
Kiefer, E.F., 305, *315*
Kilgore, S.G., 563, 564, 566, 567, *580*
Kim, C.K., 4, 19, *22*, 183, 192, 193, 194, 195, 205, 210, *216*, *218*, 220, 221, 226, 233, *234*, 253, 255, 260, 262, *263*, 268, 269, 273, 274, 276, 282, 285, *286*, 291, *307*, 381, 389, 391, 392, *396*, *399*, 495, *508*, 512, 516, 517, 518, 527, 529, 530, 531, *540*, *541*, *542–43*, 552, 555, *559*, 563, 565, *580*
Kim, H.K., 111, *118*, 422, 423, *434*
Kim, K., 363, *377*
Kimura, S., 411, *413*

King, E.G., 427, *435*
King, H., 561, *578*
King, R., 349, *359*
King, R.D., 237, *247*
King, R.E., 258, *264*, 428, *435*
King, S.A., 556, *560*
King-Thompson, N.L., 597, *601*
Kirby, H.B., 551, *559*
Kirk, R., 561, *578*
Kirkpatrick, C.H., 290, 295, *306*
Kirksey, O.W., 302, *313*, 342, 347, *356*, 633, 638, 642, *644*
Kirsch, C.M., 340, 341, *355*, 394, *400*
Kishihara, K., 229, *234*
Kishimoto, S., 299, *311*
Kishore, P., 561, *578*
Kitada, K., 411, *413*
Kitamura, D., 229, *234*
Kitamura, K., 62, *71*, 618, *628*
Kitaoka, T., 363, *377*
Klass, D.J., 303, *314*
Klatt, E.C., 363, 371, *378*, 381, 384, *395*
Klebanoff, S.J., 299, *311*
Klein, H.Z., 383, *397*
Klein, J.S., 161, 162, 163, *177*, 373, *378*, 393, 394, *400*
Klein, M.J., 163, *178*
Klein, R.S., 19, *24*, 51, *68*, 192, *218*, 492, 494, 495, *508*, 512, 527, 530, 531, *540*, *541*, 585, 586, *600*
Kleiner, D., 161, 169, 173, *177*, 363, *377*, 381, *395*
Kleinerman, J., 155, *174*
Klesius, P.H., 298, *310*
Klimpel, G.R., 298, *310*
Klimpel, K.D., 298, *310*
Klotz, S.A., 238, 241, *248*
Kluge, R.M., 512, 527, *539*
Knowles, G.K., 142, 146, *150*, 274, *285*
Knowles, M., 418, 419, 423, 424, 425, *433*
Knüsel, F., 615, *626*
Knutton, S., 239, *248*
Kobata, A., 55, 59, 63, 64, *69*, 108, 111, *118*
Kobayasi, T., 573, *582*
Kocjan, G., 155, *175*, 382, *396*

Koenig, S., 165, *178*
Kohout, E., 130, *139*, 272, *284*
Kokichi, Y., 230, *235*
Koltay, M., 440, *460*
Konan, J.B., 336, *353*
Kondo, K., 210, 222
Kopecka, M., 618, *628*
Korhonen, T., 239, *248*
Kornstein, M.J., 422, 423, *434*
Kosanke, S.D., 269, *284*
Koss, M.N., 155, 163, *174*, *175*, *178*, 381, 384, *395*
Kotas, R.V., 301, *312*
Kotasek, D., 643, *646–47*
Kovacs, A., *329*, 459, *466*
Kovacs, J.A., 4, 7, 20, 21, *22*, *23*, *24*, 25, *39*, 46–53, 59, 63, 64, *65*, *66*, *67*, *68*, *69*, 73, 74, 75, 78, 81, 83, 84, *89*, *90*, 91, 95, 99, *103*, *104*, 108, 111, 112, 114, 115, *118*, *119*, 125, 129, 130, *138*, *139*, 144, 147, *150–51*, 155, *175*, 210, 222, 260, *265*, 273, 274, 275, 279, *285*, *286*, 290, 292, 296, 305, *306–7*, *308*, *310*, *315*, 320, *328*, 332, 334, 335, 336, 337, 338, 343, 345, *350*, *352*, *353*, *357*, 381, 382, 390, 391, *395*, *399*, 408, *413*, 416, *432*, 441, 442, 444, 446, 447, *461*, *462*, *463*, 468, *483*, 488, 495, *506*, *508*, 512, 514, 515, *540*, *542*, 545, 546, 548, 549, 550, 552, 553, 555, 556, *557*, *558*, *559*, *560*, 571, *581*, 610, 611, *613*, 618, *628*, 641, 642, *646*
Kovnat, D.M., 383, *397*
Kozak, A.J., 635, *646*
Kozak, M., *90*
Koziel, H., 4, 5, 7, 9, 14, 16, 18, 20, 22, 114, *119*, 245, 250, 252, 259, 262, *265*, 280, *286*, 294, *309*
Kralove, H., 361, 363, *375*
Kramer, E.L., 428, *435*
Kramer, F., 482, *485*, 611, *613*
Krasinoki, K., 323, *328*
Kremsner, P.G., 586, *601*
Krishnan, V.L., 299, *312*

Krivan, H.C., 239, *248*
Krivisky, B., 161, *177*, 416, *432*
Krogstad, D.J., *139–40*, 267, *282*, 321, *328*, 332, 333, 336, 337, *350*, 361, *376*, 381, *395*, 440, 441, *461*, 571, *581*
Kron, M.A., 569, 571, *581*
Kronauer, C.H.M., 338, 340, 341, *355*
Kroon, M.A., 184, *217*
Kropp, H., 623, *630*, *631*
Krown, S.E., 173, *179*, 363, *376*
Krupa, D., 616, 621, 623, *627*, *630*, *631*
Kucera, K., 25, 26, 27, 30, 31, 34, 35, 37, *39*, 92, 94, *103*
Kuehner, D., 619, *629*
Kuhlman, J.E., 373, *378*, 393, *400*, 418, 419, 423, 424, 425, 426, *433*, *434*
Kuhlman, M., 294, *309*
Kuhn, M., 615, 621, *626*, *627*, *629*
Kuhn, S., 349, *359*, 451, *464*, 552, *559*
Kukayama, M., 391, *399*
Kurimoto, H., 207, *221*
Kurtz, M., 625, *632*
Kuys, D., 205, 206, *220*
Kuzma, R.J., 448, *463–64*
Kvetan, V., 349, *359*
Kwiatkowski, D., 299, *311*
Kwok, S., 363, *376*
Kyle, D.E., 561, 575, *578*
Kyuwa, S., 194, *218*, 270, 276, 278, *284*

L

Labelle, J., 173, *180*
LaBine, M., 182, 183, 184, *216*, 276, *285–86*, 290, *307*
Lachmann, B., 258, 259, 261, *264*, 348, *358*
Lack, E.E., 155, *174*, 258, *264*, 334, 338, 339, 341, 344, *352*, *354*, 409, *413*, 449, *464*, 469, *483*, 555, *560*, 634, 638, *645*
Lacoste, J.Y., 334, *352*

LaFon, S., 47, 52, 65, 610, 611, *613*
LaForce, F.M., 303, *314*, 633, *644*
Lagosky, P.A., 99, *104*
Laird, N., 641, *646*
Lambert, P., 299, *311*
Lambertus, M.W., 642, *646–47*
Lampasona, V., 563, *580*
Lancaster, D.J., 604, 606, 607, 609, 610, 611, *612*, *613*
Land, M., 610, 611, *613*
Landman, R., 290, *307*
Landry, G.J., 305, *315*
Lane, H.C., 51, 53, *68*, 258, *264*, 332, 334, 335, 338, 339, 341, 343, 344, 348, *350*, *352*, *354*, *357*, *359*, 381, *395*, 468, 469, *483*, 545, 555, *557*, *560*, 571, *581*, 610, 611, *613*
Lane, N.C., 416, *432*
Lang, O.S., 457, *465*
Lang, W., 163, *178*
Lange, M., 268, *282*, 332, 336, *350*, 381, 384, 392, *395*
Languino, L.R., 238, *247*
Lanken, P.N., 26, 30, 34, 38, *41*, 252, *262*, 291, 296, 303, *308*
Lannigan, R., 495, *508*, 512, *540*
Lanyon, H., 383, *397*
Lanza, R.P., 422, *434*
Lanzarini, P., 26, 27, 35, *40*
Lapinsky, S.E., 20, *24*, 290, *306*
LaPook, J.D., 363, *376*
LaRiviere, M., 452, 455, *465*
LaRocco, A., 642, *646–47*
Larpin, R., 348, *359*
Larson, P.H., 425, 431, *434*
Larson, S.M., 428, *435*
Laszlo, J., 555, *560*
Latorre, C.R., 4, 5, *22*
Latter, V.S., 47, *65*, 482, *485*, 495, *508*, 512, *541*, 603, 604, 605, *612–13*
Lattuada, C.P., 130, *139*, 442, *462*
Lau, W.K., 442, *461*
Laubenstein, L.J., 428, *435*, 479, *484*
Laughlin, C.A., 3, 4, *22*, 215, *222*
Laughon, B.E., 3, 4, 7, 20, *22*, 215, *222*, 488, *506*

Laughton, C.A., 571, *581*
Laurence, J., 136, *140*, 212, *222*, 334, *352*
LaVappa, K.S., 8, *23*
Lavelle, J., 457, *465*, 611, *613*
La Voie, L., 302, *313*, 342, 347, *356*, 452, *464*, 633, 638, 642, *644*
Lawler, P., 394, *401*
Lawrence, H.S., 298, *310*
Lawrence, M., 260, *265*
Lawrence, R., 323, *328*
Lawson, L.M., 302, *313*, 346, 347, 348, *357*, *358*, 384, *397*, 456, *465*, 563, *580*, 633, 634, 635, 637, 642, 643, *644*, *646*
Lazardi, K., 94, *103*
Lazzarin, A., 349, *359*, 455, *465*
Le, S.T., 563, 571, *580*
LeClair, R.A., 332, *350*
Lee, B.L., 444, *462*, 479, *484*, 553, *559*
Lee, C.H., 489, *507*, 587, 588, *601*
Lee, J.C., 237, *247*
Lee, M., 420, *433*
Lee, M.M., 165, 168, *178*
Lee, P., 348, *359*
Lee, S., 381, 391, *395*, 555, *560*
Leedom, J.M., 302, *313*, 339, 342, 347, *355*, 468, *483*
Leeuwenberg, A.D.E.M., 125, *138*, 142, 146, *150*, 252, *262*, 269, 274, 279, *283*, 320, *328*, 345, *357*
Leff, J.A., 290, *307*
Leggiadro, R.J., 321, *328*
LeGolvan, D.P., 163, 173, *178*, 361, 363, *376*, 425, *434*
Lehmann, L.K., 305, *315*
Leibovitz, E., 323, *328*, 459, *466*
Leigh, T.R., 125, 127, 128, 130, 131, 136, 137, *138*, 411, *413*
Leissring, J.D., 268, *282*
Leitman, B.S., 416, 428, *432*, *435*
Lenfant, C.J.M., 301, *312*
Lenox, T., 343, 349, *356–57*
Lenti, L., 55, 56, 58, *70*, 115, *119*, 341, *356*

Leonidas, J., 161, *177*, 416, *432*
Leoung, G.S., 338, 343, *354*, *356*, 442, 444, 447, 455, *461*, *462*, *463*, *465*, 478, 479, 481, 482, *484*, *485*, 553, *559*, 611, *613*
Leport, C., 342, *356*
Lepretre, A., 290, *307*, 457, *466*
LeRiche, J., *427*, *435*
Lerner, C.W., 332, *350*
Lerner, M., 50, 53, *69*, 78, *89*
Lerro, A.V., 193, 194, 195, 210, *218*, *221*, *226*, 233, *234*, 273, 274, 276, *285*, *286*, 291, *307*
Lesperance, E.L., 303, *314*
Lester, R.L., 302, *312*
Leterman, J.G., *328*
Leu, R.W., 299, *311*
Lev, B.I., 63, *71*
Levin, D., 347, *358*, 384, 394, *397*, 420, *433*
Levine, A.M., 637, 642, *646*
Levine, M.L., 340, 341, *355*, 394, *400*
Levine, S.J., 456, *465*
Levine, S.M., 338, *354*
Levinsky, R.J., 294, *308–9*
Levit, S., 237, *247*
Levitt, N., 633, 634, 637, 642, 643, *644*
Levy, I.L., 426, *434*
Levy, M.G., 93, *103*, 299, *311*
Lewin, S., 332, *350*
Lewis, B.J., 468, *483*
Lewis, J., 641, *646*
Lewis, M., 20, 21, *24*, 51, *68*, 292, 305, *308*, 488, *506*, 514, 515, *542*, 546, 548, 550, 552, *558*
Lewis, M.L., 281, *287*, 338, 340, 341, *354*, *355*, *356*, 391, *399*, 634, *645*
Li, X., 276, 277, *286*
Liao, S., 555, *560*
Liao, S.H.T., 604, 606, 607, 609, 610, *612*
Libby, D.M., 136, *140*, 212, *222*, 334, *352*, 643, *648*
Liberator, P.A., 62, 63, *71*, 255, *263*, 410, *413*, 619, 621, 623, *629*, *630*

Lieberman, M., 195, *219*
Liesch, J.M., 615, *626*
Liggitt, H.D., 199, *219*, 300, *312*
Light, R.B., 303, *314*
Lim, S.K., 111, *118*
Limper, A.H., 9, *23*, 26, 27, *42*, 237, 240, 245, *246*, *250*, 252, *262*, 281, *287*, 296, *309*, 337, 341, 347, *354*, 389, *398*
Lin, E.T., 476, 477, *484*, 512, *540*, 563, 569, *579*, *581*, 624, 625, *631*
Lin, H., 49, 50, *66*, 73, 74, 84, *89*, 210, *222*
Lin, J.T., 555, *560*
Lin, W., 495, *508*, 625, *631*
Linder, J., 173, *180*
Lindsay, D.S., 561, *578*, *579*
Linhartova, A., 191, *217*
Linke, M.J.A., 4, 5, 7, 13, 19, *22*, *24*, 26, 27, 36, 37, 38, *40*, 52, 53, 54, 59, 63, *69*, *71*, 108, 109, 113, 114, 115, 117, *118*, *119*, 130, 131, *139*, 144, 147, 148, *151*, 185, 186, 193, 194, 195, 210, *217*, *218*, *221*, 226, 231, 233, *234*, *235*, 245, *250*, 252, 253, 255, *262*, *263*, 268, 269, 270, 273, 274, 275, 276, 278, *283*, *284*, *285*, *286*, 291, 305, *307*, *315*, 382, *396*, 495, *508*, 512, 514, 516, 517, 518, 529, 530, 534, *541*, *542–3*, 550, 552, 555, *558*, *559*, 563, 565, *580*, 641, 642, *646–47*
Linnemann, C.C., 338, *354*, 391, 392, *399*
Linz, B.R., 394, *400*
Lipavsky, A., 258, *264*
Lipchik, G.Y., 48, 49, 52, 53, 59, 63, 64, *66*, *69*, 111, 112, *118*, 125, *138*, 144, 147, *150*, 155, 157, 158, 159, 160, 163, 164, 165, 167, 168, 169, 170, 171, 172, 173, *174*, 258, 260, *264*, *265*, 279, *286*, 296, 305, *310*, *315*
Liu, M., 471, *483–84*
Liu, Y.C., 160, 161, 162, 169, *177*, 634, *644–45*

Livingston, R.B., 333, *351*
Livingstone, C.S., 361, 363, *375*
Lloyd, D.R., 239, *248*
Lloyd, J., 205, 206, *220*
Lo, B., 349, *359*
Lodal, J., 130, *139*
Loken, M.R., 503, *509*
Lombardy, R.J., 563, 569, 570, 571, *580*
Long, E.C., 240, *249*, 252, *262*, 296, 303, *309*
Long, G.G., 209, *221*
Longo, D.L., 135, *140*, 268, *282*, 290, *306–7*, 343, *357*, 468, *483*, 545, 557, 571, *581*
Loosli, H.-R., 615, *626*, *627*
Lopes, J.N., 603, *612*
Lopez Rodriguez, C., 347, *358*
LoPresti, J.S., 336, 341, 342, *353*
Lorenz, R.R., 603, *612*
Lorenzi, P., 160, *176*
Lottin, P., 290, *307*, 456, *465*
Loudon, R.G., 392, *399*
Louie, T., 563, *580*
Loureiro, C., 637, 642, *646*
Lourie, E.M., 561, 573, *578*
Lovell, D., 201, *219*
Lowery, W.S., 419, 423, *433*
Loya, R., 302, *313*, 339, 342, 347, *355*
Lubat, E., 363, 371, *378*, 425, 426, *434*
Lucas, S., 336, *353*
Luce, J.M., 260, *265*, 302, *313*, 339, 340, 347, 348, 349, *355*, *358*, *359*, 428, *435*, 446, *462*, 468, *483*, 563, *579*, 624, *631*, 642, *646–47*
Lucet, J.C., 342, *356*
Luddy, R.E., 160, *176*, 416, 420, *432*
Lufkin, R.B., 431, *435*
Luijendijk, A., 258, 259, 261, *264*, 348, *358*
Lukes, J., 4, *22*, 319, *327*
Lum, A., 390, 391, *398*
Luna, M.A., 155, *174*, 336, *353*
Lundgren, B., 7, *23*, 49, 50, 51, 52, 53, 59, 63, 64, *66*, *67*, *68*, 69, 73,

[Lundgren, B.]
74, 75, 81, 83, 84, *89*, 98, 99, *104*, 108, 111, 112, 114, 115, *118*, *119*, 144, 147, *150–51*, 210, *222*, 275, 279, *285*, *286*, 296, *310*, 514, *542*, 549, 558, 618, *628*
Lundgren, J.D., 7, *23*, 49, 50, 51, 52, 53, *66*, 73, 74, 75, 84, *89*, 125, *138*, 144, 147, *150–51*, 210, *222*, 275, *285*
Luster, M.I., 571, *582*
Luster, W., 363, 372, *378*
Luthy, L., 470, *483*
Luthy, R., 338, 340, 341, *355*
Luyckx, B.A., 347, *358*
Lweis, V.A., 642, *646–47*
Lykens, M.G., 643, *646–47*
Lyons, H.A., 334, *352*
Lyter, D., 334, *352*

M

Maayan, S., 332, *350*
MacAdam, R.F., 573, *582*
McBride, J.D., 53, 55, *69*, 495, *508*
McCann, P.P., 573, *582*
McCarthy, T., 643, *646–47*
McCauley, D.I., 416, 428, *432*, *435*
McChesney, J.D., 598, *601*
McCleery, R., 471, *483*
McClellan, M.D., 347, *357*
McClure, H.M., 208, 209, *221*
McCook, O., 280, *286*
McCool, F.D., 416, 419, *432*
McCorkindale, N.J., 102, *104*
McCormack, F.X., 259, *265*, 296, 303, *310*, 489, *507*
McCully, R.M., 205, 206, *220*
McCune, J.M., 195, *219*
McCurdy, J.B., 303, *314*
McCutchan, A., 599, *602*
McCutchan, H.A., 302, *313*, 338, 339, 342, 345, 347, *354*, *355*
McDermott, C., 556, *560*
McDonald, C., 475, 476, *484*
MacDonald, F.M., 303, *313–14*
McDonald, J.A., 237, 239, *247*

MacDonald, M., 390, 391, *398*
McDonald, R.J., 643, *646–47*
McDougall, J.K., 238, *247*
McElvaney, G., 347, *358*, 384, *397*
McFadden, D.C., 62, 63, *71*, 189, 190, 215, *217*, 255, *263*, 512, 534, *541*, 563, *580*, 619, 620, 621, 623, 624, *629*, *630*, *631*
MacFadden, D.K., 302, *313*, 635, *646*
McGarry, T.M., 161, *177*
MacGee, J., 301, *312*
McGinley, J.R., 184, 185, 186, *217*
McGlynn, L.M., 338, 345, *354*, 635, *645*
McGowan, J.E., 633, *644*
McGuire, T.C., 208, *221*
McHardy, N., 603, *612*
Macher, A.M., 171, 172, *179*, 290, *306–7*, 336, 337, 338, 343, 345, *353*, *357*, 363, *376*, 392, *399*, 416, *432*, 441, 442, 444, *461*, 468, *483*, 545, *557*, 571, *581*, 641, 642, *646*
McIlvanie, S.K., 134, *140*, 334, *352*
Mackaness, G.B., 299, *310*
McKay, R.M., 326, *329*
McKee, K., 416, *431*
McKeen, C.R., 642, *646–47*
McKenna, R.J., Jr., 155, *175*
McKenzie, R., 155, 171, *174*
McLees, B.D., 448, *463–64*
MacLowry, J.D., 381, 391, *396*
McMechan, M.F., 479, *484*
McMeeking, A., 298, *310*
McMurtrey, M.J., 155, *175*
McNabb, P.C., 226, *234*, 442, *461*, 487, 495, *506*, 512, 527, *539*, 550, 552, *558*, 561, 562, *579*, 589, *601*
McNabb, S.J.N., 108, 112, 114, *118*, 130, *139*, 210, *221*, 269, 273, 274, *284–85*, 296, *309*
McNeish, A., 239, *248*
MacPhail, A.P., 144, 148, *151*
McPhaul, L.W., 381, 391, *396*
McQuillen, D.P., 290, *307*
McRae, D.M., 173, *179*
McSherry, G., 324, 325, *329*, 459, *466*
Macy, M.L., 8, *23*

Madalinski, K., 6, *23*, *67*, 142, 145, 272, *284*
Maddison, S.E., 107, *118*, 142, 143, 147, *150*, 269, 274, 279, *283*, 345, *357*, 382, *396*
Maehara, N., 290, *307*
Magee, D.M., 299, *311*
Magid, D., 425, 426, *434*
Magnuson, N.S., 208, *221*
Maguire, G.P., 172, *179*, 341, *355*, 373, *378*, 393, *400*, 416, 419, 425, 431, *432*, *435*
Mahan, C.T., 381, 389, *396*
Maher, M.P., 569, *581*
Maitland, N., 238, *247*
Maiuro, G., 299, *312*
Makres, T.D., 226, *234*, 442, *461*, 487, 495, *506*, 512, 527, *539*, 550, 552, *558*, 561, 562, *579*, 589, *601*
Makulu, D.R., 571, *582*
Malinverni, R., 349, *359*
Mandell, G.L., 643, *646–47*
Mandrell, R.E., 243, *249–50*, 272, *284*
Manfredi, O.L., 130, *139*
Mangos, J.A., 292, *308*
Manikumar, G., 529, *543*
Manocha, M.S., 237, *246*
Mansell, P.W., 155, *174*
Mantil, J., 394, *400–401*
Marbury, G.D., 563, 569, 570, *580*
Marcantonio, E.E., 238, 243, *248*
Marche, D., 290, *307*
Marchevsky, A., 155, *174*, 634, *644*
Marchioro, T.L., 635, *646*
Marchisio, P.C., 238, *247*
Marcial, E., 577, *583*
Margolis, D., 161, 169, 173, *177*, 363, *377*, 381, *395*
Margolskee, D., 155, *176*, 381, 382, *395*
Maridonneau-Parini, I., 299, *311*
Mariuz, P., 163, *178*, 363, 365, *377*, 393, *400*
Marks, J.D., 642, *646–47*
Marr, J.J., 19, *24*, 51, *68*, 94, 102, *103*, 492, 494, 495, *508*, 512, *541*, 585, 586, *600*

Marrack, P., 503, *509*
Marrinan, J., 620, 625, *629*, *632*
Marriott, M.S., 100, *104*
Marsh, H.M., 169, *179*
Marsh, J.C., 555, *560*
Marsh, K., 143, 147, *150*
Marshall, F., *328–29*
Marshall, G.J., 26, 27, 31, 34, 37, 38, *41*, 46, 47, 48, 52, 53, *65*, 240, *249*
Marshall, J.D., 195, 196, 197, *218*, 223, 224, 225, 231, *233*, 253, 255, 261, *263*, 634, *645*
Marshall, K.G., 26, *41*
Martel, A., 563, *580*
Martin, J.-L., 349, *359*
Martin, M.A., 343, 349, *357*
Martin, R.A., 569, *581*
Martin, R.J., 290, *307*
Martin, T.R., 184, *217*
Martin, W.J., II, 4, 6, 7, 9, 11, 20, *22*, *23*, 26, 27, *42*, 114, *119*, 182, *216*, 237, 240–43, 245, *246*, *249*, *250*, 252, 258, 259, *262*, *264*, *265*, 281, 287, 296, 297, 303, 304, *309*, *310*, 337, 341, 347, *354*, 389, *398*, 488, 489, *506*, *507*
Martin, W.R., 385, *397*
Martinet, Y., 299, *311*
Martinez, A., 49, *68*, 115, *119*
Martinez, C., 420, *433*
Martinez, G.R., 171, 172, 173, *179*
Martinez, S., 137, *140*, 149, *151*, 272, *284*, 336, 345, *353*
Martinez, A., 49, *68*, 115, *119*
Marty, B., 239, *248*
Masala, C., 55, 56, 58, *70*, 115, *119*, 341, *356*
Mascarenhas, D.A.N., 161, *177*, 336, *353*
Mascola, L., *329*
Masliah, J., 58, *70*, 258, 259, *264*, 302, 304, *312–13*
Mason, G., 475, *484*
Mason, G.R., 259, 260, *265*, 281, *287*, 341, *356*, 394, *399*, *400*, 634, *645*
Mason, R.E., 616, *627*

Masor, H., 428, *435*
Mass, J., 108, 114, *118*, 130, *139*, 144, 147, *151*, 273, 274, *285*, 320, *328*
Mastrangeli, A., 643, *648*
Mastroianni, C.M., 115, *119*, 341, *356*
Masur, H., 20, 21, *24*, 25, *39*, 46, 47, 48, 49, 50, 51, 53, *65*, *66*, *67*, *68*, 78, 83, 84, *89*, *90*, 91, 95, *103*, 108, 114, *118*, 129, 130, *138*, *139*, 144, 147, *151*, 155, *175*, 189, *217*, 243, *249*, 252, 253, 258, 260, *262*, *264*, *265*, 268, 273, 274, 280, *282*, *284*, *285*, *286*, 291, 292, 294, 305, *308*, *315*, 320, *328*, 332, 334, 335, 336, 338, 339, 341, 343, 344, 348, *350*, *352*, *354*, *357*, *359*, 373, *378*, 381, 382, 390, 391, 393, *395*, *399*, 408, *413*, 450, 456, *464*, *465*, 468, 469, 482, *483*, *485*, 488, 495, 499, *506*, *508*, *509*, 512, 514, 515, *540*, *542*, 545, 546, 548, 549, 550, 552, 555, *557*, *558*, *560*, 571, *581*, 610, 611, *613*, 618, 625, *628*, *632*
Matheron, S., 290, *307*, 342, *356*
Mathews, W.C., 338, 342, 347, *354*
Mathiesen, L., 143, 144, 146, 147, *150–51*, 269, 272, 274, 275, 279, *283*, *285*
Mathisen, G.E., 642, *646–47*
Mathre, D.J., 623, *630*
Matsubayashi, K., 209, *221*
Matsuda, S., 25, 26, 29, 34, *39*, 59, 61, 62, *70*, 173, *179–80*, 363, *377*, 618, *628*
Matsuda, T., 615, *626*
Matsumoto, Y., 25, 26, 27, 29, 31, 34, 35, 36, *39*, *40*, *41*, 49, 52, 53, 59, 61, 62, *66–67*, *69*, *70*, *71*, 82, *90*, 123, 129, *137*, *139*, 209, *221*, 255, *263*, 290, 291, 303, 304, *306*, *308*, 512, *540*, *541*, 618, 619, *628*, *629*
Matsuno, K., 210, *222*
Matsuzaki, G., 229, *234*
Matts, J.P., 457, *466*
Mavunda, K., 326, *329*
Mavunkel, B., 529, *543*
Maxfield, R.A., 348, *358*, 634, *644*

Author Index

May, D., 201, *219*
May, M., 173, *179*, 363, 371, *377–78*
Mayard, C.H., 635, *646*
Mayaud, C., 428, *435*
Mayayo, E., 173, *180*
Mayersohn, M., 477, *484*
Mazer, M.A., 46, 47, 53, *65*
Meade, J.C., 48, 49, 53, *66*, *70*, 83, *90*
Meadows, R., 361, 363, *375–76*
Meager, A., 299, *311*, *312*
Medina, I., 442, 444, *461*, *462*, 478, 479, 481, *484*, 553, *559*
Medley, S., 489, *507*
Meduri, G.U., 385, *397*
Meek, T.D., 98, *104*, 549, *558*
Megibow, A.J., 363, 371, *378*, 425, 426, *434*
Mehta, R.J., 616, *627*
Meier, J.L., 240, *249*, 252, *262*, 296, 303, *309*
Meignan, M., 428, *435*
Meijers, R., 73, 74, 78, *89*
Meisner, D., 624, *631*
Meltzer, M.S., 277, *286*
Memsic, L.D.F., 333, *351*
Mena, I., 259, *265*, 394, *400*
Mendalson, D.S., 416, *432*
Meng, T.-C., 302, *313*, 339, 342, 347, *355*
Merali, S., 52, *68*, 514, *542*, 548, 552, *558*
Mermillod, B., 349, *359*
Merola, A.J., 643, *646–47*
Merrick, W.C., 100, *104*
Meshnick, S.R., 52, *68*, 514, *542*, 548, 552, *558*, 603, *612*
Messner, R.P., 303, *314*
Metcalf, J., 334, 335, *352*
Metersky, M.L., 382, *397*
Metroka, C.E., 479, *484*
Metz, C.A., 642, *646–47*
Meuten, J., 93, *103*
Meuwissen, J.H.E.T., 25, 26, 27, 30, 34, 35, 37, *39*, *40*, *42*, 123, 125, 126, *137*, *138*, 142, 146, *150*, 252, *262*, 269, 274, 279, *283*, 320, *328*, 345, *357*

Meyer, B.C., 238, *247*
Meyer, P.R., 155, *174*
Meyer, R.D., 446, *462*, 476, *484*, 625, *632*
Meyers, J.D., 3, 4, *22*, 215, *222*, 334, *351–52*, 382, *396*
Mezger, E., 173, *179*, 625, *632*
Michael, P.F., 381, 382, *395*
Michel, F.B., 334, *352*
Michel, K.H., 621, *629*
Michelis, M.A., 268, *282*, 332, 336, *350*
Michon, C., 290, *307*
Micon, M., 336, 341, 342, *353*
Mielke, M.E.A., 277, *286*
Milberg, J., 344, *357*
Milder, J.E., 185, 190, *217*, 253, *263*, 276, *285*, 517, *542*
Miles, P.R., 338, *354*, 391, 392, *399*
Milhous, W.K., 19, *24*, 482, *485*, 492, 494, 496, 499, *507*, *508*, 512, *541*, 567, *580–81*, 586, 590, 592, 594, 595, 597, *601*
Millar, A.B., 299, *311*, 338, *354*
Millard, P.J., 240, *249*, 411, *414*
Miller, C., 272, *284*
Miller, J.J., 268, *282*
Miller, L.A., 349, *359*
Miller, L.H., 237–38, *247*
Miller, M.J., 240, *249*
Miller, R.F., 47, 50, *65–66*, 116, 117, *119*, 126, 127, 133, 137, *138*, *140*, 155, 160, *175*, *176*, 338, *354*, 382, 391, *396*, *399*, 405, 406, 408, 409, 411, *413*, 427, *435*
Miller, S.B., 347, *357*
Millet, B., 420, 421, *433*
Mille, G., 136, *140*, 336, *353*
Milligan, S.A., 394, *400*, 416, *432*
Mills, J., 226, *234*, 338, *354*, 442, 444, *461–62*, 468, 478, 479, 481, *483*, *484*, 545, 553, *557*, *559*, 562, 563, 571, *579*, 598, *601–2*, 625, *632*
Minagi, H., 347, *357*, 416, *432*
Minda, M., 26, 30, 34, 38, *41*, 252, *262*, 291, 296, 303, *308*
Mintz, L., 383, *397*
Mirelman, D., 63, *71*

Mirji, M., 423, *434*
Misasi, R., 55, 56, 58, *70*, 115, *119*, 341, *356*
Misbah, S.A., 297, *310*
Miser, J.S., 468, *483*
Mitchell, D.M., 299, *312*
Miyahira, Y., 51, *68*, 537, *543*
Mizoguchi, J., 616–17, *627*
Mizuno, K., 615–17, *626*, *627*
Modin, G., 553, *559*
Moe, K.K., 26, *41*, 207, 210, *221*, 222
Mohanty, P.K., 338, *354*
Mohsenifar, Z., 446, *462*, 476, *484*
Mojon, M., 115, *119*, 143, 146, 147, *150*, 269, 272, 274, 279, *283*, *284*
Molloy, R.M., 615, 616, 621, *626*, *629*, *630*
Momose, H., 381, 391, *395*
Monaghan, R.L., 615, *626*
Mones, J.M., 155, 161, 171, 172, 173, *175*, *177*, *179*, 373, *378*
Monk, J.P., 624, *631*
Monoz, A., 323, *328*
Montaner, J.S.G., 302, *313*, 346, 347, 348, *357*, *358*, 456, *465*, 563, *580*, 633, 634, 635, 637, 642, 643, *644*, *646*
Montealegre, F., 299, *311*
Montgomery, A.B., 446, 455, *462*, *465*, 475, *484*, 495, *508*, 512, *540*, 563, *579*, 624, 625, *631*, 642, *646*–*47*
Montgomery, J.A., 546, *557*
Morabia, A., 133, *140*
Morgan, A., 457, *465*
Morgan, R., 339, *355*
Morgenstern, G.R., 333, *351*
Morioka, H., 26, 27, 30, 31, 34, *42*, 56, 62, *70*, 296, 304, *309*
Moroson, B.A., 555, *559*, *560*
Morris, A.L., 237, *247*
Morris, H.G., 634, *645*
Morrison, S.D., 512, *540*, 561, 563, 565, 567, 573, 575, *579*
Morrissey, J.F., 303, *313*–*14*
Mosher, D.F., 238, 241, *247*
Moskovic, E., 160, *176*

Mosley, B.D., 49, 52, 53, 59, *67*, 108, *118*, 130, *139*, 210, *221*, 274, *285*, 296, *309*
Mosteller, F., 641, *646*
Mottin, D., 635, *646*
Mougeot, G., 203, *220*, 293, *308*
Mountain, C.F., 155, *175*
Moxon, E.R., 47, 50, *65*–*66*, 116, 117, *119*, 143, 147, *150*, 405, 406, 408, 411, *413*
Moyer, M.J., 269, *284*
Mugambi, M., 561, 577, *579*
Mugera, G.M., 204, *220*
Mukhopadhyay, T., 615, *626*
Mukkada, A.J., 48, *66*
Muler, I., 276, *286*
Mullen, M.P., 163, *178*, 363, 365, *377*, 393, *400*, 420, *433*
Muller, W.A., 115, *119*
Mullin, R.J., 10, 21, *23*, 52, *68*–*69*, 488, *506*, 514, 515, *542*, 550, 552, *558*, 563, 567, 568, *580*
Munger, R.G., 26, 27, 30, 34, *40*
Muniz, R.P., 603, *612*
Munoz, A., 268, *282*, 334, 335, *352*, 393, *399*, 450, *464*
Murdoch, J.K., 571, *581*
Murphy, C.F., 239, *249*
Murphy, E.D., 229, *234*
Murphy, J.W., 281, *287*
Murphy, M.J., 4, 5, 8, *22*, 27, *42*, 297, 304, *310*
Murphy, P.M., 165, *178*
Murphy, R.L., 131, *140*, 448, *463*, 481, *485*, 598, 599, *601*–*2*, 625, *631*
Murphy, R.M., 348, *358*
Murphy, S.A., 303, *314*
Murphy, T.F., 347, *358*
Murray, F.J., 428, *435*
Murray, H.W., 189, *217*, 268, *282*, 332, 336, *350*, 416, *432*, 468, *483*, 545, 557, 571, *581*, 643, *648*
Murray, J.F., 258, 260, *264*, *265*, 339, *355*, 642, *646*–*47*
Murray, K.M., 302, *313*
Murren, J.R., 336, 338, 340, 341, *353*

Murthy, A.R., 642, *646–47*
Musallan, H.A., 529, *543*
Muss, H.B., 161, 163, *177*, 418, *433*
Myerowitz, R.L., 332, *350*
Myers, C.E., 573, *582*
Myers, D., 363, *378*

N

Nacy, C.A., 277, *286*
Nadarajah, D., 348, *359*
Nadelman, R.B., 343, 349, *356–57*
Naegel, G.P., 184, *217*
Naidich, D.P., 416, 428, *432*, *435*
Nakamura, H., 363, *377*
Nakamura, Y., 49, 50, 55, 59, 63, 64, 67, *69*, 84, *90*, 100, *104*, 108, 111, *118*, 411, *413*
Nakasawa, M., 291, 303, 304, *308*
Nakata, K., 49, 50, *67*, 81, *90*, 391, *399*
Nalesnik, M.A., 333, *351*, 421, *433*
Namakura, Y., 55, 59, 64, *69*
Namikawa, R., 195, *219*
Nanos, S., 389, *398*
Narachi, M.A., 300, *312*, 512, *541–42*, 643, *648*
Nash, G., 155, *174*, 634, *644*
Nash, T., 385, *397*
Nashimoto, H., 49, 50, *67*, 81, *90*
Natanson, C., 343, *357*, 468, *483*, 545, *557*, 571, *581*
Natarajan, V., 258, 259, *264*
Nath, J., 293, *308*
Nathan, C., 238, *247*
Naude, G.E., 160, *177*
Navin, T.R., 477, *484*, 571, *581*
Naylor, B., 155, *175*
N'Dhatz, M., 336, *353*
Nealon, T.F., 385, *398*
Nedelman, M., 430, *435*
Neidle, S., 571, *581*
Nellenbogen, J., 259, *264*
Nelson, K.P., 571, *581*
Nelson, M.R., 338, *354*, 448, *463*
Nelson, N.A., 125, *138*

Nelson, N.N., 49, *68*, 115, *119*
Nelwon-Rees, W., 301, *312*
Nerurkar, L.S., 302, 303, *312*
Nes, W.D., 102, *105*
Nes, W.R., 102, *105*
Nevitt, N., 302, *313*
Newberry, G., 561, *578*
Newman, J.H., 290, 301, *307*
Newsome, A.L., 26, 34, 36, *40*
Newsome, G.S., 419, *433*
Ng, V.L., 381, 382, 390, 391, *395*, *396*
Nichol, C.A., 555, *560*
Nicholas, P., 332, *350*
Nichols, P.W., 363, *377*
Nicholson, G.L., 239, *248*
Nickodem, A., 385, *398*
Nickol, A.D., 381, 390, 391, 392, *396*
Nicks, H.L., 563, *580*
Nicod, L., 349, *359*
Nicoloff, J.T., 336, 341, 342, *353*
Nielsen, C.M., 143, 146, *150*, 269, 272, 274, 279, *283*
Nielsen, D.M., 302, *313*, 338, 339, 342, 347, *354*, *355*, 440, 441, 442, 443, *461*, 468, 469, 470, 473, 474, *483*, 633, *644*
Nielsen, J.O., 125, *138*, 143, 144, 146, 147, *150–51*, 269, 272, 274, 275, 279, *283*, *284*, *285*, 553, *559*
Nielsen, M.H., 26, 29, 30, 31, 34, 37, 38, *41*
Nielsen, P.B., 143, 146, 147, *150*, 269, 272, 274, 279, *283*, *284*
Nielsen, T., 144, 147, *150–51*, 275, *285*
Nielsen, T.N., 625, *631*
Niese, D., 363, 372, *378*
Niesel, D.W., 298, *310*
Niosi, J., 302, *313*, 339, 342, 347, *355*
Nisbet, L.J., 616, *627*
Nishiyama, Y., 586, *601*
Noah, W., 643, *646–47*
Noel, G.J., *328–29*
Nollstadt, K.H., 59, 62, *71*, 304, *314*, 495, *508*, 512, 534, *541*, 616, 618, 619, 620, 621, 622, 623, *627*, *628*, *629*, *630*, *631*

Nomoto, K., 229, *234*
Norkrans, G., 553, *559*
Norman, L.G., 4, 5, *22*, 107, 111, *118*, *119*, 142, 143, 145, 147, *150*, 269, 274, 279, *283*, 345, *357*, 382, *396*
Norrild, B., 143, 146, *150*, 269, 272, 274, 279, *283*
Northfelt, D.W., 362, 363, 371, *376*, *377*, 456, *465*, 625, *631*
Northland, R.G., 426, *434*
Norton, K.I., 416, *432*
Noskin, G.A., 348, *358*, 448, *463*, 599, *602*, 625, *631*
Notario, V., 618, *628*
Novick, W.J., 643, *646–47*
Novitzky, D., 422, *434*
Nowoslawski, A., 6, *23*, *67*, 142, 145, *149*, 272, *284*
Nüesch, J., 615, *626*
Nurre, S., 115, *119*, 268, 269, 273, 274, 275, 278, *283*, 641, 642, *646–47*
Nutter, J., 556, *560*
Nyberg, D.A., 423, *434*
Nyfeler, R., 615, *626*

O

O'Brien, R.F., 341, *356*
O'Connor, S., 334, *352*
O'Donnell, J.J., 363, *376*
O'Donoghue, 204, *220*
Odum, N., 143, 146, *150*, 269, 272, 274, 279, *283*, *284*
Ofek, I., 238, *247*
Offord, K.P., 281, *287*, 337, 341, 347, *354*, 389, *398*
Ogata-Arakaki, D., 334, 338, *352*, 468, *483*, 499, *509*, 555, 556, *560*
Ogino, K., 210, *222*, 512, *540*
Ognibene, F.P., 125, *138*, 155, 171, 172, *174*, *179*, 258, 260, *264*, *265*, 290, *306–7*, 334, 335, 338, 339, 341, 343, 344, *352*, *354*, *357*, 381, 391, 392, 393, *396*, *399*, 409, *413*, 428, *435*, 449, 450, *464*, 469, *483*, 634, 638, *645*

Ohemeng, K.A., 512, *540*, *541*, 561, 563, 564, 565, 566, 567, 573, 575, *578*, *579*, *580*
Ohfune, Y., 615, *627*
Ohga, S., 229, *234*
Ohlsen, A.S., 361, 363, *375*
Oikawa, H., 207, *221*
Oka, S., 411, *413*
Okabayashi, K., 291, 303, 304, *308*, 512, *540*
Okada, M., 363, *377*
Olbrantz, P.J., 238, 241, *247*
Oldfield, E.C., 302, *313*, 642, *646–47*
Oldham, S.A., 155, *175*
Oleske, J., 323, 324, 325, *328*, *329*
Oliver, S., 422, *434*
Olivier, J.L., 410, *413*
Olliaro, P., 26, 27, 35, *40*
O'Loughlin, B.J., 416, *432*
Olsen, G.J., 96, *105*
Olsen, G.L., 95, *104*
Omstead, M.N., 618, *629*
O'Neill, D., 556, *560*, 610, 611, *613*
O'Neill, S.J., 303, *314*
Onishi, J., 625, *632*
Onisto, M., 299, *312*
Onorato, I., 268, *282*, 332, 336, *350*
Opal, S.M., 416, 419, *432*
Opravil, M., 338, 340, 341, 349, *355*, *359*, 470, *483*
Orenstein, M., 155, *175*, 384, *397*, 416, 418, 423, 425, *432*
O'Riordan, D., 259, *265*
O'Rorke, K., 639, *646*
Orsi, R., 98, *104*
Ortmann, M., 245, *250*, 304, *314*
Ortona, E., 299, *312*
Osei, K., 571, *581*
Ossi, M.J., 51, *68*, 427, 428, *435*
Oster, C.N., 347, *358*
Osumi, M., 616, 618, *627*
Oteken, K., 173, *180*
Otten, G., 503, *509*
Otter, B.A., 192, *218*, 512, 527, 530, 531, *540*
Ouaissi, M.A., 238–39, *247*, *248*

Author Index

Ovenfors, C.O., 173, *179*
Owen, W.F., Jr., 163, *178*
Owens, D.R., 130, *139*
Oxtoby, M., *329*
Oyer, P.E., 268, *282*, 333, *351*

P

Pabst, K.M., 299, *311*
Pabst, M.J., 299, *311*
Pache, W., 615, 621, *626*, *629*
Pacht, E.R., 643, *646–47*
Padilla, M.L., 155, *175*
Page, J.E., 417, *432*
Paiva, W., 276, 277, *286*
Palat, D.S., 348, *359*
Páldy, L., 422, *434*, 440, *460*, 561, 562, 563, *579*
Palluault, F., 26, 27, 30, 31, 34, 37, *40*, *41*, 46, 47, 53, 59, 60, 62, 63, *65*, *70*, 124, *138*, 203, *220*
Palte, S., 604, 606, 607, 609, 610, *612*
Panton, L.J., 237–38, *247*
Papahadjopoulos, D., 495, *508*, 563, *579*, 625, *631*
Pappas, M.G., 14, *24*, 489, *507*
Pappas, P.G., 621, *630*
Para, M.F., 624, *631*
Paradis, I.L., 125, 127, 128, 130, 136, 137, *138*, 333, *351*, 381, 391, *396*, 420, 421, *433*, 451, *464*
Parham, D., 387, *398*
Parker, C.B., 451, *464*
Parker, M.M., 343, *357*, 468, *483*, 545, 557, 571, *581*
Parker, R., 344, *357*
Parker, R.H., 420, *433*
Parkinnen, J., 239, *248*
Parks, L.W., 102, *105*
Parks, W.P., *328*
Parquin, F., 428, *435*
Parrillo, J.E., 20, 21, *24*, 46, 47, 49, 51, 53, *65*, *67*, *68*, 108, 114, *118*, 130, *139*, 144, 147, *151*, 258, *264*, 273, 274, *285*, 292, 305, *308*, 320, *328*, 338, 339, 341, 343, 344, 348,

[Parrillo, J.E.]
354, 357, *359*, 391, *399*, 468, 469, *483*, 488, 495, *506*, *508*, 512, 514, 515, *540*, *542*, 545, 546, 548, 550, 555, *557*, *558*, *560*, 571, *581*
Parsons, P.E., 347, *357*
Parvey, R., 610, 611, *613*
Pass, H.I., 373, *378*
Pastore, L., 363, *376*
Patou, G., 338, *354*
Patten, E., 230, *234*
Patton, C.L., 573, 577, *582*
Paul, E.S., 184, *217*
Paulson, Y.J., 448, *464*
Paulsrud, J.R., 49, 53, 55, 56, *67*, *69*, *70*, 114, *119*, 243, *249*, 252, 259, *262*, *265*, 273, 274, *285*, 296, 297, 303, 304, *309*, *310*, 488, 489, *507*
Pavlica, F., 130, *139*
Pearce, D.E., 569, *581*
Pearson, M., 160, *176*
Pearson, R.D., 563, *579*
Pedersen, C., 553, *559*
Pedersen, F.K., 280, *286–87*, 293, *308*
Peglow, S.L., 115, *119*, 144, 147, *151*, 252, *262*, 268, 269, 273, 274, 275, 278, *283*, 382, *396*, 641, 642, *646–47*
Pehrson, P.O., 553, *559*
Peiperl, L., 338, *354*
Pella, J.A., 302, *313*, 635, *646*
Pennington, J.E., 634, *645*
Penny, D.P., 241, *249*
Pereira, M.E.A., 63, *71*
Pereira, W., 383, *397*
Perera, D.R., 135, *140*, 252, *262*, 333, *351*, 440, 441, *460*
Perez, P., 618, *628*
Perl, D.P., *139–40*, 267, *282*, 321, *328*, 332, 333, 336, 337, *350*, 361, *376*, 381, *395*, 440, 441, *461*, 571, *581*
Perlman, A.M., 615, *627*
Perret, C., 348, *359*
Perruquet, J.L., 268, *282*
Perryman, L.E., 208, *221*
Persson, S., 184, *217*
Peruzzi, W.T., 348, *358*

Pesanti, E.L., 4, 7, 20, 22, 24, 37, 43, 46, 47, 48, 49, 51, 53, 55, 56, 57, 59, 60, 63, 65, 66, 70, 71, 108, 114, 115, 118, 119, 184, 217, 243, 249, 259, 264, 280, 286, 290, 291, 292, 293, 296, 297, 299, 300, 301, 302, 303, 304, 305, 307, 308, 309, 310, 311, 312, 315, 488, 506, 552, 559, 643, 648
Petcher, T.J., 615, 626
Peters, S.E., 125, 127, 128, 129, 130, 131, 136, 137, 138, 139, 406, 408, 411, 413, 414
Peters, S.G., 333, 351
Petersen, C.S., 553, 559
Peters-Golden, M., 634, 645
Peterson, E.M., 390, 391, 398
Petes, T.D., 84, 90
Petitpretz, P., 441, 461
Peto, R., 641, 646
Petri, W.A., 239, 249, 363, 377
Pettinelli, C., 451, 464
Petty, B.G., 482, 485
Petuch, B.R., 623, 630
Pfaffenbach, P.I., 603, 612
Pfaller, M.A., 621, 630
Pfefferkorn, E.R., 298, 310
Pfeiffer, T.J., 93, 103
Phair, J.P., 115, 119, 268, 269, 273, 274, 275, 278, 282, 283, 323, 328, 334, 335, 348, 352, 358, 393, 399, 450, 464, 599, 602, 641, 642, 646–47
Phair, J.W.M., 144, 147, 151
Phaneuf, D., 448, 463
Phelp, R.T., 476, 484, 569, 581
Phelps, D.S., 6, 23, 258, 259, 260, 264, 265, 294, 302, 304, 309
Philip, R., 643, 647–48
Phillips, G.D., 393, 399
Phillips, J.E., 135, 140
Philp, J.R., 291, 307
Pickard, W.W., 616, 627
Pierce, P.F., 419, 433
Pierres, A., 503, 509
Pieschbacher, M.D., 238, 247

Pietra, G.G., 26, 30, 34, 38, 41, 252, 262, 291, 296, 303, 308, 422, 423, 434
Pietrzyk, B., 26, 27, 30, 31, 37, 41, 46, 47, 65
Pifer, D.D., 19, 24, 50, 59, 63, 69, 78, 89, 514, 542
Pifer, L.L., 4, 5, 8, 19, 22, 24, 27, 42, 50, 59, 63, 69, 78, 89, 126, 130, 138, 139, 142, 143, 146, 147, 150, 252, 262, 268, 269, 274, 279, 283, 286, 293, 297, 304, 308, 310, 320, 328, 345, 357, 382, 391, 396, 399, 514, 542
Piguet, P., 299, 311
Pilon, V.A., 363, 376
Pinching, A.J., 299, 312
Pincus, P.S., 160, 177
Pinsky, S., 427, 428, 435
Pinto, A.V., 603, 612
Pintozzi, R.L., 389, 398
Piras, M.M., 94, 103
Piskorowski, T.J., 333, 351
Piskura, J., 489, 507
Pitchenik, A.E., 155, 160, 175, 176, 177, 347, 358, 381, 382, 393, 395, 400, 416, 419, 423, 425, 430, 432, 434
Pittaluga, S., 155, 157, 158, 159, 160, 163, 164, 165, 167, 168, 169, 170, 171, 172, 173, 174, 258, 264
Pittarelli, L.A., 59, 62, 63, 71, 189, 190, 215, 217, 255, 263, 304, 314, 495, 508, 512, 534, 541, 618, 619, 620, 621, 623, 628, 629, 630
Pixley, F.J., 47, 50, 53, 65–66, 83, 90, 101, 104, 116, 117, 119, 126, 127, 129, 137, 138, 139, 405, 406, 408, 411, 413
Pizzo, P.A., 135, 140, 268, 282, 468, 483, 545, 557, 571, 581, 625, 632
Pizzo, S.V., 240, 249
Plata, F., 428, 435
Plattner, S.B., 25, 26, 27, 30, 31, 35, 37, 39, 92, 103
Platz, P., 143, 146, 150, 269, 272, 274, 279, 283, 284

Playfair, J.H.L., 299, *311*
Plorde, J.J., 404, *413*
Plouffe, J.F., 624, *631*
Pluda, J.M., 168, 173, *177*, *178*, 373, *378*
Poblete, R.B., 363, *377*
Pocidalo, J.J., 258, *264*, 512, *541*
Poelma, F.G., 202, *219*
Pogue, C.L., 115, *119*, 193, 194, 195, 210, *218*, *221*, 226, 233, *234*, 268, 269, 273, 274, 275, 276, 278, 279, *283*, *285*, *286*, 291, *307*, 641, 642, *646–47*
Pohle, H.D., 448, *463*, 598, *602*
Poirot, J.L., 410, *413*
Poisson, M., 448, *463*
Poletti, V., 299, *312*
Polis, M., 334, 335, *352*, 610, 611, *613*
Polk, B.F., 334, *352*
Pollack, H., 323, *328*, 459, *466*
Pomeranz, S., 416, *432*
Pomponi, C., 155, *175*
Ponticas, S., 623, *631*
Poplin, E.A., 333, *351*
Poppie, M.J., 208, *221*
Poretz, D.M., 363, *376*
Porter, R.J., 111, *118*
Porter, T., 239, *248*
Post, C., 130, *139*, 272, *284*, 422, 423, *434*
Postic, B., 160, *176*
Postma, E., 48, *66*
Potasman, I., 268, *282*, 333, *351*
Pottage, J.C., Jr., 336, 338, 340, 341, *353*, 621, *630*
Potter, D., 381, 385, *395*
Pottratz, S.T., 6, 11, *23*, 114, *119*, 182, *216*, 241–43, 245, *249*, *250*, 252, *262*, 296, 297, 304, *309*, 489, *507*
Poulsen, A.G., 143, 146, *150*, 269, 272, 274, 279, *283*
Powell, R.D., Jr., 185, 187, 188, 189, 190, 191, 194, *217*, 253, 255, *263*, 276, *285*, 517, *542*
Powles, M.A., 62, 63, *71*, 189, 190, 215, *217*, 255, *263*, 512, 534, *541*, 619, 620, 621, 623, 624, *629*, *630*, *631*
Powles, R.L., 333, *351*
Prakash, U.B.S., 169, *179*, 333, *351*
Pratt, C., 349, *359*, 552, *559*
Praz, J.O., 160, *176*
Prezant, D., 385, *398*
Price, R.A., 26, *41*, 182, *216*, 267, 272, 276, *281*, *284*, 290, *307*, 332, 333, 336, *350*, 411, *414*, 423, *434*
Proctor, R.A., 238, 241, *247*
Puchtler, H., 59, 63, *71*
Puckett, J., 623, *631*
Pudney, M., 47, *65*, 447, *463*, 482, *485*, 495, *508*, 512, *541*, 603, 604, 605, *612–13*
Pujol, J.L., 334, *352*
Pulliam, L., 390, 391, *398*
Pursey, B.A., 102, *104*
Puvanesarajah, V., 58, 59, *70*, 618, *628*
Pytela, R., 238, *247*

Q

Queener, S.F., 4, 5, 7, 8, 9, 19, *22*, *24*, 26, 27, 30, *41*, 51, 52, 53, 55, 59, 63, *68*, *69*, *71*, 191, 193, 215, *218*, 252, *261*, 448, *463*, 481, 482, *485*, 488, 489, 492, 494, 495, 496, 499, 501, *506*, *507*, *508*, *509*, 512, 514, 540, *541*, 542, 555, *560*, 567, *580–81*, 585, 586, 587, 588, 589, 590, 592, 594, 595, 597, *600*, *601*
Quigley, D.R., 618, *628*
Quigley, M.J., 162, *178*
Quinn, B.D., 363, *377*
Quinn, T.C., 144, 148, *151*

R

Rabinowitz, J.G., 416, *432*
Rachlis, A., 563, *580*
Rackow, E.C., 348, *358*
Radding, J.A., 6, 16, 19, 20, 21, *23*, *24*, 29, *43*, 52, 53, 54, 55, 59, 63, 64, *69*, *71*, 108, 111, *118*, 243, *249*, 296, 304, *310*
Rademacher, J.M., 299, *311*

Radin, D.R., 363, 371, *378*
Radio, S.J., 173, *180*
Rafdin, J.I., 239, *248*
Raffeld, M., 168, 173, *178*
Raffin, T.A., 349, *359*
Ragan, M.A., 101, *104*
Ragh, G., 333, *351*, 393, *399*
Ragni, M.V., 363, *378*
Rahal, J.J., 642, *646–47*
Rahimi, S.A., 361, 363, *376*
Rainer, C.A., 343, *356*
Raise, E., 299, *312*
Rajewsky, K., 229, *234*
Ramgopal, M., 102, *104*
Ramos, C., 155, *174*, 332, *350*
Randall, A.W., 603, *612*
Rankin, E.M., 26, 30, 35, 37, *41*
Rankin, J.A., 184, *217*, 302, *313*, 635, *646*
Ransburg, N.J., 621, *630*
Rao, C.P., 267, *282*, 290, *306*
Rao, N.A., 160, 173, *176*, 363, *377*
Rao, N.V., 643, *646–47*
Rapaport, D.M., 348, *358*, 634, *644*
Rappaport, A., 343, 349, *356–57*
Rasmussen, E.F., 361, 363, *375*
Rasmussen, P., 173, *179*, 363, *376*
Ratnam, S., 98, *104*
Rattan, S.I.S., 100, *104*
Ravalli, S., 173, *179*
Ravdin, J.I., 238, 239, *247*, *249*
Raviglione, M.C., 163, *178*, 294, *309*, 326, *329*, 362, 363, 365, *376*, *377*, 393, *400*
Rawson, P.G., *139–40*, 267, *282*, 321, *328*, 332, 333, 336, 337, *350*, 361, *376*, 381, *395*, 571, *581*
Reach, G., 571, *581*
Read, G.W., 305, *315*
Read, J.A., 143, 146, *150*, 275, *285*
Reamer, R.A., 623, *630*
Rebhun, S., 298, *310*
Rebuck, A.J., 302, *313*, 635, *646*
Receveur, M.-C., 347, *358*
Reddy, G.C.S., 615, *626*
Reddy, K.R., 363, *377*

Reddy, V.V., 512, *540*, 561, 563, 565, 567, 571, 573, 575, *579*, *580*
Redington, T.J., 182, 183, 184, *216*, 276, *285–86*, 290, *307*
Reed, C., 204, *220*
Reede, D.L., 428, *435*
Rees, A.J., 333, *351*, 374
Rehg, J.E., 202, *220*, 290, *306*
Reid, W.A., Jr., 529, *543*
Reidy, J.F., 416, 417, *432*
Reiss, E., 63, *71*
Reiss, T.F., 394, *400*
Remington, J.M., 268, *282*, 333, *351*, 442, 447, *461*, *463*, 586, *601*
Rennzi, P., 563, *580*
Reynolds, H.Y., 184, *217*, 383, 389, *397*
Reynolds, R.C., 240, *249*
Rhodes, J., 13, *23*, 27, 38, *42*
Rice, W., 259
Rice-Ficht, A., 303, *314*
Richards, F.F., 4, 5, 6, 7, 9, 14, 16, 18, 19, 20, 21, *22*, *23*, *24*, 29, *43*, 49, 50, 52, 53, 54, 55, 59, 63, 64, *66*, 69, *71*, 73, 74, 78, *89*, 108, 111, 114, *118*, *119*, 182, 185, 186, *216*, 243, 245, *249*, 250, 252, 259, *262*, *265*, 280, *286*, 294, 296, 304, *309*, *310*, 488, *506*
Richardson, C.J., 471, *483*
Richardson, J.D., 19, *24*, 26, 27, 30, *41*, 448, *463*, 481, *485*, 512, *541*, 585, 586, 588, 589, 592, *601*
Richart, C., 173, *180*
Richerson, H.B., 443, *462*
Richey, C.S., 26, 27, 29, 30, 34, 37, 38, *42*
Richie, T.L., 363, *377*
Richman, D.D., 302, *313*, 338, 339, 342, 345, 347, *354*, *355*
Richter, C.B., 208, *221*
Richter, W.J., 615, 616, *626*, *627*
Rifkin, M., 373, *378*, 411, *413*
Rifkind, D., 635, *646*
Rigaud, M., 323, *328*, 459, *466*
Riis, B., 100, *104*

Rinaldo, C., 323, *328*, 334, 335, *352*, 393, *399*
Riou, G., 573, 575, *582*
Rippon, J.W., 93, 94, *103*
Ripps, C.S., 340, *355*
Ristic, M., 299, *311*
Rivera, G.K., 451, *464*
Rizvi, F.S., 239, *248*
Road, J.D., 163, *178*
Robbins, J.B., 332, *350*
Robbins, J.F., 267, *281*
Robboy, S.J., 155, *175*
Roberts, D.D., 237–38, *247*, 303, *314*
Robeson, W.A., 339, 340, *355*
Robey, S.S., 155, *175*
Robinson, H.A., 423, 430, *434*
Robinson, J.J., 126, *138*, 334, *352*
Robinson, M.K., 391, *399*
Roca, A.N., 155, *174*
Rockstroh, J., 363, 372, *378*
Rodman, J.S., 240, *249*
Rodriguez, C.H., 302, *313*
Rodriguez, J.L., 160, *177*, 393, *400*, 416, 419, 425, *432*
Rodriguez, K., 363, *377*
Rodriguez, R.J., 102, *105*
Rogers, D.M., 604, 606, 607, 609, 610, *612*
Rogers, G.N., 239, *248*
Rogers, M., 610, 611, *613*
Rogers, M.D., 47, 52, *65*
Rogers, M.E., 16, 20, 21, *24*, 29, *43*, 59, 63, *71*
Rogers, P.L., 348, *359*
Rogers, R.M., 303, *314*
Rogers, T.S., 183, *216*
Rogers, W., 338, 342, 347, *354*
Rohde, I., 448, *463*, 598, *602*
Rollinghoff, M., 268, *282*
Romancheck, M.A., 59, 62, *71*, 255, *263*, 304, *314*, 495, *508*, 512, 534, *541*, 618, 619, 620, *628*
Romanelli, A., 420, *433*
Romano, P.A., 155, *176*, 339, 340, *355*
Romeu, J., 457, *466*
Römmele, G., 618, *627*

Ron, Y., 229, *234*
Ronco, J.J., 348, *358*
Rondanelli, E.G., 26, 27, 35, *40*
Roodman, S.T., 267, *281*, 332, 333, 334, 336, *350*
Rook, G.A.W., 299, *311*
Rorat, E., 155, *176*
Rosado, R., 205, *220*
Rose, A.G., 422, *434*
Rose, R.M., 4, 5, 6, 7, 9, 14, 16, 18, 20, *22*, *23*, 114, *119*, 245, *250*, 252, 258, 259, 260, *262*, *264*, *265*, 280, *286*, 294, 302, 304, *309*, 488, *506*
Rosen, M.J., 155, *174*, *175*, 341, 347, *356*, *358*, 416, 428, *432*, *435*, 634, *644*
Rosen, P.P., 124, 134, *137*, *140*, 149, *151*, 155, *174*, 187, 191, 194, *217*, 229, *234*, 252, *261*, 276, *286*, 290, 291, *306*, 332, 336, *350*, *353*, 416, 428, *432*, 635, *646*
Rosenbaum, D., 604, 606, 607, 609, 610, *612*
Rosenberg, Z.F., 21, *24*, 512, *541*
Rosenblatt, M.A., 173, *180*
Rosenblum, M., 173, *179*, 363, 371, 376, *377–78*
Rosenkrans, W.A., 241, *249*
Rosenkvist, J., 280, *286–87*, 293, *308*
Rosenstreich, D.L., 230, *235*
Rosenthal, G.J., 571, *582*
Rosowsky, A., 585, 586, *601*
Ross, C., 381, 391, *396*
Rossert, J., 635, *646*
Rossi, J.F., 361, 363, *376*, *378*
Rosso, J., 428, *435*
Roth, D.B., 155, *174*
Rothenberg, R., 344, *357*
Roths, J.B., 195, 196, 197, 198, *218*, *219*, 223, 224, 225, 226, 227, 229, 231, 232, 233, *233–34*, *235*, 253, 255, 261, *263*, 268, 272, 273, 278, *283*, 634, *645*
Rotstein, L., 173, *179*
Roux, P., 410, *413*
Roy, K., 615, *626*

Roy, T.M., 348, *359*
Ruben, F.L., 169, 170, *178–79*
Rubies-Prat, J., 341, *356*
Rubin, E., 155, *176*, 381, 382, *395*
Rubin, R.H., 430, *435*, 442, *461*
Rubinstein, A., 327, *328*
Rubinstein, B.E., 643, *648*
Ruebush, T.K., 135, *140*, 149, *151*, 488, 507, 585, *600*
Ruedy, J., 302, *313*, 346, 347, 348, *357*, *358*, 633, 634, 635, 637, 642, 643, *644*, *646*
Ruf, B., 448, *463*, 598, *602*
Ruffolo, J.J., 4, 5, 7, 9, 13, *22*, *23*, 25, 26, 27, 29, 30, 31, 34, 35, 36, 37, 38, *39*, *40*, 123, 131, *137*, *139*
Rummage, J.A., 299, *311*
Ruoslahti, E., 238, 241, *247*, *249*
Rush, J., 338, *354*
Ruskin, J., 276, *285*, 338, *354*, 440, 441, 442, 443, 452, 455, *461*, *465*, 468, 469, 470, 473, 474, *483*, 633, *644*
Russell, J.A., 346, 347, 348, *357*, *358*, 635, *646*
Russell, R.J., 184, 185, 186, *217*
Russi, E.W., 338, 340, 341, *355*
Russi, M.B., 302, *313*, 348, *358*
Russo-Marie, F., 299, *311*
Rutledge, M.E., 111, *118*, 185, 187, 188, 189, 190, 210, *217*, *221*, 230, *235*, 253, *263*, 269, 270, 272, 276, *283*, *284*, *285*, 517, *542*
Rutstein, R.M., 297, *310*, 387, *398*
Ruttimann, S., 349, *359*
Ryder, L.P., 143, 146, *150*, 269, 272, 274, 279, *283*, *284*
Ryo, U., 427, 428, *435*

S

Saah, A., 131, *140*, 323, *328*, 334, 335, *352*, 393, *399*
Safirstein, B.H., 347, *357*
Safrin, S., 362, 371, *376*, 444, 456, *462*, *465*, 479, *484*, *559*, 611, *613*

Sahar, E., 238, *248*
Sahebjami, H., 301, *312*
Sai, P., 571, *581*
Saiki, R.K., 404, *413*
Saimot, A., 290, *307*
Saito, T., 616–17, *627*
Sakaitani, M., 615, *627*
Salas, M., 290, 301, *307*
Saldana, M.A., 326, *329*, 387, *398*
Saldana, M.J., 155, 160, 161, 171, 172, 173, *175*, *177*, *179*, 363, 373, *377*, *378*, 393, *400*, 416, 419, 425, *432*
Sale, G.E., 381, 382, 389, *396*
Saleba, K.P., 384, 389, *397*
Salit, I.E., 635, 639, *646*
Salmeron, S., 441, *461*
Salmon, P., 619, *629*
Salvador, R.A., 638, *646*
Sampalo, M.C., 603, *612*
Sampson, J., 611, *613*
Sanchez, E., 238, *247*
Sanchez Molini, P., 347, *358*
Sanders, R.C., 427, *434*
Sanders-Laufer, D., *328–29*
Sandhu, J.S., 373, *378*, 634, *644*
Sandler, M.A., 160, *177*
Sands, M., 569, 571, *581*
Sandstrom, E., 553, *559*
Sanger, J.J., 428, *435*
Sankary, R.M., 258, *264*
Sansom, C.E., 571, *581*
Santi, D.V., 25, *39*, 49, 50, 51, *67*, 73, 74, 78, 81, 83, 84, *89*, *90*, 91, 95, 98, 99, *103*, *104*, 129, *138*, 155, *175*, 305, *315*, 408, *413*, 448, *463*, 514, *542*, 549, *558*, 618, *628*
Santoro, F., 239, *248*
Santos, I., 347, *358*
Sanyal, S.K., 51, *68*, 427, 428, *435*, 552, *559*
Sargeant, T., 259, *264–65*
Sargent, E.N., 428, *435*
Saric, M., 49, *66*, 512, *541*
Sarov, I., 305, *315*
Sastry, K., 114, *119*
Sati, M.H., 561, *578*

Author Index

Satoi, S., 615, *626*, *627*
Sattler, F.R., 302, *313*, 338, 339, 342, 347, *354*, *355*, 440, 441, 442, 443, 444, 446, 447, *461*, *462*–*63*, 468, 469, 470, 473, 474, 475, 479, 481, 482, *483*, *484*, *485*, 556, *559*, *560*, 598, *601*–*2*, 611, *613*, *633*–38, 642, 643, *644*, *646*
Sauderer, M., 113, *118*, 274, 278, *285*, 296, 297, *309*
Saulsbury, F.T., 267, *282*
Savitch, 468, *483*
Sawchuk, R., 471, *484*
Sawicki, W.L., 555, *559*, *560*
Saxon, A., 92, *103*, 268, *282*, 332, *350*
Scaife, J.G., 514, *542*, 548, *558*
Scannel, K.A., 347, *358*
Schaeffer, A., 239, *248*
Schaller, M.D., 348, *359*
Schanker, H.M., 92, *103*, 268, *282*, 332, *350*
Scharyj, M., 161, 163, *177*, 418, *433*
Schechter, M.T., 302, *313*, 633, 634, 637, 642, 643, *644*
Schein, R.M., 347, *358*
Schell, M.J., 451, *464*
Schiff, M.J., 302, *313*
Schiff, R.G., 422, 423, *434*
Schilling, J., 259, *264*
Schinella, R.A., 165, 168, *178*, 363, *376*, *377*
Schirmer, J.P., 603, *612*
Schlech, W., 563, *580*
Schlesinger, P.H., 240, *249*
Schluger, N., 373, *378*, 411, *413*
Schmatz, D.M., 59, 62, 63, *71*, 189, 190, 215, *217*, 255, *263*, 304, *314*, 495, *508*, 512, 534, *541*, 616, 618, 619, 620, 621, 622, 623, 624, *627*, *628*, *629*, *630*, *631*
Schmid, A., 27, 29, 31, 34, *42*
Schmidt, D.M., 163, *178*
Schmidt, L.H., 586, *601*
Schneerson, R., 332, *350*
Schneider, D.J., 205, 206, *220*
Schnell, V., 124, *137*, 187, 191, 194,

[Schnell, V.]
217, 229, *234*, 252, *261*, 276, *286*, 290, 291, *306*
Schnur, L.F., 573, *582*
Schoenbach, E.B., 571, 573, *581*–*82*
Schonland, M., 182, *216*, 267, 276, *281*, 290, *307*, 332, 333, 336, *350*
Schottenfeld, D., 149, *151*, 336, *353*
Schrager, L.K., 3, 4, *22*, 131, *140*, 215, *222*
Schraufnagel, D.E., 27, 29, 31, 34, *42*
Schreiber, R.D., 302, *313*
Schroff, R., 92, *103*, 268, *282*, 332, *350*
Schroy, P.C., 290, *307*
Schulman, E.S., 393, *400*
Schultz, J.A., 51, *68*, 182́, 183, 202, 203, 210, *216*, 224, *234*, 252, 253, *262*, 276, *285*, 290, *306*, 487, 495, 501, *506*, 512, *539*, 551, *559*, 563, 565, *580*, 585, *601*
Schultz, L.D., 195, *219*
Schultz, M.G., 135, *139*–*40*, 149, *151*, 267, *281*, *282*, 321, *328*, 332, 333, 336, 337, *350*, *351*, 361, *376*, 381, *395*, 440, 441, *460*, 488, *507*, 571, *581*, 585, *600*
Schumann, G.B., 389, 390, 391, *398*
Schumitzky, A., 471, *483*
Schupp, D.G., 14, *24*
Schved, J.F., 363, *378*
Schwalbe, C.H., 571, *581*
Schwartz, A.D., 160, *176*, 416, 420, *432*
Schwartz, D.A., 26, 27, 30, 34, *40*
Schwartz, J., 361, 363, *375*
Schwartz, R.E., 59, 62, *71*, 304, *314*, 495, *508*, 512, 534, *541*, 615, 616, 618, 619, 620, 621, 623, *626*, *627*, *628*, *629*, *630*, *631*
Schwarz, L., 238, *247*
Schwarz, M.I., 425, 431, *434*
Schwarzmann, S.W., 563, *580*
Schweinle, J.E., 294, *309*
Scott, G., *328*
Scott, W.T., 102, *104*

Scott, W.W., 393, *400*
Scully, C., 616, *627*
Sedaghatian, M.R., 126, *138*
Seevi, A., 333, *351*, 421, *433*, 451, *464*
Segal, E., 238, *248*
Segal, S., 229, *234*
Seigel, R., 431, *435*
Seitz, H.M., 201, *219*
Sekerak, G.F., 173, *179*, 625, *632*
Sekula, B.C., 102, *105*
Self, A., 561, *578*
Seligman, B.E., 293, *308*
Selik, R.M., 361, *375*
Selinger, D.S., 303, *314*
Selitrennikoff, C.P., 618, *628*
Selvaggi, S.M., 155, *175*
Selwyn, P.A., 642, *646–47*
Seman, M., 25, 26, 30, 31, 37, *39*
Semenzato, G., 299, *312*
Semple, S.J.G., 338, *354*, 382, *396*
Sender, J.A., 332, *350*
Sepkowitz, K.A., 336, 341, 347, *353*, 362, 373, 374, *376*, *378*, 384, 394, *397*, 411, *413*
Seru, V., 338, *354*
Sesin, D.F., 619, *629*
Sethi, K.K., 191, 199, *219*
Setia, U., 332, *350*
Settnes, O.P., 126, 127, 130, 137, *138*, *139*, 155, *174*, 183, 204, 205, 210, 212, *216*, *220*, *222*
Seymour, J., 577, *583*
Shah, B., 173, *179*
Shands, J.W., 442, *462*
Shane, L.B., 428, *435*
Shanley, D.J., 347, *358*
Shanley, J.D., 59, 60, 63, *71*, 108, 114, *118*, 296, 304, *309*
Shannon, B.J., 299, *311*
Shapiro, B.A., 348, *358*
Shapiro, H.M., 21, *24*
Shapiro, T.A., 573, 575, *582*
Shapiro, T.B., 482, *485*
Sharon, N., 239, *248*
Sharp, A.K., 299, *311*
Sharp, G.C., 50, *69*

Shaw, M.M., 4, 5, 7, 8, 9, 19, *22*, 52, 56, *69*, *70*, 191, 193, *218*, 305, *315*, 488, 489, 501, *507*, *509*, 587, 588, *601*
Shear, H.L., 300, *312*, 512, *541–42*, 643, *648*
Sheehan, P.M., 114, *119*, 258, 259, *264*, 302, 304, *313*, 643, *646–47*
Sheetz, C.T., 621, *630*
Sheffers, A., 73, 74, 78, *89*
Shein, R., 173, *179*
Sheldon, W.H., 181, 182, 191, 203, *216*, 290, *306*
Shelhamer, J.H., 155, 171, 172, *174*, *179*, 258, 260, *264*, *265*, 290, *306–7*, 334, 335, 338, 339, 341, 343, 344, *352*, *354*, *357*, 391, 392, *399*, 416, 428, *432*, *435*, 468, 469, *483*, 545, 555, *557*, *560*, 571, *581*
Shellito, J.E., 199, 200, *219*, 253, 261, 262, *265*, 268, 278, *283*, 300, *312*, 503, *509*, 634, *645*
Shenep, J.L., 387, *398*, 482, *485*, 604, 606, 607, 609, 610, *612*
Sheperd, V., 142, 146, *150*, 274, *285*
Sheppard, D., 381, 382, *395*
Sherman, M., 293, 299, *308*, 347, *358*, 384, 394, *397*, 419, 420, 427, *433*
Shermer-Avni, Y., 305, *315*
Sherwood, J.A., 237–38, *247*
Sheth, S., 427, *434*
Shimada, K., 143, *151*, 201, *219*, 411, *413*
Shimada, Y., 207, *221*
Shiota, T., 26, 27, 30, 34, 35, 36, *40*, 173, *179–80*, 202, 207, *219*, *221*, 363, *377*, 512, *540*
Shively, J.N., 26, *41*, 207, 210, *221*, *222*
Shlesinger, P.H., 239, *249*
Shramkoski, R.M., 56, *70*
Shukla, O., 561, *578*
Shultz, L.D., 188, 193, 194, 195, 210, *217*, *218*, *221*, 226, 229, 233, *234*, 273, 274, 276, *285*, *286*
Shumitzky, A., 471, *483–84*

Sidhu, G., 172, *179*, 635, 642, *646*
Sidman, C.L., *188*, 194, 195, 196, 197, 198, *217*, *218*, *219*, 223, 224, 225, 226, 227, 229, 231, 232, 233, *233– 34*, *235*, 253, 255, 261, *263*, 268, 272, 273, 278, *283*, 634, *645*
Sieben, M., 125, *138*, 142, 146, *150*, 252, *262*, 269, 274, 279, *283*, 320, *328*, 345, *357*
Sieber, S.C., 290, 301, *307*
Siebken, R.S., 332, *350*
Siegel, B., 385, *397*
Siegel, F.P., 332, *350*, 363, *377*
Siegel, S.E., 440, 441, 442, *461*
Siegelman, S.S., 373, *378*, 418, 419, 423, 424, 425, *433*
Siemsen, J.K., 428, *435*
Sierra, L.S., 390, *398*
Sigal, C.W., 555, *560*
Sigel, C., 555, *560*
Silverblatt, F., 239, *248*
Simberkoff, M.S., 338, 348, *354*, 449, *464*
Siminski, J., 393, *399*
Simmer, K., 272, 281, *284*
Simmons, J.T., 258, *264*, 334, 338, 339, 341, 344, *352*, *354*, 469, *483*, 555, *560*
Simon, G.L., 226, *234*, 394, *400*, 428, *435*, 442, *461–62*, 468, *483*, 545, 557, 563, *579*
Simon, H.B., 290, 295, *306*
Simone, J.V., 451, *464*
Simoni, L., 349, *359*
Simons, J.T., 428, *435*
Simpson, W.A., 238, *247*
Sinclair, K., 47, 49, 50, *65–66*, 83, *90*, 116, 117, *119*, 126, 127, 130, 137, *138*, *139*, 405, 406, 408, 411, *413*, *414*
Singer, C., 134, *140*, 149, *151*, 336, 353, 635, *646*
Singer, D.B., 126, *138*, 240, *249*
Singer, F., 341, *356*
Singer, M., 299, *311*
Singer, P., 349, *359*

Sinson, E.B., 268, *282*, 333, *351*
Sippel, H., 572, *582*
Siracusano, A., 299, *312*
Siratonak, F.M., 546, *557*
Sirera, G., 457, *466*
Sisko, F., 182, *216*, 267, 276, *281*, 290, *307*, 332, 333, 336, *350*
Sjoerdsma, A., 305, *315*, 448, *463*
Skolnick, M.L., 363, *378*
Skolom, J., 155, *176*
Skoutelis, A., 348, *358*
Skuza, C., 323, *328*
Slade, B.A., 382, *396–97*
Slade, J.D., 268, *282*
Sleight, P., 641, *646*
Sleight, R.G., 26, 27, 34, *40*, 56, 59, 62, *70*
Slemenda, S.B., 107, *118*, 142, 143, 147, *150*, 269, 274, 279, *283*, 345, *357*, 382, *396*
Sloan, D., 52, *68*, 514, *542*, 548, 552, *558*
Sloande, E.E., 4, 7, 20, *22*, 488, *506*
Slomianny, C., 26, 27, 30, 31, 34, 37, *41*, 46, 47, 53, 59, 60, 62, 63, *65*, *70*
Sluiters, J.F., 258, 259, 261, *264*, 348, *358*
Smaldone, G.C., 341, *356*, 577, *583*, 625, *632*
Smiddy, J.F., 383, *397*
Smith, A.B., 182, 185, 186, 197, *216*, *219*, 231, 232, *235*
Smith, B.L., 182, *216*, 276, *285*, 301, 305, *312*, *315*, *508*, 512, *539*, *540*, 552, 554, *559*, 586, *601*
Smith, B.M., 124, *138*
Smith, D.E., 338, *354*, 448, *463*, 464
Smith, D.M., 173, *179*
Smith, H.G., 299, *311*
Smith, J., 26, 27, 30, *41*
Smith, J.L., Jr., 155, *174*
Smith, J.S., 4, 5, 7, 8, 9, 13, 19, *22*, 24, 26, 27, 34, 36, *40*, 48, 49, 51, 52, 53, 55, 56, 59, 63, *66*, 67, 68, 69, *70*, *71*, 83, *90*, 114, *119*, 191,

[Smith, J.S.]
193, 215, *218*, 240, 243, *249*, 252, 261, *262*, 273, 274, *285*, 296, 297, 303, 304, 305, *309*, *315*, 448, *463*, 481, *485*, 488, 489, 492, 494, 495, 496, 499, 501, *506*, *507*, *508*, *509*, 512, 514, *540*, *541*, *542*, 550, 552, 555, *558*, *560*, 563, 564, 567, *580–81*, 585, 586, 587, 588, 589, 590, 592, 594, 595, 597, *600*, *601*
Smith, K.E., 48, *66*
Smith, L.J., 301, *312*
Smith, M.A., 363, *377*
Smith, P.D., 428, *435*
Smith, P.L., 623, *631*
Smith, R.D., 239, *249*
Smith, R.L., 238, 241, *248*, 281, *287*, 338, 340, 341, *354*, *355*, *356*, 391, *399*, 634, *645*
Smith, R.M., 443, *462*, 634, *645*
Smith, S.M., 162, *178*, 347, *357*, 425, *434*, 634, *645*
Smith, T.F., 281, *287*, 337, 341, 347, *354*, 389, *398*
Smith-McCain, B.L., 512, *540*, 553, *559*
Smithson, J., 448, *464*
Smulian, A.G., 47, 52, 53, *65*, *69*, *70*, 75, 81, 83, *89*, *90*, 115, 117, *119*, 129, 130, 137, *139*, 144, 147, 148, *151*, 192, 212, *218*, 252, *262*, 268, 269, 273, 274, 275, 278, *283*, 382, *396*, 641, 642, *646–47*
Smythe, P.M., 182, *216*, 267, 276, *281*, 290, *307*, 332, 333, 336, *350*
Sneed, S.R., 363, *377*
Snellgrove, R.L., 202, *220*, 290, *306*
Snider, G.L., 383, *397*
Sniezek, M.J., 200, *219*, 261, *265*
Snodgrass, W., 471, *483*
So, L.T., 623, *630*
Sobel, A., 340, *355*
Sogin, M.L., 25, *39*, 49, 50, *67*, 78, 83, 84, *89*, *90*, 91, 95, 96, *103*, *105*, 129, *138*, 155, *175*, 408, *413*, 618, *628*
Sohn, M., 161, *177*, 347, *357*, 634, *645*

Solleveld, H.A., 193, 194, 201, *218*
Solomon, D., 163, *178*
Solomon, R.E., 334, *352*
Soo Hoo, G.W., 446, *462*, 476, *484*
Sorenson, A.W.S., 361, 363, *375*
Sorice, M., 55, 56, 58, *70*, 115, 116, *119*, 341, *356*
Sosa, R., 322, *328*
Soulez, B., 26, 27, 30, 31, 34, 37, *40*, *41*, 46, 47, 53, 59, 60, 62, 63, *65*, *70*, 124, *138*, 203, *220*, 293, *308*
South, M.A., 280, *286*
Spain, J.A., 512, 527, *539*
Sparling, T.G., 363, *377*
Sparrow, S., 201, *219*
Spaulding, D.M., 512, 527, *539*
Spear, J., 336, 338, 340, 341, *353*
Spector, S.A., 338, 345, *354*
Speich, R., 338, 340, 341, *355*
Speights, J.W., 363, *377*
Spence, D., 639, *646*
Speziale, P., 238, *247*
Spickett, G.P., 297, *310*
Spiga, L., 299, *312*
Spitalnik, S.L., 237–38, *247*
Spouge, A.R., 419, 427, *433*
Spragg, R.G., 634, *645*
Spring, C.L., 642, *646–47*
Srimal, S., 238, *247*
Srinivasan, V., 529, *543*
Staben, C., 577, *583*
Stadhouders, A.M., 25, 26, 27, 30, 34, 35, 37, *39*, *40*, *42*, 123, *137*
Stagno, S., 126, *138*, 142, 146, *150*, 252, *262*, 269, 274, 279, *283*, 293, *308*, 320, *328*, 345, *357*, 382, *396*
Stahl, P.D., 240, *249*
Stammers, D.K., 514, *542*, 548, *558*
Staneck, J., 392, *399*
Stanforth, D., 19, *24*, 113, 115, *119*, 253, *263*, 270, 273, 274, *284*, 305, *315*, 514, 516, 517, 518, 534, *542–43*, 550, 552, *558*
Stanislawski, L., 238, *247*
Stankiewicz, M., 198, *219*, 253, *263*, 268, 270, 272, 278, *283*, 302, *313*

Starcher, E.T., 361, *375*
Stark, T., 618, *628*
Starzl, T.E., 635, *646*
Staugas, R.E.M., 272, 281, *284*
Steele, P.E., 7, *23*, 49, 50, *66*, 75, 77, 78, 84, *89*, 192, 210, 212, *218*, 222, 231, *235*, 512, 519, 523, 526, 527, 528, 529, 530, 531, 532, 533, *540*, *543*
Steensma, H.Y., 73, 74, 78, *89*
Steger, H.J., 200, *219*, 253, *262*, 268, 278, *283*, 503, *509*, 634, *645*
Stehr-Green, J.K., 473, *484*, 571, *581*
Steigbigel, R.T., 341, *356*, 373, *378*, 416, 418, *432*
Steigmsn, C.K., 363, *376*
Stein, D.S., 452, *464–65*, 604, 606, 607, 609, 610, *612*
Steinmann, U., 572, *582*
Steiss, R., 290, *306–7*, 343, *357*
Stellbrinck, K.H., 135, *140*, 336, *353*
Stenson, W.M., 348, *358*, 634, *644*
Stephens, R., 571, *581*
Stern, R.G., 423, *434*
Stern, W., 419, 425, *433*
Stevens, D.A., 615, 625, *627*, *632*
Stevens, M.F.G., 571, *581*
Stevens, R.C., 452, *464–65*
Stewart, S., 420, 421, *433*
Stewart, T.J., 143, 147, *150*
Stille, W., 616, *627*
Stiller, R.A., 125, 127, 128, 130, 136, 137, *138*
Stock, F., 49, *68*, 115, *119*
Stoeckle, M.Y., 173, *179*, 326, *329*, 362, *376*
Stoffel, 404, *413*
Stokes, D.C., 49, 59, 67, 108, 110, 114, *118*, *119*, 202, *220*, 258, 259, *264*, 290, 302, 304, *306*, *313*, 387, *398*, 428, *435*, 643, *646–47*
Stokes, J.B., 621, *630*
Stone, D.J., 172, *179*, 341, *355*, 373, *378*, 393, *400*, 416, 419, 425, 431, *432*, *435*
Stoneburner, R., 344, *357*

Stookey, J.L., 209, *221*
Stoppani, A.O.M., 603, *612*
Stouwe, R.A.V., 268, *282*, 332, 336, *350*
Stover, D.A., 155, 161, *176*, *177*, 259, 265, 333, 339, 340, *351*, *355*, 373, *378*, 381, 384, 385, 392, 394, *395*, 397, *400*, 416, *432*, 456, *465*, 468, *483*, 545, *557*, 571, *581*
Stratton, N., 390, 391, *398*
Straubinger, R.M., 495, *508*, 512, *540*, 563, *579*, 625, *631*
Strauss, H.W., 430, *435*
Strigle, S.M., 155, 163, *175*, *178*, 381, 384, 391, *395*, *396*
Stringer, J.R., 7, *23*, 25, 26, 27, 30, 31, 35, 37, *39*, 48, 49, 50, 52, 53, 55, *66*, *67*, *69*, *70*, 75, 77, 78, 80, 81, 83, 84, *89*, *90*, 91, 95, *103*, 115, 117, *119*, 125, 127, 129, 130, 136, 137, *138*, *139*, *140*, 148, *151*, 192, 193, 210, 212, 213, *218*, 222, 231, *235*, 255, *263*, 408, *413*, 618, *628*
Stringer, S.L., 7, *23*, 25, *39*, 49, 50, 53, *66*, *67*, *70*, 75, 77, 78, 80, 84, *89*, 91, 95, *103*, 129, 130, 137, *139*, *140*, 192, 210, 212, *218*, 222, 231, *235*, 408, *413*, 618, *628*
Strohofer, S.S., 381, 389, 390, 391, 392, *396*, *398*
Strumpf, J.J., 383, *397*
Stubberfield, C.R., 53, 55, *69*, 495, *508*
Stulbarg, M.S., 381, 383, 384, 392, 394, *395*, *397*, *400*, 416, *432*
Styer, C.M., 343, 349, *357*
Su, T.H., 258, 259, *264*
Suarez, M., 160, *177*, 393, *400*, 416, 419, 425, *432*
Subbarao, K., 419, 425, *433*
Sueishi, K., 26, 27, *41*, 240, *249*
Suffredini, A.F., 155, *174*, 258, 260, *264*, *265*, 268, *282*, 333, 334, 335, 338, 339, 341, 344, *351*, *352*, *354*, 409, *413*, 469, *483*
Sugar, A.M., 290, *307*
Sugar, J., 363, 365, *377*

Sugimoto, M., 292, *308*
Sullivan, D.W., 144, 148, *151*
Sullivan, G.W., 643, *646–47*
Sulzer, A.J., 135, *140*, 149, *151*, 488, *507*, 585, *600*
Sulzer, A.T., 4, 5, *22*
Sumiya, M., 294, *308–9*
Sumiyoshi, A., 26, 27, *41*, 240, *249*
Summerfield, J.A., 294, *308–9*
Summers, Q.A., 160, *176*
Sundberg, R.J., 529, *543*, 575, *582–83*
Sundelof, J.G., 623, *631*
Sundermann, C.A., 561, *578*
Sundstrom, W.R., 333, *351*
Super, M., 294, *308–9*
Suprahmanya, B., 382, *396*
Surkin, B.I., 348, *358*, 634, *644*
Suster, B., 416, 418, 423, 425, *432*
Suzara, V.V., 200, *219*, 253, *262*, 268, 278, *283*, 503, *509*, 634, *645*
Suzuki, J., 209, *221*
Svanborg-Eden, C., 237, 239, *246*, 248
Svejgaard, A., 143, 146, *150*, 269, 272, 274, 279, *283*, 284
Swan, J.C., 46, 47, 49, 51, 53, *65*, *67*, *68*, 108, 114, *118*, 130, *139*, 144, 147, *151*, 273, 274, *285*, 320, *328*, 391, *399*, 495, *508*, 512, 514, *540*, *542*, 549, 555, *558*, 560
Swartz, M., 161, *177*, 347, *357*, 634, *645*
Swartz, M.N., 442, *461*
Swensen, J.J., 389, 390, 391, *398*
Switalski, L.M., 238, *247*
Swofford, D.L., 95, 99, 100, *104*, *105*
Sypek, J.P., 237, 239, *247*
Sypherd, P.S., 100
Szakal, A., 301, *312*
Szaniszlo, P.J., 618, *628*
Szefler, S.J., 290, *307*

T

Tabona, P., 294, *308–9*
Tadao, S., 411, *413*
Taft, C., 618, *628*

Takada, M., 615, *626*
Takasaki, S., 55, 59, 63, 64, *69*, 108, 111, *118*
Takashima, T., 299, *311*
Takeda, Y., 229, *234*
Takeuchi, S., 512, *540*
Takeuchi, T., 51, *68*, 537, *543*
Talamo, T.S., 169, 170, *178–79*
Talavera, W., 341, *356*
Tamaki, K., 290, *307*
Tamburrini, E., 299, *312*
Tamisier, L., 512, *540*, 624, *631*
Tamura, T., 26, 27, 30, 31, *41*
Tan, G., 390, 391, *398*
Tanabe, K., 49, 50, 55, 59, 63, 64, *67*, *69*, 84, *90*, 100, *104*, 108, 111, *118*, 143, *151*, 201, *219*
Tanaka, H., 143, *151*
Tanaka, K., 26, 27, *41*, 240, *249*
Tanker, I., 125, *138*, 142, 146, *150*, 252, *262*, 269, 274, 279, *283*, 320, *328*, 345, *357*
Tapper, Ml., 332, *350*
Tarala, R.A., 160, *176*
Targett, G.A., 299, *311*
Tarone, G., 238, *247*
Tartar, A., 239, *248*
Tashbin, D.P., 419, 420, *433*
Taverne, J., 299, *311*
Taylor, B.C., 303, *313–14*
Taylor, F.R., 102, *105*
Taylor, G.A., 99, *104*
Taylor, M.G., 47, 53, *65*
Taytard, A., 347, *358*
Tegoshi, T., 10, *23*, 25, 26, 27, 29, 34, *39*, *42*, 59, 60, 61, 62, *70*, *71*, 209, *221*, 296, 304, *309*, 363, *377*, 512, *540*, 618, *628*
Teich, S., 173, *180*
Teirstein, A.S., 155, *175*
Telzak, E.E., 173, *179*, 256, *263*, 336, 341, 347, *353*, 362, 363, 371, 374, *376*, *377–78*, 384, 394, *397*
Tenbrinck, R., 258, 259, 261, *264*, 348, *358*
Tennant, B., 207, *221*

Author Index

Tenner, A.J., 294, *309*
Tenover, F.C., 404, *413*
Terry, D., 452, *464–65*
Tewart, T.J., 405, *413*
Thakkar, A.L., 615, 616, *626*
Thebert, P., 634, *645*
Thomas, A.H., 616, *627*
Thomas, E.D., 334, *351–52*, 382, *396*
Thomas, S.F., 164, *178*
Thompson, R., 623, *631*
Thorpe, J.E., 392, *399*
Thorssen, M., 239, *248*
Thurlbeck, W.M., 26, *42*
Tidwell, R.R., 19, *24*, 49, *68*, 448, *463*, 482, *485*, 492, 494, 496, *507*, 512, *540*, *541*, 561, 563, 564, 565, 566, 567, 569, 570, 571, 573, 575, 576, *578*, *579*, *580–81*, 586, 590, 592, 594, *601*
Tierstein, A.S., 341, 347, *356*, *358*
Tiller, R.E., 293, *308*
Tilles, J.G., 302, *313*, 339, 342, 347, *355*
Timerman, A.P., 643, *646–47*
Timms, E.S., 50, *69*
Tiu, S., 428, *435*
Tkacz, J., 618, *628*
Todaro, G., 301, *312*
Tokuomi, H., 292, *308*
Tollerud, D.J., 381, 389, 392, *396*
Toma, E., 448, *463*, 599, *602*
Tomashefski, J.F., Jr., 160, 161, 162, 169, *177*, 419, 425, *433*, 634, *644–45*
Tomford, J.W., 160, 161, 162, 169, *177*, 634, *644–45*
Tomicic, T., 297, 304, *310*
Torres, A., 155, *176*, 381, 382, *395*
Torres, R.A., 336, 338, 340, 341, *353*
Tosch, W., 615, 616, *626*
Tosteson, A.N.A., 563, *579*
Tow, T.W.Y., 155, *175*, 341, *356*
Traber, R., 615, *626*, *627*
Trager, W., 21, *24*
Train, J.S., 416, *432*
Trainor, C., 616, 620, 621, 622, 623, *627*, *629*, *630*, *631*

Tran Van Nhieu, J., 169, 170, *178*
Trats, F., 341, *356*
Travis, W.D., 155, 157, 158, 159, 160, 161, 163, 164, 165, 167, 168, 169, 170, 171, 172, 173, *174*, *177*, *178*, 258, *264*, 334, 335, *352*, 363, *377*, 381, *395*
Traxler, P., 615, 616, *626*, *627*
Treichler, H., 615, *626*
Trelstad, R.I., 638, *646*
Trenholme, G.M., 336, 338, 340, 341, *353*
Trentin, L., 299, *312*
Trento, A., 333, *351*, 421, *433*
Trinh Dinh, H., 25, 26, 30, 31, 37, *39*
Trinkle, L.S., 60, *71*, 182, *216*
Truitt, T., 347, *357*
Truman, B., 344, *357*
Tsai, I., 638, *646*
Tsang, V.C.W., 107, *118*
Tscherter, H., 615, *626*
Tsunoo, H., 411, *413*
Tsuyuguchi, I., 299, *311*
Tuazon, C.U., 155, *176*, 290, *306–7*, 334, 338, 343, *352*, *357*, 390, 394, *398*, *400*, 428, *435*, 446, *462*, 468, *483*, 499, *509*, 555, *560*, 610, 611, *613*
Tuchschmidt, J.A., 336, 341, 342, *353*
Tucker, R.M., 457, *465*
Tucker, W.S., 290, 301, *307*, 333, *351*
Tuite, M.F., 100, *104*
Tunon-de-Lara, J.-M., 347, *358*
Turbiner, E.H., 416, 428, *432*
Turek, J., 13, *23*, 27, 38, *42*
Turner, J., 258, *264*, 347, *358*, 563, *579*, 615, 616, 621, 624, *626*, *629*, *631*, 639, 642, *646–47*
Turner, M.J., 59, 62, *71*, 304, *314*, 495, *508*, 512, 534, *541*, 618, 619, 620, *628*
Turner, M.W., 294, *308–9*
Turton, C., 383, *397*
Tyers, F.O., 347, *358*
Tygstrup, I., 280, *286–87*, 293, *308*

U

Udaka, M., 290, *307*
Ueda, K., 26, 27, 30, 31, *41*, 143, *151*, 193, 194, 201, *218*, *219*, 229, *234*, 270, 272, 276, 278, *284*, *286*
Ueta, C., 299, *311*
Uhlenbruck, G., 245, *250*, 304, *314*
Ukeshima, A., 292, *308*
ul Haque, A., 25, 26, 27, 30, 31, 35, 37, *39*, 92, *103*
Ullu, E., 6, 19, *23*, 49, 50, 52, 53, 54, 55, 59, 64, *66*, *69*, 73, 74, 78, *89*, 108, 111, *118*, 243, *249*, 296, 304, *310*
Ulrich, P., 529, *543*
Unanue, E.R., 302, *313*
Ungar, B.L.P., 298, *310*
Unger, G., 562, *579*
Unger, P.D., 173, *179*, 363, 371, *376*, *377–78*
Upton, R.A., 476, 477, *484*, 569, *581*
Urata, Y., 173, *179–80*, 363, *377*
Urbina, J.A., 94, *103*
Urmacher, C., 468, *483*, 545, *557*, 571, *581*
Uys, C.J., 422, *434*

V

Vachon, F., 342, *356*
Vadas, E., 624, *631*
Vaidya, K.P., 161, *177*, 336, *353*
Valacer, D.J., 290, 295, 302, *306*
Valenski, W.R., 279, *286*
Valenta, J.R., 616, *627*
Valerius, N.H., 280, *286–87*, 293, *308*
Valladares, G., 300, *312*, 512, *541–42*, 643, *648*
van Daal, G.-J., 258, 259, 261, *264*, 348, *358*
Van Dellen, A.F., 495, *508–9*, 512, *539*
van den Akker, S., 205–6, *220*
Van den Bogert, C., 184, *217*
VandenBroek, P.J., 48, *66*
VanDerHeide, T., 390, 391, *398*
Van der Meer, G., 319, *327*, 332, *350*

Vane, R.J., 643, *646–47*
Vanek, J., 4, *22*, 319, *327*, 332, *350*, 487, *506*
Vanhems, P., 133, *140*
van Hooft, J.I.M., 193, 194, 201, *218*
VanLeeuwen, C.C., 48, *66*
Vanley, G.T., 431, *435*
Van Melle, G., 136, *140*, 336, *353*
Van Middlesworth, F.L., 59, 62, *71*, 304, *314*, 495, *508*, 512, 534, *541*, 616, 618, 619, 620, 621, *627*, *628*, *629*, *630*
van Rensburg, I.B., 205, 206, *220*
VanSteveninck, J., 48, *66*
van Zwieter, M.J., 193, 194, 201, *218*
Varma, V.M., 394, *400*, 428, *435*
Varona, R., 618, *628*
Vasconcellos, M.E., 603, *612*
Vassali, P., 299, *311*
Vasudevan, V.P., 161, *177*, 336, *353*
Vath, U., 276, *286*
Vaughn, J.T., 207, *221*
Vavra, J., 25, 26, 27, 30, 31, 34, 35, 37, *39*, 92, 94, *103*
Vendrell, J.P., 334, *352*
Venstrom, K., 259, *264*
Ventura, G., 299, *312*
Verdegem, T.D., 468, *483*
Vernazza, P., 349, *359*
Vernon, D., 326, *329*
Verra, F., 340, *355*
Vervanac, P.A., 4, 5, 13, *22*
Verzosa, M., 349, *359*, 552, *559*
Vessal, K., 130, *139*, 272, *284*, 422, 423, *434*
Vezinet, F., 25, 26, 30, 31, 37, *39*
Vidal, F., 173, *180*
Vierbuchen, M., 245, *250*, 304, *314*
Vigdorth, E.M., 131, 132, 133, *140*, 338, 339, 340, 343, 344, 349, *354*, *359*
Vincent, M.-P., 347, *358*
Vincent, R.A., 173, *179*
Vinijchaikul, K., 334, *352*
Virani, N.A., 363, *377*, 381, 391, *396*
Visscher, B., 131, *140*
Vivirito, M.C., 349, *359*

Voelker, D.R., 259, *265*, 296, 303, *310*, 489, *507*
Vogel, C.L., 625, *632*
Vojtek, A.M., 169, 170, *178*
Volberding, P.A., 347, *358*, 468, *483*
Volkan Adsay, N., 625, *632*
Volpe, F., 514, *542*, 548, *558*
Von Behren, L.A., 243, *249*, 280, *286*, 291, 292, 299, *308*
von Wartburg, A., 615, *626*, *627*
Vortel, V., 361, 363, *375*
Voser, W., 615, *626*
Vossen, M.E.M.H., 25, 26, 27, 30, 34, 35, 37, *39*, *40*, *42*, 123, *137*
Vullo, V., 55, 56, 58, *70*, 115, *119*, 341, *356*

W

Waalkes, T.P., 569, 571, *581*, *582*
Wachter, R.M., 302, *313*, 347, 348, 349, *358*, *359*
Wager, R.E., 259, *264*
Wagner, H., 268, *282*
Wajszczuk, C.P., 268, *282*, 333, *351*
Wakefield, A.E., 47, 49, 50, 53, *65–66*, 83, *90*, 101, *104*, 116, 117, *119*, 125, 127, 128, 129, 130, 131, 136, 137, *138*, *139*, 143, 147, *150*, 240, *249*, 391, 399, 403, 405, 406, 408, 409, 411, *412*, *413*, *414*
Wakefield, A.S., 126, 127, 137, *138*
Waksal, H.W., 381, *396*
Waldman, R.H., 569, *581*
Waldron, M.A., 390, *398*
Waldrop, F.S., 59, 63, *71*
Waler, P.D., 267, *282*
Walker, A.N., 26, 27, 29, 34, *40*, *43*, 59, 63, *71*
Walker, J.J., 94, *104*
Walker, R., 333, 334, 338, *351*, *352*, 555, *560*
Wall, D.A., 623, *631*
Wall, K.A., 503, *509*
Wallace, J.M., 173, *179*
Wallach, D., 305, *315*

Wallis, O.C., 561, 573, *578*
Walls, K.W., 143, 147, *150*
Wallwork, J., 420, 421, *433*
Walmsley, S., 635, 639, *646*
Walsh, T.J., 625, *632*
Walzer, D., 185, 190, *217*
Walzer, P.D., 4, 5, 7, 8, 9, 13, 19, 20, 22, *23*, *24*, 25, 26, 27, 29, 30, 31, 34, 35, 36, 37, 38, *39*, *40*, *42*, 49, 50, 52, 53, 54, 55, 56, 57, 58, 59, 60, 62, 63, *66*, *67*, *69*, *70*, *71*, 75, 77, 78, 81, 83, 84, *89*, *90*, 91, 95, *103*, 108, 109, 111, 113, 114, 115, 117, *118*, *119*, 123, 124, 125, 127, 130, 131, 136, 137, *137*, *138*, *139–40*, 144, 147, 148, 149, *151*, 182, 183, 184, 185, 187, 188, 189, 191, 192, 193, 194, 195, 201, 205, 210, 212, *216*, *217*, *218*, *220*, *221*, *222*, 226, 229, 230, 231, 233, *234*, *235*, 240, 245, *249*, *250*, 252, 253, 255, 256, 257, 258, 259, 260, *261*, *262*, *263*, 267, 268, 269, 270, 272, 273, 274, 275, 276, 278, 279, *281*, *282*, *283*, *284*, *285–86*, 290, 291, 294, 296, 304, 305, *306*, *307*, *309*, *310*, *315*, 321, 328, 332, 333, 336, 337, 345, *350*, *353*, 361, 363, *376*, *377*, 381, 391, 395, 399, 440, 441, *461*, 488, 495, *506*, *508*, 512, 514, 516, 517, 518, 519, 523, 526, 527, 528, 529, 530, 531, 532, 533, 534, *540*, *541*, *542–43*, 550, 552, 555, *558*, *559*, 563, 565, 571, 577, *580*, *581*, *583*, 618, 628, 634, 641, 642, *645*, *646–47*
Walzer, P.U., 408, *413*
Wang, C.C., 575, *582*
Wang, N.-S., 26, *42*
Ward, D.J., 419, *433*
Ward, H.D., 63, *71*
Ward, R.R., 363, *377*
Waring, M.J., 573, *582*
Warner, A., 114, *119*, 245, *250*, 252, *262*, 280, *286*, 294, *309*
Warnock, M.L., 161, 162, 163, *177*, 200, *219*, 261, *265*, 634, *645*

Waskin, H., 473, *484*
Wasserman, H.S., 363, *376*
Watanabe, J.-I., 49, 50, 55, 59, 63, 64, 67, *69*, 81, 84, *90*, 100, *104*, 108, 111, *118*, 201, *219*, 391, *399*
Watanabe, J.M., 134, *140*, 334, *352*
Watanabe, T., 615, *627*
Waterson, A.D.J., 205, 206, *220*
Watson, C.G., 363, *378*
Watson, J.G., 333, *351*
Watts, J.C., 26, 27, 34, *42*, 155, 158, *174*, *176*
Wauters, J.-P., 136, *140*, 336, *353*
Wax, M.R., 416, 418, 423, 425, *432*
Webb, W.R., 161, 162, 163, *177*, 423, *434*
Webber, B.L., 427, *435*
Webber, C.A., 155, *175*, 384, *397*
Weber, H.P., 615, *626*
Weber, R., 338, 340, 341, *355*
Weber, W.R., 156, 157, 163, 165, 169, *176*
Webster, W.P., 572, *582*
Wedgwood, J.F., 290, 295, 302, *306*
Weh, H.J., 135, *140*, 336, *353*
Wehrli, W., 618, *627*
Weil, M.H., 302, *313*, 348, 349, *358*, *359*
Weiman, D.S., 160, *176*
Weinberg, G.A., 49, *67*, 80, *89*, 212, *222*, 305, *315*
Weinberg, W., 611, *613*
Weingeist, T.A., 363, *377*
Weinstein, R.A., 135, *140*, 149, *151*, 427, 428, *435*, 488, *507*, 585, *600*
Weir, E.C., 26, *42*, 193, 194, *218*, 555, *560*
Weisman, J.D., 92, *103*, 268, *282*, 332, *350*
Weissman, I.L., 195, *219*
Weitz, C., 134, *140*, 334, *352*
Weller, I.V., 338, *354*
Weller, N.K., 296, *309*
Weller, R., 181, 182, 191, *215–16*, 487, 494, *506*
Weller, T.H., 93, *103*, 124, *137*, 495, *508*

Wendell, W.B., 603, *612*
Wentz, D., 428, *435*
Wenzel, R.P., 621, *630*
Were, J.B., 561, 577, *579*
Wertman, S.B., 573, *582*
Weseler, T.A., 381, 389, 392, *396*
Wesley, R.A., 135, *140*, 268, *282*, 334, 335, *352*, 427, *435*
Wesseler, T.A., 384, 389, *397*
Wesseler, T.W., 392, *399*
Westergaard, B.F., 143, 146, *150*, 269, 272, 274, 279, *283*
Western, K.A., 135, *140*, 252, *262*, 267, *281*, 333, *351*, 440, 441, *460*
Wharton, J.M., 440, 441, 442, 444, *461*, 468, *483*, 633, *644*
Wheeler, R., 102, *104*
Wherry, J.C., 302, *313*
Whisnant, J.K., 332, *350*
Whitcomb, M.E., 425, 431, *434*
White, D.A., 155, *176*, 339, 340, 341, *355*, 373, *378*, 381, 385, 392, 394, *395*, *400*, 634, *645*
White, J.D., 209, *221*
White, M., 192, *218*, 512, 519, 523, 526, 527, 530, 531, 532, 533, *540*, *543*
White, R., 619, *629*
White, R.F., 623, *630*
White, R.T., 259, *264*
White, T., 259, *264–65*
Whitfield, L.R., 555, *560*
Whitlock, W.L., 419, 423, *433*
Whitsett, J.A., 260, *265*
Wichmann, C.F., 615, *626*
Wiener, L., 458, *466*
Wilbur, J.R., 625, *632*
Wilde, C.E., III, 49, *67*, 273, 274, *285*
Wilde, D.B., 503, *509*
Wiley, C.A., 173, *180*
Wilkinson, R., 430, *435*
Willard, K.E., 615, 616, 621, *626*, *629*
Williams, C.D., 8, *23*
Williams, D.E., 512, *541*
Williams, D.J., 16, 20, 21, *24*, 29, *43*, 59, 63, *71*, 114, *119*, 245, *250*, 252, *262*, 280, *286*, 294, *309*

Author Index

Williams, D.M., 299, *311*
Williams, G.F., 268, *282*, 333, *351*
Williams, H., 143, 146, *150*, 275, *285*
Williams, M.H., Jr., 162, *178*, 419, *433*
Williams, R.B., 603, *612*
Williams, R.C., 303, *314*
Williams, T., 555, *560*
Williams, W.A., 161, 173, *177*, 363, *377*
Williamson, J., 573, *582*
Wilson, A.G., 417, *432*
Wilson, D.L., 53, 55, *69*, 495, *508*
Wilson, G., 623, *631*
Wilson, K.E., 59, 62, *71*, 304, *314*, 495, *508*, 512, 534, *541*, 618, 619, 620, *628*, *629*
Wilson, S.R., 419, 427, *433*
Winearls, C.G., 268, *282*, 333, *351*
Winkelstein, J.A., 267, *282*, 321, *328*
Winn, R.E., 495, *508–9*, 512, *539*
Winn, W., 416, *431*
Winston, D.J., 442, *461*
Winters, R.A., 136, *140*, 212, *222*, 334, *352*
Witorsch, P., 394, *400*, 428, *435*
Witt, K., 625, *631*
Witzbsky, F.G., 381, 391, *396*
Wixson, S.K., 193, 194, 195, 210, *218*, *221*, 226, 233, *234*, 273, 274, 276, *285*, *286*
Woelfel, M., 344, *357*
Wofsy, C.B., 226, *234*, 343, *356*, 440, 441, 442, 444, *461–62*, 468, 476, 479, 481, *483*, *484*, 545, 553, *557*, *559*, 563, 569, *579*, *581*, 633, *644*
Wold, A., 239, *248*
Wolf, B.Z., 441, *461*
Wolf, R.A., 92, *103*, 268, *282*, 332, *350*
Wolfe, L.A., 10, 21, *23*, 52, *68–69*, 488, *506*, 514, 515, *542*, 550, 552, 558, 563, 567, 568, *580*
Wolff, D., 135, *140*, 149, *151*, 488, *507*, 585, *600*
Wolff, L.J., 440, 441, 442, *461*
Wolff, M.J., 342, *356*, 426, *434*

Wolff, S.M., 230, *234*
Wolfson, J.S., 390, *398*
Wolson, A.H., 431, *435*
Wong, H., 155, *175*, 385, *397–98*
Wood, I.S., 363, *376*
Woods, D.R., 4, 5, 19, *22*, *24*, 50, 59, 63, *69*, 78, *89*, 126, 130, *138*, *139*, 142, 143, 146, 147, *150*, 252, *262*, 269, 274, 279, *283*, *286*, 320, *328*, 345, *357*, 382, 391, *396*, *399*, 514, *542*
Woods, G.L., 173, *179*
Woolfenden, J.M., 428, *435*
Wooten, O.J., 382, *396*
Worley, M.A., 49, 50, *66*, 80, 81, 84, *89*, 108, 112, 114, *118*, 130, *139*, 210, *221*, 273, 274, *284–85*, 296, *309*
Wormser, G.P., 172, *179*, 268, *282*, 332, 336, 343, 349, *350*, *356–57*, 431, *435*, 452, *465*
Wozencraft, A.O., 299, *311*
Wright, J.R., 259, *264*
Wright, S.D., 238, *247*
Wright, T.W., 53, *70*, 115, *119*
Wu, A.W., 302, *313*, 339, 342, 347, *355*
Wu, J.T., 623, *630*
Wu, T.C., 381, 391, *396*
Wu, Y.-P., 14, 15, 16, *24*, 537, *543*
Wyle, F.A., 173, *179*
Wyler, D.J., 237, 239, *247*

Y

Yagi, A., 615, *626*, *627*
Yajko, D.M., 381, 391, *396*
Yamada, J., 411, *413*
Yamada, M., 26, 34, 35, 36, *40*, 49, 59, 62, *66–67*, *71*, 82, *90*, 129, *139*, 202, 209, *219*, *221*, 291, 303, 304, *308*, 363, *377*, 512, *540*, *541*, 618, 619, *629*
Yamaguchi, E., 363, *377*
Yamaguchi, H., 615, 616, 618, *627*, *628*
Yamamoto, A., 390, 391, *398*
Yamamoto, Y., 62, *71*, 615, 618, *627*, *628*

Yamanouchi, K., 194, *218*, 270, 272, 276, *284*
Yamauchi, K., 299, *311*
Yamazaki, S., 193, 194, *218*, 276, *286*
Yancopoulos, G.D., 195, *219*
Yap, P.L., 143, 146, *150*, 275, *285*
Yapi, A., 336, *353*
Yarbro, J.W., 573, *582*
Yarchoan, R., 334, 335, *352*, 393, *399*, 450, *464*
Yazbeck, H., 341, *356*
Yeh, S.D.J., 416, 428, *432*
Yeh, Y., 114, *119*, 258, 259, *264*, 302, 304, *313*, 643, *646–47*
Yenokida, G.G., 340, 341, *355*, 394, *400*
Yeoh, C.B., 347, *357*
Yoganathan, T., 49, 50, *66*, 73, 74, 84, 89, 210, 222
Yogev, R., 323, *328*
Yoneda, K., 26, 27, 29, 30, 34, 37, 38, *42*, 184, 185, 187, 188, 189, 190, *217*, 240, *249*, 252, 253, 255, 256, 257, 258, *262*, *263*, 269, 276, *284*, *285*, 303, *314*, 517, *542*
Yorke, W., 561, 573, *578*
Yoshida, Y., 25, 26, 27, 29, 30, 31, 33, 34, 35, 36, 37, 38, *39*, *40*, *41*, *42*, 47, 49, 52, 53, 55, 56, 59, 60, 62, 63, *65*, *66–67*, *69*, *70*, *71*, 82, *90*, 123, *137*, 202, 205, 209, 210, *219*, *220*, *221*, 222, 255, *263*, 290, 291, 296, 303, 304, *306*, *308*, *309*, 363, *377*, 512, *540*, 618, *628*
Yoshikai, K., 229, *234*
Yoshikawa, H., 26, 27, 29, 30, 31, 33, 34, 35, *42*, 56, 59, 60, 62, *70*, *71*, 291, 296, 303, 304, *308*, *309*, 363, *377*, 512, *540*
Youle, M., 338, *354*
Young, C., 555, *560*
Young, E., 577, *583*
Young, K.M., 277, *286*
Young, K.R., 184, *217*
Young, L.S., 3, 4, *22*, 215, *222*, 382, *396*, 442, *461*, 625, *632*
Young, R.C., 135, *140*, 625, *632*

Young, S.A., 404, *413*
Young, T., *559*
Younker, T.D., 59, 63, *71*
Ypma-Wong, M.F., 100
Yu, B., 625, *632*
Yu, V.L., 334, *352*
Yusuf, S., 641, *646*
Yuuki, H., 229, *234*

Z

Zahtz, G., 363, *377*
Zak, O., 615, 616, *626*
Zaman, M.B., 161, *177*, 339, 340, 341, *355*, 373, *378*, 381, 382, 384, 385, 392, 394, *395*, *396*, *397*, *400*, 416, 419, 425, 431, *432*, 456, *465*, 634, *645*
Zambello, R., 299, *312*
Zambias, R.A., 621, 622, 623, *630*, *631*
Zanetti, A., 238, *247*
Zapol, W.M., 638, *646*
Zaske, D., 471, *484*
Zavala, J.V., 205, *220*
Zeckner, D.J., 615, 616, 621, *626*
Zeligs, B.J., 302, 303, *312*
Zerboni, R., 349, *359*
Zerhouni, E.A., 418, 419, 423, 424, 425, *433*
Zhang, J., 7, *23*, 53, *70*, 75, 81, *89*, 129, 130, 137, *139*, *140*, 192, 193, 210, 212, 213, *218*, 222
Zhang, Y., 52, *68*, 514, *542*, 548, 552, *558*
Zhong, M., 512, *541*
Ziefer, A., 201, *219*, 337, *354*
Zilberstein, D., 48, *66*
Zimmerman, L.E., 363, *376*
Zimmerman, P.E., 259, *265*, 296, 303, *310*, 489, *507*
Zimmerman, P.L., 160, 173, *176*, 363, *377*
Zitano, L., 619, *629*
Zuger, A., 441, *461*
Zumoff, B., 341, *356*
Zurlinden, E., 476, *484*, 569, *581*
Zweerink, M., 618, *629*
Zwi, S., 20, *24*, 160, *177*, 290, *306*

SUBJECT INDEX

A

Animal models, 181–221
  classic corticosteroid-treated rat model, 182–187
    role in research, 183
    understanding the model, 183–184
    variability in the model, 184–187
  immunodeficient mice and rats, 193
    immunodeficient mice, 194–201
      nude mouse model, 194–195
      scid mouse model, 195–199
      T-cell-depleted mouse model, 199–201
    immunodeficient rats, 201
  infection in mice, 187–190
  inoculated rodent models, 190–193
  other mammals, 202–209
    Arabian foals, 207–208
    cats and dogs, 205–207
    ferret model, 202–203
    hairless athymic guinea pig model, 204
    newborn and adult rabbit model, 203–204
    nonhuman primates, 208–209
    porcine model, 204–205
  strain and species variation, 209–213
Antigenic characteristics, 107–119
  new directions (recombinant antigens), 115–117
  other antigens, 114–115

[Antigenic characteristics]
  surface glycoprotein A (gp 120, gp 95), 108–114
    functional significance, 112–114
    host-specific antigen variation, 111–112
    isolation and characterization, 108–111
Attachment to host cells: mechanisms, 237–250
  attachment: ultrastructural studies, 240–241
  fibronectin-mediated attachment, 241–245
  lectin-mediated attachment, 245–246
  pathogen attachment mechanisms, 237–240

B

Biochemistry and metabolism, 45–71
  carbohydrates, 58–64
  intermediary and general metabolism, 46–49
  lipids, 55–58
  nucleic acids, 49–52
  proteins, 52–55

C

Cell structure, 25–43
  encystment (sporgenesis), 31–34

701

[Cell structure]
  cyst (spore case), 33–34
  intracystic bodies (spores), 34
  precyst (sporcyte), 31–33
  endogeny (thin-walled cysts), 35
  excystation (spore release), 34–35
  microscopic techniques, 26–27
  relation of structure to function and taxonomy, 35–38
    adhesion, 37–38
    motility, 35–37
    nutrition, 37
    taxonomy, 38
  trophic stages, 27–31
    large trophic form, 27–31
      cytoplasm, 30–31
      nucleus, 30
      surface, 29–30
    small tropic form, 27
Clindamycin, primaquine, and other 8-aminoquinolones, 585–602
  in vitro data, 586–589
  studies in animal models, 589–597
    intermittent dosing protocols, 594–597
    prophylaxis protocols, 593–594
    therapy protocols, 589–593
  studies in humans, 597–599
Clinical manifestations in adults, 331–359
  clinical course, 345–349
    complications, 346–349
    natural course and results of treatment, 345–346
  clinical presentation, 336–345
    clinical tests, 338–342
    history, signs, symptoms, 336–338
    influence of experience with AIDS patients, 342
    recurrence and long term prognosis, 343–345
  risk groups, 332–336
    HIV patients, 334–336
    non-HIV immunosuppressed patients, 332–334
    normal hosts, 334

[Clinical manifestations in adults]
  overview, 332
  transmission among risk groups, 336
Clinical manifestations in children, 319–329
  asymptomatic infection, 320
  extrapulmonary infection, 326
  infantile interstitial plasma cell pneumonitis, 320
  prevention, 327
  sporadic pneumonitis in the immunocompromised host, 321–326
    AIDS, 322–324
      CD4 lymphocyte count, 323–324
      prior episode, 324
      risk factors, 322
    clinical features, 324–325
    diagnostic methods, 325–326
    treatment, 326–327
Corticosteroids and other adjunctive agents, 633–648
  clinical trials, 635–641
  controversies, 641–643
  other agents, 643
  rationale, 634–635

D

Diagnosis: current methods, 381–401
  indirect diagnostic measures, 392–394
  obtaining specimens, 382–388
  stains, 388–392
Drug development, 511–543
  review of the literature, 512–514
    animal models, 512–514
      animal housing and associated microbial flora, 513
      assessment of drug efficacy, 513–514
      drug administration, 513
      experimental design, 513
      source of rats and organisms, 512–513

Subject Index

[Drug development]
University of Cincinnati experience, 514–543
  animal models, 514–534
  classification of activity, 519–520
  classification of activity by cyst counts, 520–531
  classification of activity by nucleus counts, 531
  critique of the classification system, 534
  drug prophylaxis, 519
  drugs tested in therapy, 520
  evaluation of drug efficacy, 516–519
  experimental protocol, 514–516
  prophylaxis studies, 531–534
  in vitro studies, 534–537
Drug discovery: development of models, 487–509
  animal models, 494–505
    inoculated mouse model, 501–505
    inoculated rat model, 497–501
    technical difficulties, 505
  culture method, 488–489
  culture method for drug evaluation, 489–494
  in vitro evaluation of folate antagonists, 494

E

Extrapulmonary infection and other unusual manifestations, 361–387
  case reports, 364–371
  clinical presentation, 363–364
  diagnosis and pathology, 371–372
  extrapulmonary infection: clinical reviews, 362
  frequency of extrapulmonary infection, 362–363
  outcome, 372
  pneumothorax, 374–375
  risk factors, 372–373
  unusual pulmonary manifestations, 373–374

F

Folate antagonists, 545–560
  dihydrofolate reductase, 549
  dihydrofolate reductase inhibitors, 554–556
    clinical trials, 555–556
    preclinical studies, 554–555
  dihydropteroate inhibitors, 550–554
    clinical trials, 553–554
    preclinical studies, 550–553
    other compounds, 552–553
    sulfonamides and sulfones, 550–552
  dihydropteroate synthase, 548–549
  folate metabolism: overview, 546–548
  methods for identifying new agents, 550

G

β-1,3-Glucan synthesis inhibitors, 615–632
  activity, 618–619
  activity of aerosolized echinocandins, 624–625
  history, 615–616
  mechanism of action, 616–618
  structural-activity relations and chemically modified echinocandins, 619–623
  water-soluble prodrug L-693, 989, 623

H

Host defense effector mechanisms, 289–315
  background, 289–291
  cellular immunity, cytokines, and epithelial cells, 298–303
  evasion of host defense effectors, 303–305
  functions of phagocytic cells, 291–293
  nonphagocytic mechanisms, 293–298
Humoral and cellular immunity, 267–287
  cellular immunity, 275–281
    studies in animal models, 276–279
    studies in humans, 279–281

[Humoral and cellular immunity]
humoral immunity, 269–275
studies in animal models, 269–274
studies in humans, 274–275
Hydroxynaphthoquinones, 603–613
initial studies of BW566C80 (atovaquone), 604
pharmacokinetics and safety, 604–609
therapeutic efficacy, 609–611

I

Immunodeficient mice: new animal models, 223–236
advantages, 223–225
colony maintenance, 232–233
non-scid mouse models, 227–230
organisms derived from mice vs. other species, 230–231
scid mice, 225–227
synergy with and other organisms, 231–232
In vitro cultivation, 3–24
culture systems in current use, 17–20
in vitro drug testing, 19
metabolic activity, 20
source of organisms, 19
historical background, 4
problems surrounding, 4–17
assessment of growth, 12–17
quantitation of organisms, 12–13
viability of organisms, 13–17
nature of inoculum, 6–8
influence of host contaminants, 6–7
strain differences, 7–8
viability and stage specificity, 7
properties of culture systems, 8–12
cell-free systems, 10–12
cell monolayer systems, 8–10

M

Molecular approach to diagnosis, 403–414
clinical studies, 408–411
epidemiology, 411–412
specific DNA sequences, 404–408

Molecular genetics, 73–90
genes, 83–87
mitochondrial ribosomal gene, 85
nuclear ribosomal RNA locus, 83–85
protein-encoding genes, 85–87
dihydrofolate reductase, 85–87
55-kilodalton antigen gene, 87
thymidylate synthase, 85
genome, 74–83
base composition, 81–82
electrophoretic karyotyping, 74–80
ploidy, 82–83
repetitive DNA, 80–81
transcription and translation, 87–88
Molecular phylogeny, 91–105
additional genes, 101–102
lysine biosynthesis, 101
sterol biosynthesis, 101–102
attempts at classification, 94
phylogenetic relationships, 94–101
dihydrofolate reductase sequence, 99–100
elongation factor 3 sequence, 100
5s RNA sequence, 100–101
mitochondrial DNA sequence, 101
16s-like ribosomal RNA sequence, 94–98
thymidylate synthase sequence, 98–99
relevance, 92–94

P

Pathogenic mechanisms, 251–265
changes in the alveolar microenvironment, 256–260
anatomical changes, 256–258
physiological and biochemical changes, 258–260
establishment of infection, 251–253
host inflammatory or immune response, 260–261
organism proliferation, 253–256
Pathological features, 155–180
classic histopathology, 157–158

Subject Index

[Pathological features]
concomitant processes, 171
disseminated (extrapulmonary) infection, 173
immunohistochemistry, 173
treated pneumonia, 171–173
unusual histological features, 158–171
  absence of alveolar exudate, 159–160
  alveolar proteinosis, 169–171
  cystic and cavitary lesions, 160–163
  diffuse alveolar damage, 158–159
  granulomatous lesions, 163–164
  lymphocytic-plasmacellular interstitial pneumonitis, 164–165
  marked alveolar macrophage accumulation, 168–169
  microcalcifications, 165–168
  vascular permeation and vasculitis, 169
Pentamidine and related compounds, 561–583
  drug resistance, 577
  mechanism of action, 573–577
  pharmacology, 569–571
  structure-activity studies, 563–569
  toxicity, 571–573
Pharmacokinetics and drug dosing, 467–485
  clindamycin-primaquine, 481
    clinical trials, 481
  experimental therapies, 482
    BW566C80 (atovaquone), 482
    WR6062, 482
  pentamidine, 473–478
    clinical studies, 473–476
      aerosolized pentamidine, 475–476
      parenteral therapy, 473–475
    pharmacokinetic studies, 476–477
    renal failure, 476–477
  trimethoprim-dapsone, 478–481
    clinical studies, 478–479
    dosing in renal failure, 480
    pharmacokinetic and interaction studies, 479–480
  trimethoprim-sulfamethoxazole, 468–473

[Pharmacokinetics and drug dosing]
  clinical studies, 468–470
  dosing in renal failure, 471
  pharmacokinetic studies, 470–471

R

Radiological approaches to diagnosis, 415–436
  chest radiograph, 416–423
    altered hosts, 419–422
      pentamidine and pneumothorax, 419–420
      transplantation, 420–422
    atypical patterns, 416–419
    infantile and pediatric patients, 422–423
  computed tomography and magnetic resonance imaging, 423–427
    extrapulmonary disease, 425–427
  inflammation imaging, 427–430
    dietylenetriamine pentaacetic acid scans, 430
    gallium scanning, 428–429
    immunoglobulin G scans, 430
    resolution of infection, 430–431
  ultrasound, 427

S

Serological studies, 141–151
  complement fixation assay, 145
  enzyme immunoassay, 146–147
  immunoblotting, 147–149
  indirect fluorescent assay, 145–146
  serology of outbreaks, 149

T

Therapy and prophylaxis: current methods, 439–466
  adjunctive corticosteroids, 449–450
  pediatric HIV patients, 458–459
  prophylaxis, 450–458
  treatment, 440–449
    aerosolized pentamidine, 446
    dapsone, 444

[Therapy and prophylaxis: current methods]
  other agents, 446–449
  pentamidine, 440–441
  trimethoprim-dapsone, 444–446
  trimethoprim-sulfamethoxazole, 441–444
Transmission and epidemiology, 123–140
  airborne transmission, 124–125
  epidemiology, 130–137

[Transmission and epidemiology]
  clusters of human cases, 134–137
  influence of climate or geography, 130–134
  origin of the infection, 125–130
  outside the mammalian host, 128–130
  within the mammalian host, 125–128